Handbook of Theories of Aging

About the Editors

Vern L. Bengtson, PhD, is AARP/university professor of gerontology emeritus and research professor, Edward R. Roybal Institute on Aging, School of Social Work, University of Southern California, Los Angeles, California. A senior statesman in gerontology, Bengtson is a world-recognized expert on the sociology of the life course, family sociology, social psychology, ethnicity and aging. He has been elected as president of the Gerontological Society of America and has been granted two MERIT awards for research from the National Institutes of Health. He has written or edited 17 books and published more than 260 research papers. Early in his career, Bengtson started the Longitudinal Study of Generations, a multigeneration and multidisciplinary investigation of families, aging, and social change, which now is in its 45th year of data collection from more than 350 multigenerational families. He has received research awards from the Gerontological Society of America, the American Sociological Association, the American Psychological Association, the National Council on Family Relations, and the Society for the Scientific Study of Religion. As the lead editor on the two prior editions of the *Handbook of Theories of Aging,* and coeditor of the book that preceded them, *Emergent Theories of Aging,* Dr. Bengtson has led the charge to transform gerontology into a field that is rich in both data and theories.

Richard A. Settersten, Jr., PhD, is professor of human development and family sciences, Oregon State University, Corvallis, Oregon, where he is also endowed director of the Hallie E. Ford Center for Healthy Children and Families and a member of the Center for Healthy Aging Research. Dr. Settersten is editor of numerous books and journal issues. His research spans multiple periods of the life course (especially early adulthood and late life) and multiple levels of analysis (from genomics to demography). A fellow of the Gerontological Society of America, Dr. Settersten has played leadership roles in the Gerontological Society of America as well as the American Sociological Association. His coedited book (with J. Angel), the *Handbook of Sociology of Aging,* won the 2012 Outstanding Publication Award of the American Sociological Association's Section on Aging and the Life Course. Multiple divisions of the National Institutes of Health, as well as the MacArthur and Spencer foundations, have supported his research. He has participated in activities of the National Academy of Science/National Research Council/Institute on Medicine panels on the health and well-being of young adults, and on new directions in social demography, social epidemiology, and sociology of aging.

About the Associate Editors

Brian K. Kennedy, PhD, is internationally recognized for his research in the basic biology of aging and is a visionary committed to translating research discoveries into new ways of delaying, detecting, preventing, and treating age-related conditions. He is the president and chief executive officer at the Buck Institute for Research on Aging, Novato, California, and leads a team of 20 principal investigators involved in interdisciplinary research aimed at extending health span, the healthy years of life. The inventor on several patents, Dr. Kennedy is cofounder of two U.S. companies aimed at developing treatments for age-related chronic disease. He is actively involved in aging research in the Pacific Rim, which features the largest elderly population in the world. Dr. Kennedy has published over 140 manuscripts in prestigious journals including *Science* and *Nature.* He is coeditor-in-chief of *Aging Cell* and serves as a consultant for biotech and pharmaceutical companies.

Nancy Morrow-Howell, MSW, PhD, is on the faculty of the George Warren Brown School of Social Work at Washington University, St. Louis, Missouri, and holds the Bettie Bofinger Brown Distinguished Professorship. She teaches graduate courses in gerontology and research. She is also the director of the Harvey A. Friedman Center for Aging; in that role, she promotes gerontological research and education across disciplines, schools, and departments. Dr. Morrow-Howell is a fellow of the Gerontological Society of America, and she currently is president of that national organization. Her scholarship focuses on productive engagement in later life, specifically on programs and policies to optimally engage older adults in paid and unpaid work, including working, volunteering, and caregiving.

Jacqui Smith, PhD, is professor of psychology at the University of Michigan, Ann Arbor, Michigan, and research professor at the Institute for Social Research. She has a PhD from the Macquarie University, Sydney, Australia, and a habilitation from the Free University of Berlin. She has coedited *Toward a General Theory of Expertise, Die Berliner Altersstudie* [The Berlin Aging Study], and the *Handbook of Life-Span Psychology.* Her research papers have appeared in *Psychology and Aging, Developmental Psychology, Journals of Gerontology, Health Psychology, Gerontology,* and *Journal of Population Ageing.*

Handbook of Theories of Aging

Third Edition

Vern L. Bengtson, PhD, and Richard A. Settersten, Jr., PhD
Editors

*Brian K. Kennedy, PhD, Nancy Morrow-Howell, MSW, PhD,
and Jacqui Smith, PhD*
Associate Editors

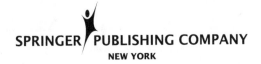

SPRINGER PUBLISHING COMPANY
NEW YORK

Springer Publishing Company, LLC
11 West 42nd Street
New York, NY 10036
www.springerpub.com

Acquisitions Editor: Sheri W. Sussman
Composition: Newgen KnowledgeWorks

ISBN: 978-0-8261-2942-0
e-book ISBN: 978-0-8261-2943-7

16 17 18 19 20 / 5 4 3 2 1

The author and the publisher of this Work have made every effort to use sources believed to be reliable to provide information that is accurate and compatible with the standards generally accepted at the time of publication. The author and publisher shall not be liable for any special, consequential, or exemplary damages resulting, in whole or in part, from the readers' use of, or reliance on, the information contained in this book. The publisher has no responsibility for the persistence or accuracy of URLs for external or third-party Internet websites referred to in this publication and does not guarantee that any content on such websites is, or will remain, accurate or appropriate.

Library of Congress Cataloging-in-Publication Data
Names: Bengtson, Vern L., editor. | Settersten, Richard A., Jr., 1964–, editor. | Kennedy, Brian K., editor. | Morrow-Howell, Nancy, 1952–, editor. | Smith, Jacqui (Professor of psychology), editor.
Title: Handbook of theories of aging / Vern L. Bengtson, Richard A. Settersten Jr., editors; Brian Kennedy, Nancy Morrow-Howell, Jacqui Smith, associate editors.
Description: Third edition. | New York, NY: Springer Publishing Company, LLC, [2016] | Includes bibliographical references and indexes.
Identifiers: LCCN 2016006253 | ISBN 9780826129420 | ISBN 9780826129437 (e-book)
Subjects: | MESH: Aging—physiology | Aging—psychology | Geriatrics | Models, Biological
Classification: LCC HQ1061 | NLM WT 104 | DDC 305.2601—dc23
LC record available at http://lccn.loc.gov/2016006253

Printed in the United States of America by Bradford & Bigelow.

Contents

PART VI. TRANSDISCIPLINARY PERSPECTIVES ON THEORY DEVELOPMENT IN AGING

PART VII. CONCLUSION

Contributors

W. Andrew Achenbaum, PhD   Professor Emeritus, University of Houston, Houston, Texas

Carolyn M. Aldwin, PhD   Jo Anne Leonard Endowed Professor, Center for Healthy Aging Research, and Professor, Human Development and Family Sciences, Oregon State University, Corvallis, Oregon

Devin Arbuthnott, PhD   Postdoctoral Fellow, Department of Pathology, University of Washington, Seattle, Washington

Monika Ardelt, PhD   Associate Professor of Sociology, Department of Sociology and Criminology & Law, University of Florida, Gainesville, Florida

Vern L. Bengtson, PhD   AARP/University Professor of Gerontology Emeritus and Research Professor, Edward R. Roybal Institute on Aging, School of Social Work, University of Southern California, Los Angeles, California

Rosemary Blieszner, PhD   Alumni Distinguished Professor, Department of Human Development, Virginia Tech, Blacksburg, Virginia

Susan T. Charles, PhD   Professor of Psychology and Social Behavior, University of California, Irvine, Irvine, California

Peter G. Coleman, PhD   Emeritus Professor of Psychogerontology, Academic Unit of Psychology, University of Southampton, Southampton, United Kingdom

Theodore D. Cosco, PhD   Postdoctoral Research Associate, Medical Research Council, University College London, London, United Kingdom

Nicholas R. DiCarlo, MSW   Research Analyst, Institute for Health & Aging, University of California, San Francisco, California

Carroll L. Estes, PhD   Professor and Founding Director Emeritus, Institute for Health & Aging, University of California, San Francisco, California

Leonid A. Gavrilov, PhD   Senior Research Scientist, Center on Aging, NORC at the University of Chicago, Chicago, Illinois; and Senior Research Scientist, WHO Collaborating Centre, Department of Statistical Analysis of Population Health, Federal Research Institute for Health Organization and Informatics, Ministry of Health of the Russian Federation, Moscow, Russia

Natalia S. Gavrilova, PhD   Senior Research Analyst, Center on Aging, NORC at the University of Chicago, Chicago, Illinois; and Senior Research Scientist, WHO Collaborating Centre, Department of Statistical Analysis of Population Health, Federal Research Institute for Health Organization and Informatics, Ministry of Health of the Russian Federation, Moscow, Russia

Denis Gerstorf, PhD   Professor, Developmental Psychology, Humboldt University, Berlin, Germany

Bethany Godlewski, MS   PhD Candidate, Human Development and Family Sciences, Oregon State University, Corvallis, Oregon

Melissa Hardy, PhD   Distinguished Professor, Department of Sociology, Pennsylvania State University, University Park, Pennsylvania

Leonard Hayflick, PhD   Professor of Anatomy, Department of Anatomy, University of California, San Francisco, San Francisco, California

Joanna Hong   PhD Candidate, Psychology and Social Behavior, University of California, Irvine, Irvine, California

Nancy R. Hooyman, MSW, PhD   Hooyman Professor of Gerontology, University of Washington, School of Social Work, Seattle, Washington

Robert B. Hudson, PhD   Professor of Social Policy, Boston University, Boston, Massachusetts

Susan L. Hughes, PhD   Professor of Community Health Sciences, School of Public Health; and Co-Director, Center for Research on Health and Aging, University of Illinois at Chicago, Chicago, Illinois

Gizem Hülür, PhD   Postdoctoral Researcher, Developmental Psychology, Humboldt University, Berlin, Germany

Heidi Igarashi, PhD   Human Development and Family Sciences, Oregon State University, Corvallis, Oregon

Derek M. Isaacowitz, PhD   Professor of Psychology, Northeastern University, Boston, Massachusetts

Heinrich Jasper, PhD   Professor, Chief Scientific Officer, Buck Institute for Research on Aging, Novato, California

Daniela S. Jopp, PhD   Professor of Psychology for Adult Development and Aging, Institute of Psychology and Swiss National Centre of Competence in Research LIVES, University of Lausanne, Lausanne, Switzerland

Matt Kaeberlein, PhD   Professor of Pathology, University of Washington, Seattle, Washington

Brian K. Kennedy, PhD   President and Chief Executive Officer, Buck Institute for Research on Aging, Novato, California

Robert G. Kent de Grey, MA   PhD Candidate, Department of Psychology, University of Utah, Salt Lake City, Utah

James L. Kirkland, MD, PhD   Noaber Foundation Professor of Aging Research; and Director of the Robert and Arlene Kogod Center on Aging, Mayo Clinic, Rochester, Minnesota

Karl D. Kosloski, PhD   Professor Emeritus, Department of Gerontology, University of Nebraska, Omaha, Nebraska

Jung Kwak, PhD   Associate Professor, Department of Social Work, University of Wisconsin–Milwaukee, Milwaukee, Wisconsin

Becca R. Levy, PhD   Associate Professor, Department of Public Health and Psychology, Yale University, New Haven, Connecticut

Kevin J. Mahoney, PhD   Professor, Boston College School of Social Work, Chestnut Hill, Massachusetts

Victor W. Marshall, PhD   Professor Emeritus, Department of Sociology, The University of North Carolina at Chapel Hill, Chapel Hill, North Carolina; and Dalla Lana School of Public Health, The University of Toronto, Toronto, Ontario, Canada

Anne Martin-Matthews, PhD   Professor of Sociology, University of British Columbia, Vancouver, British Columbia, Canada

Julie Ann McMullin, PhD   Professor of Sociology and Vice-Provost (International) at The University of Western Ontario, London, Ontario, Canada

Brad A. Meisner, PhD   Assistant Professor, School of Health and Human Performance, Dalhousie University, Halifax, Nova Scotia, Canada

Rhonda J. V. Montgomery, PhD   Professor Emerita, Helen Bader School of Social Welfare, University of Wisconsin–Milwaukee, Milwaukee, Wisconsin

Jacob A. Moorad, PhD   Lecturer, Quantitative Genetics, Institute of Evolutionary Biology, The University of Edinburgh, Edinburgh, United Kingdom

Keith Diaz Moore, PhD Dean and Professor, College of Architecture and Planning, University of Utah, Salt Lake City, Utah

Nancy Morrow-Howell, MSW, PhD Professor, George Warren Brown School of Social Work; Director, Center for Aging, Washington University, St. Louis, Missouri

Joana Neves, PhD Postdoctoral Research Associate, Buck Institute for Research on Aging, Novato, California

Nhi Ngo, MA PhD Candidate, Department of Psychology, Northeastern University, Boston, Massachusetts

Hunhui Oh, PhD, MSW Assistant Professor, School of Social Work, St. Ambrose University, Davenport, Iowa

Anthony D. Ong, PhD Associate Professor, Department of Human Development, Cornell University, Ithaca, New York

Angela M. O'Rand, PhD Professor, Department of Sociology; and Director, Center for Population Health and Aging at Duke University, Durham, North Carolina

Frank Oswald, PhD Professor of Interdisciplinary Ageing Research, Goethe University, Frankfurt, Germany

Stéphanie Pin, PhD Junior Lecturer, Institute of Social Sciences and Swiss National Centre of Competence in Research LIVES, University of Lausanne, Lausanne, Switzerland

Daniel E. L. Promislow, DPhil Professor, Departments of Pathology and Biology, University of Washington, Seattle, Washington

Tara L. Queen, PhD Assistant Research Professor, Department of Psychology, University of Utah, Salt Lake City, Utah

Nilam Ram, PhD Professor, Department of Human Development and Family Studies and Psychology, Pennsylvania State University, State College, Pennsylvania

Adriana M. Reyes, MA Doctoral Candidate, Department of Sociology, Pennsylvania State University, University Park, Pennsylvania

Karen A. Roberto, PhD University Distinguished Professor and Director, Center for Gerontology and the Institute for Society, Culture and Environment, Virginia Tech, Blacksburg, Virginia

John W. Rowe, MD Julius B. Richmond Professor of Health Policy and Aging, Robert N. Butler Columbia Aging Center, New York, New York

Molly Sands, MA PhD Candidate, Department of Psychology, Northeastern University, Boston, Massachusetts

K. Warner Schaie, PhD, ABPP, ScD (hon.), Dr. Phil. (hon.)   Affiliate Professor, Department of Psychiatry and Behavioral Sciences, University of Washington, Seattle, Washington

Andrew E. Scharlach, PhD   Kleiner Professor, School of Social Welfare, University of California, Berkeley, California

Elisabeth Schröder-Butterfill, DPhil   Lecturer, Department of Gerontology, University of Southampton, Southampton, United Kingdom

Mark Sciegaj, PhD   Professor, Department of Health Policy and Administration, Pennsylvania State University, University Park, Pennsylvania

Richard A. Settersten, Jr., PhD   Professor of Human Development and Family Sciences, Oregon State University, Corvallis, Oregon

Jacqui Smith, PhD   Professor of Psychology, University of Michigan, Ann Arbor, Michigan, Research Professor, Institute for Social Research, Ann Arbor, Michigan

Renae L. Smith-Ray, PhD   Research Scientist, Center for Research on Health and Aging, Institute for Health Research and Policy, University of Illinois at Chicago, Chicago, Illinois

Pedro Sousa-Victor, PhD   Postdoctoral Research Associate, Buck Institute for Research on Aging, Novato, California

Dario Spini, PhD   Professor of Social Psychology and the Life Course; Institute of Social Sciences, and Director, Swiss National Centre of Competence in Research LIVES, University of Lausanne, Lausanne, Switzerland

John H. Spreadbury, PhD   Senior Research Fellow, Faculty of Medicine, NIHR CLAHRC Wessex, University of Southampton, Southampton, United Kingdom

Elske Stolte, MS   PhD Candidate, Faculty of Social Sciences, Vrije Universiteit Amsterdam, Amsterdam, Netherlands

Silvia Stringhini, PhD   Senior Lecturer, Institute of Social and Preventive Medicine, University of Lausanne, Lausanne, Switzerland

Bert N. Uchino, PhD   Professor, Department of Psychology, University of Utah, Salt Lake City, Utah

Marieke Voorpostel, PhD   Senior Researcher, Swiss Centre of Expertise in the Social Sciences (FORS), Lausanne, Switzerland

Robbyn R. Wacker, PhD   Provost and Professor of Gerontology, University of Northern Colorado, Greeley, Colorado

Hans-Werner Wahl, PhD   Professor, Department of Psychological Aging Research, Heidelberg University, Heidelberg, Germany

Linda J. Waite, PhD   Lucy Flower Professor, Department of Sociology, University of Chicago, Chicago, Illinois

Jaclyn S. Wong, MA   PhD Candidate, Department of Sociology, University of Chicago, Chicago, Illinois

Ming Xu, PhD   Research Fellow, Mayo Clinic, Rochester, Minnesota

Preface

What is theory, and why are theories important in research on aging? What are the most prominent theories in contemporary gerontology? How can we nurture the development of theories to better meet the needs of the field in the decade ahead? These are some of the questions that have propelled this third edition of the *Handbook of Theories of Aging*. The need for theory-based knowledge to address problems of aging has never been greater. Yet, the ready availability of Big Data has proliferated primarily descriptive and nontheoretical research reports. Explanations of aging processes and outcomes—in other words, theories—have often taken a back seat to the generation of factual information.

With 35 chapters by some of the most highly respected researchers in gerontology today, this edition of this handbook provides a state-of-the-art overview so that researchers and practitioners can stay abreast of the latest developments. It addresses theories and concepts built on cumulative knowledge in four disciplinary areas—biology, psychology, social sciences, and policy and practice—as well as landmark advances in transdisciplinary science. Because of their explicit focus on theory, the editions of this handbook are a resource for knowledge about primary explanations of aging, whether at the level of cells or societies.

In this edition, we asked authors to place a strong emphasis on the future of theory development, assessing the current state of theories and providing a road map for how theory can shape research and how research can shape theory, in years to come. We are especially excited about a new section, "Standing on the Shoulders of Giants," which contains personal essays by four of the most senior gerontologists in our field, who share their perspectives on the history of ideas in their fields, as well as their experiences with the process and prospects of developing useful theory.

Many chapters also address connections between theories and policy or practice, especially in ameliorating problems of aging. This also means doing better by the varied populations we hope to understand and to serve. Thus we asked authors to probe matters of diversity and inequality, assessing how theories in their area address these matters and how theories might be revised or tested with diversity and inequality in mind.

Perhaps the most important feature of this edition is that its content also reflects our field's increasing commitment to transdisciplinary research that stretches across traditional disciplinary boundaries to generate more complex and comprehensive explanations of how aging processes and outcomes are intertwined.

The contributors to this handbook were asked to discuss the most exciting ideas in their areas in ways that are highly readable for a wide variety of our multidisciplinary audiences, whether researchers, practitioners, or students. On behalf of the three associate editors, 70 contributors, and ourselves, we hope you enjoy reading this handbook as much as we have enjoyed putting it together—and that you will find many ideas in its pages to stimulate your thoughts and shape your future research.

Vern L. Bengtson, PhD
Richard A. Settersten, Jr., PhD

Acknowledgments

To create a 35-chapter volume exploring the frontiers of theory development in aging is no small task, and we have been privileged to work with many creative people along the way. We want first to acknowledge the contributions of the associate editors: for the biological sciences, Brian K. Kennedy, PhD, president and chief executive officer at the Buck Institute for Research on Aging; for the psychological sciences, Jacqui Smith, PhD, professor of psychology at the University of Michigan and research professor at the Institute for Social Research; and for policy, intervention, and practice, Nancy Morrow-Howell, MSW, PhD, Bettie Bofinger Brown Distinguished Professor of Social Work at Washington University, and current president of the Gerontological Society of America.

We also want to acknowledge the extraordinary dedication of 70 contributors who share our intellectual passion for theories and concepts on aging. Whether senior, mid-career, or junior in status, the members of this cast are among the world's brightest minds in our field. We are grateful for their willingness to further strengthen their manuscripts in response to the reviews of the editors and the thought-provoking discussions that ensued. The commitment of the authors to the highest quality scholarship is evident throughout the pages of this handbook. Their chapters offer wonderful windows into their fields, and we know that readers will be as inspired as we have been by the rich and playful ideas of the authors.

On our end, the smooth production of this volume has been aided by the fine work of Bethany Godlewski, PhD candidate in Human Development and Family Sciences at Oregon State University (OSU), who efficiently managed tasks while she advanced her graduate research. We are also grateful to Laura Smith, of the Hallie E. Ford Center for Healthy Children and Families at OSU, for her assistance in preparing the manuscript in the final stretch.

On the publisher's end, Springer Publishing Company has, for several decades, maintained its status as the premier publisher of academic volumes in gerontology, thanks to the talents of editors such as Sheri W. Sussman, with whom it has again been a pleasure to work. Sheri's encouragement and support throughout the project have been exceptional from beginning to end. This is the fourth book on theories of aging that Springer has produced (the first being *Emergent Theories of Aging* and the second and third being the previous two editions of *Handbook of Theories of Aging*), and we are grateful for their investment in long-range, cumulative knowledge development in the field. Thanks are also due to Mindy Chen, who skillfully managed the production process.

We are also grateful for the support of our academic homes at the University of Southern California (USC) and OSU. The Edward R. Roybal Institute for Research on Aging at USC and the Hallie E. Ford Center for Healthy Children and Families at OSU have both provided stimulating environments for theory development, as well as support for this project and our scholarship. At USC, special thanks are due to Dr. William Vega, director of the Roybal Institute, and Dr. Marilyn Flynn, dean of the School of Social Work. At OSU, special thanks are due to Drs. Karen Hooker and Sheryl Thorburn, co-directors of the School of Social and Behavioral Health Sciences, and Dr. Tammy Bray, dean of the College of Public Health and Human Sciences, as well as to Dr. David Robinson and the Center for Humanities for a sabbatical fellowship year.

If expressions of appreciation to families are often pro forma in the acknowledgment section of books, in this case, they have special meaning. Hannah Gruhn-Bengtson was a collaborator in editing and providing helpful suggestions for Chapters 1, 5, and 35. Dan Dowhower, Maya Settersten, and Mario Settersten were encouraging and patient during the years it took to bring this volume to fruition. Both families welcomed us on several occasions so that we could work together in person in Oregon and California. They supplied us with good company, good humor, and good nourishment. We cherish the memories of our time together.

Vern L. Bengtson
Richard A. Settersten, Jr.

CHAPTER 1

Theories of Aging: Developments Within and Across Disciplinary Boundaries

Vern L. Bengtson and Richard A. Settersten, Jr.

This is the fourth handbook that is focused on theory development within aging; the first was published almost three decades ago (Birren & Bengtson, 1988). Although there have been many handbooks on aging over the past 75 years, beginning with Cowdry's (1939) *Problems of Ageing* and the three-volume *Handbooks of Aging* series two decades later (Birren, 1959; Burgess, 1960; Tibbitts, 1960), most have summarized research findings relating to specific topics or problems in aging, usually within specific scientific boundaries. By contrast, the handbooks of theories of aging (Bengtson, Gans, Putney, & Silverstein, 2009; Bengtson & Schaie, 1999; Birren & Bengtson, 1988) instead focused on *theoretical and conceptual developments* in research on aging, both within and across disciplines. This again has been the goal underlying the 35 chapters of this volume: to review current advances in theory across the wide spectrum of gerontological research today, and to spur theory-based research and interventions in research on aging in the next decade.

To ensure the scientific and humanitarian advancement of our field, we must periodically take stock of the state of the theories that undergird our knowledge and consider how we can nurture the future development of theory. In today's era of Big Data, when huge secondary data sets are readily available for rapid analysis, the temptation to churn out principally descriptive publications appears irresistible and necessary—especially when promotion, tenure, and other forms of status in the academy place a premium on empirical papers built on the latest methods and statistical procedures. However, the availability of new data and methods should be harnessed to promote the development of compelling theories as well. Recent years have brought major investments in longitudinal data, investments essential to understanding aging as a dynamic, multifaceted, and interactive process. These have been accompanied by advances in methods and statistics that make it possible to more sensitively and rigorously treat the effects of time and social contexts.

There is a natural and important synergy that links theories, methods, and data, just as there is a linkage across theories, policy, and practice. It is unfortunate that the crafts of theory, synthesis, and application often take a back seat to the more immediate and fundable work of data collection and analysis. Thinking about theory may seem too remote or too abstract to be of relevance; or too costly relative to the rewards; or discussion of theory may seem beyond the limited scope of journal pages or the appreciation of editors or reviewers relative to the data at hand. This is woefully nearsighted.

Theory has been, and continues to be, the cornerstone of scientific inquiry and the gateway to systematic knowledge development. In the following sections, we summarize what we mean by theory, and why theory is so important to advancing aging-related research, policy, practice, and intervention.

■ WHAT IS THEORY AND WHY IS IT IMPORTANT?

Theory as Explanation and Understanding

First and foremost, theories are explanations—explanations that lead to, and are driven by, cumulative knowledge. Theories guide the questions we ask and the research we design. Theories answer the "why" and "how" behind what we find in data. Such explanations can be formal or informal, long or short, but they should be clear and explicit. Most often, they assume the form of a causal statement: X occurs because Y caused it, in conjunction with (or because of the absence of) Z.

Theories also provide understanding, which is somewhat different from explanation. We can posit a theory about the causal relationship between two variables without knowing the mechanism that underlies the relationships; a theory that includes mechanisms achieves a deeper level of understanding. In some fields of the social sciences it can be said that there are two primary types of theory: (a) theories of *explanation* of *why* and *how* something occurs—for example, cumulative advantage/disadvantage theories that explain *why* variability among older people partly reflects social inequalities, and *how* social processes generate those inequalities over time; and (b) theories of *orientation* that provide a worldview and even a set of explicit assumptions or propositions, which lead us to see and interpret aging phenomena in particular ways—for example, postmodern theory, feminist theory, critical gerontology, or the life-course perspective. Although the latter are often called "theories," they are, from another perspective, more often broader "paradigms" than theories. However, the frame and propositions they provide are extremely useful in developing more specific theories. In any case, both types are represented in gerontology today.

"An attempt to explain," perhaps also adding "for now," is probably the simplest and most direct way to define theory. This expression has the advantage of reminding us that theories are provisional and embedded in a process that involves rejections, refinements, and reconsiderations over time as we are confronted with new knowledge and data, and with changing people in a changing world. Another useful phrase, "theorizing," turns the noun into a verb that reflects the ongoing dynamic of *building* explanations. Advances in methods, and in the identification of problems to be studied, are dependent on the knowledge—theorizing—that preceded them, just as they in turn shape the resulting knowledge.

The principal value of theory, then, lies in building knowledge in a systematic and cumulative way, such that empirical efforts will lead to integration with what is already known and help us to see gaps or inconsistencies in existing knowledge or between new knowledge and old. The principal use of theory is to provide a set of lenses through which we can view aging phenomena and make and interpret observations.

Barefoot Empiricism, Empirical Generalizations, and Models

Theory should not be confused with other steps in the process of knowledge development or the terms that have been used to describe them. For example, what James Birren, one of the founders of the psychology of aging, described as *barefoot empiricism*

(Birren, 1973, p. 11) is particularly problematic. This can be seen in papers presenting table after table of data with little interpretation as to why these results occurred or why they matter. Many articles like this can still be found in gerontology journals today, but it is unclear what lasting contribution they make beyond mere description.

What have been called *empirical generalizations* represent a conceptual step up from barefoot empiricism: statements that describe findings that have been repeatedly observed across multiple data sources. Empirical generalizations are usually anchored in extensive reviews of previous research on a given problem, and are often the grounds for explicit and even competing hypotheses. The research process involves collecting data through methods intended to reduce sources of bias, especially reliable and valid approaches to measurement and, in the social sciences in particular, sound sampling. In all scientific fields, the statistical handling of data is highly scrutinized by reviewers.

These steps, taken together—a thorough review of previous knowledge, an explicit statement of the research problem, a concern for unbiased collection of data, and state-of-the-art statistical analysis—can produce empirical generalizations about a research problem that look impressive. Nevertheless, too many journal articles still consist of empirical generalizations that are basically accounts of covariation across or between variables. This limits knowledge development to a description of observations and relationships at a certain point in time, with little interpretation concerning mechanisms of *why* and *how* they are related—in other words, no theorizing.

Models represent another process in knowledge development. A model is a way to *depict* a theory. It portrays the relationships among the complex variables suggested by a theory. It is a prototype of how empirical generalizations might be related to each other. The development of models and approaches to model *fitting* are recent contributions of 20th-century statistical and engineering applications of basic science. However, a model is not yet a theory.

Why Theory Is Important

In the history of science, theory has proven to be of great importance. In addition to explanation and understanding, there are pragmatic reasons for investing in efforts to develop theory.

First, in fostering explanation through specifying *why* and *how* empirically observed phenomena are related, theory contributes to the *integration of knowledge* over time. A good theory identifies the problem and its most important components (concepts) based on the separate findings and empirical generalizations from research. It also describes the linkages among the concepts in a causal sequence, based on previous knowledge. A good theory does this in a way that is clear, concise, and testable. This enables future investigators to test, refine, or refute it, thus advancing future knowledge development.

Prediction is another pragmatic contribution of theory. Theory-driven studies can point to new research directions based on findings that are partial, unexpected, or even anomalous and might otherwise remain hidden. Predictions based on theory can create radical shifts in the way we understand human life and the world around us. This is most obvious in the natural and biological sciences: Darwin's theory of natural selection led to a revolution in human biology; Mendeleev's theory led to the prediction of new elements in the periodic table; Einstein's theory of relativity led to the discovery of new planets and eventually to the atomic bomb.

Theories also guide *interventions to improve human conditions*. Theory is valuable when we attempt to apply or advance existing knowledge in order to solve problems or alleviate undesirable human conditions. This can be seen in most organizations whose structures and actions are guided by popular theories about effective management, leadership, and communication. At a global level, the usefulness of theory in technological intervention is obvious in applications related to communication. In little over a century, communication has developed from the telegraph to Internet connections that can connect refugees in rural Somalia to reporters in London in a few seconds.

Other interventions are behavioral and social, though these have less often been informed by rational theories. At the *macro*-social level are the actions of governments, whose interventions through public policy are intended to ameliorate problems, such as subsidies meant to keep people above poverty in old age or supports meant to delay the institutionalization of older persons through the delivery of home health care and meals. These interventions can sometimes be evidence based, but they are rarely based on strong theory. At the *micro*-social level are interventions by practitioners who serve older people. These daily provide help and assistance to elders in need. Their efforts, which are routinely touted as being anchored in "best practice" models, most often reflect empirical generalizations concerning practices employed in the past.

The difficult task of implementing effective public policy and service delivery is exacerbated by the fact that little funding is available for the evaluation of these efforts. What is clear is that these interventions rarely rest on strong theory. If we do not understand the *theory* (the why and the how) of the problem, how can we best set up an intervention to fix it?

■ THE DEVELOPMENT OF THEORY IN GERONTOLOGY

In looking back through previous handbooks on aging, one can see that the theories of aging have undergone several pendulum shifts during the relatively short history of gerontology. In the first handbooks, there was still an emphasis on "grand" theory, from Edmund Vincent Cowdry's (1939) biological theory of aging as a disruption in homeostasis (see Park, 2008), to Ernest Burgess's (1960) sociological theory of modernization as creating a "roleless role" for the aged (see Chapter 5), and to James Birren's (1960) "counterpart" theory of psychological decrement. Later, the pendulum shifted back to an era that was "data rich but theory poor"—what C. Wright Mills (1959) would have called "abstracted empiricism" or Robert Merton (1968) "strict empiricism," in which too much attention was given to data over theory. And the pendulum seems to be swinging back again today, as the chapters throughout this edition attest, to what Merton (1968) once called theories of the "middle range," built around circumscribed topics and adequate, if not ample, data.

The first of the four volumes to date on theories of aging (Birren & Bengtson, 1988) was not called a "handbook." With "only" 20 chapters, 480 pages, and 23 contributors, the publisher felt that it was not hefty enough to warrant such a designation; so it was more modestly titled *Emergent Theories of Aging*. It was also the most philosophical of the four editions, with chapters on basic assumptions in theories of aging, dynamics related to aging and time, heuristics and metaphors in aging research, and contributions from the humanities. The chapters were thoughtful and often speculative, and there were far fewer studies to review than in later editions.

Over a decade passed before the next edition (Bengtson & Schaie, 1999) appeared as the *Handbook of Theories of Aging*. This volume contained 25 chapters and 524 pages, representing the work of 49 authors. In it, one can see the movement of the field toward greater specialization, a narrowing of focus on research topics, and a more problem-oriented perspective. For example, the biological and biomedical section contained a chapter on stress theories of aging; the psychology section, a chapter on everyday competence and aging; and the social sciences section, a chapter on political economy and aging.

The 2009 edition (Bengtson et al., 2009) expanded significantly, with 40 chapters, 789 pages, and 79 authors. In it, the editors observed one major theoretical development in the years since the previous edition: a significant increase in theories and research that crossed traditional disciplinary boundaries. Indeed, that edition also contained a new section on "Translating Theories of Aging," with chapters on topics such as jurisprudential gerontology, spirituality, a wisdom-based model of psychotherapy, and educational gerontology. Commitments to theory-based translational research have continued to grow, with this section of the current edition being the strongest to date.

In this 2016 edition, readers will find a strong emphasis again on theories related to health, but this time with greater attention to health-related processes and a wider range of health outcomes. This reflects movements in medicine, public health, and health sciences that are focused on prevention and treatment and on health disparities. Research in sociology and psychology, too, has more rigorously examined broader conceptions of well-being and the influences of close relationships, wider social networks, and life-course dynamics. Much of the action in biology has similarly shifted away from longevity and toward "health span" and aging well, not just aging long. Health and well-being are clearly central nodes around which scholars are fostering theories that bridge disciplines and levels of analysis, from cells to societies. The trend toward transdisciplinary work is also very apparent in this edition. In fact, it is now the longest section, and one can see the influence of transdisciplinary commitments in the disciplinary sections and in the section on policy, intervention, and practice as well.

■ AN OVERVIEW OF THIS EDITION
Goals and Emphases

Since the previous edition of this handbook, important developments have occurred within each of the disciplinary areas reflected in gerontology—the biology, psychology, and social sciences of aging, as well as in policy, intervention, and practice. A primary goal of this edition—with 35 chapters, 718 pages, and 70 contributors—is to update researchers, professionals, and students of aging on the latest theoretical developments across these traditional areas of gerontology.

A second goal is to foster "transdisciplinary" theories of aging by expanding concepts and explanatory systems across traditional boundaries. Critical advances have been made in transdisciplinary theories on circumscribed topics. Indeed, this is where much of the action in theory now resides and will continue to move.

A third goal is to increase attention to matters of variability and diversity in aging processes, from the cellular level of biological aging to the societal level of public policy. We asked chapter authors to consider the following issues: How sensitive are theories and concepts to matters of variability and diversity in aging—for example, to differences by gender, race and ethnicity, social class, or culture? How might theories and concepts be revised or tested with these matters in mind? In an effort to treat matters of globalization, we have also increased the coverage of international topics and the roster of international authors.

A fourth goal is to be a catalyst for developing future theories. To this end, we have asked contributors to contemplate common questions that bridge past, present, and future:

- *The state and evolution of theories*: What is the current state of theories and concepts and how far have they come? What theories and concepts have generated excitement? Which have fallen away, and which might be reclaimed but reshaped in light of contemporary conditions or intellectual currents?
- *The synergy between theories and research*: How have key theories and concepts shaped research and the current knowledge base? What research needs to be done to ensure vibrant theories in the decade ahead? What steps need to be taken in order to propel theory development in these directions?

Organization

The body of this handbook is organized into seven sections, six of which have its own introduction by an editor or associate editor. The section introductions not only highlight the key contributions of the specific chapters therein, but also provide a global orientation to the theories in that area and an integrated story about the section as a whole.

The next chapter provides an overview of the volume and an examination of age and aging as our central theoretical constructs. Part I—"Standing on the Shoulders of Giants: Personal Perspectives on Theory Development in Aging"—is a new feature of this edition. This part contains chapters from four of the most senior gerontologists of our day from the fields of biology, psychology, social sciences, and the policy and practice of aging. The essays give readers an intimate backstage view into history of theory development in their respective fields. They share their personal experiences with the process and prospects of developing good theory: disappointments and victories, barriers and opportunities, and solutions and advice.

Parts II, III, and IV—on biological, psychological, and social science theories and concepts of aging—have been mainstays of this handbook since its initiation. Each discipline has an important set of theoretical traditions of its own. In this edition, we have built up the section on policy, intervention, and practice theories and concepts (Part V) to reflect commitments their field is making in theory-based, in addition to evidence-based, application.

Part VI highlights the surge in transdisciplinary theory development. Despite the challenges of bridging disciplines, and of working with different research paradigms and methods, researchers have made significant breakthroughs in explanations of aging phenomena that crossed and integrated disciplinary perspectives. This cross-pollination has been fostered by interdisciplinary graduate programs and training grants, as well as by funding agencies, which have placed a premium on interdisciplinary team science. It is exciting to see the emergence of theories and models that have as centerpieces concepts around which multiple scientific disciplines can collaborate.

Part VII, the conclusion, discusses some of the challenges of theory building in gerontology and advances an agenda for the development of theories in the future. As the field of gerontology and research on aging continue to rapidly expand, the need for a strong theory will only grow.

REFERENCES

Bengtson, V. L., Gans, D., Putney, N. M., & Silverstein, M. (2009). *Handbook of theories of aging* (2nd ed.). New York, NY: Springer Publishing Company.

Bengtson, V. L., & Schaie, K. W. (1999). *Handbook of theories of aging* (1st ed.). New York, NY: Springer Publishing Company.

Birren, J. E. (1960). Behavioral theories of aging. In N. W. Shock (Ed.), *Aging: Some social and biological aspects* (pp. 305–332). Washington, DC: American Association for the Advancement of Science.

Birren, J. E. (1973). Methods and models in the study of aging. In R. H. Davis & M. Neiswender (Eds.), *Aging: Prospects and issues* (pp. 1–17). Los Angeles, CA: Andrus Gerontology Center, University of Southern California.

Birren, J. E., & Bengtson, V. L. (1988). *Emergent theories of aging.* New York, NY: Springer Publishing Company.

Burgess, E. W. (1960). *Aging in Western societies.* Chicago, IL: University of Chicago Press.

Cowdry, E. V. (1939). *Problems of ageing.* Baltimore, MD: Lippincott Williams & Wilkins.

Merton, R. (1968). *Social theory and social structure* (3rd ed.). New York, NY: Free Press.

Mills, C. W. (1959). *The sociological imagination.* London, UK: Oxford University Press.

Park, H. W. (2008). Edmund Vincent Cowdry and the making of gerontology as a multidisciplinary scientific field in the United States. *Journal of the History of Biology, 41*, 529–572.

Tibbitts, C. (1960). *Handbook of social gerontology: Societal aspects of aging.* Chicago, IL: University of Chicago Press.

CHAPTER 2

Concepts and Theories of Age and Aging
Richard A. Settersten, Jr., and Bethany Godlewski

Gerontology has an uneasy and codependent relationship with chronological age. On one hand, age lies at the heart of scholarship on aging, consuming a major space in our scientific lenses. It is such a taken-for-granted part of our worldview that we fail to notice it or question its presence as it snuggles comfortably in the models and equations of most empirical articles. On the other hand, some of the most dominant rhetoric of the field, and the messages that gerontologists perpetuate, sends quite a different signal—that age is not something to be embraced as much as it is something to be transcended.

In this chapter, we chart the meanings and uses of age in research on aging, focusing mainly on concepts and theories but also making a few observations on methods. We follow two major strands of inquiry, reviewing selected research and generating ideas that are ripe for theory development. The first strand of inquiry relates to age as a property of individuals and groups. It addresses age as a proxy for statuses and experiences, age as relative personal time, subjective age, and age as an index for different types of time. The second strand of inquiry relates to age as a property of social organization and dynamics. It addresses age and life phases; ageism and age stereotypes; age and the timing and allocation of social roles; age integration and cooperation versus age segregation and conflict; age as a right and benefit; and the intersections among age, gender, and culture.

We find two opposing trends: For many aspects of individual aging, age may not matter as much as researchers assume it does, at least not directly. To advance theories of individual-level phenomena, investigators should think more critically about *why* and *how* age might or might not matter for their topics of interest. For many social aspects of aging, in contrast, age may matter much more than researchers realize. To advance theories of social phenomena, investigators must reveal the relevance and irrelevance of age in contemporary social life. In addition, to advance multilevel and transdisciplinary theories, investigators must reveal how larger social forces related to age have both direct and indirect effects on individual aging.

■ AGE AS A PROPERTY OF INDIVIDUALS AND GROUPS

Age is an identifiable yet somewhat intangible property of individuals. It is hard to find a study that does not include age, especially as a means for classifying people into groups. These are the most common methodological uses of age, to which we will return later. Age is at times connected to possibilities of various kinds of growth (e.g., wisdom, emotion regulation, or mental health) or it becomes a protective factor of some type (e.g., accumulated experiences may bring a wider repertoire of coping strategies or human capital).

However, more often than not, age is posited to bring decline or risk in various domains (e.g., cognitive or physical health). The senior author was reminded of this not long ago when, in reporting some health symptoms to his doctor, the doctor replied, "Well, *at your age*, what do you expect?"

Age as Proxy for Statuses and Experiences

Chronological age has long been recognized as an "empty" independent variable. Researchers often use age as a proxy for things that are highly age-related but have not been measured—say, some biological, psychological, or social aspect of development. Age *itself* is not the cause of an outcome. Instead, it is whatever age presumably indexes that matters. For example, chronological age might be a proxy for individuals' emotional maturity (psychological age), roles and responsibilities (social age or legal age), position in their potential life spans (biological age), or ability to function in daily life and adapt to their environments (functional age). There have been approaches to measuring and validating each of these types of age. But rather than rely on age, researchers might think more critically about what it is standing in for and whether those things might be measured more directly. These are old debates, but the problems persist.

It is easy to see why chronological age has great appeal. It is convenient and practical as a research variable and as an administrative gauge (for a classic discussion, see Neugarten & Hagestad, 1976). It is easily and objectively measured, and it is universal—everyone has one. Even more, chronological age is enmeshed with aging because aging seems to be about advancing *in* age. When push comes to shove, however, gerontologists often have difficulty distinguishing between age and aging, and between aging and age-related disease. Theoretical advances rest on moving beyond age as an "instrumental property of measurement," to use Jan Baars's phrase (2010), and on interrogating *why* and *how* age becomes meaningful in explaining particular phenomena.

Age as Relative Personal Time

Chronological age is ultimately an index of *absolute* time (years since birth) that stems from a human-made calendar (see also Fry, 2009). It serves as a crude gauge for where an individual is in life. Experientially, however, age prompts both internal and external comparisons that are really about *relative* time. Internally, individuals use age to assess the present and then judge the past and anticipate the future. Externally, individuals make judgments about themselves relative to their age peers ("At the reunion, many of my classmates looked much older than me") or relative to people who are younger or older ("He's 30 years older than me, but he works just as much. I hope I'm able to keep working at that level when I'm his age"). Individuals also use age to make the same kinds of assessments of *other* people ("They're the same age, but our parents couldn't be more different; mine are so active and yours are couch potatoes").

Age can similarly be understood as *duration* in that it may be used to estimate time *to* an event ("I will be 53 when my daughter graduates high school, just 2 years from now"), time *in* a role ("I retired at 67 after being a professor for 40 years"), or time *between* experiences ("I had my daughter at 26 but waited 3 years before I had my son"). A common experience in this regard is for individuals in middle age to begin thinking less about how many years have passed since birth, and to start thinking more about how many years they have before death (Neugarten, 1968). This insight propelled a vibrant field of inquiry on "future time perspective" (e.g., Carstensen, 2006), in which the goals, behaviors, and emotions of people of any age are understood to be shaped by how much time they think they have left (see also Chapter 12 by Ngo, Sands, & Isaacowitz). As with age, these duration experiences can involve internal or external comparisons. For example, serious illness brings the feeling that one is running out of time in having his or her own life or time with loved ones cut short (Hagestad, 1996).

Subjective Age

These internal and external comparisons underlie another major tradition of research since the 1960s: subjective age. Research on subjective age identification examines how old a person feels, into which age group an individual categorizes himself or herself, or how old one would like to be, regardless of his or her actual age. This body of research is important in that it generally does not anchor age in simple chronological terms, but instead in phenomenological terms. It does, however, often make comparisons between the actual chronological ages of people versus those they give for a variety of dimensions: such as physical appearance (look age), activity level or types of behaviors (act age), how old one feels (feel age) or would like to be (desired age), or the ages other people would give them (assigned age) (for a review, see Settersten & Gannon, 2006). These subjective ages have been linked to health, personality, and social behavior, and the kinds of goals people set and pursue (for illustrations, see a recent collection of papers edited by Diehl & Wahl, 2015).

New developments have also been made in the area of subjective *aging* and "awareness of age-related change" (AARC; Diehl & Wahl, 2010; Diehl, Wahl, Brothers, & Miche, 2015). The model emphasizes the fact that a person's AARC is based on his or her "*conscious* perceptions of changed behavior, performance, or reflected experience," and that, in perceiving these changes, the person "attributes them to his or her *increased chronological age* and not to other conditions" (Diehl et al., 2015, p. 12). Diehl and colleagues (2015) proposed that AARC can occur in five separate domains: (a) health and physical functioning, (b) cognitive functioning, (c) interpersonal relationships, (d) social–cognitive and social–emotional functioning, and (e) lifestyle and engagement.

Although subjective age and aging are often construed to be "personal" experiences, they are inherently interpersonal and therefore social phenomena (Settersten & Hagestad, 2015). They largely rest on how individuals see themselves relative to their younger selves and relative to other people; how others see the individual and respond to his or her aging; and how individuals see and respond to the aging of others.

Age and Other Kinds of Time

Chronological age takes on unique social meanings in a society, a theme to which we will return. These meanings underlie *social time*: what age means for the social roles an individual holds, the events and transitions an individual experiences, or the behaviors that are expected of an individual. Age can also be tangled up in other kinds of time: family time, organizational time, and historical time. *Family time* designates the generation within which an individual is located in an extended family structure (for classic discussions, see also Bengtson & Black, 1973; Hagestad, 1982). As generations "turn over" (i.e., as older generations die and new generations are born), individuals' locations in family structures change, bringing new identities, roles, and responsibilities. Family time can also refer to the interwoven nature of family relationships, and the degree to which individual time meshes with family time. Occurrences in the lives of one family member often have repercussions for other family members, and the scheduling of family events and transitions in one generation affects other generations, whether difficult experiences such as divorce or terminal illness, or joyful experiences such as marriages or births.

Individuals and groups are also affected by *organizational time*. Educational programs require the completion of a specific number of credit hours; courses must be tackled at a specific pace and in a specific sequence; ultimate time limits are set for obtaining a degree. Work organizations similarly operate on specific shifts; hours are clocked; production is timed; deadlines are set; sick, personal, and holiday time is monitored and negotiated; timetables are set for promotional tracks. The rhythm of experiences in medical institutions marches to the clock, as stays are time bound, patients and treatments are scheduled, and rounds are made. Each of these environments can also be highly age graded, such that individuals who are younger or older than the typical populations may not have the same opportunities and may feel "out of sync" relative to their peers.

Finally, individuals and the collective lives of whole cohorts are framed and shaped by *historical time* (for classic discussions, see Bengtson & Cutler, 1976; Rosow, 1978; Ryder, 1965). Historical time is accompanied by both short- and long-term changes in economic, political, and social life that may gradually or abruptly alter life circumstances. Just as age is a simple index for lifetime, cohort is a simple index for historical time and brings similar concerns. To advance theories of aging, investigators must interrogate *why* and *how* cohort becomes meaningful in explaining particular phenomena, as well as clarify the relationship between cohort and age, which are often confounded or confused. Age-based explanations are about maturation, but cohort-based explanations are about historical events and social change.

These "times of our lives," to use Joe Hendricks and Calvin Peters's (1986) phrase, call attention to the *dynamic* and linked nature of human aging—as individuals and groups move through the age strata of the population, generations within their families, social settings and institutions, and the course of history. These types of time offer important gateways to theoretical advances in gerontology. They bring attention to the "sociocultural" realm, and to powerful, but often invisible, social forces that structure aging experiences, to which we now turn.

■ AGE AS A DIMENSION OF SOCIAL ORGANIZATION AND DYNAMICS

Basic "ascribed" social categories, like age, often conceal subtle, complicated processes and take on complex social meanings (i.e., influencing attitudes, behaviors, and language). Social scientists begin their work with the assumption that lives are socially structured, and in most Western societies, age is a meaningful dimension of social organization. Chronological age is embedded in social systems, including age-homogeneous or "age-graded" social institutions (e.g., schools and residential facilities), age-based policies (e.g., compulsory schooling, adult rights and duties that come at 18 and 21 years, work promotion prospects, retirement and pension rules), public discourse, and face-to-face interactions.

Age seems more salient in the economic and political spheres than in the family sphere. Within the economic sphere, age structuring has been linked to the emergence of the market; and in the political sphere, age structuring has been linked to the emergence of the nation-state, citizenship, and the welfare state (Dannefer & Settersten, 2010). These spheres run on linear "man-made" clock time that is predictable and both future- and goal-oriented. The qualities of chronological age noted earlier have made it appealing and useful in a historical process of what sociologists, dating back to Max Weber (1904–1905), call "rationalization"—a process in which human action has increasingly been subject to administrative calculation and control in order to help society and its systems run more efficiently.

The family sphere, on the other hand, may not be as age-structured because it runs on time that is less linear. The time binds in managing and integrating work and family life exist in part because these spheres operate on different kinds of time. The needs of the body and of other people (sickness, childbirth, or child rearing) limit the ability to plan. However, dramatic changes in mortality and morbidity have also made patterns of chronic illness and death among family members more predictable—that is, they are generally confined to old age. Of course, women's fertility is also highly bound to biological clocks that place lower and upper age limits on reproduction.

Age and Life Phases

Age is tied to the social construction of broader life phases. It shapes how members of a culture splice up the life course, give names to different periods and define their beginnings and ends, and organize institutions and professions around them—including gerontology. Individuals are aware of their movement, and the movement of others, into and out of these life phases. Identities, relationships, and expectations are based on them.

The increasing differentiation of life phases has been a historically emergent property of modern societies, beginning with "childhood," "adulthood," and "old age" (Settersten, 1999). Childhood was eventually differentiated into "early childhood," "middle childhood," and "youth and adolescence." Adulthood was segmented into "early adulthood," "midlife," and "old age." As the phase immediately preceding old age, midlife has grown to be of special interest to research on aging (see Lachman, 2015). Old age was further split into the "young-old" and the "old-old" (Neugarten, 1974, 1979/1996) or the "third age" and "fourth age" (Baltes, 1997; Laslett, 1989), with people in the "fourth age" sometimes called the "oldest-old" (Suzman & Riley, 1985). In light of the prolonged transition to adulthood today, it would not surprise us if "early adulthood" were soon split into the "young-young" and the "old-young" to distinguish the front and back ends of the 20s, which are very different (Settersten & Ray, 2010).

The terms "young-old" and "old-old" have become permanent fixtures in aging research since Bernice Neugarten first coined them in the 1970s. Since then, researchers have defined them in purely chronological terms, with the young–old traditionally defined as 65 to 74 years old and the old–old as 75 years and older. With the advent of the "fourth age" and the "oldest old" amid greater longevity, these terms now often refer to those 80 or 85 years and older, leaving investigators to sometimes reconfigure the boundaries of the younger group(s).

From the vantage point of theory, however, it is important to note that Neugarten's original use of these terms was explicitly *not* about chronological age. It was instead to separate elders who are relatively healthy, affluent, and active from those who are not—regardless of their ages—precisely because people of a given age are so highly variable. For this reason, the field of gerontology should move away from defining these classes in terms of chronological age. The spirit beneath Neugarten's use of these terms is important. It is this same spirit that drove Leonard Cain (2003, p. 301) to argue that the study of those who are considered "elderly" or "senior" should be differentiated for both scientific and policy purposes into the "go-go," the "slow-go," and the "no-go," or into the "frisky," the "frail," and the "fragile."

The traditional starting point for defining "old age" is also a cultural and historical property in that it is tied to eligibility thresholds for social security and other government programs. And yet, research on subjective age has also repeatedly revealed that many people who have passed this threshold do not classify themselves as "old" (Settersten & Hagestad, 2015).

Social change, too, continues to "blur the lines" between life phases, to use Jack Levin's (2012) phrase, and life as it is experienced is clearly more transitional than discrete. That is, people do not wake up one day and suddenly feel as if they are in a new phase, and certainly not based on age alone. Instead, they gradually experience an accumulation of changes that may raise their awareness, some of which may be related to chronological age, but many of which are not (for illustrations, see Settersten & Hagestad, 2015).

Ageism and Age Stereotypes

Larger life phases can be the basis for ageism and age stereotypes—common images or perceptions of people of different ages, and their physical, psychological, and social characteristics. Through these images and perceptions, age enters into and shapes everyday social interaction, affecting the expectations and evaluations of the individuals involved in those exchanges.

Age is, to use Boyd and Dowd's (1988) phrase, a "diffuse status characteristic." Individuals use cues about others' ages to make assumptions about their attributes and abilities, a practice which seems especially likely when little else besides other "master status" characteristics, like sex or race, are known. Like these other characteristics, age is portable—it always accompanies the individual. However, the appearance of age, in contrast, is something that can be more easily manipulated for those with the desire and resources (see also Biggs, 2005). Indeed, the large over-the-counter cosmetic market, which peddles "regenerative" "anti-aging" products, has been built around the manipulability of age (see also Mykytyn, 2006). The desire to look or act younger should occur more often in environments in which age and aging are devalued, although looking or acting *too* young might also carry negative judgments.

Stereotype embodiment theory (SET) has advanced recent research on ageism and age stereotypes (see Chapter 14 by Meisner and Levy). This theory posits that individuals internalize age stereotypes throughout life, and that stereotypes can exist outside of an individual's awareness, being reinforced whenever an individual's lived experience matches the stereotype and manifest psychologically, behaviorally, and physiologically.

Some researchers further theorize that confronting negative stereotypes depletes the limited amount of strength an individual has to regulate thoughts, feelings, and behaviors (Emile, d'Arripe-Longueville, Cheval, Amato, & Chalabaev, 2015), forcing older adults to switch their mindset from one of achieving gains to avoiding losses (Barber, Mather, & Gatz, 2015). Others have explored whether experiencing stressful life events in older adulthood, such as the death of a family member or hospitalization, strengthens existing negative stereotypes of aging and, consequently, the ill effects of aging (Levy, Slade, Chung, & Gil, 2015). SET implicitly builds on Robert Butler's (1969) comparison of ageism to sexism and racism, in which age represents an accumulation of exposure to negative stereotypes, thereby increasing the likelihood of internalization.

Individuals' personal stereotypes about aging are associated with physical, cognitive, and mental health outcomes in later adulthood. Those who have held over many years negative personal beliefs about aging, and/or who live in environments that reinforce these stereotypes, have poorer memory function and are more likely to experience health concerns such as anxiety, cardiac events, suicidal ideation, and posttraumatic stress disorder (Horton, Baker, Pearce, & Deakin, 2008; Levy, Pilver, & Pietrzak, 2014).

Many stereotypes of aging are negative, but they need not be. Positive stereotypes also exist, such as stereotypes that older people are wise, dignified, nurturing, friendly, patient, or giving. These positive stereotypes are important counterparts to the negative stereotypes that many gerontologists deem as "ageist." Theories of ageism must probe the positive end of the continuum, as age stereotypes can also provide social advantages, not just disadvantages.

What makes age different from sex or race as a dimension of stratification and inequality is that, eventually, "everyone becomes vulnerable to ageism if they live long enough" (Palmore, 2015, p. 873). This is not to say, however, that ageism is experienced uniformly by sex or race. Ageism is also relatively invisible relative to other kinds of "isms." Individuals are often unaware of ageism in their attitudes or behavior, or of when they tacitly support the ageist attitudes and behaviors of others. Ageism is enjoying renewed attention in gerontology, as reflected in 2015 special issues of the *Journals of Gerontology: Social Sciences* and *Generations*. However, ageism is not the exclusive domain of gerontology. Ageism can exist for young people too, especially in settings where there is competition (or perceived competition) for employment and public resources. Advances in theory will be found in probing how ageism is transmitted and its full range of outcomes, as well as how theory-based social interventions might be designed to interrupt or stop it.

Theoretical advances are also to be found in clarifying the relationship between negative age stereotypes and ageism, on one hand, and successful aging, on the other (see Chapter 27 by Rowe & Cosco and Chapter 35 by Settersten & Bengtson). One might be tempted to attempt to overturn negative stereotypes by simply replacing them with positive stereotypes, such as those advanced in the successful aging tradition. Yet, overly positive portrayals can be both unrealistic and dangerous models of aging that may not be attainable for many individuals, and negative and positive stereotypes may have distinct sources, mechanisms, and consequences.

Age and the Timing and Allocation of Social Roles

Social roles and activities are allocated on the basis of age or life phase. For societies, as noted earlier, this is reflected in the age-based organization of education, work, and retirement and leisure institutions. This "tripartite" division of the life course, to use Martin Kohli's (2007) phrase, largely frontloads education, confines work to the middle, and keeps leisure and the absence or reduced level of work for the end. Family experiences, in contrast, exist across the whole of life, although the nature of family experiences and the constellation of family forms change over time. Opportunities in education, work, leisure, and family life are also age-based because institutions and markets cater to particular age groups. This line of thinking has been central to the "age stratification" framework begun by Matilda White Riley and colleagues in the late 1960s (see Riley, 1987), but which was preceded by Cain's (1964) often overlooked work.

Life trajectories are conceptualized as being calibrated by a sequence of age-linked role transitions: times when social personae change; when new rights, duties, and resources are encountered; and when identities are in flux. Members of groups share informal notions about the "normal, expectable life," to use Neugarten's (1969) phrase: social and cultural expectations—"age norms"—for the timing and sequencing of major life transitions such as leaving home, finishing school, finding full-time work, partnering and parenting, or retiring (for a review, see Settersten, 2003). Age norms are social prescriptions for, or proscriptions against, involvement in particular activities or roles at particular ages.

Individuals use these age-linked scripts to organize their own lives and their expectations for the lives of others. In orienting behavior, these maps serve an important human need for order and predictability. For individuals, this is reflected in a sense of being on time, off time, or out of time with respect to accomplishing these transitions. When experiences come early, late, or never—or when experiences come along that have never been in our minds as possibilities—we are caught off guard and unprepared.

Age norms are similarly central to many sociological theories because adherence to these expectations is taken to be important for maintaining social order and the division of labor in society, and for allocating resources. From this vantage point, there must be consensus about these age-based prescriptions or proscriptions, and they must be enforced through social sanctions that reward people for staying "on track" or penalize them for deviating.

In the face of an increasingly individualized or "de-standardized" life course today, age may have diminished strength as a regulator of transitions. Nonetheless, individuals may cling to old ideas about what constitutes a normal, expectable life even if the reality is that their lives will not or cannot match those ideals.

Age Integration and Segregation, Age Cooperation and Conflict

The fact that societies often allocate opportunities and roles based on age brings the possibility that various age "strata" in the population might be too segregated from one another. As a result, a strand of research has called for a thorough examination of the costs of age segregation and the benefits of age integration for individuals and societies (Hagestad & Uhlenberg, 2005, 2006). So, too, has it called for the design of social interventions to more often put people of different ages together as they learn, work, and live in order to foster deeper relationships across generations within a society. Otherwise, the only meaningful cross-cohort relationships are those that are found in the family, and age segregation outside the family can be the root of ageism.

Age segregation or integration can give way to themes of conflict versus cooperation among age strata (Henretta, 1988), although research has seldom examined these dynamics. A working assumption is that age segregation generates conflict across cohorts, and that age integration generates cooperation. That is, if people are embedded in age-similar networks, they will act in ways that promote the interests of their age group, and if people are embedded in age-diverse networks, they will act in ways that transcend the interests of their age group. Alternatively, one could argue that being embedded in age-diverse networks makes it more possible to have age-based conflict. In addition, processes of "cohort flow" mean that members of all cohorts will, eventually, have the experience of being in a particular age stratum. Older cohorts have already passed through many life phases and therefore have an understanding of what those phases are like; younger cohorts have not. These differences in experience and worldview can be significant sources of intergenerational conflict within families and across social generations.

It is important to note that age segregation is not simply the result of structural forces outside of one's control. It is sometimes about personal choice. Many older people, for example, actively decide to live in "55+" or "65+" communities that are, by design, meant to facilitate social engagement and integration among age peers, and to respond to the emerging health needs of aging individuals (for a classic discussion, see Rosow, 1967). Although such communities may bring important amenities and benefits, they necessarily restrict interaction with people of younger ages, perhaps even regulating the presence of children, youth, and young adults. At the early end of adult life, the same can be said about college dormitories, which have similar functions and consequences for students. These examples serve as reminders that one cannot assume that integration brings uniformly positive effects, or that segregation brings uniformly negative ones. Both scenarios come with costs and benefits.

The reality is that life in any society will involve both age-based cooperation and conflict. Classic debates in gerontology about generational equity (Bengtson & Achenbaum, 1993; Quadagno, 1989; Williamson, Kingson, & Watts-Roy, 1999), triggered by Preston (1984), are related to the theme of conflict. If different age groups have disproportionate slices of the public resource pie, the assumption is that this will create conflict. This leads to the uses of age in law and policy, to which we now turn, and to any age divisiveness that might stem from it.

Age as a Right and Benefit

The state often relies on, and even creates, conceptions of age and life phases. These create cross-national variability in the structure and experience of the life course. General references to age-related categories, without clearly specified ages, are common in legislation ("minors," "adult," "the elderly"). Specific age rules or preferences are embedded within laws, policies, and institutions that relate to education, work, family, or health (for classic discussions, see Cain, 1964; Mayer & Müller, 1986). In most countries, determining the rights and responsibilities of "adult" status are explicitly structured by chronological age—for example, regulations regarding compulsory schooling, driving, drinking, voting, consensual sex, working, marrying, or seeking public offices. Eligibility for pensions, social services, or social insurance is often determined by age. Many discussions about legal ages are centered on questions of how soon in life individuals should be granted adult rights and obligations, and on how late in life these rights and obligations should be maintained, or the conditions under which they should be revoked (see also Cain, 2003).

In the United States, there is extensive scaffolding of government-sponsored social programs and services in the first and last few decades of life. This scaffolding is based on assumptions about risk and dependence on others during these years. In the case of childhood, it relates to the need to invest in and protect children and, in recent years, young adults, because of their longer *dependence* on parents or guardians. In the case of old age, it relates to the need to protect and promote the security of older adults because of their increased health and economic risks (and the risk of *becoming* dependent). It also makes retirement viable and rewards elders for their prior contributions to society (see also Skocpol, 2000).

Age and Its Intersection With Gender and Culture

Age operates together with gender as "twin statuses" of social organization, to use Ralph Linton's (1940) phrase (see also Parsons, 1942). That is, age and sex are often coupled. There are not generic old *people*; there are old *men* and old *women* (Settersten & Hagestad, 2015). Yet, theories are often created and research often conducted as if age and aging are unisex phenomena. This is true of many of the issues described thus far, and it is true of many of the chapters of this handbook.

With respect to age, for example, men and women probably attach different social meanings to age, use different guidelines to measure the progress of their lives, and are subject to different expectations and evaluations (Settersten & Hagestad, 2015; see also Calasanti, 2010; Levy & Widmer, 2013). For instance, there are strong and persistent cultural differences related to aging bodies, including the "double standard" of aging for men and women—that the physical signs of aging often accentuate a man's social capital but for women take it away (Bell, 1970; Sontag, 1972).

Similarly, some have suggested that men and women may have different needs for predictability and order, and that they may experience different kinds of time—with the rhythms of men's lives being more linear (and therefore more regulated by chronological age), and women's being more nonlinear (and therefore less regulated by chronological age). This has to do with the fact that work and family spheres, to which men and women have traditionally been differentially attached, run on different kinds of time, as discussed earlier.

Age and sex are two prominent dimensions of social organization and differentiation, but there are others. Every society simultaneously classifies its members using multiple dimensions. In the United States, social class and race work alongside and interact with age and gender as major sources of inequality. These, too, are important for theories of aging to take into account. For example, social class and race are associated with the different types and levels of cultural, social, and economic capital. These, in turn, lead to different aging outcomes through mechanisms such as differential access to health care, education, and housing. Exposure to risks and opportunities in these domains accumulates over individuals' lifetimes, promoting resilience or magnifying risks in the face of continued adversity (see also Dannefer, 2003; DiPrete & Eirich, 2006; Chapter 19 by O'Rand).

Concepts and theories of age should similarly be sensitive to culture. Most cultures and societies have their own frameworks for understanding age, age periods, and the life course as a whole; yet little is known about these frameworks. For example, the landmark study Project AGE from the 1990s, the only study of its kind, mapped the meanings of age and aging in seven different cultural contexts (Keith et al., 1994). It is a compelling case for theory development because it explicitly targeted the "how" and "why" culture matters in determining the structure, experience, and meaning of aging (see also Chapter 20 by Marshall, Martin-Matthews, & McMullin).

The Project AGE team explored three types of meanings of age: cognitive, evaluative, and social participation. *Cognitive* meanings of age are related to whether age is relevant as a dimension of social organization, the age categories that members of a culture perceive, and how they define, indicate, or signal these categories. Age had more significance in environments that were larger and more stable, that had higher levels of education and greater predictability in life experiences, as well as in cultures in which the life course is strongly organized by work, the economy, and the state and its policies.

Evaluative meanings of age are related to the value attached to different ages and age categories. Here, investigators found old age to be the least desirable time in life in all settings, but the least negative evaluations were found in cultures where individuals' livelihoods are not as highly determined by health and vigor and where independence can be maintained.

Age as a criterion for *social participation* relates to norms for formal and informal interaction between people of different ages. Here, too, investigators unveiled significant variability across communities in the age "borders" on interaction and behavior, ranging from sites where it was difficult to find any situation in which people of only one age category are present, to tight and fine-grained social boundaries that separate people into distinct age-graded social contexts.

Today, "age explicit life courses" or "staged life courses," to use Fry's (2010) terms, are typical in many societies. Age is used to manage people, to organize life stages, and to allocate privileges, power, access to goods and services, and social support. It is ultimately culture that gives meaning to both age and gender. To advance theories of age and aging, researchers must therefore probe *why* and *how* gender and culture matter for phenomena under study.

■ CONCLUSION

We have described two major strands of concepts and theories of age. The first strand addressed age as a property of individuals and groups. Here, we examined age as a proxy for statuses and experiences. We discussed age as it enters matters of self and identity, through comparisons within oneself and to others, and through facets of subjective age. We illustrated how age makes its way into experiences of time in family life, in organizations, and in history.

Each of these fronts is ripe for advancing person-centered theories of aging. The passing of time is related to aging phenomena. When theories actually address age, they often stop at the description stage and do not reveal mechanisms of change. Age itself is generally not a mechanism that causes changes in cognition, behavior, emotion, or motivation. It is a "carrier" variable for processes associated with chronological age that may cause age-related differences. Individual aging is poorly indicated by higher chronological ages, but scientific practices ignore this fact.

Progress in theories of aging, then, rests on stronger theoretical and methodological treatments of *age* (see also Barrett, Redmond, & Rohr, 2012). Rather than automatically including age in models and equations—whether as a continuous or categorical independent variable or as a covariate—investigators must provide a theoretical justification as to *why* and *how* age might matter for the phenomena under study. Deeper thought is generally given to questions for which age is a moderator or mediator because inquiry demands it.

The pervasive practice of using age as a dimension for grouping and then comparing individuals across those groups, without any justification, is especially problematic from the vantage point of theory development. In these cases, investigators are often trying to infer something about maturational changes based on age-group differences, even making artificial growth curves by stacking up age groups. In making comparisons across age groups, investigators may also be trying to infer cohort differences based on them—but then the point of entry in searching for an explanation should be found in the realm of historical time, not developmental time.

When age differences are in focus, a well-formulated theory is needed to identify which age-related processes bring about which age-related differences. Advances are to be found in experimental approaches that target the theory-based causal mechanisms that drive change (or stability) with aging, and in including stimuli that represent the natural environment of the person's ecology (Freund, 2015). Statistical models produce information on age that is difficult to interpret, prompting the need for a better theory to justify age categories or to create alternative classifications based on dimensions other than age.

Age can also be an outcome variable. As Schaie (Chapter 4) notes, this practice began as scientists realized that the study of age or duration as a dependent variable could be operationalized via methods of survival or event–time analysis. Modeling the age at an event (widowhood or diagnosis of cognitive impairment) or status at a particular age (health status) are good examples. Modern methods of multilevel modeling have also made it possible to disaggregate individual growth curves (and typologies of growth curves) from the group averages that had previously been a primary focus of inquiry.

Some age-related phenomena have also gotten attention as dependent variables in more substantive ways, such as inquiry into subjective age, or into social phenomena such as age discrimination, age stereotypes, or age integration and segregation. In these cases, there is more theoretical treatment as to *why* and *how* age matters because, as a dependent variable, it is demanded.

The second strand of inquiry addressed age as a dimension of social organization and dynamics. Here, we examined a number of important issues that are ripe for theory development. Those working in more person-centered traditions often do not have these phenomena in view, or they assume that the effects of forces *outside* of people are already represented on the *inside* of people and need not be probed. The burden is on social scientists, especially those working within what Dannefer and Settersten (2010) call the "institutional paradigm," to make age-related social phenomena more visible, and to demonstrate the relevance and irrelevance of age in contemporary social life. We have described how age undergirds the social construction of life phases, how social roles and activities are allocated based on age, how age enters into social interactions and expectations, and how age underlies the organization of institutions, policies, and programs. To advance transdisciplinary theories that cross individual and social levels of analysis, scientists must probe how larger forces related to age may have both direct and indirect effects on individual aging.

A recent 30-year review of scientific journals on aging (Settersten & Angel, 2011) included an observation related to the language of age that is particularly relevant here: that terms such as "old people," "old age," and "elderly," which were once so prevalent, have virtually vanished and have been replaced by neutral language intentionally meant to avoid the sense of becoming "old." We now speak only of "older" people and "later" life. The word "old" is taboo in our science and in society.

The salience of age in gerontology's theoretical lenses has diminished over time, despite the fact that age is so central to our methodological practices. This has occurred in tandem with the emphasis on *successful* aging among gerontologists and in our society. The field of gerontology has, ironically, perpetuated a sense that age and aging are things to be defied, or at least neutralized, which creates its own strand of ageism. In lauding the potentials of age and aging, the field has deemphasized the social problems *of* aging—and aging *as* a social problem—that early captured the attention of the field, problems that researchers of aging are uniquely positioned to help solve.

Gerontology is therefore in the awkward position of wanting to overcome one of the central dimensions that has traditionally been at its core: chronological age (see also Andrews, 1999). Thinking cautiously and critically about age is an important task for building theories of age, aging, and the relationship between them. It is hard to imagine a science of aging without age, but many aspects of aging are not ultimately about age. We may sometimes need to liberate ourselves from age in order to understand aging. However, it is also clear that many aspects of age, especially social ones, are terribly consequential for the aging experiences of individuals and groups.

REFERENCES

Andrews, M. (1999). The seductiveness of agelessness. *Ageing and Society, 19*, 301–318.

Baars, J. (2010). Time and ageing: Enduring and emerging issues. In W. D. Dannefer & C. Phillipson (Eds.), *International handbook of social gerontology* (pp. 367–376). London, UK: Sage.

Baltes, P. B. (1997). On the incomplete architecture of human ontogeny: Selection, optimization, and compensation as foundation of developmental theory. *The American Psychologist, 52*(4), 366–380.

Barber, S. J., Mather, M., & Gatz, M. (2015). How stereotype threat affects healthy older adults' performance on clinical assessments of cognitive decline: The key role of regulatory fit. *The Journals of Gerontology, Series B, 70*(6), 891–900.

Barrett, A., Redmond, R., & Rohr, C. (2012). Avoiding aging? Social psychology's treatment of age. *American Sociologist, 43*, 328–347.

Bell, I. P. (1970). The double standard. *Transaction/Society, 8*, 75–80.

Bengtson, V. L., & Achenbaum, W. A. (1993). *The changing contract across generations.* Hawthorne, NY: Aldine de Gruyter.

Bengtson, V. L., & Black, K. D. (1973). Inter-generation relations and continuities in socialization. In P. Baltes & K. W. Schaie (Eds.), *Life-span developmental psychology: Personality and socialization* (pp. 207–234). New York, NY: Academic Press.

Bengtson, V. L., & Cutler, N. E. (1976). Generations and inter-generational relations: Perspectives on age groups and social change. In R. Binstock & E. Shanas (Eds.), *Handbook of aging and the social sciences* (pp. 130–159). New York, NY: Van Nostrand Reinhold.

Biggs, S. (2005). Beyond appearances: Perspectives on identity in later life and some implications for method. *The Journals of Gerontology, Series B, 60*, 118–128.

Boyd, J. W., & Dowd, J. J. (1988). The diffusiveness of age. *Social Behaviour, 3*, 85–103.

Butler, R. (1969). Ageism: Another form of bigotry. *The Gerontologist, 9*, 243–246.

Cain, L. D. (1964). Life course and social structure. In R. E. Faris (Ed.), *Handbook of sociology* (pp. 272–309). Chicago, IL: Rand McNally.

Cain, L. D. (2003). Age-related phenomena: The interplay of the ameliorative and the scientific. In R. A. Settersten, Jr. (Ed.), *Invitation to the life course: Toward new understandings of later life* (pp. 295–326). Amityville, NY: Baywood Publishing Company.

Calasanti, T. (2010). Gender relations and applied research on aging. *The Gerontologist, 50*, 720–734.

Carstensen, L. L. (2006). The influence of a sense of time on human development. *Science, 312*, 1913–1915.

Dannefer, D. (2003). Cumulative advantage/disadvantage and the life course: Cross-fertilizing age and social science theory. *The Journals of Gerontology, Series B, 58*, S327–S337.

Dannefer, W. D., & Settersten, R. A., Jr. (2010). The study of the life course: Implications for social gerontology. In W. D. Dannefer & C. Phillipson (Eds.), *International handbook of social gerontology* (pp. 3–19). London, UK: Sage.

Diehl, M., & Wahl, H.-W. (Eds.). (2015). Subjective aging: New developments and future directions (*Annual Review of Gerontology and Geriatrics*, Vol. 35). New York, NY: Springer Publishing Company.

Diehl, M., Wahl, H.-W., Brothers, A., & Miche, M. (2015). Subjective aging and awareness of aging: Toward a new understanding of the aging self. In M. Diehl & H.-W. Wahl (Eds.), Subjective aging: New developments and future directions (*Annual Review of Gerontology and Geriatrics*, Vol. 35, pp. 1–28). New York, NY: Springer Publishing Company.

Diehl, M. K., & Wahl, H.-W. (2010). Awareness of age-related change: Examination of a (mostly) unexplored concept. *The Journals of Gerontology, Series B, 65*(3), 340–350.

DiPrete, T. A., & Eirich, G. M. (2006). Cumulative advantage as a mechanism for inequality: A review of theoretical and empirical developments. *Annual Review of Sociology, 32*, 271–297.

Emile, M., d'Arripe-Longueville, F., Cheval, B., Amato, M., & Chalabaev, A. (2015). An ego depletion account of aging stereotypes' effects on health-related variables. *The Journals of Gerontology, Series B, 70*(6), 876–885.

Freund, A. M. (2015). Getting at developmental processes through experiments. *Research in Human Development, 12*, 261–267.

Fry, C. L. (2009). Out of the armchair and off the veranda: Anthropological theories and the experiences of aging. In V. L. Bengtson, M. Silverstein, N. M. Putney, & D. Gans (Eds.), *Handbook of theories of aging* (2nd ed., pp. 499–516). New York, NY: Springer Publishing Company.

Fry, C. L. (2010). Social anthropology and ageing. In W. D. Dannefer & C. Phillipson (Eds.), *International handbook of social gerontology* (pp. 48–60). London, UK: Sage.

Hagestad, G. O. (1982). Parent and child: Generations in the family. In T. M. Field, A. Huston, H. C. Quay, L. Troll, & G. E. Finley (Eds.), *Review of human development* (pp. 485–499). New York, NY: John Wiley & Sons.

Hagestad, G. O. (1996). On-time, off-time, out of time? Reflections on continuity and discontinuity from an illness process. In V. L. Bengtson (Ed.), *Adulthood and aging: Research on continuities and discontinuities* (pp. 204–221). New York, NY: Springer Publishing Company.

Hagestad, G. O., & Uhlenberg, P. (2005). The social separation of old and young: A root of ageism. *Journal of Social Issues, 61*, 343–360.

Hagestad, G. O., & Uhlenberg, P. (2006). Should we be concerned about age segregation? Some theoretical and empirical explorations. *Research on Aging, 28*, 638–654.

Hendricks, J., & Peters, C. B. (1986). The times of our lives. *American Behavioral Scientist, 29,* 662–678.

Henretta, J. C. (1988). Conflict and cooperation among age strata. In J. E. Birren & V. L. Bengtson (Eds.), *Emergent theories of aging* (pp. 385–404). New York, NY: Springer Publishing Company.

Horton, S., Baker, J., Pearce, G. W., & Deakin, J. M. (2008). On the malleability of performance: Implications for seniors. *Journal of Applied Gerontology, 27,* 446–465.

Keith, J., Fry, C. L., Glascock, A. P., Ikels, C., Dickerson-Putnam, J., Harpending, H. C., & Draper, P. (1994). *The aging experience: Diversity and commonality across cultures.* Newbury Park, CA: Sage.

Kohli, M. (2007). The institutionalization of the life course: Looking back to look ahead. *Research in Human Development, 4,* 253–271.

Lachman, M. (2015). Minding the gap in the middle: A call to study midlife. *Research in Human Development, 12,* 327–334.

Laslett, P. (1989). *A fresh map of life: The emergence of the third age.* London, UK: Weidenfeld and Nicolson.

Levin, J. (2012). *Blurring the boundaries: The declining significance of age.* London, UK: Routledge.

Levy, B. R., Pilver, C. E., & Pietrzak, R. H. (2014). Lower prevalence of psychiatric conditions when negative age stereotypes are resisted. *Social Science and Medicine, 119,* 170–174.

Levy, B. R., Slade, M. D., Chung, P. H., & Gill, T. M. (2015). Resiliency over time of elders' age stereotypes after encountering stressful events. *The Journals of Gerontology, Series B, 70*(6), 886–890.

Levy, R., & Widmer, E. D. (Eds.). (2013). *Gendered life courses: Between standardization and individualization.* Zürich, Switzerland: Lit Verlag.

Linton, R. (1940). A neglected aspect of social organization. *American Journal of Sociology, 45,* 870–886.

Mayer, K. U., & Müller, K. (1986). The state and the structure of the life course. In A. B. Sørensen, F. E. Weinert, & L. R. Sherrod (Eds.), *Human development and the life course: Multidisciplinary perspectives* (pp. 217–245). Hillsdale, NJ: Lawrence Erlbaum Associates.

Mykytyn, C. E. (2006). Anti-aging medicine: A patient/practitioner movement to redefine aging. *Social Science and Medicine, 62*(3), 643–653.

Neugarten, B. L. (1968). The awareness of middle age. In B. L. Neugarten (Ed.), *Middle age and aging* (pp. 93–98). Chicago, IL: University of Chicago Press.

Neugarten, B. L. (1969). Continuities and discontinuities of psychological issues into adult life. *Human Development, 12*(2), 121–130.

Neugarten, B. L. (1974). Age groups in American society and the rise of the young-old. *Annals of the American Academy of Political and Social Science, 187,* 187–198.

Neugarten, B. L. (1979/1996). The young-old and the age-irrelevant society. In D. Neugarten (Ed.), *The meanings of age: Selected papers of Bernice L. Neugarten* (pp. 47–55). Chicago, IL: University of Chicago Press.

Neugarten, B. L., & Hagestad, G. O. (1976). Age and the life course. In R. Binstock & E. Shanas (Eds.), *Handbook of aging and the social sciences* (pp. 35–55). New York, NY: Van Nostrand Reinhold.

Palmore, E. (2015). Ageism comes of age. *The Journals of Gerontology, Series B, 70*(6), 873–875.

Parsons, T. (1942). Age and sex in the social structure of the United States. *American Sociological Review, 7*, 604–616.

Preston, S. H. (1984). Children and elderly: Divergent paths for America's dependents. *Demography, 25*, 44–49.

Quadagno, J. S. (1989). Generational equity and the politics of the welfare state. *Politics and Society, 17*, 353–376.

Riley, M. W. (1987). On the significance of age in sociology. *American Sociological Review, 52*, 1–14.

Rosow, I. (1967). *Social integration of the aged.* New York, NY: Free Press.

Rosow, I. (1978). What is a cohort and why? *Human Development, 21*, 65–75.

Ryder, N. B. (1965). The cohort as a concept in the study of social change. *American Sociological Review, 30*(6), 843–861.

Settersten, R. A., Jr. (1999). *Lives in time and place: The problems and promises of developmental science.* Amityville, NY: Baywood Publishing Company.

Settersten, R. A., Jr. (2003). Age structuring and the rhythm of the life course. In J. T. Mortimer & M. J. Shanahan (Eds.), *Handbook of the life course* (pp. 81–98). New York, NY: Springer Science.

Settersten, R. A., Jr., & Angel, J. (2011). Trends in the sociology of aging: Thirty-year observations. In R. A. Settersten, Jr., & J. Angel (Eds.), *Handbook of sociology of aging* (pp. 3–15). New York, NY: Springer Science.

Settersten, R. A., Jr., & Gannon, L. (2006). Age identity. In G. Ritzer (Ed.), *Blackwell encyclopedia of sociology* (pp. 49–51). Oxford, UK: Blackwell Publishing.

Settersten, R. A., Jr., & Hagestad, G. O. (2015). Subjective aging and new complexities of the life course. In M. Diehl & H.-W. Wahl (Eds.), Subjective aging: New developments and future directions (*Annual Review of Gerontology and Geriatrics*, Vol. 35, pp. 29–54). New York, NY: Springer Publishing Company.

Settersten, R. A., & Ray, B. (2010). What's going on with young people today? The long and twisting path to adulthood. *The Future of Children, 20*(1), 19–41.

Skocpol, T. (2000). *The missing middle: Working families and the future of American social policy.* New York, NY: W. W. Norton.

Sontag, S. (1972, September 23). The double standard of aging. *The Saturday Review*, pp. 29–38.

Suzman, R., & Riley, M. W. (1985). Introducing the "oldest old." *Milbank Memorial Fund Quarterly, 63*, 177–186.

Weber, M. (1904–1905/1930). *Protestant ethic and the spirit of capitalism* (translated by T. Parsons, with an introduction by A. Giddens). New York, NY: Routledge.

Williamson, J. B., Kingson, E. R., & Watts-Roy, D. M. (1999). *The generational equity debate.* New York, NY: Columbia University Press.

PART I

Standing on the Shoulders of Giants:
Personal Perspectives on Theory Development in Aging

STANDING ON THE SHOULDERS
OF GIANTS IN GERONTOLOGY
Richard A. Settersten, Jr.

The third edition of this handbook includes a new feature: "Standing on the Shoulders of Giants: Personal Perspectives on Theory Development in Aging." This part comprises chapters written by four senior scholars in gerontology today: Leonard Hayflick, Warner Schaie, Vern Bengtson, and Carroll Estes. These scholars represent major sections of the Gerontological Society of America (GSA), the primary research organization of our field: biological sciences (Hayflick); behavioral and social sciences (Bengtson and Schaie); and social research, policy, and practice (Estes). Each of these authors is either a past president of the Society (Bengtson, Estes, and Hayflick) or winner of the Robert W. Kleemeier Award (Bengtson, Hayflick, and Schaie) or the Donald P. Kent Award (Estes), representing the highest recognitions of the GSA for science and its application in policy and practice.

These senior researchers reflect on the history of theory development in their areas, from the beginning of gerontology as a scientific field. They also share their personal experiences with the process and prospects of developing good theory. Thus, this section gives readers an intimate backstage view into how the central theories of our field were developed and into the persons—the "giants" of gerontology—who developed them. The essays have an intimate feel, as the careers of these scholars emerged and grew alongside gerontology itself. Their stories remind us that the field of aging is remarkably young.

Their essays reveal common themes. For one thing, the authors describe their challenges in coming into a new field, gerontology, which was in its infancy. Their motivations to study aging were often tied to personal experiences with aging individuals, to (often chance encounters with) mentors or others who pulled them in, and to the intrigue of aging as a then-unconquered field that posed complex scientific puzzles.

Second, they reveal some of the uncertainties they faced as they developed their careers. These included struggles to carve out a niche, to find money to support research, to publish, and to find status and honor in a field that was, in its early years, marginalized. Their careers unfolded within a shifting set of opportunities; an evolving infrastructure of professional organizations, journals, and funders; and an expanding landscape of undergraduate and graduate programs and postdoctoral training.

Third, in each of these chapters, we see the powerful role of social networks and relationships in science—of being mentored and mentoring others, of observing in-groups and out-groups in research and professional leadership, of being accepted or dismissed, and of the ways in which individual careers are enmeshed with colleagues and collaborators near and far.

Finally, in these accounts, we glimpse the inevitable ups and downs that mark careers, working with or against the changing theoretical, topical, and methodological tides of science. We hear stories of not only personal hardship and dogged determination that pioneers of a field inevitably confront, but also the satisfaction of having notable productivity and ideas that are widely recognized today.

In Chapter 3, Leonard Hayflick describes his accidental entry into the biology of aging, which began with an equally accidental discovery that he made in his laboratory, one that defied explanation. At that time, he says, to be a young scientist who admitted to working on aging was tantamount to committing professional suicide. And few resources were available. He recounts how he discovered the "Hayflick Limit," for which he is so well known. This is the concept that cells have a limit in the number of divisions they can make before death, and a system for counting the number of times they can divide.

Hayflick tells about the sting of rejection when a paper based on years of research was rejected by a top journal—and the triumph when it was instead published by another journal. That paper has by now been cited more than 6,000 times. He discusses his pioneering research on telomeres as longevity determinants, and the 6 years of lawsuits that followed the confiscation of the cells in his experiments by administrators in the National Institutes of Health, who believed that government was the sole owner of the cells. His litigation was successful: The government agencies settled out of court. Hayflick concludes with an impassioned plea for more resources to support basic research on understanding the causes of biological aging—funding that has been elbowed out by an emphasis on Alzheimer's disease and research on longevity determinants or age-associated diseases.

In Chapter 4, K. Warner Schaie discusses major paradigm shifts that occurred as the psychology of aging progressed over the course of the 20th century. He also considers the consequences of increased interdisciplinary for psychological studies of aging. Schaie describes his start in gerontology, influenced by his escape from Nazi Germany at the age of 6 and his family's internment in Shanghai during World War II, and his work as a printer while starting night-school classes in psychology. Finally entering the University of California, Berkeley, for undergraduate studies, and then the University of Washington for graduate studies, his dissertation research became the basis for the long-term Seattle Longitudinal Study, which is still ongoing.

Schaie discusses four developments that have influenced geropsychology over the past six decades: (a) methodological advances, such as considering chronological age as a dependent rather than an independent variable; (b) increasing interdisciplinary, for example by incorporating independent variables from domains of neighboring disciplines, such as sociology, to explain psychological phenomena; (c) rising and crucial roles of longitudinal studies in unveiling developmental mechanisms; and (d) recent interest in psychological interventions directed toward the enhancement of cognitive competence, self-efficacy, and caregiving.

In Chapter 5, Vern Bengtson traces seven themes that defined early theory development in the sociology of aging. These include the importance of age and the roles of the "aged" in society, conceptualizations of successful aging and its outcomes, the tension between social structure and individual agency (especially as reflected in controversies surrounding activity and disengagement theories), the social meanings of generations and cohorts, age stratification and cohort flow, families and intergenerational relationships, and social dimensions of the life course.

Bengtson also describes his unlikely route into gerontology and how he became interested in families and aging, interests that led him to start the Longitudinal Study of Generations, which is presently in its 45th year of data collection. He recounts his interactions with a number of the founding figures, including Ernest Burgess, Talcott Parsons, Robert Havighurst, Bernice Neugarten, Elaine Cumming and William Henry, and Robert Butler.

In Chapter 6, Carroll Estes, with Nicholas DiCarlo, provides a perspective on the foundations of theory development in aging policy and practice. She emphasizes both the people and the historical conditions that propelled these developments. She begins with two early practitioners who reflect the social work and social welfare origins of social gerontology, Ollie Randall and Louis Lowy. She then describes the influence of several prominent academics who were early champions of policy and practice: Wilma Donahue, Clark Tibbitts, Ethel Shanas, Walter Beattie, and Robert Binstock.

Estes highlights the diversity of leadership in the policy-and-practice sphere, not only researchers but also public intellectuals and activists. Here, Estes examines the contributions of Elaine Brody, Maggie Kuhn, Bernice Neugarten, and Jacquelyne Johnson Jackson. She also discusses the formation of her own career and her commitments to the aging "enterprise," especially the political economy of aging and critical gerontology.

It is important to know—and remember—the history of theory in our field and the giants on whose shoulders we stand. This is important for several reasons. First, although many of these scholars have been forgotten, a remarkable number of the concepts and theories they developed are still alive, though under different guises and often without attribution to their originators. Second, without proper appreciation of the foundations that have been laid in our field, we run the risk of not learning from past mistakes or, worse, thinking that we have discovered what has already been known for some time. Third, the careers and life stories of these giants provide wonderful examples of how science is both personal and social; and how even the most prominent and productive have struggled with self-confidence, rejection, and failure. But their biographies also show the rewards of having courageous ideas that, with perseverance, came to be recognized and ultimately changed the course of gerontology.

CHAPTER 3

Unlike Aging, Longevity Is Sexually Determined
Leonard Hayflick

For having a very ardent desire to see and observe the state of America a hundred years hence, I should prefer to any ordinary death being immersed in a cask of Madeira wine, with a few friends, till that time, to be then recalled to life by the solar warmth of my dear country.

Benjamin Franklin (as cited in Gruman, 1966/2003, p. 84)

Efforts to understand the biology and cause of human aging are as old as recorded history. Evidence exists in the 3,000 BCE Babylonian epic poem in which King Gilgamesh seeks to conquer aging and achieve immortality (Gruman, 1966/2003). The thousands who joined Gilgamesh's search in subsequent millennia are members of either the first or second oldest profession.

Today, the most conservative seekers simply wish to slow the aging process, less cautious believers wish to stop or reverse it, and a small but vocal minority—like King Gilgamesh—seeks immortality.

The most complete and well-documented history of efforts to understand the biology of aging is, perhaps, the work of Gruman (1966), who documents ideas about prolonging life from recorded history to 1800. Even during the Age of Enlightenment, and the major discoveries made in biology in the 20th century, the fundamental cause of aging is still a mystery.

In the late 1950s, when I accidently found myself in the field of aging, theories of causation were dominated by phenomena that occurred outside of the fundamental unit of life—cells. Radiation, stress, failure of nutrients to enter cells, waste system congestion, and poorly defined "wear and tear" theories dominated the speculations.

Significantly, research in the field was avoided by mainstream scientists; so for a young scientist to admit working on aging was tantamount to committing professional suicide. Few National Institutes of Health (NIH) resources were available and those were buried in the tiny Aging Branch of the National Institute on Child Health and Human Development. In the United States, the most noteworthy descriptive studies were undertaken by Nathan Shock and his group at the Baltimore City Hospitals, an extramural arm of the National Institute on Child Health and Human Development. Here the important Baltimore Longitudinal Study on Aging was launched.

Until the mid-20th century, and even to this day, most research on aging was predominantly descriptive. Studies on causation and cures were mostly the provenance of the huge lunatic fringe that has historically bedeviled science-based researchers in the field. For centuries, this fringe has exploited the ignorance of the general public by offering nostrums and lifestyle changes that claimed, without evidence, to slow, stop, or even reverse human aging. Even in today's era of scientific enlightenment, mainstream biogerontologists (scientists who do research on the biology of aging) have collectively endorsed the fact that we know about no intervention that will perturb the fundamental process of aging (Olshansky, Hayflick, & Carnes, 2002). The huge industries that market products to cover up the clinical manifestations of aging depend on the differences in how much we value young people more than we value old people. These industries are a major economic force in many nations.

It has been argued that there are as many theories of the cause of aging as there are biogerontologists but this cynical observation is now fading with the increasing understanding that like all matter—both animate and inanimate—the etiology can be found at the molecular level or even below. I will return to this notion later.

My assignment is to discuss "How did you become so curious? Get to a great university? Why science and not banking?" and in respect to aging "not only the *content* of the most current theories but,...also the *development* of theories of aging..." from "...the time you came into the field" and "...some of the debates as theories emerged and were refined (or discarded)..." and "how the 'Hayflick Limit' came about and has evolved over time."

■ EXPLOSIVES AND ROCKETS AND FLARES, OH MY!

At about the age of 10 years, and living in a Southwest Philadelphia row house, a favorite uncle presented me with a Gilbert chemistry set (I still have the small book that describes suggested experiments). I was fascinated with names of the chemicals, the enormous variety of experiments that could be done with them, and the knowledge of how they worked and what that revealed about how the world worked. Today, almost all of the chemicals that were in my set are forbidden to be sold to the lay public. My passion grew to the point where my liberal parents allowed me to build a chemistry laboratory in the basement of our house. In addition to more tame experiments, I made gun powder, flares, and then rockets that I learned how to explode in various colors.

After a similarly inquisitive friend and I befriended a clerk at a scientific supply house next to the University of Pennsylvania campus, we were determined to buy metallic sodium from him. Elemental sodium is a soft buttery material sold in a closed can of kerosene. If metallic sodium is exposed to the oxygen in air, it explodes in a violent burst of yellow flame.

The clerk insisted that to sell it to me would require a note from my mother. Her trust in my knowledge and abilities was such that she consented. I designed an apparatus using metallic sodium as fuel to propel rockets higher and higher. But the noise and erratic paths of the ascending rockets did not please our neighbors. I was forced to end my budding career as a rocket scientist.

My increasing knowledge of basic chemistry also caused my high school chemistry teacher to banish me to the chemistry laboratory stock room for embarrassing him by publicly correcting some of his lecture statements.

However, the ban benefited me by providing access to chemicals that I did not already have. My home laboratory expanded, additional shelving for the chemicals became necessary, and the labeling and storage of my growing collection became more and more time consuming. By this time a college decision had to be made (www.webofstories.com).

■ A SKINNY, 110-POUND HIGH SCHOOL STUDENT GRADUATES, MATRICULATES TO PENN, IS INTIMIDATED BY MILITARY OFFICERS, JOINS THE ARMY, RETURNS TO PENN, MAJORS IN MICROBIOLOGY, AND ESCAPES THE KOREAN WAR

I was an excellent high school student and this qualified me to take a written test to compete for a scholarship to Temple University in Philadelphia. I won and then rejected the scholarship because I was determined to go to Penn, whose impressive reputation was a magnet for me. I was the only high school student admitted to Penn in January 1946 because most places were given to returning servicemen. All were several years older than me. I became intimidated by having classmates who were officers, pilots, military leaders, and professionals in many other occupations. It also became apparent that my parents could not afford the $350 costs for each semester of my 4-year university education.

I took leave of absence from Penn to accept an 18-month enlistment in the army, where I rose to staff sergeant. I returned to Penn and with the GI Bill I paid for my tuition and living expenses. Perhaps the greatest benefit was as a veteran (I won the World War II Victory Medal because, unknowingly, I enlisted 2 days before the war legally ended on May 15, 1946). Even more significant was the fact that, as a veteran, I escaped being among the first to be drafted later to serve in the Korean War.

A critical event occurred in my junior year that steered me from chemistry to a passion for microbiology. On my return to Penn, and during the first week of an introductory course in microbiology, the laboratory technician walked by me carrying a tray of several dozen test tubes. Each contained a gelatin-like substance called "agar". On the surface of these gelled surfaces there grew visible colonies of different species of microorganisms, each displaying a different color. Why, I thought, do bacteria have different colors? I was hooked! This electrified me and initiated my interest in microbiology, which then became my undergraduate major.

With my BA in hand, I began work at the research laboratories of Merck, Sharp, and Dohme in a Philadelphia suburb. This further excited my interest in biology generally and microbiology specifically. I decided to return to Penn to pursue master's and PhD degrees, where I worked on the smallest free-living microorganisms now called "mycoplasmas". When my advisor returned full of enthusiasm from taking the first national course in cell culture, he persuaded me to do my PhD dissertation on the growth of mycoplasmas in cell cultures (Hayflick & Stinebring, 1960). This preceded the discovery that these microorganisms are, to this day, common contaminants of cell cultures.

■ ON BEING ACCIDENT PRONE

My accidental entry into the field of research on biological aging began with an equally accidental discovery that I made in my laboratory and that defied explanation.

I was fascinated by the fact that living cells could be removed from an animal or human and cultured in glassware just like bacteria. I pursued this interest by building and operating my own primitive cell culture facilities to undertake my graduate studies at the University of Pennsylvania where I was also given a laboratory at the Wistar Institute encircled by the Penn campus. This institute is the oldest private biological research facility in the United States. Here I discovered that a mycoplasma was the etiological agent of a middle ear infection that was an enzootic disease in the famous colony of albino Wistar rats. After graduation, I accepted a postdoctoral appointment at the University of Texas's Galveston laboratory of Charles M. Pomerat, an internationally known expert on culturing cells. Pomerat's laboratory provided me with significant additional expertise. Other accidental circumstances arose that led me back to the Wistar Institute for the second time in 1958.

I returned to the newly refurbished Wistar Institute to establish a cell culture laboratory and provide cultures to other institute scientists. This left me with ample time to pursue my own research interests unfettered with the need to seek grant support and to be engaged in the onerous attendant paperwork. The excess cell cultures and associated materials that I used were purchased by the institute with overhead funds because mine was a service laboratory. These inexpensive materials would have been discarded but I found them to be useful for my research interests.

The work that led to my accidental observations did not have as its goal an effort to understand the aging process. At that time, several oncogenic (cancer-causing) viruses had been isolated from lower animals so it seemed reasonable to expect that humans should not be an exception. My naive idea was to determine whether extracts, or treated fluids, from cultured human cancer cells would have some detectable effect on cultured human normal cells. An effect, if found, might be evidence for the presence of a cancer virus. At that time, efforts to transform normal cells into cancer cells with chemicals, viruses, or radiation were just emerging as an important concept.

Human cancer tissue was easy to obtain from hospital operating rooms for my studies. For normal cells, I wanted fetal tissue because adult human tissue has a greater likelihood of containing unwanted known viruses that would have confounded my work. I obtained aborted human embryonic tissue locally and from Sweden.

It was a central dogma in cell culture from its beginning (Harrison, 1907) that all cultured cells have the potential to replicate indefinitely and when they fail to do so, it simply reflected ignorance of how best to cultivate them. Thus, it was no surprise when I found that the cultures of fibroblasts (connective tissue cells) that I grew from human fetal tissues luxuriated for some months and then stopped dividing. They stopped, I was taught, because no one knew what culture conditions were required to grow normal human or animal cells indefinitely.

Ever since the first cell culture was set, with one alleged and celebrated exception, every culture of normal cells ultimately would stop dividing and die. I will return to this alleged exception later.

It was not until 1943, when Wilton Earle, at the National Cancer Institute, isolated the abnormal mouse L929 cell line, that the first immortal cell line was discovered (Earle et al., 1943). However, no proven normal human or animal cells had ever been shown to replicate indefinitely.

Simultaneously, with my cancer virus studies, I made an unrelated discovery of the cause of another human disease. Again, I did not have a grant to do this research work and I even suffered the indignity of receiving from the institute director a disturbing memo. It read, "You have been hired to run a tissue culture laboratory and not to work with microorganisms. You must stop this work immediately." Of course, I ignored him.

The research that I was asked to stop was my experiments designed to discover the cause of a common human disease called "walking pneumonia," medically known as "primary atypical pneumonia."

For years, it was believed to be caused by a virus that was never found.

Because my PhD dissertation described my work on mycoplasmas, I knew that they caused pneumonia in lower animals. So, I thought that they also might be the cause of this similar human pneumonia disease.

I succeeded in isolating the organism that causes "walking pneumonia" and I named it *Mycoplasma pneumoniae* (Chanock, Hayflick, & Barile, 1962). It was the first human disease found to be caused by mycoplasmas.

This discovery was so important that it was described in an article on the front page of the *New York Times*, and of course gave welcomed publicity to the Wistar Institute. The next day, the director boldly appeared in my lab with his hand outstretched to congratulate me on the work that he had previously demanded I stop.

■ CELL CULTURE 101

In order to understand what follows, it is important to know the simple techniques used to culture cells.

All activities are conducted under conditions that prevent contamination with microorganisms and usually include the use of antibiotics in the nutrient fluid. Tissue removed from aborted embryos were minced and exposed to an enzyme that dissolves the cement-like substance that holds cells together. It is much like dissolving the mortar in a brick wall that would then release individual bricks. The individual cells released from a match-head-size piece of tissue will number in millions. They are then introduced into a rectangular glass bottle (plastic vessels did not exist in the 1960s) with a small amount of nutrient medium.

When the upright rectangular bottle is turned on its side, what ordinarily would be called the wall of the upright bottle now becomes the floor. The small amount of fluid nutrient medium now bathes the cells, approaches the shoulder, but does not enter the mouth of the stoppered bottle. The bottle is incubated at body temperature. The cells in the fluid medium now fall to the bottle's floor, attach to the glass, and begin to divide. Within a week or so, the cells have divided to the point where they cover the floor of the bottle. This condition causes the cells to stop dividing. The cells are now called "confluent" because they have multiplied to cover the entire surface. If more cells are required, then the medium is removed and, for example, one million cells stuck to the floor of the bottle are removed using the enzyme mentioned earlier. Two equal portions (500,000 cells in each portion) are then put into two new daughter bottles of the same dimensions as the first, or primary, culture. Thus, the one million cells taken from the first bottle will double to two million cells when the 500,000 cells in each daughter bottle reach confluency. This is called a "population doubling." If this operation (called a "subcultivation") is performed weekly, the cell population doubles each week. Soon, so many bottles of cells will be made to allow for freezing the excess cultured cells at each doubling. The normal human cells will remain alive in the frozen state indefinitely as I later found.

■ HOW I REACHED MY LIMIT

After setting cell cultures from several embryos that had arrived in my laboratory at random times, it was my habit to examine them daily. One day I found that one culture looked unusual and the cell division seemed to have slowed.

I gave this little thought assuming that this unique event was caused simply by some unknown technical error or microbial contamination. Later, I observed that other cell cultures were behaving similarly. When I looked at my research notebook, I found something very strange. Only the oldest cultures that were set 10 months or so earlier and were at about the 40th population doubling were the ones in which the cells had stopped dividing. The younger cultures, at doublings less than 40, were luxuriating. All were cultured in the same lot of nutrient medium, same group of bottles, and all were cultured by the same person.

This was not the proverbial "Eureka Moment" but it was, for me, the "that's funny moment."

My curiosity was piqued. I doubted that this finding was the result of a culturing error or contamination, because only the older cultures exhibited the phenomenon and, critically, the younger cultures also showed cessation of cell division only when they also reached about the 40th population doubling. But, it was necessary to provide proof that a mistake had not been made. I conducted several experiments to answer this question, all of which supported the view that no error had been made.

But, the definitive experiment was conducted with my colleague, Paul Moorhead, who was a skilled cytogeneticist and our results came close to proving beyond doubt that not only had an error not been made but that a finite capacity to divide is a fundamental property of normal human (and later animal) cells.

Our experiment was possible because Paul could distinguish between cultured male and female cells by identifying the sex chromosomes in the cells.

■ THE "DIRTY OLD MAN" EXPERIMENT

I mixed the same number of male cells at the 40th doubling level with an equal number of female cells at the 15th doubling level. After 20 more doublings of the mixture, we found that the only cells present were female. Both unmixed control cultures of cells of both genders stopped dividing at the anticipated times. Obviously, the older male cells in the mixture stopped dividing and vanished while the younger female cells continued to flourish. Clearly, the presence of any virus, toxin, nutrient deficiency, or any other cultural condition that might have eliminated the male cell component could not be expected to spare the younger female cells nor were the young female cells capable of somehow rescuing the older male cells. In fact, any theory that might be suggested to cause the elimination of the male cell component in the mixture must be capable of discriminating between male and female cells—a possible, but highly improbable event (Hayflick & Moorhead, 1961). We called this the "dirty old man" experiment. However, the "dirty old lady" experiment gave the same result. To me these results meant that the dogma was dead. Nevertheless, it was so well entrenched that it took years for other scientists to agree.

It is a well-known phenomenon in science that the length of time necessary to accept a new discovery is directly proportional to how much that discovery is thought to defy received knowledge.

Our results led us to three general conclusions, the most important of which was that the limited replicative capacity of normal human cells might be telling us something about aging and the determinants of longevity. Second, that there are two classes of cultured cells—mortal cell strains and immortal cell lines. I realized that, having discovered that normal cells are mortal, it was now possible for me to claim that only cancer cells are immortal (Hayflick, 1965). These properties are also found in vivo (in the body) where most cancer cells can be shown to be immortal and, of course, our normal cells are mortal.

The third conclusion that my work revealed was that the normal human cells were exquisitely sensitive to virtually all of the then-known human viruses, and free of contaminating viruses. Consequently, I reported that they would make an excellent alternative to the use of virus-contaminated primary monkey kidney cells that were then used in the manufacture of the Sabin and Salk poliomyelitis vaccines and in other human virus vaccines (Hayflick, 1965; Hayflick & Moorhead, 1961; www.webofstories .com).

▨ THANKS FOR THE MEMORIES

Other discoveries followed. After a few months of frozen storage, I was stunned to discover that, on thawing, the cells had a memory. When they were thawed months after freezing and then cultured, they remembered at what doubling level they were frozen and then underwent only that number of doublings remaining from the total of 50 that was possible. Clearly, the cells had a system for counting the number of times that they could divide. One of the normal human fetal cell strains that I developed, called WI-38, has been stored frozen for 53 years and the memory of the cells is as good today as it was in 1962. This is the longest time that normal human cells have ever been frozen in the living state.

▨ THE IMPORTANCE OF BEING NORMAL

Paul Moorhead had the expertise to establish what I thought was essential. That was to determine that the cell strains I had isolated consisted of chromosomally normal human cells. It had just been discovered a few years earlier that, unlike what was formerly believed, humans have 46 and not 48 chromosomes. It had also been discovered how the shapes and sizes of normal human chromosomes should appear. Paul undertook this study and showed that my human cell strains were chromosomally normal.

I realized that it was essential to prove that my cell strains were normal in order to make the novel claim that immortal cultured cell lines differed by having abnormal or cancer cell properties. For example, at this time, the HeLa cancer cell line had been cultured continuously since 1952 (Gey, Coffman, & Kubicek, 1952) and after a decade of continuous culturing could be considered to be immortal. A few other immortal cancer cell lines also existed at this time. All were chromosomally abnormal, grew when inoculated into laboratory animals, and were abnormal in other ways. The fact that my cultured cells were chromosomally normal, did not grow in laboratory animals, and were normal in all other respects would demonstrate the critical insight that cell immortality is a property only of abnormal cancer cells (Hayflick, 1965; www.webofstories.com).

My additional finding in 1965 that the normal cells from adults replicated fewer times than those from fetuses seemed to support our earlier suggestion that my discovery may bear directly on problems of aging, or more precisely, "senescence" (Hayflick & Moorhead, 1961). These observations compelled me to abandon my cancer virus research plans and motivated me to make an excursion into the question of why normal human cells stopped dividing after a specific number of population doublings.

What I thought would be a brief expedition lasted for more than 40 years. I never did return to the cancer virus project.

▨ IS IT AGING?

The time soon arrived when we were obligated to write a paper that described our work and to interpret the meaning of our results.

Our experiments had shown that the dogma was dead and that normal cells had an intrinsic mechanism that limited their replicative ability. After excluding all obvious explanations for our findings, we were left with the novel idea that our results were telling us something about senescence or aging.

We wrote,

> The third possible explanation for entry into Phase III (when normal cells stop dividing) may bear directly upon problems of ageing, or more precisely, "senescence." This concept, although vague at the level of the whole organism, may have some validity in explaining the phenomenon at the cellular level, at least as an operational concept. (Hayflick & Moorhead, 1961, p. 614)

Biological aging was such a mysterious process, it seemed safe to explain our findings by speculating that aging could be invoked as a cause. At that time only a few dozen intrepid people in the world did research in what was later called "biogerontology." In the late 1950s and early 1960s, the study of the aging process commanded little scientific respect because for centuries it was considered to be a black art that defied understanding and was dominated by charlatans and snake oil merchants.

Furthermore, those using cell cultures in their research, as I was, were doubly damned because cell culture itself was just emerging from a 50-year shadow of condemnation as a black art.

Because the central dogma claimed that all cultured cells were potentially immortal, those researchers on aging who preceded us logically concluded that the ultimate causes of aging did not have an intracellular origin. This was clear to them because, if cultured normal human cells are immortal in the absence of the body's normal control mechanisms, then aging could not be the result of intracellular events. It was for this reason that the focus of attention on what little fundamental work was done in biogerontology during the 60 years before our work was directed to extracellular causes of age changes like radiation, changes in the extracellular matrix, stress, and many other putative nonintracellular causes. Therefore, our suggestion that we found aging to have its origins within the cell was revolutionary.

Of the tens of thousands of papers published in this field in the last 42 years (which I subsequently named "cytogerontology"; "cyto" means cell), none has disproved our suggestion. In fact, most independent studies made during these years have added significant weight to our suggestion that the cessation of normal cell replication is telling us something about one or both aspects of the finitude of life, that is, aging or longevity determination, each of which is discussed subsequently.

■ OVERCOMING INTIMIDATION BY DOGMA

Yet, so intimidated were we by the dogma, that we were still fearful of publishing our results. Paul and I were both recent postdoctoral students, so to make a stupid mistake while challenging a central dogma in cell biology would have torpedoed any hope of a successful scientific career. I decided to do one more experiment. It does not appear in the methods section of the published paper but it had a simple and effective design. I decided to send cultures to three or four of the giants in the field of cell culture who had expressed grave doubts about our work and cautioned us not to publish our results.

I reasoned that if these experts could culture the cells indefinitely under their alleged superior culture conditions, we would know that we had made a serious error. Cultures at an early population doubling level were sent to several leaders in the field with instructions to call me 6 months hence when I predicted that the flourishing cultures would cease replicating. All of the recipients called at the predicted time to confirm our prediction. We reasoned that, if we were subsequently proven to be fools, then we would have some highly respectable company to accompany us as we went down in flames. We decided to publish our results.

■ THE ALLEGED EXCEPTION

Earlier I indicated that, ever since the development of cell culture techniques at the beginning of the 20th century, with one possible exception, every culture of normal cells ever set ultimately died. The apparent exception was well known in the early 1960s when we conducted our studies and it demanded an explanation.

Interest in vertebrate cell immortality reached a zenith in the early part of the 20th century when, Alexis Carrel, a noted French cell culturist, surgeon, fascist, and Nobel laureate, described experiments purporting to show that supposedly normal fibroblasts derived from chick heart tissue could be cultured serially indefinitely. Carrel did this work in what was then called the Rockefeller Institute in New York City. The alleged immortal chick cell strain was voluntarily terminated after 34 years in continuous culture (Ebeling, 1942; Parker, 1961). Carrel's associate, Albert Ebeling, who cultured the cells for most of the 34 years, discarded them in 1946, 2 years after Carrel's death in Vichy, France, where Carrel had returned as a fascist sympathizer (Friedman, 2007; Witkowski, 1979, 1980, 1985).

The Carrel–Ebeling experiment was of enormous importance in concepts about the origin of aging because, if true, and as stated earlier, it implied that cells released from in vivo controls could divide and function normally for a period of time greater than the life span of the species. Carrel's results, and his interpretation, were of great importance because his findings strongly suggested that an alleged normal cultured chick cell population was immortal. Therefore, aging must not be the result of intracellular events and this flew in the face of our findings. However, neither Carrel nor Ebeling attempted to show that their cultured chicken cells were normal.

I suggested that, although perhaps unknown to them, Carrel and Ebeling made a serious technical error. The alleged immortal chick heart cell culture was fed in those years with an extract of chick embryo tissue prepared daily and extracted under conditions that permitted the addition of fresh living cells to the alleged immortal culture at each feeding (Hayflick, 1965).

Witkowski (1979, 1980, 1985) has published a series of papers based on a thorough investigation that documents his belief that Carrel may have known about this error. Also, the periodic addition of fresh cells may have been done purposely to avoid the embarrassment that Carrel would have suffered because news of the alleged immortal cells was encouraged by Carrel and popularized by the news media worldwide. Some published annual articles to celebrate the culture's birthday.

■ THE AGONY OF REJECTION

The dogma that we thought we had overturned was so well entrenched that our manuscript was rejected in 1960 by *The Journal of Experimental Medicine*, chosen because it had previously published most of the work reported by Alexis Carrel. In more recent years, it published several articles by authors who had worked with cultured human cells but did not realize that their cells were mortal (Marcus, Cieciura, & Puck, 1956; www.webofstories.com).

The letter of rejection read, in part,

The inference that death of the cells...is due to "senescence at the cellular level" seems notably rash. The largest fact to have come out from tissue culture in the last 50 years is that cells inherently capable of multiplying will do so indefinitely if supplied with the right milieu in vitro.

The letter was signed by Peyton Rous, discoverer of the Rous sarcoma virus, the use of trypsin in cell culture, and soon to be awarded a Nobel Prize in Physiology or Medicine.

Paul Moorhead and I were crushed because we both thought that our 3 years of work were a significant contribution. The paper was then sent to Experimental Cell Research and within 2 months it was accepted for publication without change (Hayflick & Moorhead, 1961). The paper has been cited about 6,000 times according to Google Scholar (Garfield, 1980; Hayflick, 1978b) and was one of the 200 most cited papers in the world for the 21-year period from 1961 to 1982 when the total number of citations reached 1,560 (Garfield, 1984). Its sister paper, published in 1965, has been cited about 5,000 times according to Google Scholar (Hayflick, 1990).

Only 0.4% of all scientific papers receive more than 100 citations (Pendlebury, personal communication, Institute for Scientific Information, 1999). Today, citations to both articles number more than ten thousand according to Google Scholar (www .researchGate.net).

Despite the mounting citations to our publications and confirmation by others of our work, overturning the dogma took a decade or more. Full acceptance of my phenomenological findings did not occur until the molecular mechanism was discovered 30 years later (discussed later).

Two observations led me to the notion that normal, mortal, human cells must contain a replication-counting mechanism. First was the reproducibility of our finding that normal human fibroblasts from different embryonic donors underwent a finite number of population doublings that spanned a narrow range between 40 and 60. Second, cells frozen at any population doubling level from 1 to 50 retained "memory" of that level until reconstitution so that the total number of population doublings traversed, both before and after freezing, totaled 50 (Hayflick, 1965; Hayflick & Moorhead, 1961).

The replication-counting mechanism should not be called a clock or chronometer because time is not measured but cell doublings, or more precisely DNA replications, are. I named the unknown mechanism that I predicted a "replicometer" because it counts replication events.

In 1975, we made the first effort to determine the location of the putative replication counter. By employing enucleation and fusion techniques in which nuclei removed from old and young cultured cells were fused to opposite aged enucleated cytoplasts, we concluded that the counter was located in the nucleus (Muggleton-Harris & Hayflick, 1976; Wright and Hayflick, 1975).

There are four aspects of the finitude of life—aging, longevity determinants, age-associated diseases, and death. All but the latter are discussed here.

■ AGING AND THE DETERMINANTS OF LONGEVITY

Biological aging can be defined at many levels of organization from population aging to aging at the molecular level or below.

Age changes can occur in only two fundamental ways—either by a purposeful program driven by genes or by stochastic or random events.

It is a cornerstone of modern biology that a purposeful genetic program drives all biological processes that occur from conception to reproductive maturation. But, once reproductive maturation is reached, thought is divided with respect to whether the aging process results from a continuation of the genetic program or whether it occurs by the accumulation of dysfunctional molecules. Yet, there is no direct evidence that genes drive age changes—a claim made because of the failure to distinguish age changes from longevity determinants.

The aging phenotype is expressed after reproductive maturation and is driven by random events in animals that reach a fixed size in adulthood. No gene that codes for a universal biomarker of aging has been found. Analogously, inanimate objects also require no instructions to age. Evidence for the belief that aging is a random or stochastic process is that, (a) everything in the universe changes or ages in space–time without being driven by a purposeful program; (b) there is no direct evidence that age changes are governed by a genetic program; and (c) there is a huge body of knowledge indicating that all age changes are characterized by the accumulation or expression of dysfunctional molecules.

The common denominator that underlies all causes of aging is change in molecular structure and, hence, in function. It is caused by the intrinsic thermodynamic instability of complex biomolecules, or the manifestations of the Second Law of Thermodynamics. Entropy increase was, until recently, dismissed as a cause of biological aging because biological systems are open. The recent reinterpretation of the Second Law states that "Entropy is the tendency for concentrated energy to disperse when unhindered regardless of whether the system is open or closed. The 'hindrance' is the relative strength of chemical bonds" (Blackshear, 2014; Lambert, 2013). The capacity to repair chemical bond breakage or to replace dysfunctional molecules until reproductive maturation is the *sine qua non* for the maintenance of life and species continuity. This is the role of longevity determinants or maintenance, repair, and synthesis systems. All ultimately suffer the same effects of the Second Law as do other molecules.

Thus, biological aging can be defined as the random, systemic accumulation of dysfunctional molecules that exceeds repair or replacement capacity. This occurs throughout life, but in youth the balance favors the bodies' enormous capacity for repair, turnover, and synthesis—otherwise individuals would not live long enough to reproduce and the species would vanish. After reproductive maturation the balance shifts to slowly favor the accumulation of irreparable, dysfunctional molecules, including those that compose the maintenance and disposal systems themselves. The balance shifts because natural selection does not require life to extend beyond reproductive maturation. It is unnecessary for species survival. The repair shops also age. Then the myriad decrements that produce the aging phenotype become slowly revealed. This accumulation of dysfunctional molecules increases vulnerability to age-associated diseases.

Blueprints contain no information to instruct a car, or other inanimate object, how to age. Yet, in the absence of blueprints, molecules composing these objects also obey the Second Law as their molecules dissipate energy and incur structural and functional losses over lengths of time that vary from picoseconds to light years. Analogously, the genome also does not contain instructions that determine age changes because, like the car, instructions are unnecessary to drive a spontaneous process.

■ GENES DO NOT GOVERN AGING

Because aging is not a programmed process, it is not governed directly by genes. On the contrary, aging is a stochastic process. The many studies in recent years in which invertebrates have been used have led to the view that genes are involved in aging. Yet, none of these experiments has shown a reversal or arrest of the inexorable expression of molecular dysfunction that is the hallmark of aging. These studies are more accurately interpreted to increase our understanding of longevity determination (discussed as follows). Most of the experimental results using invertebrates, and allegedly thought to modify age changes, alter physiological capacity well before the aging process begins. Furthermore, most experiments with invertebrates use an "all-cause mortality" end point that is interpreted to be exclusively aging but does not exclude causes of death attributable to disease, pathology, predation, or accidents. Finally, as there are no generally accepted biomarkers for aging in these or any other animals, the effects of experimental manipulations on their fundamental aging process can only be speculated on.

Another argument against the direct role of genes in programming the aging process is that animals do not age at the same rate nor are the patterns of age changes identical. This results in the great variations found in the location and timing of the acquisition of pathology and the subsequent differences in the chronological age of death. When these random events, which characterize the aging process, are compared with the orderly, virtually lockstep, changes that occur during genetically driven embryogenesis and development, that orderliness and precision stand out in stark contrast to the quantitative and qualitative disorder of age changes. The variability in the manifestations of aging differs greatly from animal to animal but the variability in normal developmental changes from animal to animal differs trivially. Humans from conception to adulthood are virtually identical with respect to the stages and timing of biological development but from about age 20 years on, age changes make humans much more heterogeneous.

■ THE DETERMINANTS OF LONGEVITY

The second aspect of the finitude of life is longevity determination—a completely different process from aging. Longevity is determined by the length of time that the synthesis, turnover, disposal, and repair processes can maintain the biologically active state of molecules. These processes are governed by the genome.

Unlike the stochastic process that characterizes aging, longevity determination is not a random process. It is governed by the enormous excess of physiological reserve produced before and during the time of reproductive maturation and evolved through natural selection to better guarantee survival to that age.

Life does not end immediately after reproductive maturation in most species because it does not benefit species survival. Also, the energy necessary to produce a mechanism that would cause death immediately after reproductive maturation in higher animals is too costly. Exceptions are semelparous "big bang animals" like salmon, and some insects. But it is rare in vertebrates other than some bony fish.

Thus, the determination of longevity is incidental to the main goal of the genome, which is to reach reproductive maturity.

After reproductive success, feral animals soon die as a result of predation, disease, or accidents. But humans have learned how to substantially eliminate or slow many of these causes of death, allowing us and the animals we choose to protect to experience greatly increased life expectancy. Aging in its extreme manifestations is unique to humans and our protected animals.

Longevity determination is an entirely different process from aging and is independent of it. One might think of longevity determination as the energy state of molecules before they incur age changes. This energy state is part of the answer to the question: "Why do we live as long as we do?"

One might think of aging as the state of molecules after they incur irreparable damage that leads to the aging phenotype. This condition answers the question: "Why do things eventually change or go wrong?"

Aging is a catabolic (destructive) process that is chance driven. Longevity determination is an anabolic (constructive) process that, indirectly, is genome driven. They are opposing forces.

The genome directs events until reproductive maturation after which the aging process dominates. Thus, the genome only indirectly determines potential longevity by governing the levels of excess physiological capacity, repair, synthesis, waste disposal, and turnover. No specific genes determine longevity but, collectively, they all govern aspects of biological processes that increase the likelihood of survival to reproductive maturity. The quantitative variation in physiological capacity, repair, and turnover accounts for the differences in longevity both within and between species.

Because longevity is indirectly governed by the genome it is sexually determined. Because aging is a stochastic process, it is not.

■ GOOD HEALTH IS MERELY THE SLOWEST POSSIBLE RATE AT WHICH ONE CAN DIE FROM AN AGE-ASSOCIATED DISEASE

Absent any discussion of death, the third and last of the four aspects of the finitude of life to be discussed is age-associated diseases. The distinction between the aging process and age-associated disease is critical and it is rooted in several practical observations:

Unlike any disease, age changes: (a) occur in every animal that reaches a fixed size in adulthood; (b) cross virtually all species barriers; (c) occur in all members of a species only after the age of reproductive maturation; (d) occur in all animals protected by humans even when that species probably has not experienced aging for thousands or even millions of years; (e) occur in virtually all animate and inanimate objects; and (f) have the same universal molecular etiology, that is, thermodynamic instability.

There is no disease or pathology that has all of these properties.

Age-associated disease is the research and care provenance of geriatric medicine. The fundamental biology of aging is the research provenance of biogerontology.

■ WHAT WOULD LIFE EXPECTANCY BE IF ALL CAUSES OF DEATH WERE RESOLVED?

In 2001, life expectancy at birth was 77 years (Arias, Heron, & Tejada-Vera, 2013). If cardiovascular diseases would be resolved, life expectancy would increase by about 5.48 years, stroke 0.65 years, and cancer 3.2 years. If all of the causes of death legally allowed on death certificates (*International Classification of Diseases, 10th Revision* [*ICD-10*]) were resolved, average human life expectancy could not exceed more than about 12 years. Or, age 89 years would be the maximum life expectancy for humans if all of the present causes of death would be resolved (Arias et al., 2013; Beltrán-Sánchez, Preston, & Canudas-Romo, 2008; Hayflick, 2003a; Olshansky, Carnes, & Cassel, 1990). Curiously, and contrary to what frequently appears in the media, it is illegal for anyone to die from either "natural causes" or "old age" in the United States or in other developed countries that have adopted the *ICD-10*.

For age-associated diseases the fundamental question is: "Why are old cells or those near the end of a lineage more vulnerable to pathology than are young cells?" Regrettably, little research is—or has been—done in an effort to answer this important question.

■ HOW THE DISCOVERY OF TELOMERE ATTRITION AND THE ENZYME TELOMERASE EXPLAINED MY FINDINGS

In 1989, Calvin Harley, who had worked for several years with my system of senescent human cells, had a fortuitous discussion with Carol Greider and found that chromosome ends (telomeres) decreased in length at each round of normal human cell division (Harley et al., 1990).

The remaining critical question was: "How does that class of cells that we identified as immortal avoid telomere shortening that, if it occurs, would lead to their loss of replicative capacity?"

In 1985, Greider and Blackburn discovered the enzyme "telomerase" that, in cancer cells, adds the missing molecules onto the telomeres at each division. Thus, the telomeres do not shorten to a critical length and provide cancer cells with the immortality that we conjectured they had. The Nobel Prize in medicine or physiology was awarded to Blackburn, Greider, and Szostak in 2009 for their discovery of the telomere protection of chromosome ends and of telomerase (Gilson & Ségal-Bendirdjian, 2010). This had the effect of eliminating all of the doubt about my phenomenological discoveries that were now explicable by their findings at the molecular level. It also provided enormous interest in my interpretation 48 years earlier that these findings might be associated with aging when the Nobel Committee announcements associated the prize with illuminating knowledge about the biology of aging (Hayflick & Moorhead, 1961).

The suggestion that telomere attrition in cultured normal human cells is associated with biological aging was a conclusion quickly reached by many. However, that conclusion is spurious because biological aging, as defined earlier, is a stochastic process that is not governed by the genome. The attrition of telomeres and the subsequent downstream DNA events that trigger the cessation of cell division and other changes is more likely to be associated with longevity determination than it is with the stochastic process of aging.

■ HOW CULTURED NORMAL HUMAN CELLS BENEFITED BILLIONS

In the 1960s, one of the major research areas at the Wistar Institute was the development of human virus vaccines. Many scientists, including the director, were engaged in these studies; so I was immersed in knowing about this work because of the usual interactions with colleagues who worked in this area. This resulted in my efforts to determine whether my normal human cell strains would grow human viruses. I found that they grew all of the major human viruses then known (Hayflick & Moorhead, 1961).

Of equal importance was my finding that the normal human cell strain WI-38, on which I decided to focus, did not contain any contaminating viruses. This was contrary to the many new and dangerous viruses found in primary monkey kidney cells then used for the manufacture of the widely used Salk and Sabin poliomyelitis vaccines.

WI-38 also soon became a standard cell culture in virus diagnostic laboratories worldwide for the detection of viruses from human clinical specimens. In fact, we isolated a new common-cold virus using these cells (Tyrrell, Bynoe, Buckland, & Hayflick, 1962). This resulted in our suggestion that normal human cells would be a better and safer substrate for human virus vaccine preparation than the then-existing and dangerous primary monkey kidney cells (Hayflick & Moorhead, 1961). Two years later, we reported that a safe and efficacious poliomyelitis vaccine had been produced in these cells (Hayflick, Plotkin, Norton, & Koprowski, 1962).

After a 10-year struggle over objections made by the Division of Biologics Standards (DBS, NIH), now a part of the Food and Drug Administration (FDA), WI-38 became the first subcultivated culture and the first normal human cell strain to be used for human virus vaccine production (Hayflick, 1989; Hayflick, 2001). Today, more than one billion people have received virus vaccines produced in WI-38 or similar normal human cell strains developed later by others. These include vaccines against poliomyelitis, adenovirus types 4 and 7, rubella, measles, varicella, mumps, hepatitis A, and rabies (Fletcher, Hessel, & Plotkin, 1998).

There is no other cell substrate, including the HeLa cell line, that has benefited so many people. These benefits occurred without any of the putative side effects predicted for the use of these cells that had been feared by early detractors from both within and without the DBS U.S. Control Authority. These baseless fears caused a 10-year delay in the use of WI-38 as a human virus vaccine substrate in the United States until, in 1972, Pfizer Laboratories received the U.S. approval for their poliomyelitis vaccine grown in WI-38. During the preceding decade, WI-38 was widely used for vaccine manufacture in many other countries, but, in the same decade, several people in the United States and elsewhere either died or became permanently comatose from working with virus-contaminated primary monkey kidney cells. Also, before 1972, millions of people received poliomyelitis vaccines grown in primary monkey kidney cells and were later found to be contaminated with the Simian virus 40 (SV40), now suspected to be associated with some human cancers (Bookchin & Schumacher, 2004; Hayflick, 1984, 1989, 2001).

■ A NOVEL TECHNIQUE FOR TRANSFORMING THE ALLEGED THEFT OF HUMAN CELLS INTO PRAISEWORTHY FEDERAL POLICY

Other interesting events in the history of the discovery of the replicative limit of normal human cells include the confiscation of WI-38 from my Stanford University laboratory by NIH, FDA, and Department of Health, Education, & Welfare (DHEW) zealots (Hayflick, 1984, 1990, 1998) who believed that the government was the sole owner of the cells. The irony of this belief occurred after the decades that the FDA fought against the use of these cells for vaccine manufacture (Hayflick, 1989, 2001). The government's astonishing reversal of position is only understandable when WI-38 began to be used for vaccine manufacture in Yugoslavia, Russia, Germany, France, and the United Kingdom.

The reversal of position might also be seen as revenge for my congressional testimony in which I asserted that it was a conflict of interest for the FDA to be in the same business of vaccine development in competition with private enterprises that it controls. Who would you think would win in the competition for an FDA license of a new rubella vaccine between the FDA and Merck? When the FDA's annual appeal for funds is made before Congress, and in which its rubella vaccine research progress is used as a basis for its appeals, the outcome of its competition with a private enterprise is guaranteed. My testimony before a congressional committee in which these facts were exposed resulted in the director of the DBS being removed and the agency itself moved from the NIH to the FDA where I proposed that it obviously belonged. This infuriated the DBS scientists then stationed at the NIH and who saw themselves as research scientists and not wanting the lesser valued title of "controllers."

The belief by the NIH, FDA, and DHEW that they were the sole owners of WI-38 was held despite the fact that the government did not provide grant or contract support for my discovery of the cell strains. I have always maintained that there are four stakeholders for the title to WI-38. These include the institute where the work was done, the institution that may have provided support, the estate of the donor, and the scientists who gave value to the cells. In my absence at a conference, NIH and FDA employees gained entrance to my Stanford University laboratory and confiscated all of my ampules of WI-38 and its precursor, WI-26. I decided to sue.

During the 6 years of litigation, several significant events occurred that forced the Department of Justice, which represented the defendants, to ask me for an out-of-court settlement. First, amicus briefs were offered by the nascent biotechnology industry, which, unlike my laboratory, were directly founded using materials developed on government grants, funded by taxpayers, and awarded to academic laboratories. Second, the Supreme Court ruled that living cells could be patented. Third, a presidential executive order declared that federally supported research resulting in novel cells or microorganisms could be commercially exploited. Finally, the passage of the Bayh–Dole Act made the executive order law (35 USC 200–212). We negotiated an out-of-court settlement that returned many of the WI-38 ampules to me. The funds that I had placed in an escrow account for shipping WI-38 cultures to scientists was not requested by the defendants and all of it was given to my attorneys. More importantly, the settlement of my lawsuit established that biologists have intellectual property rights. Eighty-three scientists published a letter in *Science* damning the conduct of the government and supporting my position (Hayflick, 1978b, 1998; Strehler et al., 1982; Wadman, 2013; www .webofstories.com).

■ WI-38'S OTHER ADVENTURES IN WONDERLAND

The history of WI-38 also includes the picketing of Cape Kennedy by antichoice people in an unsuccessful effort to thwart the National Aeronautics and Space Administration (NASA) 1973 launch of Skylab 2, which contained an elaborate experiment designed to determine whether the chromosomes in normal human WI-38 cells were affected by zero G. WI-38 was chosen because it was the most well-characterized normal human cell strain in the world. The objectors to orbiting WI-38 believed that it was wrong to undertake an experiment on cells removed from an aborted fetus. This objection was held despite the fact that the tissue would otherwise have been incinerated. However, after the launch director spoke with me and learned that the legal, voluntary abortion occurred in Sweden, the protesters ultimately dispersed and the launch succeeded (Montgomery et al., 1978).

■ OLD THINGS CONSIDERED

It is only within the past 40 years or so that the field of research on the biology of aging has emerged as a legitimate area for scientific inquiry. Today, the science of biogerontology flourishes but it still has far to go before it escapes completely from what is analogous to alchemy in the middle ages. The popular belief that the goal of biogerontologists is to stop, slow, or reverse the aging process or to make us all immortal is equivalent to the belief that the goal of modern chemists is to turn base metals into gold.

Adding to the stigmatization of the field is the belief by a gullible public, at least in the United States, that some nostrum or lifestyle will soon be found to slow or stop the aging process in humans. The fact is that we know of no intervention that has been proven to alter the aging process in humans nor is one likely to be found (Hayflick, 1996, 2000; Olshansky, Hayflick, & Carnes, 2002). The goal of biogerontology research is not different from the goals of research in, for example, embryology and childhood development, that is, to understand the processes with no intention of reversing, slowing, or stopping them. Satisfying curiosity itself is a legitimate goal in scientific research. In fact, it is the only goal in most scientific research.

There are several impediments to our understanding of the aging process. Perhaps the most important is the belief that our present understanding of fundamental biological mechanisms is sufficient to understand its cause and to interfere in the process. This same belief, which has been held during many previous decades, also did not result in an understanding. Research on the etiology of aging in the 19th century or later, and before our understanding of the structure of complex biomolecules, DNA activity and biological pathways failed, although researchers had the chutzpah to believe that the state of knowledge at those times was sufficient to succeed. Those who pursue the etiology of aging today are likely to fall again into the same trap because we still fail to understand that major discoveries bearing on the biology of aging are yet to be made. Worse is the failure to focus on increasing health span and not increasing life span. Even worse is the present lack of support to conduct research on the fundamental biology of aging.

A second impediment to understanding the aging process is the failure to distinguish aging from the determinants of longevity and from age-associated diseases. Finally, the terminology used in this field has resulted in the misdirection of most of the funds that might be available for research on the etiology of aging into other fields. This aspect of research on biological aging is discussed later.

Fifty or 60 years ago, a review of the status of research on the etiology of biological aging could have been done in a few pages because most work was descriptive. I do not intend to review the present state of what is commonly called "Research on Aging" because the misleading use of this term has seriously compromised the field for the last half century.

"Research on Aging" is rarely defined to mean the study of the biology of the fundamental cause of aging. Many would assume that the rubric "Research on Aging" would be defined this way. It is not. And, it has resulted in a "One Billion Dollar Misunderstanding" (Hayflick, 2003b).

■ THE ONE BILLION DOLLAR MISUNDERSTANDING

"Research on Aging" should not apply to geriatric medicine because that is the provenance of research on, or treatment of, age-associated pathologies and the decrements of old age in humans.

One good example of the present widespread abuse of the term "aging" is how it is used in the titles of institutes, centers, departments, and similar organizations. Rarely do any members of these organizations conduct research on the etiology of aging. Research is either focused on the geriatric aspects of aging, descriptive events that occur during the aging process, age-associated diseases, or longevity determination.

When questioned, most leaders of these organizations will reply that appeals for funding research on the fundamental biology of aging rarely produce results. However, an appeal for the support of research on age-associated diseases or pathology is significantly more productive because most decision makers have had direct, or indirect, experience with at least one of these diseases or pathologies. The importance of the highly probable link between the biology of old cells, where the increased vulnerability to all age-associated pathologies actually occurs, has gone unappreciated.

Furthermore, the rubric "Research on Aging" could involve research on virtually every time-dependent aspect of human, animal, microbial, or plant life. It could also reasonably include the aging of inanimate objects. These enormous areas would also be increased if we incorporate research from the molecular level to the whole animal, object, and groups of each.

This universal embrace is one of the most serious past and present problems in the field called "Research on Aging." It is also one of the least understood or appreciated problems. Yet, the impact that this language failure has had on the field, and will continue to have, is extraordinary.

■ THE ALZHEIMERIZATION OF AGING

One excellent example of another major, and still present, conceptual error in the field of research on aging is the strange association of Alzheimer's disease with "Research on Aging."

Since the establishment of the National Institute on Aging in 1974, support for research on Alzheimer's disease has increased dramatically. One consequence of this has been the phenomenon in which, at almost every meeting or conference on aging that has been held in the last 40 years, a session on Alzheimer's disease has been almost obligatory. This phenomenon has been called "The Alzheimerization of Aging" (Adelman, 1998).

The resolution of Alzheimer's disease as a cause of death would add about 2 months onto human life expectancy (Arias et al., 2013). In the last 5 years, $450,000,000 has been added to the Alzheimer's disease research budget. The budget for research on the "Biology of Aging" has remained almost static.

It is remarkable that this minor pathology that is not a leading cause of death has become so inseparable from "Research on Aging" that its importance has eclipsed the three major causes of death—cardiovascular disease, stroke, and cancer. These rarely appear as a separate part of conferences on the biology of aging. Yet, these major causes of death require as much, or more, from caregivers and from researchers as does Alzheimer's disease.

■ THE TYRANNY OF WORDS

Decision makers who direct and/or fund "Research on Aging" usually have little understanding of the imprecision of terms used in the field. With respect to biology, the term usually means research on longevity determinants or age-associated diseases. It rarely means research on understanding the cause of biological aging, which should be its only meaning. Biologists have attempted to distinguish themselves from geriatricians and nonbiologists in the field of "Research on Aging" by characterizing themselves as biogerontologists or cytogerontologists. However, these labels are not universally used. Calling those who do research on the nonbiological aspects of aging as "Researchers on

Aging" is misleading because it includes everything from economics, sociology, politics, psychology, and architecture to geriatric medicine and anything old.

Research funds that may be appropriated under the rubric "Research on Aging" are largely expended for research on longevity determinants or age-associated diseases because of the failure to understand that increasing the longevity of animals or curing diseases by manipulating repair, synthesis, or anabolic processes will tell us little about the dysfunctional molecules that characterize the destructive or catabolic process of aging.

Further evidence for this misunderstanding is that the availability of funds for research on age-associated diseases is several orders of magnitude greater than what is available for research on the fundamental biology of aging. What is far more meaningful is that most decision makers believe that the resolution of age-associated diseases will tell us something about the fundamental biology of aging. It will not.

This belief is comparable to the notion that resolving childhood diseases will enlighten us about the fundamental biology of embryogenesis or childhood development. The resolution of childhood diseases, like poliomyelitis, Wilms' tumors, and iron deficiency anemia, added nothing to our fund of knowledge about embryogenesis or the biology of human development. Likewise, the resolution of age-associated diseases has not in the past, nor will it in the future, add to our understanding of the fundamental biology of aging.

A century ago, the leading cause of death in old age was pneumonia, often called "the old man's friend" (with its sexist overtones). Pneumonia is no longer one of the leading causes of death in old age but its resolution did not advance our knowledge of the biology of aging. Nor will the resolution of any other age-associated cause of death or pathology. If the goal of research on aging is to understand the fundamental process at the molecular level, little, if any, progress has been made in the last 50 years.

The irony of these observations is that the common mantra uttered and published by most geriatricians, and also by many biogerontologists, is that "The greatest risk factor for cancer, cardiovascular disease, stroke, or Alzheimer's disease is aging."

It does not take a great leap of intellect to conclude: "Then why are we not doing research on the fundamental biology of aging?"

REFERENCES

Adelman, R. C. (1998). The Alzheimerization of aging: A brief update. *Experimental Gerontology, 33*(1–2), 155–157.

Arias, E., Heron, M., & Tejada-Vera, B. (2013). United States life tables eliminating certain causes of death; 1999–2001. *National Vital Statistics Reports, 16*(9), Hyattsville, MD: National Center for Health Statistics.

Bayh–Dole Act, 35 U.S.C.§ 200–212 (1980).

Beltrán-Sánchez, H., Preston, S. H., & Canudas-Romo, V. (2008). An integrated approach to cause-of-death analysis: Cause-deleted life tables and decompositions of life expectancy. *Demographic Research, 19*, 1323–1350.

Blackshear, H. (2014). *Six*. Retrieved from http://entropysite.oxy.edu

Bookchin, D., & Schumacher, J. (2004). *The virus and the vaccine: The true story of a cancer-causing monkey virus, contaminated polio vaccine, and the millions of Americans exposed*. New York, NY: St. Martin's Press.

Chanock, R. M., Hayflick, L., & Barile, M. F. (1962). Growth on artificial medium of an agent associated with atypical pneumonia and its identification as a PPLO. *Proceedings of the National Academy of Sciences, 48*, 41–49.

Earle, W. R., Schilling, E. L., Stark, T. H., Straus, N. P., Brown, M. F., & Shelton, M. (1943). Production of malignancy in vitro. IV. The mouse fibroblast cultures and changes seen in living cells. *Journal of the National Cancer Institute, 4*, 165–212.

Ebeling, A. H. (1942). Dr. Carrel's immortal chicken heart. *Scientific American, 166*, 22–24.

Fletcher, M. A., Hessel, L., & Plotkin, S. A. (1998). Human diploid cell strains (HDCS) viral vaccines. *Developments in Biological Standardization, 93*, 97–107.

Friedman, D. M. (2007). *The Immortalists: Charles Lindbergh, Dr. Alexis Carrel, and their daring quest to live forever*. New York, NY: Echo.

Garfield, E. (1980). Current comments: Most cited articles of the 1960s. 3. Preclinical basic research. *Essays of an Information Scientist, 4*, 370–378.

Garfield, E. (1984). Current comments: The articles most cited in 1961–1982. 2. Another 100 citation classics. *Essays of an Information Scientist, 7*, 218–227.

Gey, G. O., Coffman, W. D., & Kubicek M. T. (1952). Tissue culture studies of the proliferative capacity of cervical carcinoma and normal epithelium. *Cancer Research, 12*, 264–265.

Gilson, E., & Ségal-Bendirdjian, E. (2010). The telomere story or the triumph of an open-minded research. *Biochimie, 92*(4), 321–326.

Greider, C. W., & Blackburn, E. H. (1985). Identification of a specific telomere terminal transferase activity in Tetrahymena extracts. *Cell, 43*(2, Pt. 1), 405–413.

Gruman, G. J. (2003). *A history of ideas about the prolongation of life*. New York, NY: Springer Publishing Company. (Reprinted from *A history of ideas about the prolongation of life* by G. J. Gruman, 1966, Philadelphia, PA: American Philosophical Society)

Harley, C. B., Futcher, A. B., & Greider, C. W. (1990). Telomeres shorten during ageing of human fibroblasts. *Nature, 345*(6274), 458–460.

Harrison, R. G. (1907). Observations on the living developing nerve fiber. *Proceedings of the Society for Experimental Biology and Medicine, 4*, 140.

Hayflick, L. (1965). The limited in vitro lifetime of human diploid cell strains. *Experimental Cell Research, 37*, 614–636.

Hayflick, L. (1978a). Hayflick's reply. *Science, 202*(4364), 127–136.

Hayflick, L. (1978b). Citation classics: Serial cultivation of human diploid cell strains. *Current Contents/Life Sciences, 26*, 12.

Hayflick, L. (1984). The coming of age of WI-38. *Advances in Cell Culture, 3*, 303–316.

Hayflick, L. (1989). History of cell substrates used for human biologicals. *Developments in Biological Standardization, 70*, 11–26.

Hayflick, L. (1990). Citation classics: WI-38—From purloined cells to national policy. *Current Contents, 3*, 14.

Hayflick, L. (1996). *How and why we age*. New York, NY: Ballantine Books.

Hayflick, L. (1998). A novel technique for transforming the theft of mortal human cells into praiseworthy federal policy. *Experimental Gerontology, 33*(1–2), 191–207.

Hayflick, L. (2000). The future of ageing. *Nature, 408*(6809), 267–269.

Hayflick, L. (2001). A brief history of cell substrates used for the preparation of human biologicals. *Developments in Biologicals, 106*, 5–23; discussion 23.

Hayflick, L. (2003a). *Has anyone ever died of old age?* New York, NY: International Longevity Center Occasional Publications.

Hayflick, L. (2003b). The one billion dollar misunderstanding. *Contemporary Gerontology, 10*, 65–69.

Hayflick, L., & Moorhead, P. S. (1961). The serial cultivation of human diploid cell strains. *Experimental Cell Research, 25*, 585–621.

Hayflick, L., & Stinebring, W. R. (1960). Intracellular growth of pleuropneumonia-like organisms (PPLO) in tissue culture and in ovo. *Annals of the New York Academy of Sciences, 79*, 433–449.

Hayflick, L., Plotkin, S. A., Norton, T. W., & Koprowski, H. (1962). Preparation of poliovirus vaccines in a human fetal diploid cell strain. *American Journal of Hygiene, 75*, 240–258.

Lambert, F. L. (2013). *Entropy is simple—If we avoid the briar patches!* Retrieved from http://entropysimple.oxy.edu/content.htm

Marcus, P. I., Cieciura, S. J., & Puck, T. T. (1956). Clonal growth in vitro of epithelial cells from normal human tissue. *Journal of Experimental Medicine, 104*, 615–632.

Montgomery, P. O., Cook, J. E., Reynolds, R. C., Paul, J. S., Hayflick, L., Stock, D.,...Campbell, D. (1978). The response of single human cells to zero gravity. *In vitro, 14*(2), 165–173.

Muggleton-Harris, A. L., & Hayflick, L. (1976). Cellular aging studied by the reconstruction of replicating cells from nuclei and cytoplasms isolated from normal human diploid cells. *Experimental Cell Research, 103*(2), 321–330.

Olshansky, S. J., Carnes, B. A., & Cassel, C. (1990). In search of Methuselah: Estimating the upper limits to human longevity. *Science, 250*(4981), 634–640.

Olshansky, S. J., Hayflick, L., & Carnes, B. A. (2002). No truth to the fountain of youth. *Scientific American, 286*(6), 92–95.

Parker, R. C. (1961). *Methods of tissue culture.* New York, NY: Harper and Row.

Strehler, B. L., Abraham, S., Bayreuther, K., Bienenstock, A., Binstock, R., Birren, J.,...Zatz, L. M. (1982). Hayflick-NIH settlement. *Science, 215*(4530), 240–242.

Tyrrell, D. A. J., Bynoe, M. L., Buckland, F. E., & Hayflick, L. (1962). The cultivation in human embryo cells of a virus (D.C.) causing colds in man. *The Lancet, 280*, 320–322.

Wadman, M. (2013). Cell division. *Nature, 422*, 498.

Witkowski, J. A. (1979). Alexis Carrel and the mysticism of tissue culture. *Medical History, 23*(3), 279–296.

Witkowski, J. A. (1980). Dr. Carrel's immortal cells. *Medical History, 24*(2), 129–142.

Witkowski, J. A. (1985). The myth of cell immortality. *Trends in Biochemical Sciences, 10,* 258–260.

Wright, W. E., & Hayflick, L. (1975). Nuclear control of cellular aging demonstrated by hybridization of anucleate and whole cultured normal human fibroblasts. *Experimental Cell Research, 96*(1), 113–121.

CHAPTER 4

The Psychology of Aging

K. Warner Schaie

The purpose of this chapter is to consider the major paradigm shifts that have occurred in geropsychology as it has progressed over the course of the 20th century. I also consider the consequences of increased interdisciplinarity for studies of aging within the discipline of psychology. From my perception of the consequences of these shifts, I then try to project what future directions might look like in the new century. This account will, of course, reflect heavily those influences that have shaped my own views of adult development as they have grown over the past six decades (cf. Schaie, 1996, 2000, 2005, 2008a, 2011, 2016). These conceptions were shaped largely by myself being engaged throughout my career in a set of large-scale longitudinal studies designed to systematically identify those influences that distinguish between those lucky individuals who age successfully (cf. Rowe & Kahn, 1987; Siegler et al., 2009) and those exposed to a variety of hazards likely to lead to early decline and low levels of functioning in their last years (cf. Schaie, 1989, 1996, 2005, 2008a, 2013; Schaie & Willis, 2000). But they were also influenced by shifts in methodological paradigms, and perhaps even more by the increasing interdisciplinarity that has characterized the development of modern geropsychology.

I begin this account by describing how I came to become a geropsychologist. I next comment on the beginnings of the psychology of aging in the first half of the 20th century. I then trace the methodological and interdisciplinary influences and summarize the impact of longitudinal studies on the body of knowledge of geropsychology (also see Schaie, 2011; Schaie & Hofer, 2001). I also consider the recent interest in research-based psychological interventions in the aging process, and of the more recent influence of advances in neuroscience. Finally, I make some prognostications as to the proximal future of the field. I should also indicate that many of the thoughts expressed in this chapter came from my review of the eight editions of the *Handbook of the Psychology of Aging*, all of which I coedited with Birren (Birren & Schaie, 1977, 1985, 1990, 1996, 2001, 2006) and more recently with Willis (Schaie & Willis, 2011, 2016). Each of these volumes contains at least one or several chapters on the history, concepts, and theories in the psychology of aging, and hence would be of interest to readers of the present volume (cf. Baltes & Willis, 1977; Birren & Birren, 1990; Birren & Cunningham, 1985; Birren & Renner, 1977; Birren & Schroots, 1996, 2001; Dixon, 2011; Riegel, 1977; Salthouse, 2006; Schaie, 2011, 2016).

■ A BRIEF BIOGRAPHICAL NOTE

I was born in 1928 in Stettin, Germany (now in Poland), as the child of Jewish middle-class parents. My parents had a store that sold specialized clothing and accessories for the then-beginning-to-burgeon crowd of motorcyclists. Because my mother helped in the store, I was taken care of by a teenage nanny. During my fourth year, I went to a German Kindergarten, but when it was time to enter the public school at the age of 6, the Nazis had come to power and it became difficult for Jewish children. I was therefore sent to a private school that had been organized by the Stettin Jewish Community, where I studied the typical German curriculum until the middle of the fifth grade. Nazi hoodlums destroyed my parents' store during *Kristallnacht* in November 1938. My father thereupon decided that we were no longer safe and had to leave Germany as soon as possible and he was able to book passage on an Italian cruise ship from Trieste to Shanghai. We were finally able to leave Germany in May 1939, just barely before the start of World War II.

In Shanghai, I was able to resume my education in a school for refugee children staffed by British and American teachers, where I was taught to speak and write proper English. But when I reached about middle school level, the Japanese attacked Pearl Harbor and promptly interned our teachers. Hence, although I am technically a high school dropout, it was not I who dropped out, but rather my school dropped out on me! Finally, in 1943, the Japanese occupation army required all European refugees to live in a restricted area, although many of us (including me) were often permitted to go to work outside of our area.

I subsequently attended a private business school, where I learned typing, shorthand, and bookkeeping, followed by jobs as a clerk, a switchboard operator, and finally an apprentice to a printer in a small print shop. After the American troops liberated Shanghai, I learned to operate linotype machines at the American-owned *Shanghai Evening Post* and *Mercury*. I worked several months for the American Jewish Joint Distribution Committee as an untrained social worker, writing up life histories for refugees seeking sponsors for their emigration to the United States. Finally, in November 1947, I found sponsors for my mother and myself and set sail on the General Gordon, a converted troop ship.

In San Francisco, I soon found work as a printer, first in small print shops, and eventually at the *San Francisco Chronicle*, where I worked night shift throughout my college years and where, I must mention, as a printer I learned to read and type upside down. One night I saw an article about a high school program for adults at the San Francisco City College. Having nothing better to do in the morning, I signed up and after one semester obtained my high school diploma from the San Francisco Unified School District, which also operated the junior college. I liked the college setting and then continued to my Associate in Arts degree. In California at the time, if one obtained an average of C or better at a junior college for one's lower division college courses, one was entitled to automatic admission to any of the state-operated colleges or universities. So, in the spring of 1951, I became a commuter to the Berkeley campus of the University of California from which I graduated with a BA in psychology in the class of 1952.

■ HOW I BECAME A GEROPSYCHOLOGIST

As an undergraduate in the Department of Psychology of the University of California at Berkeley, I was introduced to the seminal work of L. L. Thurstone on what he called the "building blocks of intelligence" by the stimulating lectures of Professor Read Tuddenham, who eventually became my undergraduate advisor. Having discovered that Thurstone's primary mental abilities had never been studied in adults, I conducted a directed study with Tuddenham in which I administered the Primary Mental Abilities tests to some 70 adults, most of whom were recruited from the geriatric practice of my family physician,

Robert M. Perlman. The latter encouraged me to submit an abstract for a presentation at the Second International Congress of Gerontology in 1951 in St. Louis, Missouri. Here I first met many of the early players in American gerontology, including James Birren, Jack Botwinick, Robert Butler, and Robert Kleemeyer. I was encouraged to submit my paper, which eventually became my first scientific publication (Schaie, Rosenthal, & Perlman, 1953). Having a paper "in press" may have been a major factor in myself being accepted for graduate study in clinical psychology at the University of Washington.

To survive as a psychology graduate student in the early 1950s at the University of Washington, one had to have one of the department's powerful senior faculty as a mentor as well as some special interests that distinguished you from the crowd. I soon became known as that fellow Schaie who was interested in old folks (why doesn't he do something mainstream?), but I was lucky to also interest Charles Strother, then director of clinical training, in my concerns. Not only did he become my formal mentor, but he also encouraged my continuing concern with the psychology of aging. He not only obtained a faculty grant for a pilot study to be conducted by me of the intellectual performance of a group of well-educated elders, but he also helped me organize an interdisciplinary seminar on adult development, and persuaded the dean of the graduate school to appoint an interdisciplinary Committee on Gerontology, of which he became the chair, and I became the executive secretary.

After first trying to interest me in applying Flanagan's critical incident technique to the study of the psychoanalytic process for my dissertation research, he allowed me to return to my interest in cognitive aging. At that time, Strother was chairman of the board of one of the first American health maintenance organizations (HMOs), the Group Health Cooperative of Puget Sound. He worked out a deal by which I was allowed to give the Thurstone tests to a random sample drawn from the HMO membership in return for also collecting and analyzing a consumer satisfaction survey. My dissertation research (Schaie, 1958), of course, was the eventual basis for the long-term Seattle Longitudinal Study (Schaie, 1996, 2000, 2005, 2013).

My interests in geropsychology became enhanced when I moved to West Virginia University and, during the 1960s, I actively pursued geropsychology within the context of a life-span developmental psychology program that included a National Institutes of Health (NIH)-funded doctoral program and started the series of West Virginia conferences on life-span developmental psychology (Baltes & Schaie, 1973; Schaie, 1968). Finally, James Birren recruited me in 1973 to join him at the Andrus Gerontology Center, where I served as director of the Gerontology Research Institute, a position I also held for many years at the Pennsylvania State University. In the latter role, I also conducted a series of 20 conferences exploring the many interfaces of the psychology of aging with the humanities and biological, and social sciences and edited published proceedings thereof. I retired from active academic service at Penn State in 2008, but I am still active in several ways as an affiliate professor of psychiatry and behavioral sciences at the University of Washington.

I have also served as president of the division of adult development and aging of the American Psychological Association (APA), and have served four terms as a representative of that division on the APA governing council. For additional later biographical information, see Schaie (1996, 2000).

■ HOW THE PSYCHOLOGY OF AGING BEGAN

The first American account of what was then known about the psychology of aging is represented by G. Stanley Hall's book *Senescence: The Second Half of Life*, published in

1922. Hall suggested early but gradual decline of all faculties, but maintained a developmental point of view.

Early work with intelligence tests such as the Binet tests or the intelligence test used to screen inductees into the American army in World War I suggested wide individual differences, but work on age differences was mostly cross sectional in nature (e.g., Jones & Conrad, 1933; Kallman & Sandez, 1949). For more details, see Birren and Birren, 1990; Riegel, 1997.

The next systematization of the psychology of aging may be found in Cowdry's (1942) *Problems of Aging*. In the introduction to that book, Dewey (1939) discussed the illogical confusion about considering adult development to involve maturation and eventual debilitation. However, the psychology of aging was not reviewed in detail until the publication of Birren's *Handbook of Aging and the Individual* (1959).

The study of aging, however, was early on recognized in the context of American psychology, and the division of adulthood and aging was one of the first 20 substantive divisions of the APA. Besides, the APA recognized two of the early gerontological research psychologists (Birren and Schaie) with its award for distinguished psychological research. Psychologists also became some of the major actors in the section of behavioral and social science of the Gerontological Society.

Geropsychologists published a variety of psychological journals. From its beginning in 1946, the *Journal of Gerontology* soon established a psychological science section. In 1985, the APA recognized the marked increase in research on adult development and aging by establishing a new journal called *Psychology of Aging* (Willis, 1996).

■ THE INFLUENCES OF METHODOLOGICAL ADVANCES ON THE PSYCHOLOGY OF AGING

Perhaps the most noteworthy development to impact geropsychology over the last six decades can be found in methodological advances that shape our understanding of adult development (cf. Ferrer & Ghisletta, 2011; Hofer & Sliwinski, 2006; McDonald & Stawski, 2016; Schaie, 1977, 1988; Schaie, Campbell, Meredith, & Rawlings, 1989; Schaie & Hertzog, 1985). Here it was largely the paradigmatic shift from predominance of cross-sectional studies of age differences to the understanding that antecedent–consequent relationships in development can be elicited only by following the same individuals over time. No less important, a second paradigmatic shift occurred when confirmatory factor analysis became a common method for hypothesis testing (McArdle & Anderson, 1990; Nesselroade & Lavouvie, 1985; Rudinger & Rietz, 2001; Schaie, Maitland, Willis, & Intrieri, 1998). This method made it possible to assess the invariance of the relation between observed variables and the latent constructs of primary interest to science, a prerequisite for conducting studies comparing individuals and groups over long periods of time, or the comparison of groups differing in salient characteristics such as gender or ethnicity. In addition, emphasis shifted from assessing singular variables to multiply marked constructs. Also added was a move from laboratory-based tests and questionnaires to measures of performance on everyday problems (see Willis, 1985).

A third important methodological development was the paradigmatic shift to consider chronological age as a dependent rather than an independent variable. First introduced conceptually by Wohlwill (1973), behavioral scientists soon began to realize that the study of age or duration time as a dependent variable could be operationalized via methods of survival or event–time analysis (Schaie, 1989; Singer & Willett, 1991). Modern methods of multilevel modeling (MLM; Bryk & Raudenbush, 1987) have also made it possible to disaggregate individual growth curves (and typologies of growth curves) from the group averages that had previously been almost the primary focus of inquiry.

Finally, the development of structural and functional MRI has had a revolutionary enhancement of neuroscience, allowing for the first time the conduct of direct tests of the relationship between age changes in behavior and brain changes during normal and pathological aging (cf. Borghesani et al., 2012; Kramer, Rabiant, & Colcombe, 2006; Nyberg & Bäckman, 2011; Schaie, 2013).

■ THE INCREASING INTERDISCIPLINARITY OF GEROPSYCHOLOGY

A second major shift I have encountered during my career as a gerontologist (Schaie, 2000) has been the ever-increasing prevalence of interdisciplinarity in geropsychological research. I have come to recognize that behavioral change can be understood (and predicted for that matter) only by examining behavioral change in the context of societal change (Bengtson, Kaschau, & Ragan, 1977; Fry, 1985; Lowenthal, 1977; Moos & Lemke, 1985; Plomin & McClearn, 1980; Riley, Foner, & Riley, 1999), giving due recognition to lasting heritable influences (cf. Schaie, Plomin, Willis, Gruber-Baldini, & Dutta, 1992; Schaie & Zuo, 2001), as well as to the obvious age-related changes in the efficiency of the physiological infrastructure (Deeg, Kardaun, & Fozard, 1996; Elias, Elias, & Elias, 1990; Marsh & Thompson, 1977; Siegler & Costa, 1985). Over the course of this century, the many relevant variables from the social and biological sciences have required behavioral scientists to become less parochial and more comfortable in considering the convergence of scientific findings from adjacent disciplines. Hence, although outcome (dependent) variables for the discipline of psychology must always be sought in the domain of behavior, the predictor (independent) variables are increasingly located in domains where the collaboration of colleagues from neighboring disciplines is often essential. On the other hand, behavioral assessments have become increasingly important in the assessment of risk and the prediction of onset and severity of late-life chronic diseases and the dementias (e.g., DeFrias, Schaie, & Willis, 2014).

An understanding of development from early adulthood to old age must include embedding what we know about development within the context of changing environmental influences and changes in individuals' physiological infrastructures. The initial basis for adult behavior must, of course, be attributed to both heritable (genetic) influences and early environmental influences typically experienced within the home of the biological parents (Schaie, 2002). The early environmental influences will, of course, also exert influences on midlife social status. Genetic factors are also likely to be implicated in the rate of age-related decline in competence with increasing age (Kremen & Lyons, 2011; Reynolds & Finkel, 2016). Thus far, the best-studied gene in this context is the Apo-E gene, one of whose alleles is thought to be a risk factor for Alzheimer's ailment (cf. DeFrias et al., 2014).

■ THE ROLE OF LONGITUDINAL STUDIES IN GEROPSYCHOLOGY

It is interesting to note that, from the very beginning of empirical inquiry on development beyond adolescence, substantive concerns were limited primarily to the areas of intellectual development and personality traits. Investigators interested in age-related aspects of learning and memory largely adopted the paradigms popular in early experimental child psychology and thus limited themselves to age-comparative studies of young and old adults. Only recently have we seen an interest in this area in studies that would investigate the developmental mechanisms by use of longitudinal paradigms (see Salthouse, 1999). But for the areas of intellectual development and cognition as well, cross-sectional studies predominated until the late 1930s and clouded our understanding of adult development because of the confusion of age-related development with secular changes expressed as cohort effects (also see Collins, 1996; Hofer & Sliwinski, 2006; Schaie, 1965, 2011; Parmelee and Lawton, 1890).

The initial longitudinal studies that have informed our understanding of adult development were of two types. First, there were studies that began with a focus on early childhood and child-rearing practices, but whose participants were followed into adulthood. A prime example of such a study is the follow-up of the Berkeley Growth and Guidance studies (Eichorn, Clausen, Haan, Honzik, & Mussen, 1981). A second group of studies traced participants who had been assessed as young adults as part of their college experience and reassessed in midlife or later. An example of such studies is Owens's (1966) follow-up of persons in their 50s who had first been assessed as Reserve Officers' Training Corps (ROTC) members during World War I.

The earlier cross-sectional studies had placed peak performance in intelligence and other positive psychological attributes in late adolescence or early young adulthood with linear decline thereafter (Omen, 1977). By contrast, the longitudinal follow-up studies suggested that psychological growth continued generally into early midlife and for some variables (notably the verbal abilities) at least into the 50s.

In the early 1960s, I became convinced that the cross-sectional versus longitudinal issue needed to be confronted directly by following a structured cross-sectional sample covering most of the adult life span over time. I therefore designed a study that converted my original cross-sectional study into a series of short-term longitudinal studies of mental abilities each extending over a simultaneous 7-year period. My replicated cross-sectional findings were quite similar to the original findings, but the longitudinal data showed later ages of peak performance, maintenance of average function on most abilities until the 60s, and only modest decline through the 70s. Further extensions of these studies (with some longitudinal data over as long as 49 years) over the past several decades have consistently replicated these findings, with dramatic declines not experienced until the 80s are reached (Schaie, 2005, 2013).

The early work on adult development was pretty much oriented within the context of a life span development framework, but the field of geropsychology soon divided into at least two rather different orientations. Some researchers remained committed to the notion that an understanding of the aging process required the careful charting of human development at least across the entire adult life span. This orientation, which I share, holds that our primary interest should be directed to the understanding of the mechanisms that contribute to the behavioral differences between youth and old age within a process that extends across the life span (Schaie, 2016). The other orientation, sometimes labeled the "clinker method" (after the residue that remains when charcoal is produced), considers the characteristics of the elderly as their primary interest, and would investigate the aging process only from that period of life when a categorical transformation has begun (e.g., leaving the world of work, or family dissolution caused by death of a spouse).

The second orientation argued for longitudinal studies of the elderly that begin at an advanced age, anywhere from the 60s to the 80s, and follow individuals through the remainder of their lives. Perhaps the most prominent of studies begun in late life has been the Duke Longitudinal Study (Palmore, Busse, Maddox, Nowlin, & Siegler, 1985). But many others can be found in the literature conducted in various industrialized societies (see Schaie & Hofer, 2001, for a general review of longitudinal studies).

These studies generally find less behavioral decrement than would be suggested by cross-sectional data: only small average decline in the 60s, with increasingly steep decrement for each successive age decade. There is also a strong suggestion that decline accelerates as a precursor of eventual death. But most importantly, all of these studies call attention to vast individual differences in rate of change occurring for individuals of all levels of original functioning and socioeconomic status. Thus, although the frequency of individuals who show some decline increases at a near logarithmic rate once the 60s are passed, there are still rare individuals to be found even in the mid-80s who function exceedingly well. What many of these studies also suggest is that there may be an individualized pattern of developmental trajectories. For example, in the case of mental abilities, most individuals by the time they reach the 60s will have experienced a significant drop in one of their abilities, but that ability will be specific to the individual (Schaie, 1989, 2013). But some characteristics identify groups of individuals who show greater and lesser decline. Thus, individuals with advanced education decline more slowly than grade-school graduates; those who have pursued professional occupations decline more slowly than those who spent their lives in unskilled pursuits; and those postponing retirement from challenging jobs seem to be at an advantage (cf. Schaie, 2008b, 2011; Wang & Shi, 2016; Willis, 1985). It is only from the longitudinal study of adult development that it is possible to inquire into possible mechanisms and/or causes of these vast individual differences in developmental progressions through adulthood.

■ SOME FINAL THOUGHTS

A final development worth mentioning is an increasingly important shift from studies designed to understand behavioral aging to the programming of research-based interventions that attempt to gain partial control over the aging process. These studies involve behavioral interventions that are designed to remediate age-related declines or to slow the rate of decline and maintain independent functioning in older persons.

In a number of laboratories (primarily in the United States and in Germany) training programs have been developed that have been applied in the laboratory, and more recently in cooperative multisite intervention trials. These interventions have been directed toward the enhancement of cognitive competence, to increase self-efficacy, or train caregiving behaviors. In contrast to training young children, where it can be assumed that new skills are conveyed, older adults are likely to have had access to the skills being trained, but through disuse have lost their proficiency. Information from longitudinal studies is therefore particularly useful in distinguishing individuals who have declined from those who have remained stable. In the former, training is directed toward remediation of loss, while in the latter, the enhancement of previous levels of functioning is sought with the intention of compensating for possibly cohort-based disadvantage of older persons (see Schaie, 2013; Stein-Morrow & Basak, 2011; Willis, 2001; and Willis & Belleville, 2016 for greater detail).

There also has been continued recognition that the course of development over the adult life span is markedly affected by the environmental context, including the work environment within which both behavioral and biological aging occurs (Lawton, 1977; Schaie, 2016; Scheidt & Windley, 1985; Wang & Shi, 2016; Whitbourne, 1985). The environmental context, of course, differs markedly depending on the cultural setting, and cross-cultural studies are therefore increasing in importance (Fung & Jiang, 2016; Guttmann, 1977).

The significant increase in life expectancy has led to increasing numbers of the very old, increasing research in issues involving the very old (Smith & Ryan, 2016). Very old age often also involves an increase of concern with religious views and religious practices and activities (Krause, 2006; McFadden, 1996). Finally, it has been realized that death in advanced age involves different issues from those prominent at earlier life stages (Biak, 2016; Hülür, Ram, Willis, Schaie, & Gerstorf, 2015; Kastenbaum, 1985; Lawton, 2001).

■ SUMMARY

The study of adult psychological development is increasingly informed by relevant neighboring disciplines that investigate the genetic basis, physiological infrastructure, and societal context of the developing individual. Hence, I would predict that the study of the life course of single psychological variables that was common in the first two thirds of the past century will be largely replicated or displaced by multivariate multi-disciplinary efforts (Nesselroade, 1977). Indeed, many of the more recent longitudinal studies of adults already display these characteristics. Cross-sectional investigations, except as exploratory pilot studies or as the first stage of a prospective longitudinal study, will become far more rare. They will be replaced by more programmatic long-range investigations that may frequently include experimental paradigms and in par-ticular interventions designed to modify the rate of developmental change (Bengtson, Reedy, & Gordon, 1985; Willis, Schaie, & Martin, 2009).

With our increasing sophistication in psychological measurement, we will take advan-tage of the work on structural invariance to develop better scales, perhaps applying item response theory, for those robust marker variables that seem to do well in measuring behavior across the entire adult life span. Common archives are being developed that will make available web-based access to large data sets from many different populations that cover a wide range of psychological attributes. This development calls even more urgently for the development of "gold standards" for a core set of measures that can then be used to link disparate data sets and provide the basis for substantively meaningful meta-analyses.

The investigation of adult development will increasingly turn to the identification of mechanisms and processes that underlie developmental interventions and that are rel-evant to public policy questions. Hopefully, we can expect the development of a strong applied psychology of adult development, one that will find ways to enhance the qual-ity of our existence in that large portion of the life span that we call "adulthood."

Finally, it is my hope that future researchers will indeed fulfill my expectation that I first expressed more than 40 years ago (Schaie, 1968) that the future of aging research lies in the continuous integration of research methods with conceptual development and theory as they ask ever more sophisticated questions about one of the major issues of all mature societies.

REFERENCES

Baltes, P. B., & Schaie, K. W. (Eds.). (1973). *Life-span developmental psychology: Personality and socialization*. New York, NY: Academic Press.

Baltes, P. B., & Willis, S. K. (1977). Towards psychological theories of aging and development. In J. E. Birren & K. W. Schaie (Eds.), *Handbook of the psychology of aging* (pp. 128–154). New York, NY: Van Nostrand Reinhold.

Bengtson, V. L., Kaschau, V. L., & Ragan, P. K. (1977). The impact of social structures on aging individuals. In J. E. Birren & K. W. Schaie (Eds.), *Handbook of the psychology of aging* (pp. 327–354). New York, NY: Van Nostrand Reinhold.

Bengtson, V. L., Reedy, M. N, & Gordon, C. (1985). Aging and self-conceptions: Personality processes and social contexts. In J. E. Birren & K. W. Schaie (Eds.), *Handbook of the psychology of aging* (2nd ed., pp. 544–593). New York, NY: Van Nostrand Reinhold.

Berg, S. (1996). Aging, behavior, and terminal decline. In J. E. Birren & K. W. Schaie (Eds.), *Handbook of the psychology of aging* (4th ed., pp. 323–337). San Diego, CA: Academic Press.

Biak, D. (2016). The psychology of death and dying in later life. In K. W. Schaie & S. L. Willis (Eds.), *Handbook of the psychology of aging* (8th ed., pp. 475–489). San Diego, CA: Elsevier.

Birren, J. E. (Ed.). (1959). *Handbook of aging and the individual.* Chicago, IL: University of Chicago Press.

Birren, J. E., & Birren, B. A. (1990). The concepts, models, and history of the psychology of aging. In J. E. Birren & K. W. Schaie (Eds.), *Handbook of the psychology of aging* (3rd ed., pp. 3–20). San Diego, CA: Academic Press.

Birren, J. E., & Cunningham, W. (1985). Research on the psychology of aging: Principles, concepts and theories. In J. E. Birren & K. W. Schaie (Eds.), *Handbook of the psychology of aging* (2nd ed., pp. 3–34). New York, NY: Van Nostrand Reinhold.

Birren, J. E., & Renner, V. J. (1977). Research on the psychology of aging: Principles and experimentation. In J. E. Birren & K. W. Schaie (Eds.), *Handbook of the psychology of aging* (pp. 3–38). New York, NY: Van Nostrand Reinhold.

Birren, J. E., & Schaie, K. W. (Eds.). (1977). *Handbook of the psychology of aging.* New York, NY: Van Nostrand Reinhold.

Birren, J. E., & Schaie, K. W. (Eds.). (1985). *Handbook of the psychology of aging* (2nd ed.). New York, NY: Van Nostrand Reinhold.

Birren, J. E., & Schaie, K. W. (Eds.). (1990). *Handbook of the psychology of aging* (3rd ed.). San Diego, CA: Academic Press.

Birren, J. E., & Schaie, K. W. (Eds.). (1996). *Handbook of the psychology of aging* (4th ed.). San Diego, CA: Academic Press.

Birren, J. E., & Schaie, K. W. (Eds.). (2001). *Handbook of the psychology of aging* (5th ed.). San Diego, CA: Academic Press.

Birren, J. E., & Schaie, K. W. (Eds.). (2006). *Handbook of the psychology of aging* (6th ed.). San Diego, CA: Academic Press.

Birren, J. E., & Schroots, J. J. F. (1996). History, concepts and theory in the psychology of aging. In J. E. Birren & K. W. Schaie (Eds.), *Handbook of the psychology of aging* (4th ed., pp. 3–23). San Diego, CA: Academic Press.

Birren, J. E., & Schroots, J. J. F. (2001). History of geropsychology. In J. E. Birren & K. W. Schaie (Eds.), *Handbook of the psychology of aging* (5th ed., pp. 3–28). San Diego, CA: Academic Press.

Borghesani, P., Weaver, K. E., Aylward, E. H., Richards, A. L., Madhyastha, T. M., Kahn, A. R., . . . Willis, S. L. (2012). Midlife memory improvement predicts preservation of hippocampal volume in old age. *Neurobiology of Aging, 33,* 1148–1155.

Bryk, A. S., & Raudenbush, S. W. (1987). Application of hierarchical linear models to assessing change. *Psychological Bulletin, 101,* 147–158.

Collins, L. M. (1996). Measurement of change in research on aging: Old and new issues from an individual change perspective. In J. E. Birren & K. W. Schaie

(Eds.), *Handbook of the psychology of aging* (4th ed., pp. 38–58). San Diego, CA: Academic Press.

Cowdry, E. V. (1942). *Problems of ageing*. Baltimore, MD: Lippincott Williams & Wilkins.

Deeg, D. J., Kardaun, W. P. F., & Fozard, J. L. (1996). Health, behavior and aging. In J. E. Birren & K. W. Schaie (Eds.), *Handbook of the psychology of aging* (4th ed., pp. 129–149). San Diego, CA: Academic Press.

DeFrias, C. M., Schaie, K. W., & Willis, S. L. (2014). Hypertension moderates the effect of APOE on 21-year cognitive trajectories. *Psychology and Aging, 29,* 431–439.

Dewey, J. (1939). Introduction. In E. V. Cowdry (Ed.), *Problems of aging* (pp. XXVI–XXXIII). Baltimore, MD: Lippincott Williams & Wilkins.

Dixon, R. A. (2011). Enduring theoretical themes in psychological aging: Derivation, functions, perspectives and opportunities. In K. W. Schaie & S. L. Willis (Eds.), *Handbook of the psychology of aging* (7th ed., pp. 3–24). San Diego, CA: Academic Press.

Eichorn, D. H., Clausen, J. A., Haan, N., Honzik, M. P., & Mussen, P. H. (1981). *Present and past in middle life*. New York, NY: Academic Press.

Elias, M. F., Elias, J. W., & Elias, P. K. (1990). Biological and health influences on behavior. In J. E. Birren & K. W. Schaie (Eds.), *Handbook of the psychology of aging* (3rd ed., pp. 80–102). San Diego, CA: Academic Press.

Ferrer, W., & Ghisletta, P. (2011). Methodological and analytical issues in the psychology of aging. In K. W. Schaie & L. Willis (Eds.), *Handbook of the psychology of aging* (7th ed., pp. 25–40). San Diego, CA: Academic Press.

Fry, C. L. (1985). Culture, behavior and aging in the comparative perspective. In J. E. Birren & K. W. Schaie (Eds.), *Handbook of the psychology of aging* (2nd ed., pp. 216–244). New York, NY: Van Nostrand Reinhold.

Fung, H., & Jiang, D. (2016). Cross-cultural psychology of aging. In K. W. Schaie & S. L. Willis (Eds.), *Handbook of the psychology of aging* (8th ed., pp. 323–337). San Diego, CA: Elsevier.

Guttmann, D. (1977). The cross-cultural perspective: Toward a comparative psychology of aging. In J. E. Birren & K. W. Schaie (Eds.), *Handbook of the psychology of aging* (pp. 302–326). New York, NY: Van Nostrand Reinhold.

Hall, G. S. (1922). *Senescence: The second half of life*. New York, NY: Appleton.

Hofer, S. M., & Sliwinski, M. J. (2006). Design and analysis of longitudinal studies of aging, In J. E. Birren & K. W. Schaie (Eds.), *Handbook of the psychology of aging* (6th ed., pp. 17–40). San Diego, CA: Academic Press.

Hülür, G., Ram, N., Willis, S. L., Schaie, K. W., & Gerstorf, D. (2015). Cognitive dedifferentiation with increasing age and proximity to death. *Psychology and Aging 30,* 311–323.

Jones, H. E., & Conrad, H. S. (1933). The growth and decline of intelligence: A study of a homogenous group between the ages of ten and sixty. *Genetic Psychology Monographs, 13,* 223–298.

Kallman, F. J., & Sandez, H. (1949). Twin studies of senescence. *American Journal of Psychology, 106,* 29–36.

Kastenbaum, R. (1985). Death and dying: A life-span approach. In J. E. Birren & K. W. Schaie (Eds.), *Handbook of the psychology of aging* (2nd ed., pp. 361–646). New York, NY: Van Nostrand Reinhold.

Kramer, A. F., Rabiant, M., & Colcombe, S. J. (2006). Contributions of cognitive neuroscience to the understanding of behavior and aging. In J. E. Birren & K. W. Schaie (Eds.), *Handbook of the psychology of aging* (6th ed., pp. 57–84). San Diego, CA: Academic Press.

Krause, N. (2006). Religion and health in late life. In J. E. Birren & K. W. Schaie (Eds.), *Handbook of the psychology of aging* (6th ed., pp. 500–518). San Diego, CA: Academic Press.

Kremen, W. S., & Lyons, M. J. (2011). Behavior genetics of aging. In K. W. Schaie & S. L. Willis (Eds.), *Handbook of the psychology of aging* (7th ed., pp. 93–108). San Diego, CA: Academic Press.

Lawton, M. P. (1977). The impact of the environment on aging and behavior. In J. E. Birren & K. W. Schaie (Eds.), *Handbook of the psychology of aging* (pp. 276–301). New York, NY: Van Nostrand Reinhold.

Lawton, M. P. (2001). Quality of life and the end of life. In J. E. Birren & K. W. Schaie (Eds.), *Handbook of the psychology of aging* (5th ed., pp. 592–616). San Diego, CA: Academic Press.

Lowenthal, M. F. (1977). Toward a sociological theory of change in adulthood and old age. In J. E. Birren & K. W. Schaie (Eds.), *Handbook of the psychology of aging* (pp. 116–127). New York, NY: Van Nostrand Reinhold.

Marsh, G. R., & Thompson, L. R. (1977). Psychophysiology of aging. In J. E. Birren & K. W. Schaie (Eds.), *Handbook of the psychology of aging* (pp. 219–248). New York, NY: Van Nostrand Reinhold.

McArdle, J. J., & Anderson, E. (1990). Latent variable growth models for research on aging. In J. E. Birren & K. W. Schaie (Eds.), *Handbook of the psychology of aging* (3rd ed., pp. 21–44). San Diego, CA: Academic Press.

McDonald, S., & Stawski, R. (2016). Methodology, attrition, missingness, meta-analysis and data imputation. In K. W. Schaie & S. L. Willis (Eds.), *Handbook of the psychology of aging* (8th ed., pp. 6–41). San Diego, CA: Elsevier.

McFadden, S. H. (1996). Religion, spirituality, and aging. In J. E. Birren & K. W. Schaie (Eds.), *Handbook of the psychology of aging* (4th ed., pp. 162–180). San Diego, CA: Academic Press.

Moos, R. H., & Lemke, S. (1985). Specialized living environment for older people. In J. E. Birren & K. W. Schaie (Eds.), *Handbook of the psychology of aging* (2nd ed., pp. 864–890). New York, NY: Van Nostrand Reinhold.

Nesselroade, J. R. (1977). Issuing in studying developmental change from a multivariate perspective. In J. E. Birren & K. W. Schaie (Eds.), *Handbook of the psychology of aging* (pp. 39–69). New York, NY: Van Nostrand Reinhold.

Nesselroade, J. R., & Labouvie, E. W. (1985). Experimental design in research on aging. In J. E. Birren & K. W. Schaie (Eds.), *Handbook of the psychology of aging* (2nd ed., pp. 35–60). New York, NY: Van Nostrand Reinhold.

Nyberg, L., & Bäckman, L. (2011). Memory changes and the aging brain: A multi-modal imaging approach. In K. W. Schaie & S. L. Willis (Eds.), *Handbook of the psychology of aging* (7th ed., pp. 123–132). San Diego, CA: Academic Press.

Omen, G. E. (1977). Behavior genetics. In J. E. Birren & K. W. Schaie (Eds.), *Handbook of the psychology of aging* (pp. 190–218). New York, NY: Van Nostrand Reinhold.

Owens, W. A. (1966). Age and mental abilities: A second adult follow-up. *Journal of Educational Psychology, 57*, 311–325.

Palmore, E., Busse, E. W., Maddox, G. L., Nowlin, J. B., & Siegler, I. C. (1985). *Normal aging III*. Durham, NC: Duke University Press.

Parmelee, P. A., & Lawton, M. P. (1990). The design of special environments for the aged. In J. E. Birren & K. W. Schaie (Eds.), *Handbook of the psychology of aging* (3rd ed., pp. 465–489). San Diego, CA: Academic Press.

Plomin, R., & McClearn, G. E. (1990). Human behavior genetics of aging. In J. E. Birren & K. W. Schaie (Eds.), *Handbook of the psychology of aging* (3rd ed., pp. 67–79). San Diego, CA: Academic Press.

Reynolds, C. A., & Finkel, D. G. (2016). Cognitive and physical aging: Genetic influences and gene-environment interplay. In K. W. Schaie & S. L. Willis (Eds.), *Handbook of the psychology of aging* (8th ed., pp. 125–146). San Diego, CA: Elsevier.

Riegel, K. F. (1977). History of psychogerontology. In J. E. Birren & K. W. Schaie (Eds.), *Handbook of the psychology of aging* (pp. 70–102). New York, NY: Van Nostrand Reinhold.

Riley, M. W., Foner, A., & Riley, J. W., Jr. (1999). The aging and society paradigm. In V. L. Bengtson & K. W. Schaie (Eds.), *Handbook of theories of aging* (pp. 327–343). New York, NY: Springer Publishing Company.

Rowe, J. W., & Kahn, R. L. (1987). Human aging: Usual and successful. *Science, 237*, 143–149.

Rudinger, G., & Rietz, C. (2001). Structural equation modeling in longitudinal research on aging. In J. E. Birren & K. W. Schaie (Eds.), *Handbook of the psychology of aging* (5th ed., pp. 329–352). San Diego, CA: Academic Press.

Salthouse, T. (1999). Theories of cognition. In V. L. Bengtson & K. W. Schaie (Eds.), *Handbook of theories of aging* (pp. 196–208). New York, NY: Springer Publishing Company.

Salthouse, T. (2006). Theoretical issues in the psychology of aging. In J. E. Birren & K. W. Schaie (Eds.), *Handbook of the psychology of aging* (6th ed., pp. 4–16). San Diego, CA: Academic Press.

Schaie, K. W. (1958). Rigidity-flexibility and intelligence: A cross-sectional study of the adult life span from 20 to 70. *Psychological Monographs, 72*(462), Whole No. 9.

Schaie, K. W. (1965). A general model for the study of developmental problems. *Psychological Monographs, 64*, 92–107.

Schaie, K. W. (Ed.). (1968). *Theories and methods of research on aging*. Morgantown, WV: West Virginia University Press.

Schaie, K. W. (1977). Quasi-experimental research designs in the psychology of aging. In J. E. Birren & K. W. Schaie (Eds.), *Handbook of the psychology of aging* (pp. 39–58). New York, NY: Van Nostrand Reinhold.

Schaie, K. W. (1988). The impact of research methodology on theory-building in the developmental sciences. In J. E. Birren & V. L. Bengtson (Eds.), *Emergent theories of aging: Psychological and social perspectives on time, self and society* (pp. 41–58). New York, NY: Springer Publishing Company.

Schaie, K. W. (1989). The hazards of cognitive aging. *The Gerontologist, 29*, 484–493.

Schaie, K. W. (1996). The natural history of a longitudinal study. In M. Merrens & G. Brannigan (Eds.), *The developmental psychologists* (pp. 233–249). New York, NY: McGraw-Hill.

Schaie, K. W. (2000). Living with gerontology. In J. E. Birren & J. J. F. Schroots (Eds.), *A history of geropsychology in autobiography* (pp. 233–248). Washington, DC: American Psychological Association.

Schaie, K. W. (2002). The impact of longitudinal studies on understanding development from young adulthood to old age. In W. Hartup & R. K. Silbereisen (Eds.), *Growing points in developmental science: An introduction* (pp. 307–328). Cambridge, UK: Psychology Press.

Schaie, K. W. (2005). *Intellectual development in adulthood: The Seattle Longitudinal Study.* New York, NY: Oxford University Press.

Schaie, K. W. (2008a). A lifespan developmental perspective of psychological aging. In K. Laidlaw & B. G. Knight (Eds.), *Handbook of emotional disorders in late life: Assessment and treatment* (pp. 3–32). Oxford, UK: Oxford University Press.

Schaie, K. W. (2008b). Historical processes and patterns of cognitive aging. In S. M. Hofer & D. F. Alwin (Eds.), *Handbook on cognitive aging: Interdisciplinary perspective* (pp. 368–383). Thousand Oaks, CA: Sage.

Schaie, K. W. (2011). Historical influences on aging and behavior. In K. W. Schaie & S. L. Willis (Eds.), *Handbook of the psychology of aging* (7th ed., pp. 41–55). San Diego, CA: Academic Press.

Schaie, K. W. (2013). *Intellectual development in adulthood: The Seattle Longitudinal Study* (2nd ed.). New York, NY: Oxford University Press.

Schaie, K. W. (2016). Theoretical perspectives for the psychology of aging in a lifespan context. In K. W. Schaie & S. L. Willis (Eds.), *Handbook of the psychology of aging* (8th ed., pp. 3–15). San Diego, CA: Elsevier.

Schaie, K. W., Campbell, R. T., Meredith, W., & Rawlings, S. C. (Eds.). (1989). *Methodological issues in aging research.* New York, NY: Springer Publishing Company.

Schaie, K. W., & Hertzog, C. (1985). Measurement in the psychology of adulthood and aging. In J. E. Birren & K. W. Schaie (Eds.), *Handbook of the psychology of aging* (2nd ed., pp. 61–94). New York, NY: Van Nostrand Reinhold.

Schaie, K. W., & Hofer, S. M. (2001). Longitudinal studies in research on aging. In J. E. Birren & K. W. Schaie (Eds.), *Handbook of the psychology of aging* (5th ed., pp. 55–77). San Diego, CA: Academic Press.

Schaie, K. W., Maitland, S. B., Willis, S. L., & Intrieri, R. C. (1998). Longitudinal invariance of adult psychometric ability factor structures across seven years. *Psychology and Aging, 13*, 8–20.

Schaie, K. W., Plomin, R., Willis, S. L., Gruber-Baldini, A., & Dutta, R. (1992). Natural cohorts: Family similarity in adult cognition. In T. Sonderegger (Ed.), *Psychology and aging: Nebraska Symposium on Motivation, 1991* (pp. 205–243). Lincoln: University of Nebraska Press.

Schaie, K. W., Rosenthal, F., & Perlman, R. M. (1953). Differential mental deterioration of factorially "pure" functions in later maturity. *Journal of Gerontology, 8*, 191–196.

Schaie, K. W., & Willis, S. L. (2000). A stage theory model of adult cognitive development revisited. In B. Rubinstein, M. Moss, & M. Kleban (Eds.), *The many dimensions of aging: Essays in honor of M. Powell Lawton* (pp. 175–193). New York, NY: Springer Publishing Company.

Schaie, K. W., & Willis, S. L. (Eds.). (2011). *Handbook of the psychology of aging* (7th ed.). San Diego, CA: Academic Press.

Schaie, K. W., & Willis, S. L. (Eds.). (2016). *Handbook of the psychology of aging* (8th ed.). San Diego, CA: Elsevier.

Schaie, K. W., & Zuo, Y. L. (2001). Family environments and cognitive functioning. In R. J. Sternberg & E. Grigorenko (Eds.), *Cognitive development in context* (pp. 337–361). Hillsdale, NJ: Lawrence Erlbaum.

Scheidt, R. J., & Windley, P. G. (1985). The ecology of aging. In J. E. Birren & K. W. Schaie (Eds.), *Handbook of the psychology of aging* (2nd ed., pp. 245–260). New York, NY: Van Nostrand Reinhold.

Siegler, I. E., & Costa, P. T., Jr. (1985). Health behavior relationships. In J. E. Birren & K. W. Schaie (Eds.), *Handbook of the psychology of aging* (2nd ed., pp. 144–168). New York, NY: Van Nostrand Reinhold.

Siegler, I. E., Poon, L. W., Madden, D. J., Dilworth-Anderson, P., Schaie, K. W., Willis, S. L., & Martin, P. (2009). Psychological aspects of normal aging. In D. G. Blazer & D. Steffens (Eds.), *Textbook of geriatric psychiatry* (4th ed., pp. 137–156). Arlington, VA: American Psychiatric Publishing.

Singer, J. D., & Willett, J. B. (1991). It's about time: Using discrete-time survival analysis to study duration and the timing of events. *Journal of Educational Statistics, 18*, 155–195.

Smith, J., & Ryan, L. H. (2016). Psychological vitality in the oldest old. In K. W. Schaie & S. L. Willis (Eds.), *Handbook of the psychology of aging* (8th ed., pp. 303–322). San Diego, CA: Academic Press.

Stein-Morrow, E. A., & Basak, C. (2011). Cognitive interventions. In K. W. Schaie & S. L. Willis (Eds.), *Handbook of the psychology of aging* (7th ed., pp. 153–174). San Diego, CA: Academic Press.

Wang, M., & Shi, J. (2016). Work, retirement and aging. In K. W. Schaie & S. L. Willis (Eds.), *Handbook of the psychology of aging* (8th ed., pp. 339–359). San Diego, CA: Elsevier.

Whitbourne, S. J. (1985). The psychological construction of the life span. In J. E. Birren & K. W. Schaie (Eds.), *Handbook of the psychology of aging* (2nd ed., pp. 594–618). New York, NY: Van Nostrand Reinhold.

Willis, S. L. (1985). Towards an educational psychology of the older learner. In J. E. Birren & K. W. Schaie (Eds.), *Handbook of the psychology of aging* (2nd ed., pp. 818–847). New York, NY: Van Nostrand Reinhold.

Willis, S. L. (1996). Everyday problem solving. In J. E. Birren & K. W. Schaie (Eds.), *Handbook of the psychology of aging* (4th ed., pp. 287–308). San Diego, CA: Academic Press.

Willis, S. L. (2001). Methodological issues in behavioral intervention research with the elderly. In J. E. Birren & K. W. Schaie (Eds.), *Handbook of the psychology of aging* (5th ed., pp. 78–108). San Diego, CA: Academic Press.

Willis, S. L., & Belleville, S. (2016). Cognitive interventions, neural processes and outcomes. In K. W. Schaie & S. L. Willis (Eds.), *Handbook of the psychology of aging* (8th ed., pp. 220–243). San Diego, CA: Elsevier.

Willis, S. L., Schaie, K. W., & Martin. M. (2009). Cognitive plasticity. In V. Bengtson, M. Silverstein, N. Putney, & D. Gans (Eds.), *Handbook of theories of aging* (2nd ed., pp. 95–322). New York, NY: Springer Publishing Company.

Wohlwill, J. (1973). *The study of behavioral development*. New York, NY: Academic Press.

CHAPTER 5

How Theories of Aging Became Social: Emergence of the Sociology of Aging

Vern L. Bengtson

There were relatively few sociologists conducting research in aging in 1963, the year I began my career in gerontology. The Gerontological Society of America (GSA) was still small and comprised mostly of psychologists, biomedical researchers, and practitioners. The first GSA annual meeting I attended was conducted in St. Petersburg, Florida, and it was intimate enough that some sessions were held in the First Baptist Church next to the hotel.

Despite these signs of modest beginnings, by 1963 a foundation had already been established for theories about the social forces of later life, and soon serious debates about theory would energize growing numbers of social scientists interested in aging. I came on the scene just as those debates were heating up at the University of Chicago where Ernest W. Burgess, who should rightly be regarded as the founder of the sociology of aging, had written some foundational theorizing about aging and social structures decades earlier.

In this chapter, I want to provide a perspective on how the theory developed in the sociology of aging from its earliest stages through the early 1970s. I hope to demonstrate how today's researchers are standing "on the shoulders of giants," as Aldous Huxley put it, in their conceptualizations about society and aging, because these pioneers developed many of the concepts and outlined many of the problems that are the basis of sociological research in aging today. Although many of these scholars have by now been forgotten along with their pioneering work in aging, a remarkable number of the concepts they developed are still alive, though under different guises and without attribution to their founders—concepts related to aging in changing societies, successful aging, the meanings of age, and inequalities of aging that accumulate over the life course.

This chapter is organized around seven concepts and issues that defined the early development of theory in the sociology of aging and the giants in gerontology (their names are shown in bold within the text) whose work is identified with them:

1. The importance of age in social structure and the place of the aged in changing societies
2. "Successful aging": How to define, measure, and achieve it
3. Social structure versus individual agency in the activity versus disengagement controversy
4. The social meanings of age and generations
5. Families, intergenerational relations, and aging
6. Cohorts, generations, and age stratification
7. The life course as a socially constructed process

This will also be a personal account, because I was privileged to know personally and be influenced by many of the giants identified with these developments. As my own research career developed, it followed themes similar to these pioneers and has been situated on the shoulders of these giants in the sociology of aging.

I came to gerontology by an unlikely route, as recounted in an earlier biographical essay (Bengtson, 2011). I grew up in a series of small farming towns where my father was pastor of evangelical congregations. My dad, born in Sweden, was part of a large evangelical family whose fervent Pietistic tradition, dating back to the 1840s, had been transmitted across many generations. In college, I became aware of the powerful social forces of family transmission, for better or worse, a theme that would eventually follow me throughout my research career. My parents' devout hope was that I would follow my dad in the ministry, or at the very least become a medical missionary doing godly deeds in some far-off place. I was the only kid in my high school class to go on to college, and going from a farm community to the cultural adventures of Chicago was an awesome experience. Hedging my bets, I determined to major in both philosophy and biology at North Park College (arguing that I could then be a well-rounded physician) and then applied for graduate school to the University of Chicago where there was a combined MD–PhD program.

However, there were no fellowships available in that program, though there was one in something called gerontology, which combined biology, psychology, and sociology. I went for an application interview with Bernice Neugarten, who was later to become my mentor. It was the most terrifying interrogation of my life. I said I was interested in "geh-ron-tol-ogy" (pronounced with a *g* like in "guess"; I had read the word, but never actually heard it pronounced). She informed me that it was "jeh-ron-tol-ogy," and implied that, if I knew so little about gerontology that I could not even pronounce the word correctly, why should I think I wanted to become a gerontologist (Bengtson, 2011)? Despite this gaffe, I gained admission to the University of Chicago's Committee on Human Development program, where I was introduced for the first time to the ideas of age, social structure, and the life course.

■ THE IMPORTANCE OF AGE IN SOCIAL STRUCTURES AND THE POSITION OF THE AGED IN CHANGING SOCIETIES

The first issue concerning age and aging to attract attention by American sociologists involved the role or status of older people in societies that were changing rapidly in the wake of the Industrial Revolution. The first sociologist to recognize this was **Ernest W. Burgess** (1886–1966), one of the most prominent figures in early American sociology and a founding member of the GSA in 1945.

Burgess was an impressive presence in American sociology from 1916 through the 1960s. His book with Robert Park, *Introduction to the Science of Sociology*, was the standard textbook for three decades of American sociology students. He helped to develop what became the American Sociological Association as well as the *American Sociological Review*, *Journal of Marriage and Family*, and *Social Problems*. Burgess was codirector of what became the first major social science survey of older individuals in America, *Personal Adjustment in Old Age* (Cavan, Burges, Havighurst, & Goldhamer, 1949). Elected president of the Gerontological Society in 1952, he was part of the group that, with James Birren, Clark Tibbitts, and Wilma Donahue, edited the first *Handbook of Gerontology* series (Burgess, 1960).

Burgess was truly an innovator in sociology. He inherited a tradition of 19th-century sociological thinking based on moral and political philosophy, and adapted this to focus on the social problems encountered by early–20th-century Americans—urbanization, poverty, crime, dislocation, and the like. Because so little systematic social research had preceded him, he became a pioneer in almost every field he entered, from the methodology of social surveys (Burgess, 1916) to the study of families (Burgess, 1926) and the place of the aged (Burgess, 1960). Burgess was a bridge builder, and, as a theorist, he built bridges between structural functionalism, which he inherited from Durkheim, and symbolic interactionism, building on the ideas of Weber and his colleague George Herbert Mead at Chicago in developing a new perspective on family processes. He wrote about the family transitioning "from institution to companionship" (Burgess, 1926).

In gerontology, one of the things Burgess is remembered for is the concept of the "roleless role of the aged." Burgess intended this as a caricature: an "ideal type" in Weberian terms, to describe the effect that rapid social change can have on older people. Because of industrialization, urbanization, and migration, many people approach old age in unfortunate circumstances:

> The retired older man and his wife are imprisoned in a roleless role. They have no vital function to perform as they had in rural society…This roleless role is thrust by society upon the older person at retirement, and…the effect of economic and social trends which capitulated old people from the family-oriented rural society to the organization-centered urban society are still in operation. (Burgess, 1960, pp. 20–21)

He used the "roleless role of the aged" as a term of advocacy, to call attention to the problem of the lack of cultural and policy provisions for elderly people in industrial societies, notably the United States.

Burgess was briefly my teacher at the University of Chicago, several years after his own formal retirement. I remember him as a courtly and diminutive gentleman, peering over the lectern as he talked, apparently without notes, in Bernice Neugarten's class. Shortly thereafter, he became increasingly frail and unable to live on his own. This led to a situation of profound irony. This giant of American gerontology, this pioneer in family studies, had never married, had outlived all his biological kin, and had no family to take care of his needs in his declining years.

In 1965, unable to live independently, Burgess quietly checked himself into a neighborhood board and care home for the elderly that turned out to be in deplorable condition. When they discovered this, Bernice Neugarten, Robert Havighurst, and other University of Chicago faculty arranged for his transfer to the superb Drexel Home for the Aged, a Jewish facility (Burgess, a lifelong Presbyterian, had been unaware that he would qualify for admission). He died there in December 1966 at the age of 80 years, without family except for the "fictive kin" of the Drexel Home staff and his University of Chicago colleagues. It was an ironic departure for one of the pioneers in family sociology and gerontology.

The theme of status and roles related to age and aging was also pioneered by **Ralph Linton** (1893–1953), an anthropologist who developed enduring concepts of social structure and cultural organization. After doing fieldwork in the American southwest and Guatemala, he published what became the most popular textbook in anthropology for several decades, *The Study of Man* (Linton, 1936). In it, he presented his classic distinction between status and role, a structural analysis that influenced gerontology. Turning his attention to aging, he also described age grading, movement upward through the course of life through the process of aging, which he described as a universal feature of both preliterate and modern societies (Linton, 1942).

Linton's concepts were picked up by sociologists focusing on aging starting a decade or so later, most importantly by Leonard Cain (1959, 1964), who applied them for the first time to a sociology of aging, as will be described later in this chapter. The ideas about age status and the life course percolated and were carried forward by Bernice Neugarten and Glen Elder to the "life course perspective," and by Matilda White Riley to the "age stratification" or "aging and society" perspective in decades to come.

A third important contributor to the theme of age as an important dimension of social structure was **Talcott Parsons** (1902–1979). These days Parsons is sometimes discounted as an outmoded structural functionalist, but it is worth remembering what he did to call the attention of mainstream sociologists to age as a sociological parameter. In an *American Sociological Review* article, Parsons (1942) wrote about age as a crucial dimension of American social structure, equating it with sex as a way to understand social stratification. This elevated age from the status of a conditional to an analytical variable. His emphasis on age as a sociological variable was not visible in his other publications, but it created a lasting impact on the sociology of aging through his mentorship at Harvard of some creative students such as John W. Riley, Matilda White Riley, Fred W. Cottrell, and Irving Rosow.

Parsons influenced my career in two ways. In addition to convincing me that age was an important independent (not just a control) variable, I learned a great deal from his focus on the dynamics (not just the structure) of families. At Chicago, I worked with his student, Fred Strodtbeck, on a project observing conflict resolution among adolescent–mother–father triads. From coding those interchanges, I got my ideas of solidarity and conflict as orthogonal dimensions of family interaction, concepts that were to later dominate my career (Bengtson, Giarrusso, Mabry, & Silverstein, 2002; Bengtson, Olander, & Haddad, 1976; Bengtson & Roberts, 1991).

My only interaction with the great man himself was something of a surprise. He was awarded an honorary doctorate at the same University of Chicago commencement when I received my PhD degree in June 1967. I wanted to tell him that his work had been instructive in my graduate career in studying aging and family intergenerational relationships. The line of PhD graduate students moving to congratulate him was surprisingly short. When I introduced myself, and started telling him how I appreciated his work, he looked over my head and muttered something like, "Aging, yes, thank you..." and quickly moved to shake the hand of the next person in line. I think Talcott Parsons, the person who so dominated American sociological theory for more than three decades, may have been a very shy man.

■ "SUCCESSFUL AGING": HOW TO DEFINE, MEASURE, AND ACHIEVE IT

The second theme that emerged early in the sociology of aging focused on the life satisfaction of aging individuals and the social conditions associated with it. The originator of this line of inquiry, **Robert J. Havighurst** (1900–1991), was truly a Renaissance man. The son of missionaries to China, he got a PhD in chemistry, did postdoctoral training in physics, joined the University of Chicago faculty in education, and became prominent in both developmental psychology and gerontology. He was instrumental in founding the GSA in 1945 and was elected president in 1957.

Havighurst became interested in aging as he watched his grandparents grow old. He watched his grandfather struggle with forced retirement at age 65 from the factory where he worked, and his grandmother attempt to adjust to a long period of widowhood and living alone. He listened to his colleague Ernest Burgess talk about the "roleless role" of elders in American society as a consequence of losing the social roles of midlife, but he also observed that some individuals did very well in their retirement years. Why?

With Burgess and a graduate student interested in the family, Ruth Cavan, Havighurst conducted what became the first social science survey to investigate the social psychology of aging. The central finding of the study was that older individuals who had high levels of social activity and psychological engagement also had high levels of morale, or life satisfaction (Cavan et al., 1949). Havighurst followed this up with a larger, community-based study with another student, Ruth Albrecht (Havighurst & Albrecht, 1953), and developed an elaborate system of measuring role activity, based on role theory and social life space, and life satisfaction. The positive relationship between social activity and life satisfaction remained strong; this formed the basis for what came to be called the "activity theory of aging."

Havighurst was a theorist, or more properly an empiricist whose work was characterized by concepts and typologies that he went on to examine with data. Early in his career in aging, he developed a typology of "social and psychological needs of the aging" (Havighurst, 1952), in which he suggested four needs common to all people: (a) emotional security and affection; (b) social recognition and status; (c) a sense of worth and self-respect; and (d) adequate food, clothing, and shelter. Whenever these needs are not met, there is a social problem; and for many older people in America, several of these needs are not met.

> The aging body conspires with society's youth-favoring attitudes and practices to create special needs of older people. It is well to call them "developmental needs" and regard them in the same positive light with which we regard the developmental needs of youth and middle adulthood. (Havighurst, 1952, p. 12)

Almost a decade later, in the very first issue of *The Gerontologist*, Havighurst published his theory of successful aging. He began by suggesting that a major aim of gerontology was "to provide society and individuals with advice on the making of societal and individual choices" about such things as retirement policy, housing, and what to do with spare time (Havighurst, 1961, p. 8). Moreover, "in order to provide good advice, *it is essential that gerontology have a theory of successful aging*" (italics mine). He suggested four operational definitions of successful aging that could be empirically tested: (a) a way of life that is socially desirable for this age group—one that is regarded by society as appropriate for older people; (b) maintenance of middle-age activity; (c) a feeling of satisfaction with one's present status and activities; and (d) a feeling of happiness and satisfaction with life. Note that two of the four involve perceptions and feelings—subjective or interpretive aspects of aging on the part of the individual—while the first involves social acceptance. These social and subjective components are absent from today's models of successful aging, as pointed out by critics, and Havighurst's definition of successful aging is substantially different from that of Rowe and Kahn (1998; see also Chapter 28).

Havighurst was chair of my graduate committee at Chicago until his retirement in 1965, when Bernice Neugarten took over. I remember him as a genial grandfather type, always supportive, always saying to me, "Yes, of course, that's all right," and giving me the affirmation to proceed with whatever wild ideas I had, whereas Bernice Neugarten always stopped me short with: "What? What do you mean?" I remember him seeming to doze through my MA thesis meeting and coming awake to say, "Yes, that's fine. We're agreed then. OK." I needed that affirmation, insecure as I was. When he retired and Bernice took over as my mentor, I found I needed her challenges, too. Havighurst died at the age of 91 years, of dementia, having outlived his wife Jean, who had held his domestic and social life together, by almost two decades.

■ SOCIAL STRUCTURE VERSUS INDIVIDUAL AGENCY IN THE ACTIVITY VERSUS DISENGAGEMENT THEORY CONTROVERSY

I had arrived at the University of Chicago shortly after the start of the first and probably the most exciting theoretical controversy in social gerontology. Earlier, survey data collected by Havighurst and his students had linked what he called "successful aging," indicated by high scores on measures of life satisfaction scores, to the maintenance of high levels of activity in the social roles of adult life, such as parent, grandparent, friend, neighbor, citizen, spouse, and the like. This came to be known as the "activity theory of aging" (high activity leads to high life satisfaction) and it became popular with gerontological practitioners working with elderly patients, because it provided justification for what they had been doing to keep them active.

However, Havighurst was not satisfied with this formulation, nor with the data at his disposal—too shallow in its focus on social roles and opinions, too limited in the sample on which it was based. Therefore, with a sizable grant from the Carnegie Foundation, he went to Kansas City with a multidisciplinary research team to select a stratified probability sample of middle-aged and elderly residents. The Kansas City Study design involved collecting not only survey data on activities and attitudes but also extensive psychological data, including projective psychoanalytic techniques to measure dimensions of inner life, such as interiority of experience and ego involvement.

Among this team were two young and ambitious researchers, Elaine Cumming and William Henry. Cumming was a Harvard-trained sociologist, a student of Talcott Parsons and functionalist theory on the influence of social structure on individual behavior. Her previous work had been on kinship relations (Cumming & Schneider, 1961). Henry was a psychoanalyst interested in psychosocial aspects of human development who had done pioneering work on the analysis of fantasy (Henry, 1956). Together they analyzed the Kansas City data and very soon, after Cumming arrived at Chicago, proposed a theory of successful aging that was quite the opposite of the dominant "activity theory" of the day. They called it the "disengagement theory of aging" (Cumming & Henry, 1961).

Disengagement theory posited that withdrawal by the individual, in both social and psychological involvement, was a normal part of the aging process over time. The theory posited that biological, psychological, and social disengagement was universal and inevitable. It was adaptive in that it prepared both individuals and those in their social networks for their subsequent and inevitable leave taking through death. Moreover, disengagement was functional: satisfying for the aging individual, because it enhanced life satisfaction by freeing him or her from the increasingly unrealistic demands and expectations of middle age; and useful for the social system because it helped the group maintain equilibrium while preparing younger members to fit into the retiree's position. The theory was also multidisciplinary, based on Cumming's sociological analysis of the Kansas City interviews on social relationships and Henry's psychodynamic analysis of the psychological data. Finally, it was an elegant theory, if judged by the criteria of scientific theory—explicit, parsimonious, even axiomatic, everything a logic-based scientific theory should be, according to textbooks.

However, it immediately created controversy and drew severe criticism within the gerontological community. Disengagement theory clashed with activity theory that implicitly assumed that aging involved declines and losses that must be "adjusted to" by replacing or maintaining the levels of social activity in midlife. This "keep active!" formula of successful aging was much more in keeping with American values of individualism, autonomy, and agency than was the concept of disengagement, and much more in keeping with gerontological practice. It was a rationale for the development of senior citizen centers and the emerging "silver market" of Leisure World–type retirement communities.

The scholarly community criticized disengagement activity for other reasons. **George Maddox** (1925–2012), who later became one of the giants in gerontology and medical sociology while at Duke University, published as his first paper in the sociology of aging a critique of disengagement theory (Maddox, 1965). He argued that the theory was flawed because of its reliance on functionalist assumptions of universality and inevitability of disengagement. **Arnold Rose** (1918–1968), one of the proponents of symbolic interactionist theory who came to the sociology of aging late in his career, criticized disengagement theory for not considering cultural values and meanings of aging, which are always changing—not universal, as disengagement theory posited (Rose, 1965). **Irving Rosow** (1922–2001), who deserves much more attention than he has received in the sociology of aging, was critical of both disengagement and activity theory. He developed the concepts of "social integration of the aged" and "socialization to old age," which in many ways bridged them (Rosow, 1974).

It was in the middle of this conflict that I launched my dissertation, a brave effort to test both theories and specifically to refute the postulate of "universality" in the functionalist disengagement theory of aging. The data were from another of Havighurst's ambitious projects, a cross-national study of retired and middle-aged school teachers and steelworkers from urban centers in six nations—Vienna, Bonn, Milan, Warsaw, Nijmegen, and Chicago. These data provided support neither for disengagement theory's postulates (Havighurst, Neugarten, & Bengtson, 1966) nor for activity theory. Although the retired Americans—particularly teachers—did show a high correlation between activity and life satisfaction in a manner supporting activity theory, the Dutch and Italians showed low activity and high satisfaction, supporting disengagement theory. Several years later, my students and I developed a formal test of activity theory of aging (Lemon, Bengtson, & Peterson, 1972). Our data provided no support for the proposition that maintaining high levels of social activity is related to high levels of well-being in aging. There was too much variation across individuals, income groups, and between men and women to support such a sweeping model as suggested in activity theory.

Yet, despite criticism and lack of empirical support, remnants of both activity theory and disengagement theory are found today, though in different forms from their original formulation. This is because each reflects observable patterns of normal aging. Activity theory, for example, can be seen (though it is never referenced) as a basic premise of current "successful aging" models: Stay active! Control your aging as much as possible! Avoid disease, eat healthy, exercise, and be active mentally and socially (see Chapter 28). Although critics may argue that this prescription is both stereotypic and unrealistic for many older individuals, activity reflects a cultural value that resonates with many Americans, though staying active, eating healthy, and avoiding disease are impossible to achieve for many, particularly minority elderly. In turn, disengagement is an assumption of Socioemotional Selectivity Theory (Carstensen, Isaacowitz, & Charles, 1999). In this developmental theory, aging individuals gradually reduce and select the relationships and activities in which they invest emotional energy, and this brings satisfaction. This seems similar to the major premise of disengagement theory: "We can conclude that approval and love-seeking, the appropriate rewards of the instrumental world of work and the socio-emotional world of social relationships, fall off during disengagement, and that a new freedom to choose among relational rewards emerges" (Cumming & Henry, 1961, p. 83).

■ THE SOCIAL MEANINGS OF AGE AND THEIR EFFECTS ON AGING

A different perspective on the sociology of aging was provided by those operating from the phenomenological perspective in sociology, what Berger and Luckman (1966) had termed the "social construction of reality." Here the focus was on the meanings of age, for individuals and society, and how these—particularly those that were negative—influenced the status or well-being of those who were old. One example of the phenomenological perspective was the work of **Jabar Gubrium** (1942–), whose *Living and Dying in Murray Manor* (Gubrium, 1975) is an ethnography of a nursing home with insights as to how both residents and staff dealt with the end stages of life. Another was the work of Glaser and Strauss (1968), whose *Time for Dying* showed that even the temporal parameters of death were socially constructed, a finding extended by Victor Marshall (1945–), whose work on the sociology of death and dying solidified the interpretive perspective in gerontology (Marshall, 1978).

Bernice Neugarten (1916–2001) approached the social meanings of age and aging from a slightly different direction. Her early research, with Robert Havighurst, had convinced her that many perceptions of old age were stereotypic—most older adults were satisfied with their lives (Neugarten, Havighurst, & Tobin, 1961). She examined social perceptions of age norms, what she called "prescriptive timetable(s) for the ordering of major life events" (Neugarten, 1996, p. 13), and found remarkable agreement in public opinion on the ages around which an individual would be "on time" for events such as marriage, the launching of a family, and retirement (Neugarten, Moore, & Lowe, 1965). She pursued these themes throughout her career and attacked the perception that the elderly constituted a homogeneous group. In one of her most enduring contributions (Neugarten, 1974), she differentiated them as the "young old" (age: 55–75 years) and the "old old" (75 years and older), a distinction that was to find its way into public policy formation.

Neugarten chaired my doctoral committee, and I was perpetually in awe of her quick intelligence and scathing critiques. It turned out that she and I shared a highly unlikely pre-Chicago connection. She had grown up in Norfolk, Nebraska, a farming center of about 5,000, where she must have been the only Jewish kid for miles around. Her father owned a women's dress shop, and years later, when I was in graduate school, my mother told me she used to shop at the Neugarten store when we lived in a small farm town nearby. However, that was long after Bernice had escaped at the age of 16 years to study at the University of Chicago. After teaching in the U of C's Committee on Human Development for three decades, she went on to Northwestern University, where she founded the program in Human Development and Social Policy. She was elected president of the GSA in 1969. A collection of her most influential papers has been published in

The Meanings of Age: Selected Papers of Bernice L. Neugarten (Neugarten, 1996). A volume of papers written in her honor by her former students and colleagues (Bengtson, 1996) was appropriately titled *Adulthood and Aging: Research on Continuities and Discontinuities.*

"Ageism" is one of the most important contributions to the social meanings of age. The term was introduced by a friend of Neugarten's, **Robert Butler** (1927–2010), the giant of geriatric psychiatry and founding director of the National Institute on Aging. I first met him in a swimming pool at the University of Chicago, where he was playfully splashing us graduate students (see the full story in Bengtson, 2015; Butler's contributions to gerontology are told in a masterful biography by Andrew Achenbaum [2013]). The origins of "ageism," one of the most notable terms in gerontology's history (Butler, 1969, 1975), makes an interesting story. In 1969, opposition had arisen in downtown Washington, DC, against a proposal to build senior housing. A young reporter from the *Washington Post* by the name of Carl Bernstein (later to gain fame by breaking open the Watergate political scandal touching the Nixon White House) interviewed Butler about this. In an off-hand comment, Butler said that this situation showed negative stereotyping against the elderly—not unlike the evils of racism and sexism. "It's sort of like ageism," he said. The term became a headline in the news story (Bernstein, 1969). It stuck, and it was a theme he would return to again and again in his career.

I was intrigued by "ageism" and negative perceptions being related to problems of aging, because this fit well with other ideas such as Robert Lemert's labeling theory, Alfred Schutz's phenomenology, and Thomas Saasz's notion of the social construction of mental illness. Taken as a whole, these seemed to me to help explain the problems that aging individuals encountered in a society that devalued age, explanations that bridged micro- and macro-social levels. Together with Joseph Kuypers, my graduate school friend from the University of Chicago, I began to construct a theory that would explain why social competence broke down in older adults and how interventions might help restore it. What we came up with was the Social Competence/Breakdown Model of Aging (Bengtson & Kuypers, 1984; Kuypers & Bengtson, 1973). The origins of the model came from an interpretive theoretical perspective (in those days, it was called "symbolic interactionist") based on labeling theory, but drew on elements of Marxism and exchange theory as well.

The Social Competence/Breakdown Model of Aging posits that an older individual's sense of self, as well as her social world's assessment of her worth and competence, are both related to the kind of valuing, or labeling, that she experiences in the course of aging. This can be viewed as a cycle, or spiral, of social competence or incompetence that starts (stage 1) with the vulnerability that characterizes many old persons because of a health crisis, widowhood, or lowered income. It can set in motion a downward spiral with additional crises (stage 2) concerning role losses (loss of social contacts, immobility) that lead to loneliness, depression, and anomie. This creates dependence on external sources of self-labeling (stage 3), many of which reflect stereotypical images of elderly people as dependent, incapable, and incompetent. The older individual who accepts such negative labeling is then inducted into the negative, dependent situation of the final stages of life (stage 4), learning to act like very old, dependent people are supposed to act. This reduces her social and psychological competence even more, with a corresponding atrophy of skills involving social and cognitive coping (stage 5). This, in turn, makes her even more vulnerable to even greater debilitation, thus setting the stage for another round of the vicious spiral of the Social Breakdown syndrome.

However, the cycle of competence breakdown can be broken through the efforts of practitioners (Bengtson & Kuypers, 1984). For example, the model can help gerontological social workers assist families with practical interventions at each stage to: (a) clarify the nature of the crisis event; (b) suggest roles of short-term involvement for each potential family caregiver; (c) discuss unrealistic expectations and guilt; (d) suggest some quick, short-term successes; and (e) follow up and develop external supports.

■ FAMILIES, INTERGENERATIONAL RELATIONS, AND AGING

Families and aging were a focus of interest among the pioneer sociologists in aging, as is evidenced in the first two handbooks of aging. There chapters written by Ernest Burgess (1960) and **Gordon Streib** (1918–2011) reflected two quite different perspectives on families and aging at the time. Burgess focused on family structure and relationships and the forces of social change. He contrasted the family before the industrial revolution and after, writing that "Family and kinship ties still persist but they are no longer central and vital. The result is that the older person feels dethroned and devalued in the realm of family relations where he once reigned supreme" (Burgess, 1960, p. 272). He went on to review studies from four nations to support his point, particularly research in England. Streib took a different approach. Based on data from Streib's own ongoing panel research, the Cornell Study of Occupational Retirement (Streib, 1958), he suggested that "Among the most important of the older person's interests and activities, his family still serves as a significant source of gratification and personal satisfaction" (Streib & Thompson, 1960, p. 485).

A few years later, two British scholars produced work on the family life of older people that were highly influential on American gerontologists. **Peter Laslett** (1915–2001) was a social demographer who later took issue with those, like Burgess and others, who he felt glorified the supposedly age-friendly family structure of the past. Laslett decried those who romanticized "the world we have never lost" (Laslett, 1965). He later became known for his term "the third age." **Peter Townsend** (1928–2009) produced a landmark study of kinship and families creating social structures in Bethnel Green, a working-class community in postwar London in which families showed significant intergenerational contact (Townsend, 1957).

At about the same time, **Ethel Shanas** (1914–2005) began her influential career in social dimensions of health and family relationships in aging. Shanas had studied under Ernest Burgess and Robert Havighurst at the University of Chicago. She partnered with Townsend in a five-nation survey on the health and family relationships of older adults (Shanas et al., 1968). Results indicated that families were the major caretakers of older people in all countries, and that contact between older parents and adult children were high—even in the United States and Britain, contrary to initial expectations. In an earlier study, Shanas had found in a national survey of Americans that, although most older adults reported being in good health, the general public perceived old age as similar to illness, and feeling lonely or isolated. Shanas later broke decisively with the position of her mentor, Burgess, in her Kleemeier Award address on "Social Myth as Hypothesis" (Shanas, 1979). The "myth" was the popular belief that older people were isolated from or abandoned by their families, and that industrialization had resulted in the demise of familial support of elders.

I first became aware of the excitement in research on families and intergenerational relationships in Bernice Neugarten's classes during my first year at Chicago, and this was to become my professional preoccupation for the next 45 years. Our class assignment was to study a three-generation family; I was fascinated by the continuities and differences I saw in this African-American family who were coping with poverty following their post–World War II migration from Alabama. Then in 1966 as I was finishing my dissertation, I became intrigued by a project down the hallway in Cobb Hall, the "Activism" study directed by sociology professor Richard Flacks. These were the days of mounting student protest, and Flacks and his students were interviewing students who had been arrested in protests against the Vietnam war and also interviewing their parents. The aim of the research was to examine value and personality differences between young radicals and their parents in politics, morality, and religion. Much to the researchers' surprise, results showed that few of the young radicals were rebelling against their parents' values—many of the parents themselves had been radicals in the 1920s labor movements.

I went from the University of Chicago to the University of Southern California (USC) to join James Birren, the giant in the psychology of aging who had been recruited from the National Institutes of Health (NIH) to build a center for research on aging at USC. In my youthful optimism, I quickly submitted a proposal to National Institute of Mental Health (NIMH) for a study to test the "generation gap" across not two, but three generations, on a sample much larger than the Chicago activists' study and based on extended families to allow examination of mental health issues related to family interactions. Astonishingly, the research was funded, and it went on to become the 35-year Longitudinal Study of Generations (LSOG). The study has been supported by NIH over eight waves of data collection from 1970 to 2005 (see Bengtson, Putney, & Harris, 2013) and has recently been refunded for a ninth wave under the direction of Merril Silverstein. Data will be available from these multigeneration families for over a 45-year span.

Two enduring contributions to theory came out of the initial wave of the LSOG. First was the Intergenerational Stake concept, also called the "developmental stake theory" (Bengtson & Kuypers, 1971). While Wave 1 of the study did show differences between generations in attitudes and political orientations (Bengtson, 1975; Glass, Dunham, & Bengtson, 1986), the more surprising contrast was between parents and youth in describing their common relationship. Parents as a whole overestimated the closeness, similarity, and contact compared with their children's ratings. This was true whether the children were 18 or 48 years old. Why? From the Intergenerational Stake theory, each generation has an investment in the other generation, but these cross-generational investments were unequal. Parents' investments were large over time, involving significant commitments of time, support, and finances, and parents might justify this, according to dissonance theory, by perceiving warmth and similarity in the relationship. Children, by contrast, have a higher psychological investment in individuation and autonomy. This leads to less investment in the intergenerational relationship, leading perhaps to devaluing or underestimating the closeness, similarity, and contact. Their differing "developmental stake" has caused different perceptions of their common relationship. Longitudinal data have shown that this intergenerational bias persists for many years and is still reflected between aging parents and their children (Giarrusso, Feng, & Bengtson, 2004). The Intergenerational Stake theory too has persisted over time: It has been used as an explanation by researchers for more than 40 years now (see Birditt, Hartnett, Fingerman, Zarit, & Antonucci, 2015).

The second theoretical contribution from the first wave of this longitudinal study was the Intergenerational Solidarity model and/or theory (Bengtson et al., 1976; Bengtson & Schrader, 1982). This posited that family intergenerational relationships, particularly in aging, were based on not only frequency of interaction and support received or given but also on affect, shared values, and norms or expectations of solidarity. This we called "intergenerational solidarity," measured in six dimensions of interaction (Bengtson &

Schrader, 1982; Mangen, Bengtson, & Landry, 1988). This typology has been widely used by other investigators (see Rossi & Rossi, 1990) and with regard to grandparent–grandchild relationships (Bengtson, 2001). In the Wave 1 data, we found that higher levels of solidarity were associated with mental health indicators, such as depression and self-esteem, a finding that has been subsequently replicated in many other studies that have used this theory (see Szydlik, 2008, 2016). The theory has also helped explain why intergenerational transmission is more effective in some families than others: It is not so much the example of the parent (role modeling, teaching), as the quality of the relationship (solidarity), that predicts high parental influence (Bengtson et al., 2013).

■ COHORTS, GENERATIONS, AND AGE STRATIFICATION

Both the age stratification and the life-course perspectives began in gerontological theory with the insights of **Leonard D. Cain** (1926–). He drew from sociologists (e.g., Mannheim and Eisenstadt) on the importance of generations and anthropologists (e.g., Van Gnepp and Malinowski) for the concept of age grading and age statuses in preliterate societies, to build a persuasive case that stages of life were important phenomena in modern American society. He may have been the first to coin the phrase "the life course" (Cain, 1959) and outlined its sociological determinants (Cain, 1964).

Cain was something of a maverick in the gerontological establishment. After receiving his PhD in sociology from the University of California, Berkeley, he did not go on to take a position at a prestigious university with graduate students whose research would follow up on his ideas. Rather he went to the newly established Sacramento State College, where, for years, he taught general sociology classes to undergraduates. He published nothing until a decade later when he did work on aging and the law (Cain, 1979). Unfortunately, he is largely unrecognized in today's gerontological literature.

However, Cain's work and the concepts he developed had lasting effects in the sociology of aging. They were most obvious in Glen Elder's model of the life course (discussed in the following section) and Matilda White Riley's development of what she at that time called the "age stratification model" (Riley, 1971; Riley, Johnston, & Foner, 1972). **Matilda White Riley** (1911–2009) studied at Harvard under Talcott Parsons, where she was his teaching assistant and picked up on his interest on age and social structure. She also met, and married, Jack Riley, another promising young sociologist (her frequent coauthor in later publications, he is also remembered as Matilda's effervescent companion in tennis shoes at GSA meetings). She became pregnant and dropped out of graduate school in the 1930s to raise her family. It is amazing that she was able later to rise to superstardom in universities, in the American Sociological Association, and in the National Institute of Aging without having attained a PhD, though she was awarded honorary doctorates later in her career.

Matilda White Riley's model of age stratification and the life course quickly became the most widely used conceptualization in the 1970s of how social structures and cohort flow interface with the aging of individuals in ways that produced variations in populations of the aged. The model used concepts such as age cohorts, age roles, age-graded social structures, age segregation/integration, and structural lag. Structural lag occurs when social structures cannot keep pace with the changes in population dynamics and individual lives—for example (Riley, Kahn, & Foner, 1994) it is the discordance between the increasing numbers of elderly parents for caregiving support, concurrent reductions in available state resources to provide long-term care services, and the increasing demands this places on families to provide parent care, creating conflicts with demands of their jobs. Using this theoretical perspective, Riley and Loscocco (1994) argued that a more age-integrated society brought about by policy changes can compensate for structural lag and improve the lives of older adults. Restructuring the social institutions of work, education, and the family, through such policies as extended time off for education or caregiving, can bring social structures in balance with individuals' lives.

My own work on generations and cohorts was influenced by Lenard Cain's (1964) article, though mine had a more political focus. The 1960s were years of protest, with the Civil Rights Movement, the Student Rights Movement, the Anti-Vietnam War movement, and the counter-culture gaining more and more publicity month by month. I was interested in these youth protest movements, and it appeared to many that the "generation gap" was wide and deeply rooted in radically different political and economic values between youth and their parents. At the same time as I became involved in anti-war protests, I was reading the work of Karl Mannheim (1952) on generational units being a force in social change, Benet Berger (1960) on youth representing a new *Zeitgeist*, and Seymour Eisenstadt (1956) on the succession of generations. In Wave 1 of the LSOG, I included a variety of items to test perceptions of individuals and age groups across generations.

The results were somewhat surprising. Despite the great amount of publicity that had been given to differences between age groups and generations, respondents saw less of a "gap" between generations than anticipated, and there were fewer value differences between generations than expected (Bengtson, 1971, 1975). There was little evidence of a "generational consciousness" among youth participating in protests during the late 1960s (Kasschau, Ransford, & Bengtson, 1974). We could find little empirical support for Mannheim's thesis concerning the development of generational units out of the youth involved in protest demonstrations (Laufer & Bengtson, 1974). This led us to argue that we should stop using the term "generation" as applied to age groups—it was too vague and impossible to operationalize (Bengtson & Cutler, 1976). Instead, "cohort" was the appropriate concept, with the term "generation" reserved for families and lineages.

■ THE LIFE COURSE AS A SOCIALLY CONSTRUCTED PROCESS

The life-course perspective has become the most widely used theoretical framework in social gerontology today. It is based on the premise that, to understand the present circumstances of elderly people, we must take into account the social and psychological forces operating throughout the earlier course of their lives, as well as the changing historical context in which they are aging (George, 1996). In the first systematic statement of the life-course perspective, Cain (1964) described individuals situated in a context of structural and historical factors that influenced their development. However, it was Glen Elder's work, starting with his classic *Children of the Great Depression* (Elder, 1974), that brought the life-course perspective into the mainstream of sociology, psychology, and gerontology (George, 1996; Settersten & Gannon, 2005).

Glen Elder (1935–) had not intended to be a sociologist. His first degree was in agricultural science at Pennsylvania State University, but he had a growing interest in developmental psychology. He went to graduate school at the University of North Carolina and became interested in family sociology. His dissertation on family cohesion between adolescents and their parents caught the attention of John Clausen at the University of California, Berkeley, who invited him to join the group at the Institute of Human Development analyzing the unmined data sets of the Berkeley and Oakland longitudinal studies that were started in the 1920s. Elder jumped at the chance and began to work on data focusing on the later life consequences of children who grew up during the Great Depression. His analysis highlighted the historical and social structural contexts of development to make it a uniquely sociological study. As he went on to other academic positions, he picked up an ever-expanding cadre of talented graduate students who have continued to publish with him noteworthy contributions to the literature on human development, families, and aging. We collaborated on several projects, starting with a piece on "Values, Personality, and Social Structure: An Intergenerational Analysis" (Bengtson & Lovejoy, 1973) that I contributed to one of his earlier projects up to a more recent application of the life-course perspective to aging and families (Bengtson, Elder, & Putney, 2005).

The life-course perspective, as Elder crystallized it, is based on five premises: (a) development and aging are lifelong processes; (b) lives are linked interdependently over time, and "linked lives" (his term) such as in families powerfully influence individual development; (c) individuals make choices (aging) that affect development; (d) historical and social structural contexts are important influences on individual development; and (e) the nature and timing of life transitions affect individuals' development (Elder, 1992, 1995). These principles have formed the basis for hundreds of empirical articles in developmental psychology and the sociology of aging. They have influenced the work of subsequent life-course theorists and aided the development of several important theoretical perspectives in our field. These include the Cumulative Advantage and Disadvantage theories put forth by Dannefer (1984), O'Rand (1996), and Ferraro, Shippee, and Shafer (2009); George's (1996) research on the social psychology of the life course, especially related to stress and health trajectories; Hagestad's (2003; Hagestad & Neugarten, 1985) conceptualizations of the life course and social time, particularly concerning family relationships; Kohli's (1986) and Marshall's (Marshall, Heinz, Krueger, & Verma, 2001) work on the institutionalization of the life course, especially through work; and Heinz and the Bremen group's activities on the life course and the risk society (Heinz, 1991; Heinz & Marshall, 2003).

■ CONCLUSION

That "we stand on the shoulders of giants" in scholarship and science may be a cliché; nevertheless, it is true. So too it is true that we tend to forget the contributions as well as the names of the giants who have shaped our field. This is particularly unfortunate in gerontology, for ours is a young field with a history spanning less than a century. However, without a proper appreciation of the foundations that have been laid and of the conceptual developments that have preceded us, we run the risk of not learning from past insights or, worse, of rediscovering the wheel.

This chapter has traced the development of concepts and theories in the sociology of aging from the 1940s through the mid-1970s (for a review of the last 30 years, see Settersten & Angel, 2011). I have organized this review around several themes that became prominent in this new field during that time, and cited those individuals who stood out as making foundational contributions in these areas. I began with the earliest theme in the sociology of aging: the importance of age in social structure and the place of the aged in changing societies. Here the giants were Ernest Burgess, Ralph Linton, and Talcott Parsons.

Next came the issue of "successful aging"—how to define, measure, and achieve it, with Robert Havighurst the prime mover. A third development highlighted the tension between social structure and individual agency in the activity versus disengagement theory controversy that involved Elaine Cumming, William Henry, George Maddox, Arnold Rose, and Irving Rosow. Shortly thereafter, a fourth theme emerged concerning the social meanings of age, age cohorts, and generations, as well as interactions between age groups, with Bernice Neugarten, Robert Butler, and others.

Although pioneering work on the fifth theme of families, aging, and intergenerational relations had been established earlier, research in this area burgeoned in the late 1960s and early 1970s under Gordon Streib, Peter Townsend, Peter Laslett, and Ethel Shanas. At the same time, a growing body of work coalesced around a sixth theme of age stratification, the interplay between cohort succession and the aging of individuals (Leonard Cain and Matilda White Riley). A seventh emerging development during this time involved the life course as a socially constructed process (Glen Elder and others). Since the mid-1970s, many scholars have entered the field of the sociology of aging and left their mark. I have not been able to acknowledge them here. However, they, as emerging giants in our field, will be the subject of similar essays in the future.

Taken together, the founders cited earlier as giants in the sociology of aging should be recognized more than they are today, for they have left behind them many of the central concepts and theories that are still evident in our field. Younger scholars should be courageous in standing on the shoulders of their predecessors, because the conceptual innovations these pioneers have bequeathed will allow them to see much farther as they peer at the complex interplay of social forces on later life.

REFERENCES

Achenbaum, A. (2013). *Robert Butler, M.D.: Visionary of healthy aging.* New York, NY: Columbia University Press.

Bengtson, V. L. (1971). Inter-age perceptions and the generation gap. *The Gerontologist, 11*, Suppl:85–Suppl:89.

Bengtson, V. L. (1975). Generation and family effects in value socialization. *American Sociological Review, 40*(3), 358–371.

Bengtson, V. L. (1996). *Adulthood and aging: Research on continuities and discontinuities* (pp. 271–303). New York, NY: Springer Publishing Company.

Bengtson, V. L. (2001). Beyond the nuclear family: The increasing importance of multigenerational relationships in American society. *Journal of Marriage and Family, 63*(1), 1–16.

Bengtson, V. L. (2011). Gerontology with a "J": Personal reflections on theory building in the sociology of aging. In R. A. Settersten, Jr. & J. A. Angel (Eds.), *Handbook of the sociology of aging.* New York, NY: Springer Publishing Company.

Bengtson, V. L. (2015). From ageism to the longevity revolution: Robert Butler, pioneer. *The Gerontologist, 54*(6), 1064–1074.

Bengtson, V. L., & Cutler, N. E. (1976). Generations and inter-generational relations: Perspectives on age groups and social change. In R. Binstock & E. Shanas (Eds.), *Handbook of aging and the social sciences* (pp. 130–159). New York, NY: Van Nostrand Reinhold.

Bengtson, V. L., Elder, G. H., Jr., & Putney, N. M. (2005). Ch. 6.1. The life course perspective on aging: Linked lives, timing and history. In M. Johnson, V. L.

Bengtson, P. Coleman, & T. Kirkwood (Eds.), *The Cambridge handbook of age and ageing* (pp. 619–626). Cambridge, UK: Cambridge University Press.

Bengtson, V. L., Giarrusso, R., Mabry, J. B., & Silverstein, M. (2002). Solidarity, conflict and ambivalence: Complementary or competing perspectives on intergenerational relationships? *Journal of Marriage and Family, 64*, 568–576.

Bengtson, V. L., & Kuypers, J. A. (1971). Generational difference and the "developmental stake." *Aging and Human Development, 2*(1), 249–260.

Bengtson, V. L., & Kuypers, J. A. (1984). Toward competence in the older family. In T. H. Brubaker (Ed.), *Family relationships in later life* (pp. 211–228). Beverly Hills, CA: Sage.

Bengtson, V. L., & Lovejoy, M. C. (1973). Values, personality, and social structure: An intergenerational analysis. *American Behavioral Scientist, 16*(6), 880–912.

Bengtson, V. L., Olander, E. B., & Haddad, A. A. (1976). The "generation gap" and aging family members: Toward a conceptual model. In J. E. Gubrium (Ed.), *Time, roles and self in old age* (pp. 237–263). New York, NY: Human Sciences Press.

Bengtson, V. L., Putney, N. M., & Harris, S. C. (2013). *Families and faith: How religion is passed down across generations.* London, UK: Oxford University Press.

Bengtson, V. L., & Roberts, R. E. L. (1991). Intergenerational solidarity in aging families: An example of formal theory construction. *Journal of Marriage and Family, 53*, 856–870.

Bengtson, V. L., & Schrader, S. S. (1982). Parent–child relations. In D. Mangen & W. Peterson (Eds.), *Handbook of research instruments in social gerontology* (Vol. 2, pp. 115–185). Minneapolis, MN: University of Minnesota Press.

Berger, B. (1960). How long is a generation? *British Journal of Sociology, 2*, 10–23.

Berger, P. L., & Luckman, T. (1966). *The social construction of reality.* New York, NY: Doubleday.

Bernstein, C. (1969, March 7). Age and race fear seen in housing opposition. *Washington Post*, A12.

Birditt, K. S., Hartnett, C. S., Fingerman, K. L., Zarit, S., & Antonucci, T. C. (2015). Extending the intergenerational stake hypothesis: Evidence of an intraindividual stake and implications for well-being. *Journal of Marriage and Family, 77*(4), 877–888.

Burgess, E. W. (1916). *The function of socialization in social evolution.* Chicago, IL: University of Chicago Press.

Burgess, E. W. (1926). The family as a unity of interacting personalities. *The Family, 7*, 3–9.

Burgess, E. W. (1960). Aging in Western culture. In E. W. Burgess (Ed.), *Aging in Western societies* (pp. 3–38). Chicago, IL: University of Chicago Press.

Butler, R. N. (1969). Age-ism: Another form of bigotry. *The Gerontologist, 9*(4), 243–246.

Butler, R. N. (1975). *Why survive? Growing old in America.* New York, NY: Harper and Row.

Cain, L. D. (1959). The sociology of aging: A trend report and bibliography, *Current Sociology, 8*, 57–133.

Cain, L. D. (1964). Life course and social structure. In R. E. L. Faris (Ed.), *Handbook of modern sociology.* Chicago, IL: Rand-McNally.

Cain, L. D. (1979). The impact of Manhart of pension payment and the legal status of the elderly. *Aging and Work, 2*, 147–160.

Carstensen, L. L., Isaacowitz, D. M., & Charles, S. T. (1999). Taking time seriously. A theory of socioemotional selectivity. *The American Psychologist, 54*(3), 165–181.

Cavan, R. S., Burgess, E. W., Havighurst, R. J., & Goldhamer, J. (1949). *Personal adjustment in old age*. Chicago, IL: Science Research Associates.

Cumming, E., & Henry, W. E. (1961). *Growing old: The process of disengagement*. New York, NY: Basic Books.

Cumming, E., & Schneider, D. M. (1961). Sibling solidarity: A property of American kinship. *American Anthropologist, 63*, 498–507.

Dannefer, D. (1984). Aging as intracohort differentiation: Accentuation, the Matthew Effect, and the life course. *Sociological Forum, 2*, 211–36.

Eisenstadt, S. N. (1956). *From generation to generation: Age groups and social structure*. Glencoe, IL: Free Press.

Elder, G. H., Jr. (1974). *Children of the Great Depression*. Chicago, IL: University of Chicago Press.

Elder, G. H., Jr. (1992). Life course. In E. Borgata & M. Borgata (Eds.), *The encyclopedia of sociology* (pp. 1120–1130). New York, NY: Macmillan.

Elder, G. H., Jr. (1995). The life course paradigm: Social change and individual development. In P. Moen, G. H. Elder, Jr., & K. Luescher (Eds.), *Examining lives in contest: Perspectives on the ecology of human development*. Washington, DC: American Psychological Association.

Ferraro, K. F., Shippee, T. P., & Shafer, M. H. (2009). Cumulative inequality theory for research in aging and the life course. In V. L. Bengtson, D. Gans, N. Putney, & M. Silverstein (Eds.), *Handbook of theories of aging* (2nd ed., pp. 413–433). New York, NY: Springer Publishing Company.

George, L. K. (1996). Missing links: The case for a social psychology of the life course. *The Gerontologist, 36*(2), 248–255.

Giarrusso, R., Feng, D., & Bengtson, V. L. (2004). The intergenerational stake phenomenon over 20 years. *Annual Review of Gerontology and Geriatrics, 24*, 55–76.

Glaser, B. G., & Strauss, A. L. (1968). *Time for dying*. Chicago, IL: Aldine Press.

Glass, J., Bengtson, V. L., & Dunham, C. C. (1986). Attitude similarity in three-generation families: Socialization, status inheritance, or reciprocal influence. *American Sociological Review, 51*, 685–698.

Gubrium, J. F. (1975). *Living and dying in Murray Manor*. Charlottesville, VA: University Press of Virginia.

Hagestad, G. O. (2003). Interdependent lives and relationships in changing times: A life-course view of families and aging. In R. A. Settersten, Jr. (Ed.), *Invitation to the life course: Toward new understandings of later life* (pp. 135–160). Amityville, NY: Baywood.

Hagestad, G. O., & Neugarten, B. L. (1985). Age and the life course. In E. Shanas & R. Binstock (Eds.), *Handbook of aging and the social sciences* (2nd ed., pp. 36–61). New York, NY: Van Nostrand Reinhold.

Havighurst, R. J. (1952). Social and psychological needs of the aging. *Annals of the American Academy of Political and Social Science, 279*, 11–17.

Havighurst, R. J. (1961). Successful aging. *The Gerontologist, 1*, 4–7.

Havighurst, R. J., & Albrecht, R. (1953). *Older people*. New York, NY: Longmans, Green.

Havighurst, R. J., Neugarten, B. L., & Bengtson, V. L. (1966). A cross-national study of adjustment to retirement. *The Gerontologist, 6*(3), 137–138.

Heinz, W. R. (1991). *Theoretical advances in life course research*. Weinheim, Germany: Deutscher Studien Verlag.

Heinz, W. R., & Marshall, V. W. (2003). *Social dynamics of the life course: Transitions, institutions, and interrelations*. New York, NY: Aldine de Gruyter.

Henry, W. E. (1956). *The analysis of fantasy*. New York, NY: Wiley.

Kasschau, P. K., Ransford, E. A., & Bengtson, V. L. (1974). Generational consciousness and youth movement participation: Contrasts in blue-collar and white-collar youth. *Journal of Social Issues, 30*(3), 69–94.

Kohli, M. (1986). The world we forgot: A historical review of the life course. In V. W. Marshall (Ed.), *Later life: The social psychology of aging* (pp. 271–303). Beverly Hills, CA: Sage.

Kuypers, J. A., & Bengtson, V. L. (1973). Social breakdown and competence: A model of normal aging. *Human Development, 9*(4), 345–58.

Laslett, P. (1965). *The world we have lost*. London, UK: Methuen.

Laufer, R. S., & Bengtson, V. L. (1974). Generations, aging and social stratification: On the development of generational units. *Journal of Social Issues, 30*(3), 181–205

Lemon, B. W., Bengtson, V. L., & Peterson, J. A. (1972). An exploration of the activity theory of aging: Activity types and life satisfaction among in-movers to a retirement community. *Journal of Gerontology, 27*(4), 511–523.

Linton, R. (1936). *The study of man*. New York, NY: Appleton Century.

Linton, R. (1942). Age and sex categories. *American Sociological Review, 7*, 589–603.

Maddox, G. L. (1965). Fact and artifact: Evidence bearing on disengagement theory from the Duke Geriatrics Project. *Human Development, 8*, 117–130.

Mangen, D. J., Bengtson, V. L., & Landry, P. H. Jr. (Eds.) (1988). *The measurement of intergenerational relations*. Beverly Hills, CA: Sage.

Mannheim, K. (1952). The problem of generations. In K. Mannheim (Ed.), *Essays in the sociology of knowledge*. New York, NY: Oxford University Press.

Marshall, V. W. (1978). No exit: A symbolic interactionist perspective on aging. *International Journal of Aging and Human Development, 9*(4), 345–358.

Marshall, V. W., Heinz, W., Krueger, H., & Verma, A. (Eds.) (2001). *Restructuring work and the life course*. Toronto, Canada: University of Toronto Press.

Neugarten, B. L. (1974). Age groups in American society and the rise of the young-old. *Annals of the American Academy of Political and Social Science, 415*, 187–198.

Neugarten, B. L. (1996). *The meanings of age: Selected papers of Bernice L. Neugarten*. Chicago, IL: University of Chicago Press.

Neugarten, B. L., Havighurst, R. J., & Tobin, S. S. (1961). The measurement of life satisfaction. *Journal of Gerontology, 16*, 134–143.

Neugarten, B. L., Moore, J. W., & Lowe, J. C. (1965). Age norms, age constraints, and adult socialization. *American Journal of Sociology, 70*, 710–717.

O'Rand, A. M. (1996). The precious and the precocious: Understanding cumulative disadvantage and cumulative advantage over the life course. *The Gerontologist, 36*(2), 230–238.

Park, R. A., & Burgess, E. W. (1918). *Introduction to the science of sociology.* Chicago, IL: University of Chicago Press.

Parsons, T. (1942). Age and sex in the social structure of the United States. *American Sociological Review, 7*, 604–616.

Riley, M. W. (1971). Social gerontology and the age stratification of society. *The Gerontologist, 11*(1), 79–87.

Riley, M. W., Johnson, M., & Foner, A. (1972). *Aging and society: Vol. 3. A sociology of age stratification.* New York, NY: Russell Sage Foundation.

Riley, M. W., Kahn, R. L., & Foner, A. (Eds.) (1994). *Age and structural lag: Society's failure to provide meaningful opportunities in work, family, and leisure.* New York, NY: Wiley.

Riley, M. W., & Loscocco, K. A. (1994). The changing structure of work opportunities: Toward an age-integrated society. In R. P. Abeles, H. C. Gift, & M. G. Ory (Eds.), *Aging and the quality of life* (pp. 235–252). New York, NY: Springer Publishing Company.

Rose, A. (1965). A subculture for the aging: A framework for research in social gerontology. In A. Rose & W. Peterson (Eds.), *Older people and their social world* (pp. 12–19). Philadelphia, PA: F. A. Davis.

Rosow, I. (1974). *Socialization to old age.* Berkeley: University of California Press.

Rossi, A. S., & Rossi, P. H. (1990). *Of human bonding: Parent–child relationships across the life course.* New York, NY: Aldine de Gruyter.

Rowe, J. W., & Kahn, R. L. (1998). Successful aging. *Aging (Milan, Italy), 10*(2), 142–144.

Settersten, R. A., Jr., & Angel, J. L. (Eds.) (2011). *Handbook of sociology of aging.* New York, NY: Springer Science.

Settersten, R. A., Jr., & Gannon, L. (2005). Structure, agency, and the space between: On the challenges and contradictions of a blended view of the life course. *Advances in Life Course Research, 10*, 35–55.

Shanas, E. (1979). Social myth as hypothesis: The case of family relations of old people. *The Gerontologist, 19*, 3–9.

Shanas, E., Townsend, P., Wedderburn, D., Fris, H., Milhoj, P., & Stehouwer, J. (1968). *Old people in three industrial societies.* New York, NY: Atherton Press.

Streib, G. F. (1958). Family patterns in retirement. *Journal of Social Issues, 14*(2), 46–60.

Streib, G. F., & Thompson, W. E. (1960). The older person in a family context. In C. Tibbitts (Ed.), *Handbook of social gerontology* (pp. 477–488). Chicago, IL: University of Chicago Press.

Szydlik, M. (2008). Intergenerational solidarity and conflict. *Journal of Comparative Family Studies, 39,* 97–114.

Szydlik, M. (2016). *Sharing lives: Adult children and parents.* London, UK: Routledge.

Townsend, P. (1957). *The family life of old people.* London, UK: Routledge & Kegan Paul.

CHAPTER 6

Social Movements and Social Knowledges: Gerontological Theory in Research, Policy, and Practice

Carroll L. Estes with Nicholas R. DiCarlo

This chapter provides a perspective on the development of theory, research, policy, and practice through 1960 to 1980. During these decades, social movements uprooted conventional theory and methodology in the social sciences. Serious questions about the possibility of value-free social science, problems of objectivity, and the ideological commitments and assumptions in traditional approaches were subject to criticism and interrogation.

Activist students and university scholars of the 1960s questioned the most revered mainstream thinking. Several thinkers discussed in this chapter exemplify the challenges of "received theory" in social sciences, raising the question of what constitutes a theory. Postmodernism—breaking with the Enlightenment project, which failed to provide emancipation (Habermas, 1980)—reflected thinkers' dissatisfaction with the fragmented worldview of balkanized disciplines and their obvious failure to anticipate or explain the civil rights, peace, or feminist movements. Narrow conceptions of the state, its authority and legitimacy, were identified by critical theorists as intellectual straitjackets, and the structural functionalist theories of the political and social order became the object of critical challenge (Gouldner, 1971; Mills, 1959).

Social gerontology was not immune to this turbulent period, as criticism and revised thinking of many gerontologists reviewed here illustrate. Cumming and Henry's classic work on *Disengagement Theory* (Cumming & Henry, 1961) fell from grace as the universality of its assumptions and predictions were faulted as White Middle America. It is no surprise that there was a cascading effect of work on the sociology of knowledge: *The Coming Crisis of Western Sociology* (Gouldner, 1971); *The Structure of Scientific Revolutions* (Kuhn, 1962); *The Sociology of Science* (Ben-David & Sullivan, 1975), *Conflict Sociology: Toward an Explanatory Science* (Collins & Annett, 1975), and the first translations and broad awareness of the Frankfurt School through American immigrant intellectuals, Herbert Marcuse and others (e.g., Antonio Gramsci's *Prison Notebooks* [Gramsci, 1971], and his concept of "ideological hegemony"). Fast approaching, yet discounted by many, were new Black consciousness; feminism; the Delano grape boycott of immigrant farm workers; lesbian, gay, bisexual, and transgender (LGBT) struggles for political power; and pushback by those in poverty (*Poor People's Movements*, Piven & Cloward, 1979).

This chapter begins with two early, leading practitioners who reflect the social work and social welfare origins of social gerontology: Ollie A. Randall and Louis Lowy. They were direct practitioners framing early discussions of vulnerability and difference.

Second, we turn to disciplinary thought, giving credit to those who institutionalized gerontology in the academy, establishing credibility, funding, and growth of this respected discipline. Wilma Donahue, Clark Tibbitts, Ethel Shanas, Walter M. Beattie, and Robert H. Binstock were fundamental in this process. Third, we focus on the diverse epistemological standpoints and social contexts of scholars, not just as multidisciplinary thinkers (psychologists, sociologists, and political scientists), but as public intellectuals and activists (Black, feminist, and critical contributors) to an evolving critical discipline. In this section, we examine the advances made by Jacquelyne Johnson Jackson, Betty Friedan, Bernice Neugarten, Elaine Brody, Maggie Kuhn, and Carroll Estes (chapter author). The chapter concludes with a critical commentary on developments through the 1980s to the present, the tenuous footholds of social movements, and advances in critical theory.

■ THE SOCIAL WORK ORIGINS OF SOCIAL GERONTOLOGY

Social gerontology evolved from a relationship between direct practice with older adults, the organizations and institutions that served them, and policy advocates. Often, a gerontologist of the era participated in multiple roles. **Ollie A. Randall** (1890–1984) is one such gerontologist who laid a path for the work of those to follow.

A 1912 graduate of the Women's College of Brown University, Randall's life, publications, and editorials illustrate a deep understanding of the changing landscape of aging over the 20th century. Born in 1890, Randall witnessed women gaining the right to vote in 1920, the economic devastation of the Great Depression in the 1930s, and the introduction of programs and policies, such as home care and Social Security, which facilitated a gradual shift away from "indigent elderly" ending up mainly in poorhouses (incarceration of debt). Randall locates the ideological constraints that follow money. She writes:

> The depression economy brought into being the Social Security program of the federal government with its financial participation in state programs. This has had a lasting influence on the philosophy and practice in social welfare services, administered by either public or voluntary agencies, at state and local levels. The agency controlling the purse strings has much to say about policies. (Randall, 1965, p. 44)

Randall worked for the Association for Improving the Condition of the Poor (AICP) and Community Service Society (CSS) for four decades. She also directed the Women's Division of the Emergency Work Bureau, a volunteer organization of the Great Depression. She drafted the invitation list to the first Conference on Aging (organized by the Social Security Administration) in 1950, which became the model for the 1961 White House Conference on Aging (WHCoA). Most pivotal, she was the principal consultant on aging to the Ford Foundation (1959–1969), which provided $6.7 million to aging between 1956 and 1963. Randall was the first female president of the Gerontological Society of America (GSA) in 1955.

Randall (1951) describes the personal and social aspects of aging in the *Journal of the American Medical Association*, balancing concern with the growing burden on the younger generation to care for elders without resources with the concern that the elders would be pushed out of participating in life. Randall (1951) rails against the social exclusion in old age, describing, "oldsters who find themselves committed, willy-nilly, to a life of leisure and, for far too many, one of idleness and utter boredom" (p. 1326).

Louis Lowy (1920–1991) was a social worker engaged in multiple levels of gerontological intervention. As a student of philosophy and philology in Prague, Lowy had exposure to a variety of thinkers and disciplines, including sociologists and psychologists such as Weber, Freud, Jung, and Piaget. Lowy had wanted to be a professor, first earning an elementary education diploma where he learned interactive practices called "social pedagogy." However, in 1939, Nazi forces invaded Czechoslovakia and interned Lowy, his family, and 55,000 Jews to the disease-riddled Terezin Ghetto, followed by Auschwitz. Holocaust survivors, Lowy and his wife came to the United States soon after the war.

Lowy's BS and Master in Social Work (MSW) degrees were from Boston University (BU) and after graduation he worked in Bridgeport, Connecticut, as activities director at the Jewish Community Center. He joined the social work faculty at BU in 1957, received his EdD from Harvard University in 1966, and cofounded BU's Gerontology Center in 1974.

Surviving war and genocide, Lowy adamantly reminded those around him to question prejudice, racism, and injustice. Each year he returned to Germany as an ambassador for international social work, developing curriculum rooted in group work and social gerontology. In *The Gerontologist*, he stated the goal of social work education: "Expose all students to ultimate philosophical questions of the meaning of life and death, which are irrevocably raised when the life of older people is the subject of study and practice" (Lowy & Miller, 1974, p. 467).

Lowy lived in several countries that exposed him to social welfare policy and raised his consciousness. Lowy notes that it is "ironic that social work study has not accorded economic and political theory a foremost place among the disciplines that condition human existence and influence the social environment of man" (Lowy in Gardella, 2014, p. 18). Social gerontology can both identify appropriate, needed services and inform how to implement and organize service plans (Lowy, 1972). Lowy's thinking resonates with the Marxist–Weberian theoretical focus on a reflexive interplay between theory and practice, known as "praxis" (Freire, 1970; and the Frankfurt School scholars).

Lowy did not speak of the Holocaust until his last years, and no other Jewish gerontologists involved here wrote about how their identities directly affected their work. Nevertheless, we believe that it important to locate the Jewish roots of gerontologists and acknowledge their epistemological standpoint. Much of social welfare history locates the helping tradition as Judeo-Christian lineage, conflating Jewish and Christian traditions of charity. The Holocaust brutally renders these identities as separate—identities engendering stark contrasts of hope, trauma, and doom. Although an analysis of these epistemological inflections is beyond the scope of this chapter, we dutifully note that the Jewish focus on the aged stands against the incomprehensible loss of a generation.

■ LEGITIMIZING SOCIAL GERONTOLOGY AND THE ACADEMY

Gerontological thought required a place and space to develop and financing to flourish. Two academicians played an integral role in legitimizing the discipline, navigating the politics of institutions of higher learning, and negotiating congressional recognition of the field with funding from government sources.

Wilma Donahue (1900–1993) and **Clark Tibbitts** (1903–1985), both at the University of Michigan, produced key compilations of gerontological texts, institutionalizing the academic knowledge of gerontology. Together they wrote and edited: *Planning the Older Years* (Donahue & Tibbitts, 1950), *Growing in the Older Years* (Donahue & Tibbitts, 1951), *The New Frontiers of Aging* (Donahue & Tibbitts, 1957), *Aging in the Modern World* (Donahue & Tibbitts, 1957), *Handbook of Social Gerontology* (Tibbitts, 1960), and *Processes of Aging* (Vols. I and II, Williams, Tibbitts, & Donahue, 1963). In 1946, Donahue cofounded Division 20 of the American Psychological Association, establishing gerontology as a subject in the discipline's largest professional body. Donahue founded and directed the University of Michigan's then Division of Gerontology in 1951 and 1966, respectively, with funding from the Older American's Act (OAA) of 1965. Donahue transformed this into the Institute of Gerontology. Tibbitts was pivotal in securing and guiding federal support for gerontology through the OAA.

Ethel Shanas (1914–2005), a statistician trained at the University of Chicago, demonstrated the importance of national health surveys and advanced the field of "health services research." She employed the best large-scale statistical sampling and survey research methodologies, inspiring the first cross-national gerontological collaboration. With the exception of medical sociology and Shanas's work, there was little disciplinary commitment in the academy to applied health economics, political science, or sociology. Such work was generally denigrated until two large philanthropies (The Robert Wood Johnson Foundation and The Pew Charitable Trusts) invested millions in elite universities (1980s–2000s) to seed the health services policy and research in the academy, particularly within economics, political science, sociology, public health, and social work.

In a prescient move, Shanas called for research on family forms that deviate from "the norm" and on the "special situation of the childless elderly" (Shanas, 1979a). With declining birth rates, she foresaw a large proportion of old people with no or only one child. She argued for research to investigate how individuals establish and use helping relationships, and how human service systems and personnel may assist in "helping relationships with child substitutes" (Shanas, 1979b, p. 8).

Shanas was on the U.S. National Committee on Vital and Health Statistics, chairperson of its Technical Consultant Panel on Long-Term Care, delegate to the 1960 WHCoA, and a member of the United Nations' North American Expert Committee for the World Assembly on Aging. In 1974, she became the third female president (of 30) of the GSA. She also led the Illinois Sociological and the Midwest Sociological Societies, was vice president of the International Sociological Association's Research Committee on Aging, secretary of the International Association of Gerontology, and chaired the American Sociological Association's Section on Aging. Shanas's disciplinary perspective established quantitative and survey research as integral to aging and the social sciences. Robert H. Binstock and she coedited the first and second editions of the classic handbook (Binstock & Shanas, 1976, 1985).

Walter M. Beattie (1923–2007) notably contributed to gerontological research, policy, and practice in the United States and internationally. At the University of Chicago, he studied under Ollie A. Randall, who encouraged his development of "action-research" in long-term health care. In the first study of its kind, Beattie followed the local elderly population for the Health and Welfare Council of Metropolitan St. Louis from 1959 to 1963. In 1972, Beattie founded and directed the Gerontology Center (now the Aging Studies Institute) at Syracuse University, funded by the Administration on Aging (AoA). Working with the UN Center for Social Development and Humanitarian Affairs (1972–1979), he served on the board of the International Center for Social Gerontology in Paris. Drawing on his international work, Beattie proposed "A Framework of Characteristics and Considerations for Cooperative Efforts Between Developing and Developed Regions of the World"(Beattie, 1978; U.S. Senate Special Committee on Aging, 1978).

When most gerontologists (predominately Caucasian) were not writing explicitly about race, Beattie offered distinct contributions with his 1960 article "The Aging Negro: Some Implications for Social Welfare Services" (using the term for African Americans that was common at the time "later we will discuss historical shifts in language"). Beattie questions "whether the patterns of health, welfare and leisure-time services which are emerging for our aging population throughout the United States have relevance or meaning for the aging Negro and his family" (Beattie, 1960, p. 131). Examining disparities in longevity, the labor market where the Negro is "last hired and the first fired," and housing, where conditions are often poor, Beattie identifies the precariousness of this population and the challenges of aging in place. This prompted the Urban League to develop a program focusing on aging.

In "The Design of Supportive Environments for the Life-Span," Beattie (1970) argues that, for the aging adult, social planning must consider how environmental forces impede or facilitate meeting developmental needs. Blending developmental and eco-logical theoretical approaches, Beattie rejects the idea of intrinsic behavior and under-scores the dynamic interplay between environment and individual.

Beattie insists the gerontologist must examine his or her own stakes in the process of assessing need. In his strongest editorial, "Promises. Promises. Promises." in *The Geron-tologist* (Beattie, 1973), he lambasts the dissipation of "vision" at the 1971 WHCoA and the lack of progress in higher education. He wonders if the discipline's failure to effect change lies in an "inability of gerontologists to link their identities and capabilities to those of the elderly in the communities." Beattie's leadership at the Syracuse University and as GSA president in 1963 were two platforms where he articulated his concerns about the shortcomings of and his hopes for the field to study long-term health across the life span and to develop international perspectives on aging.

Robert H. Binstock (1935–2011) played a crucial role in building political and social science in gerontology. A Harvard-educated political scientist, who served on the faculty at the Heller School of Social Welfare at Brandeis University and later at Case Western Reserve University, he quickly became a key influential person in bridging policy and gerontology. Binstock served as a key policy adviser to the White House for President Lyndon B. Johnson and the 1971 WHCoA. His early published work on aging is a Ford Foundation study (*Feasible Planning for Social Change*, Morris, Binstock, & Rein, 1966), coauthored with Brandeis professor and former National Association of Social Workers (NASW) and GSA president, Robert Morris. This research indicated the marginalization of community planning agencies from local power elites and structures.

Binstock is known for promulgating the conceptual–theoretical use of "interest group liberalism" in analyzing the politics of aging, applying and adapting the theoretical framework of Theodore Lowi's book, *The End of Liberalism* (Binstock, 1972; Lowi, 1969). Lowi's formulation is that private interest groups, rather than citizens, are the ones through which democracy is carried out. Lowi's point is that interest group liberalism does not represent the people, nor is it likely to produce social justice for the people. Also building on Lowi, Binstock opines that government and aging interest groups work as "middle men" with legislators and policy makers, bargaining and brokering to shape and implement aging policy and services that they may direct. Binstock projects that aging-based interest groups will be limited to "incremental gains." He asserts that aging interest groups "rarely present details on means through which problems of the disadvantaged aged might be solved" (Binstock, 1974, p. 208; see also Estes, 1979, 2011). Strikingly, he shows that national aging organizations are only peripherally involved in the big income programs of Social Security and Medicare. Yale's leading Medicare scholar, Ted Marmor, argues that aging organizations played no significant role in Medicare's passage.

Binstock studied the voting behavior of older persons, and whether they were (or could be become) a voting bloc. Based on the multiple analyses of election data, he contributes the theory and concept of the "electoral bluff." He asserts that the old are *not* a voting bloc and that the prospects for senior power are dim if not mythical.

> There is no sound reason to expect that in the immediate or remote future the aging will wield decisive power in determining the outcome of national elections [....] Are there alternatives for increased senior power in national politics? No, not very strong ones. (Binstock, 1974, p. 211)

Theories of the social construction of reality, the "self-fulfilling prophecy," and the "looking glass self" were being employed in gerontology (e.g., Estes, 1979; Estes & Freeman 1976; Rose, 1962; Rose & Peterson, 1965). Estes saw the potential negative effects (e.g., a self-fulfilling prophecy) of Binstock's repeated, vigorous denial of the realities of older persons' collective power. In a little-referenced publication, Estes (1979) challenged the validity of Binstock's "discounting the salience of old age in American politics." On a parenthetical note, the last time Estes heard Binstock speak at GSA, he cited the possible dawning of a senior voting bloc in view of the increasing attacks on Social Security and Medicare and his last presidential election analysis.

Binstock understood that "public policy issues may be debated increasingly in age distribution terms" (Binstock, 1974, p. 205). Later he writes, "The Aged as Scapegoat: The Donald P. Kent Memorial Lecture" (Binstock, 1983). Nevertheless, the writings of Robert H. Binstock were solidly mainstream. He raised important questions of need and justice; yet he did not speak to, for, or, as empathic to, the budding critical, structural, and reflexive intellectual perspectives breaking out between 1960 and 1980. Binstock's work reflected the core disciplines of political science, social work, and later, public health.

Binstock publicly acknowledged his indebtedness to the earliest cadre of strong female gerontologists: Ollie A. Randall, Wilma Donahue, Ethel Shanas, Bernice Neugarten, and Dorothy Wedderburn. Binstock was the GSA president in 1976, and he mentored and collaborated with the current leading political scientist, Rob Hudson.

■ DIVERGING VOICES OF THE GERONTOLOGICAL IMAGINATION

Social movements of the 1960s included Vietnam and student anti-war and anti-draft protests with some university campuses resembling battlefields (e.g., Kent State shootings and the 1964 Berkeley Free Speech movement; see Estes, Binney, & Culbertson, 1992). The civil rights movement reached a fever pitch of civil disobedience, Black Power and militant resistance and self-defense by Black Panthers, and the nonviolent resistance of Martin Luther King, Jr. The media and TV camera lenses catapulted violent local skirmishes into a national moral struggle. Chicano activists, such as Cesar Chavez, organized and protested for the labor rights of farm workers in California. In 1969, Native peoples occupied Alcatraz Island for 19 months, resisting the federal government's perpetual discrimination and treaty breaking. In 1969, New York erupted as transwomen and gay men fought against police in the Stonewall Riots. Unheralded, Black women went on strike against Black men doing civil rights work in Macomb, Mississippi, as members of the Student Nonviolent Coordinating Committee (SNCC). SNCC Spellman College student, Ruby Doris Smith, spoke against being relegated to routine office duties, highlighting the crucial protest work of women of color who risked their lives on the front lines.

In its midst, President John F. Kennedy was assassinated in 1963, and Lyndon B. Johnson became the U.S. president. Johnson's legacy is unforgettable: (a) his full expansion of the disastrous Vietnam war that produced an anti-war movement; (b) the civil rights struggle in full bloom, followed by the enactment of the Civil Rights and Voting Rights Acts (signed by President Johnson in 1965 and 1968, respectively); and (c) the most significant legislation for the old and the poor since Social Security: The 1965 passage of Medicare, Medicaid, and the Older Americans Act (OAA).

Emerging Black scholars and activists held federally supported forums (e.g., WHCoA) to account, explicitly denouncing the GSA's repeated failure to address aging minorities and oppressed populations. In 1970, Hobart Jackson spoke at the Symposium on Research Goals and Priorities in Gerontology addressing the indignity of racial unconsciousness and the overwhelming Whiteness of the Gerontological Society (GS). As a Black man, he shared his frustration at the lack of meaningful progress and raised awareness of the importance of "an activist component" in gerontological research. He argued that "we cannot achieve wholeness and fulfillment for the elderly until we achieve it for other deprived segments of our society" (Jackson, 1971a, p. 89). Hobart Jackson's attention to the stagnation of White liberal thought stands out as a valuable insight, but how did the GS respond to his bold dissent? The WHCoA in 1971 failed to focus on policy addressing the Black aged, especially those in poverty. In 1972, Hobart Jackson and Robert Kastenbaum formed the National Caucus on the Black Aged (NCBA). Their colleague, Jacquelyn Johnson Jackson, joined them, directing the NCBA's first years and its AoA grant.

Jacquelyne Johnson Jackson (1932–2004), born in Winston-Salem, North Carolina, received her bachelor's and master's degrees at the University of Wisconsin–Madison and her PhD at Ohio State in 1960. She taught at Louisiana State University–Baton Rouge (1959–1962), and then at the historically Black schools, Jackson State University and Howard University. She did her postdoctoral work as a National Institutes of Health (NIH) fellow at Duke, where she served as an assistant professor of medical sociology (1966–1968) as well as at the University of North Carolina at Chapel-Hill (1977–1978). She returned to Howard as a full professor from 1975 to 1985, and then returned to Duke where she remained until 1998 as assistant professor (Achenbaum & Albert, 1995).

Jacquelyne Johnson Jackson provided a Black woman's perspective of civil rights. Her prolific scholarship includes more than 30 articles on aging in dozens of journals, many centered on the landscape of the civil rights movement of the 1960s, the adversity facing Black aging populations, and the struggle to adequately study this population (*Black Aging* and *The Black Scholar*). She was associate editor and editor of the *Journal of Health and Social Behavior, Journal of Minority Aging, Social Problems, International Journal of Aging and Human Development,* and *Journal of Social Service Research.* Jackson filled multiple leadership positions, as chair of the Caucus of Black Sociologists and president of the Association of Social and Behavioral Scientists (an organization of scholars from historically Black colleges and universities).

In "Negro Aged: Toward Needed Research in Social Gerontology," Jackson (1971c) summarized the scant scholarship on the Negro population, concluding that existing research neglected the aging process, requiring further study. She argued there is no uniform experience of aging for older Negroes, and that longitudinal research must explore the contexts of these various populations. Research should locate its goals and objectives with an awareness of subgroups within racial demographics, and studies must reflect on the cultural competency of testing methodologies. Jackson located the importance of examining social change and how Negro protest movements influence and shape the experience and futures of the Negro aged.

Dr. Jackson built on the theory of "double jeopardy" (first named and written about in 1969 by Frances M. Beal, to describe the experience of a Black woman, exploited by both racism and sexism [Beal, 1969]). In "The Blacklands of Gerontology," Dr. Jackson (1971b) developed the concept of "quadruple jeopardy"—being Black, female, old, and living in poverty—which exponentially poses risks of being failed by society and social welfare support. She identified mental health and nursing home use by the Black aged as critical areas of research.

Historian Andrew Achenbaum locates Jackson's book, *Minorities and Aging* (Jackson, 1980), as "the most complete work on minority aging" of its time (Achenbaum & Albert, 1995, p. 173). Jackson coined the term "institutionalized victimization," to depict how structural barriers to equal care invariably erode the aging experience. She was a critical lens of activity and disengagement theory, noting that they cannot be equally applied to non-Whites:

> ... those of lower status, such as American Indian, Asian-American, or black women, have constrained opportunities for active involvement outside their familial and kinship circles. Institutionalized victimization, which earlier reduced their life chances for educational and occupational mobility, later restricts their activity levels, perhaps heightening their psychological and psychiatric problems. (Jackson, 1980, pp. 110–111)

Jackson operated outside the institutional mainstream, voicing marginalized analysis, thought, experience, and the urgency of change. She was an organic intellectual (Gramsci, 1971). Contrasted with traditional ivory tower scholars, the quest of organic intellectuals is the creation of "a grounded, radical hegemonic re-thinking and politics" aimed at social change (Sassoon, 2000). Organic intellectuals openly see, speak, identify, and act with oppressed classes, races, genders, and other oppressed (subaltern) groups and identities. Their work is extraordinarily difficult because it requires transforming the "pessimism of the intellect" into the "optimism of the will" (Sassoon, 2000). This framework informs an understanding of how feminist thinking gained academic ground in gerontological thought. The figures here—Jackson, Neugarten, Brody, Estes, and Kuhn—reflect how women of the era, conscious of institutional oppression, began to name and organize gerontological theory research and *praxis* as resistance.

Betty Friedan's (1921–2006) *The Feminine Mystique* (Friedan, 1963) on "the problem that has no name" challenged the status quo of the era. Friedan's standpoint was that of an educated White middle-class housewife, living through her husband and children. As an organic intellectual, Friedan fomented feminist standpoint theory, challenging the "taken for granted" and dominant "structural functionalist theory" that depicted women's domestic and caregiving roles in terms of their positive functions for all: society, economy, culture, and the nuclear family (Talcott Parsons). Friedan offered rage laced with the positivity of possibility, a way forward. Her "get out of jail" card for women activated feminist work in and out of the academy, social gerontology included. Friedan's work reconsidered sex roles and socialization at all stages of the life course—providing opportunities to challenge normative and essentialist theories such as Cumming and Henry's Disengagement Theory (Cumming & Henry, 1961). In her late career, Friedan addressed GSA conferences on *The Fountain of Age* (1993).

Bernice Neugarten (1916–2001) received her MA in educational psychology and her doctorate through the Multidisciplinary Committee on Child Development at the

University of Chicago. In 1943, she was the first PhD in the new field, human development. During her dissertation on personality development in later life, under the tutelage of Robert Havighurst, Neugarten discovered that many stereotypes of old age were untrue. Traditional understandings of midlife crisis and the phenomenon of empty nest syndrome depicted older adults with a diminished experience of later life. These did not match the reported experience of many older adults Neugarten studied. Her research showed that most older adults had meaningful and satisfying lives. This more realistic portrait of how older adults, especially women, adapted to their changing roles illustrated the failure of stereotypes.

Born in a small town in Nebraska, Neugarten (nee Levin), like several of the other outstanding gerontologists in this section, was Jewish. Her husband, also a Jew, escaped Nazi Germany in 1936. After her doctorate, Neugarten left academia to raise her children. She reentered the University of Chicago in 1951 to teach in the graduate program. In 30 years leading the department, she trained many notable gerontologists, including Vern Bengtson. On retirement in 1980, she founded the doctoral program in human development and social policy at Northwestern University. She held countless positions of leadership in the field. Neugarten served as the second female president of the GSA in 1969 (of 25), where she established the first public policy committee and marshaled resources for the first special project on "Aging and Social Policy."

Neugarten and Havighurst's 1961 study on "The Measurement of Life Satisfaction" set a standard for gerontological research and remains one of the most frequently cited social science articles in the field (Ferraro & Schafer, 2008). In "Age Norms, Age Constraints, and Adult Socialization," Neugarten, Moore, and Lowe (1965) investigated social convention and age norms, which she conceptualized as a "prescriptive timetable for the ordering of major life events," such as marriage, family, and retirement (p. 711). She reported that beliefs in norms vary across the life span, although there is more congruence between opinions and experiences of old age. Instead of using these results to essentialize the experience of old age, Neugarten questioned whether the socialization resulting from cumulative years of speculated stereotypes across the life span produced "internalization" and "crystallization" of age norms for older adults (Neugarten, 1965, p. 717). These distinctions, anchored in psychometric evaluations of the quality of life, broke down stereotypes and widened understandings of the lived experiences of older adults.

In "Age Groups in American Society and the Rise of the Young-Old," Neguarten (1974) interrogated the practice of grouping all elderly people homogeneously. For social policy, the treatment of old age as a homogeneous category, she noted, collapsed and blurred distinctions between the different needs and resources of the "young-old" (ages 55–75 years) and the "old-old" (ages 75 years and older). In "Age and the Life Course," Neugarten (1976) offered a critical perspective, rejecting the ability of chronological criteria to measure experience, urging researchers to examine age with a cultural awareness: "Chronological age is meaningless unless there is knowledge of the particular culture" (Neugarten & Hagestad, 1976, p. 36).

In her book *Policy for the 1980s: Age or Need Entitlement?*, Neugarten wrote that public policy "may have the unintended effect of ... stigmatizing rather than liberating older people" (Neugarten, 1979, p. 27). Questioning the soundness of social welfare that protects only a percentage of the population, Neugarten advocated for a guaranteed base income, such as called for by Martin Luther King (*Chaos or Community*, King, 1968) and the 1,200 economists who petitioned Congress in 1968.

Elaine Brody (1923–2014), president of GSA in 1980 (fourth woman of 36), connected strongly to Friedan's feminist thinking, citing her as an influence in her theoretical perspective of "women in the middle" (Brody, 1981, 1990). Her term describes the experience of women straddling the care needs of two generations. As a social worker with the Jewish elders at the Philadelphia Geriatric Center, Brody's work involved family systems where the brunt of care rested on the shoulders of daughters who also were mothers. This double-care bind invariably affects how women enter the work force, while simultaneously meeting their family care needs. Brody's spouse and fellow social worker, Stanley Brody, collaborated in her work and both served as Social Research, Policy, and Practice (SRPP) section chairs of the GSA.

Brody's reflection piece in *The Gerontologist*, "On Being Very, Very Old: An Insider's Perspective" (Brody, 2010), speaks to how the Great Depression influenced her understanding of poverty and the precariousness of the family. She writes that "Social Security, Medicare, and subsequent legislation benefitted not just old people but all generations" (p. 3). Her ability to connect the intersections of gender and economic pressure offers insights for research, policy, and practice. Brody's connection to the realities of long-term care informed her resistance to the family propaganda, which accompanied New Federalism and the push for austerity. She rejected President Reagan's simple, saccharine sound bites, offering strong words of her own:

> Right now, the Reagan administration is sort of cheering the family on. You know, "Let's go back to the good old days when families did more." Well, families did not do more in the good old days. They did less. There weren't as many elderly people, and the needs were not as great. (Brody quoted in Hacker, 1986)

Maggie Kuhn (1905–1995), a self-proclaimed "wrinkled radical," was an early theorist in the Sociology of Knowledge of Aging, producing provocative critiques of the scientific pursuits of gerontologists. Estes, Portacolone, and Kuhn posted (in every media possible of her day) creative opposition to what she described as the objectification, individualization, and trivialization of the condition of old age in America and the culpability of gerontologists in such portrayals. She and the Gray Panthers implemented a "media watch," as she railed against the dominant discourse portraying old age as weak and diminished. As senior centers were touted by some as positive spaces for older adults, Kuhn attacked policy that supported (in her words) "play pens" and other pacification techniques. She rejected the infantilization and dehumanization of older adults: "We are not wrinkled babies, succumbing to trivial, purposeless waste of our years and our time" (Kuhn in Hessel, 1977, p. 14).

Kuhn worked on stages and platforms with Dr. Robert Butler, first director of the National Institute on Aging and author of the 1975 Pulitzer Prize book, *Why Survive? Being Old in America*. Both Kuhn and Butler are credited with the concept of "agism." Kuhn denounced "society [as] agist....It is also racist and sexist. Agism is the arbitrary discrimination against people on the basis of their chronological age" (Kuhn in Hessel, 1977, p. 15).

Anti–Vietnam War rallies drew Maggie Kuhn in, with a commitment to peace and to "elders of the tribe" to take the risks of arrests that young students could not. She blazed a parallel path built on trenchant structural analysis and critical left theorizing while attracting overflowing public audiences to hear her. In scholarly and professional convocations, she challenged the dominant gerontological and medical practices. In 1972, she cofounded the activist group, the Gray Panthers, committed to "a strong ethical-moral base in our social analysis and social strategy" (Kuhn in Hessel, 1977,

p. 123). Kuhn was a television hit on the *Tonight Show Starring Johnny Carson*, talking frankly about the sexual and intellectual vitality she enjoyed as an old woman. Maggie was committed to the common welfare by undoing the institutionalized racist, sexist, classist, and ageist forces governing social policy and public perception. It required a process to radicalize and increase political awareness.

In the 24 years following her forced retirement from the Presbyterian Church, Maggie Kuhn not only contributed to social gerontology, but also forwarded the work of younger scholars, including Carroll Estes (chapter author). It is impressive that Kuhn's theoretical insights are deeply inscribed in the contemporary academic discourse in six areas: (a) identity politics, (b) intersectionality, (c) cultural and media studies in the cognitive sciences, (d) the political economy of aging, (e) the sociology of knowledge of gerontology, and (f) critiques of globalization and imperialism (Estes & Portacolone, 2009).

Maggie Kuhn fits the profile of Buroway's "organic public sociologist" (Burawoy, 2005, p. 11), immersed in her causes and vigorously interacting with counterpublics. As an organic intellectual, working on the ground with and from the people, she was all about *praxis* and social justice. She delivered not only critiques of the paradigms and theories employed by gerontologists (including disengagement and activity theories), but also critiques of the disempowering and distancing research methods focused on the individual level and in ways that objectify human beings who are old. Instead, she suggested studies of the social consequences of victim blaming and investigation to reveal the injurious acts of the power elites, profiteers, and "knowledge definers" (Kuhn, 1978, pp. 423–424).

Tangible successes of Kuhn's social movement include the 1978 amendment to the Age Discrimination in Employment Act, raising the mandatory retirement age from 65 to 70 years. Nevertheless, as Horowitz (1970) notes, revolutionaries sustain themselves by their therapeutic stance of struggle, not the tangibility of results, as outcomes are never certain or sustained. Kuhn exemplified this stance by rejecting the traps of the centralization of power and bureaucratic elitism in her movement, while sharing the joys and sorrow of wins and losses in the cause.

Carroll L. Estes (1938–), my work, to this very moment, is profoundly influenced by my early immersion in social and philosophical thought during graduate school(s) and sabbaticals. With degrees in sociology, my teaching and sabbaticals spanned sociology, social work, economics, public health, and nursing at the University of California, San Diego (UCSD) campuses, the London School of Economics, and the Sorbonne in Paris. I was privileged and profoundly influenced by theorists, including Max Weber, Emile Durkheim, Karl Marx, George Herbert Mead, Antonio Gramsci, Herbert Blumer, Alvin Gouldner, Jurgen Habermas, Randall Collins, and James O'Connor. While in PhD study, UCSD was a hothouse of radical empiricism and ontological critiques of positivism and deductive research. The new–new included ethnomethodology (Cicourel) and grounded theory (Glaser & Strauss, 1967). My PhD methods courses were taught as theory and techniques of inquiry.

My first job (1963–1967) at Brandeis University (Heller School for Advanced Studies in Social Welfare) was formative in becoming a gerontologist. In this policy-wonk environment, I learned welfare-state debates surrounding The New Deal and The Great Society. Daily conversations covered the War on Poverty, Aid to Families With Dependent Children, medical insurance, housing, and Social Security. I cowrote my first federal grant and coauthored my first international paper (Vienna, Austria) on "Differences Between Current Gerontological Theories: Implications for Research Methodology." I was privileged to meet and learn from Bernice Neugarten and Powell Lawton. From Howard

Freeman, I saw institutional building of a think tank; as well as learned survey research, probability sampling, and how to get statistical analyses from the huge Massachusetts Institute of Technology (MIT) computing building. Equally significant, I witnessed and participated in social movements on the streets of Boston and Columbia, South Carolina (volunteering in voter education with the Southern Christian Leadership Conference).

I arrived at Brandeis with an MA thesis that became my first book, *The Decision-Makers: The Power Structure of Dallas* (Estes-Thometz, 1963). This research identified a "power-elite" (consistent with C. Wright Mills), as opposed to the then-dominant "pluralist"—structural functionalist theories of democracy of Robert Dahl (political scientist) and Talcott Parsons (sociologist). As a 23-year-old research assistant, I was way too intimidated to discuss this with Bob Binstock, the newly hired Harvard PhD political scientist at Brandeis. Bernice Neugarten and Powell Lawton were much less fearsome! After my PhD (1970–1973) and my appointment at the University of California, San Francisco (UCSF), I published my first book in gerontology, *The Aging Enterprise* (Estes, Lee, Gerard, & Noble, 1979), that focused on the OAA with the subtitle: *A Critical Examination of Social Policies and Services for the Aged.*

My original theoretical contribution is to develop and bridge two disparate theoretical strands in my research on old age politics and policy: The macro and micro perspectives, respectively, building on the macro Conflict Theory (Max Weber) and the micro Social Constructionist Theory (Symbolic Interactionist) (Blumer, 1969/2012). As a Randall Collins– and Alvin Gouldner–trained Weberian, my focus is the organizational, political, and sociocultural processes and forces in policy and politics. As a Herbert Blumer–trained interactionist, I examined the contested social construction(s) of social problems (e.g., old age and aging) that become the subject of the debates and battles in policy and politics—and the effects of these on the self-esteem and personal control of older persons and groups. Using the conflict and constructionist theoretical lens, my analyses concern (a) the power struggles and disparate rewards (win or lose) of different definitions of "the problem," while studying (b) the ongoing conflicts (symbolic and material) that reside in class, status, race, age, gender, ability, and power dynamics, and (c) the effects of these on the old as individuals and collectivities. My PhD dissertation did just that. My theoretical and empirical approach (Conflict Theory) is distinctly *oppositional* to the structural functionalist (Consensus Theory) that portrays the integrated social systems and believes in a "neutral" state characterized by accommodative relations among state, citizen, and society.

The political economy of aging theory that I introduced in 1979 and have elaborated on since then assesses not only the social construction of old age and aging, and the political economy of aging, but also (a) the aging enterprise; (b) austerity and aging; (c) legitimacy and crisis in the state, capital, and democracy; and (d) the distributive effects of policy by race, class, gender and sexuality, ethnicity, (dis)ability, and age.

Since 1976, I have emphasized the social construction of reality and symbolic interaction framework. Powerful, coercive messages of futility and worthlessness reside in social labeling surrounding ageist epithets such as "kooky," "senile," "greedy," and "worthless" (Estes & Freeman, 1976). Such labeling does not occur in a vacuum—it is a product and mechanism of experts, institutions, economic and political systems that benefit from such labels. Much of my scholarship attends to the meso-institutional level of practice and ideologies attendant thereto.

Concepts and theories of "the looking glass self" and "self-fulfilling prophecy" denote the potential effects of how others view us or how we view ourselves and our self-esteem and (dis)empowerment. Research in sociogenics and biosocial interactions affirms relationships between immune systems, telomeres, other genetic changes, and social class, race, education, income, and wealth. This hints at the serious health and mental health consequences of institutional processing and stigmatizing labeling of individuals and groups. Concepts of "resilience" and "allostatic load" are similarly relevant. This work is integral to the political economy of aging since its introduction in the 1970s.

Drawing from critical theory, there is a commitment (both scientific and normative) to identifying and eradicating oppression in all forms and faces. This is a *subaltern* perspective, historically contentious in the academy, which intellectual critics argue resides in the ideological underpinnings of positivism and hegemonic theorizing in economics, sociology, and other disciplines.

My work speaks to:

- The socially and structurally produced nature of old age and aging and the lived experience of these phenomena as they vary by class, gender, generation, race, ethnicity, and (dis)ability
- Ideology as a central element in the social, economic, and political processing of the old and old age in society (globally and within nation-states)
- The social construction, social control, and management of elder dependency by organizations, professions, and institutions including the state and capital
- The types of social interventions (including research) that are legitimated and delegitimated by the dominant, competing, and repressed, social construction(s) of aging
- The role, function, and social relations of the state, employers, and employees, and how they affect the "life chances" of the old, especially their economic and health security
- The "aging enterprise" and its largest component, the global medical–industrial complex comprising industries, professionals, and multinationals that seek control of the definitions, interventions, and markets designed to treat the problems of old age and aging
- The policy effects of inequalities in sociogenetics and biosocial interactions, and
- The critical and reflexive examination of gerontological knowledge and the role of intellectuals, practitioners, the state, corporations, elders and their families in producing it

I examined the national, state, and local policy in aging, as well as global developments—including the transitions from Creative Federalism (Kennedy and Johnson presidencies of 1961–1969) to New Federalism (Nixon and Carter presidencies of 1970–1979), through Reagan, Clinton, Bush I and II, and Obama. I study social movements seeking to dismantle Social Security, Medicare, and social insurance—and resistance movements organizing in opposition to these attacks.

I am privileged to experience mentorship and community with women: my mother Carroll Cox Estes, Maggie Kuhn, Tish Sommers, and Betty Friedan. Bound by the injuries of gender, we understood that our "private troubles" were indeed public issues. Each made imperative the urgency for feminism. Bernice Neugarten convinced me that I was doctoral material, when I had neither confidence nor voice. Every day my daughter, Duskie Lynn Estes, shows me that nothing is impossible (see Estes, 2008).

▪ CLOSING COMMENTARY
The Perspective of a Critical Public Gerontologist

We introduce leading figures in gerontological theory, research, policy, and practice during 1960 to 1980. The decades are not simply "context" or "environment" in which science and knowledge(s) progressed; historical events and social movements are the cauldron in which substantive topics, theories, and methods were contested, reconstructed, and/or reproduced.

The dominant theoretical problems of the 1960s resonated with a view of older persons as vulnerable and "deserving" within the assumed frames of the collective and legitimate state role in assisting old people and others vulnerable (e.g., OAA, Medicare, and Medicaid). Theoretical and conceptual developments timidly acknowledged diversity, race, women, and old-age poverty.

During the 1970s, with the brief exception of one-term President Carter, a conservative backlash against the nation-state was led by presidents Nixon, Ford, and H. W. Bush. Beginning with President Nixon's New Federalism, policy and theoretical-ideological discourses shifted to the transfer of federal funding to subsidize the commodification and privatization of the previously public and nonprofit services (e.g., home health care). The rhetoric of cost containment and budgetary concerns (deficit hysteria) combined with the rhetoric of a demographic "tsunami" as the rationale for shifting government subsidies to the theoretically "more efficient" private sector, particularly with respect to billions of dollars in Medicare and medical insurance. In the home disciplines of gerontologists, theoretical and empirical work advanced welfare-state crisis theories, theories of risk and uncertainty, postmodernism, critical theory, and epistemological standpoints and knowledge in the social sciences and humanities. Competing methodological paradigms (positivism, postpositivism, critical theory, constructivism, and radical microsociology) were examined *as theory*, while *theory* was examined *as resistance* (Collins, 2004; Guba & Lincoln, 1994).

The 1970s hosted robust anti-state discourse, with think tanks dedicated to the cause of redirecting the welfare state: taxpayer revolt, individual responsibility, and preference for market solutions. Government is the problem. Older persons are now "the problem," with extended life expectancy seen as threatening to a prosperous economy and society. Greedy Geezers alarm bell sounds.

Scholars in gerontological theory and practice witnessed, experienced, and reflected the challenges to the theoretical, methodological, and empirical "givens" in their respective disciplines of psychology, social psychology, social work, sociology, political science, and economics. Feminist and Black theorizing confronted dominant mainstream social thought. The contributions of the 12 gerontologists featured are substantial (see Table 6.1).

In the social gerontology mainstream, the more influential disciplines of psychology and sociology were eclipsed by the rise of classic *laissez faire* economics embedded within ideologies of market fundamentalism and individualism.

Since the 1980s, and especially from the 1990s forward, gerontologists intensified research on *cumulative advantage and disadvantage.* Concepts of "allostatic load" (McEwen & Stellar, 1993) link chronic stress to deleterious effects on morbidity and mortality. Risk factors are: low socioeconomic status, low education, and lived realities of cumulative inequality including race, ethnicity, gender and sexuality, (dis)ability, income, and wealth. Investigating *biosocial interactions* is integral to the "cells to society" intellectual

TABLE 6.1   Social Gerontologists in the Lead: 1960 to 1980

Name	Years	Contributions
Ollie A. Randall	1890–1984	Orchestrated Ford Foundation commitment in aging; aging as exclusion and burden on families
Wilma Donahue	1900–1993	Academic legitimizer (University of Michigan) of gerontology as an academic field
Clark Tibbitts	1903–1985	Architect of federal funding of aging education, training, and research via Older Americans Act
Ethel Shanas	1914–2005	Statistician, laid foundation for health services research in aging and cross-national health surveys, concept of "social myth as hypothesis"; theory of family relations as primary basis of security of old people
Bernice Neugarten	1916–2001	Dispelling myth of empty nest and menopause madness, life course theory, off-time/on-time, age norms, age grades, young-old/old-old/very-old; debate of age versus need in old age policy
Louis Lowy	1920–1991	International development of field, Group Work in Aging, advocated for "belonging"—the idea that interdependence of children and parents is a family goal
Walter M. Beattie, Jr.	1923–2007	Supportive environments for the life span, and long-term health care
Elaine Brody	1923–2014	The family and long-term care, "women in the middle"
Jacquelyne Johnson Jackson	1932–2004	Identifying research needs in minority aging, theories of "institutionalized victimization" and "quadruple jeopardy"
Robert H. Binstock	1935–2011	Theories of interest group liberalism, the "electoral bluff," the aged as scapegoat
Maggie Kuhn	1905–1995	Organic intellectual, Gray Panthers, ageism, racism, and sexism, common stakes of youth and aging; Standpoint Theory of Age, media analysis, gorilla theater
Carroll L. Estes	1938–present	Social construction and political economy theories of aging; crisis, the state, capital, and aging; distributive effects of policy by race, class, gender, and age; the "aging enterprise," and biomedicalization of aging

revolution. Nobel prizes, theory, and research on telomeres, chronic stress, and health elevate their prominence (Blackburn & Epel, 2012).

"Risks" are no longer conceptualized solely as individual attributes, but rather are seen as "built into the ways we do things; built into the system." The quest for causation is institutional, structural, and cultural forces in the streets, neighborhoods, and geo-political and identity spaces that comprise the *habitus* of human beings (in Pierre Bourdieu's sense of the term). Concepts of *plasticity* and *resilience* amplify the urgency of identifying forces, including policy, that predict quality years in old age and aging and who lives and thrives (or not).

Following the 1960 to 1980 period highlighted in this chapter, scholars produced an avalanche of theorizing and large-scale empirical work on the welfare state and aging, public welfare expenditures, globalization, and the construction and manage-ment of crisis in old age policy (Estes, 2011). Critical perspectives in gerontology emerged and flourished in the 1980s in the United States (Carroll Estes, Laura Katz Olson, and Jill Quadagno), Canada (John Myles and Victor Marshall), and Europe (Peter Townsend, Alan Walker, Chris Phillipson, Anne Marie Guillemard, and Jan Baars) in response to limited (microfication; Dale Dannefer) social gerontology per-spectives on the aging process, individual life-course development, disengagement, life satisfaction, and dependency. Work in critical gerontology has developed under the rubrics of radical gerontology, political gerontology, the moral economy of aging, cultural and humanistic gerontology, and perhaps most well recognized, the political economy of aging.

Accumulating work on health and economic disparities, globally and locally, is occurring in tandem with the mainstreaming of critical gerontology. There is a deep bench of *subaltern* critical gerontological work on globalization and political economy, social movements, and the life course, particularly in the European Union (EU) and Canada—Alan Walker, Chris Phillipson, Jan Baars, Robin Blackburn, John Myles—and in the United States—Dale Dannefer, Jill Quadagno, and my own work among others. Postcolonial, Black feminist, and systemic racism; (dis)ability; and LGBT/queer theoret-ical work moves forward on the margins.

Simultaneously, there is inculcation in national and global institutions like the WHO, the United Nations (UN), the World Bank, and the EU of the distinctively American con-cepts of "productive aging," "successful aging," and "positive aging"—along with goals of diminishing health inequalities. Global woes are defined as the socially constructed demographic "gray tsunami" raising pandemic fears of billions living too long—with Alzheimer's disease and cognitive and chronic impairments, blotting the future of all developed and developing countries.

To a critical observer, the magnitude of scholarship on successful aging is contradic-tory to the deepening chasm of social, psychological, health, and wealth inequalities that are associated with welfare state austerity policies. The dislocating and decentering effects of the suffering of vulnerable peoples is visual and virtual via multiple media platforms. Progressive new-revitalized social movements connect in the U.S. Black Lives Matter, the War on Women's health and reproductive care, Social Security, Medi-care, and Medicaid defenders, equality for LGBTQ (lesbian, gay, bisexual, transgender, queer), with global warming, and immigration movements blooming.

Public intellectuals in sociology, gerontology, economics, psychology, and political science are vital in linking the professional–science–policy nexus to address the enor-mous challenge of individual, societal, and global aging.

A NOTE ON LIMITATIONS

Today, economics is a (if not the) dominant discipline shaping the policy and practice agenda of consequence for the old and aging societies. The gerontologists featured here do not include an economist, primarily due to the descriptive work of gerontological economists during this period. Of special acclaim are James Schultz, Brandeis professor emeritus, and Juanita Kreps, Duke University professor and secretary of commerce under President Carter.

As intergenerational collaborators and cowriters, we wish to locate our respective individual epistemological advantages and disadvantages. We are both Caucasian and carry with us a history of White privilege and the intellectual gifts of exposure to elite higher education. Carroll Estes, now in her mid-70s, was born and raised as a girl in Texas who endured injuries attendant to her sex and gender. Nicholas DiCarlo is a queer male in his late 20s who hails from Appalachia and contributes existential, gerontological imaginings in part to secure a foothold in academia and also to dream of what his own aging may be.

REFERENCES

Achenbaum, W. A., & Albert, D. M. (1995). *Profiles in gerontology: A biographical dictionary.* Westport, CT: Greenwood Publishing Group.

Beal, F. M. (1969). *Double jeopardy: To be black and female.* New York, NY: Third World Women's Alliance.

Beattie, W. M. (1960). The aging Negro: Some implications for social welfare services. *Phylon, 21,* 131–135.

Beattie, W. M. (1970). The design of supportive environments for the life span. *The Gerontologist, 10*(3), 190–193.

Beattie, W. M. (1973). Promises. Promises. Promises. *The Gerontologist, 13*(2), 133.

Beattie, W. M. (1978, April). *Aging: A framework of characteristics and considerations for cooperative efforts between the developing and developed regions of the world.* In a background paper prepared for the Expert Group Meeting on Aging.

Ben-David, J., & Sullivan, T. A. (1975). Sociology of science. *Annual Review of Sociology, 1,* 203–222.

Binstock, R. H. (1972). Interest-group liberalism and the politics of aging. *The Gerontologist, 12*(3), 265–280.

Binstock, R. H. (1974). Aging and the future of American politics. *Annals of the American Academy of Political and Social Science, 415,* 199–212.

Binstock, R. H. (1983). The aged as scapegoat: The Donald P. Kent Memorial Lecture. *The Gerontologist, 23,* 136–143.

Binstock, R. H., & Shanas, E. (Eds.). (1976). *Handbook of aging and the social sciences.* New York, NY: Van Nostrand Reinhold.

Binstock, R. H., & Shanas, E. (Eds.). (1985). *Handbook of aging and the social sciences* (2nd ed.). New York, NY: Van Nostrand Reinhold.

Blackburn, E. H., & Epel, E. S. (2012). Telomeres and adversity: Too toxic to ignore. *Nature, 490,* 169–171.

Blumer, H. (2012). Symbolic interactionism. In C. Calhoun, J. Gerteis, J. Moody, S. Pfaff, & I. Virk (Eds.), *Contemporary sociological theory* (pp. 46–89). West Sussex, UK: John Wiley & Sons. (Original work published 1969)

Brody, E. M. (1981). "Women in the middle" and family help to older people. *The Gerontologist, 21*(5), 471–480.

Brody, E. M. (1990). *Women in the middle: Their parent-care years.* New York, NY: Springer Publishing Company.

Brody, E. M. (2010). On being very, very old: An insider's perspective. *The Gerontologist, 50*(1), 2–10.

Burawoy, M. (2005). 2004 American Sociological Association Presidential address: For public sociology. *British Journal of Sociology, 56*(2), 259–294.

Butler, R. N. (1975). *Why survive? Being old in America.* New York, NY: Harper & Row.

Collins, R. (2004). *Interaction ritual chains.* Princeton, NJ: Princeton University Press.

Collins, R., & Annett, J. (1975). *Conflict sociology: Toward an explanatory science.* New York, NY: Academic Press.

Cumming, E., & Henry, W. E. (1961). *Growing old, the process of disengagement.* New York, NY: Basic Books.

Donahue, W. T., & Tibbitts, C. (Eds.). (1950). *Planning the older years.* Ann Arbor, MI: University of Michigan Press.

Donahue, W. T., & Tibbitts, C. (Eds.). (1951). *Growing in the older years.* Ann Arbor, MI: University of Michigan Press.

Donahue, W. T., & Tibbitts, C. (Eds.). (1957). *The new frontiers of aging.* Ann Arbor, MI: University of Michigan Press.

Donahue, W. T., & Tibbitts, C. (Eds.). (1957). *Aging in the modern world.* Ann Arbor, MI: University of Michigan Press.

Estes, C. L. (1979). Toward a sociology of political gerontology. *Sociological Symposium, 26*, 1–25.

Estes, C. L. (2011). Crises and old age policy. In R. A. Settersten & J. L. Angel (Eds.), *Handbook of sociology of aging* (pp. 297–320). New York, NY: Springer Publishing Company.

Estes, C. L., Binney, E. A., & Culbertson, R. A. (1992). The gerontological imagination: Social influences on the development of gerontology, 1945–present. *International Journal of Aging & Human Development, 35*(1), 49–65.

Estes, C. L., & Freeman, H. (1976). Strategies of design and research for intervention. In R. H. Binstock & E. Shanas (Eds.), *Handbook of aging and the social sciences* (pp. 536–560). New York, NY: Van Nostrand Reinhold.

Estes, C. L., Lee, P. R., Gerard, L. E., & Noble, M. (1979). *The aging enterprise.* San Francisco, CA: Jossey-Bass.

Estes, C. L., & Portacolone, E. (2009). Maggie Kuhn: Social theorist of radical gerontology. *International Journal of Sociology & Social Policy, 29*, 15–25.

Estes-Thometz, C. L. (1963). *The decision-makers: The power structure of Dallas.* Dallas, TX: Southern Methodist University Press.

Ferraro, K. F., & Schafer, M. H. (2008). Gerontology's greatest hits. *The Journals of Gerontology, Series B, 63*(1), S3–S6.

Freire, P. (1970). *Pedagogy of the oppressed*. Myra Bergman Ramos (Trans.). New York, NY: Continuum.

Friedan, B. (1963). *The feminine mystique*. London, UK: Penguin.

Friedan, B. (1993). *The fountain of age*. New York, NY: Simon & Schuster.

Gardella, L. G. (2014). *The life and thought of Louis Lowy: Social work through the holocaust*. Syracuse, NY: Syracuse University Press.

Glaser, B. G., & Strauss, A. L. (1967). *The discovery of grounded theory: Strategies for qualitative research*. Piscataway, NJ: Transaction.

Gouldner, A. W. (1971). *The coming crisis of Western sociology*. London, UK: Heinemann.

Gramsci, A. (1971). *Selections from the prison notebooks*. Quintin Hoare and Geoffrey Nowell Smith (Trans. and Ed., p. 62). New York, NY: International Publishers.

Guba, E. G., & Lincoln, Y. S. (1994). Competing paradigms in qualitative research. In N. K. Denzien & Y. S. Lincoln (Eds.), *Handbook of qualitative research*. Thousand Oaks, CA: Sage.

Habermas, J. (1980). *Legitimation crisis*. London, UK: Heinemann.

Hacker, K. (1986, January 8). A career of aiding the aging: Elaine Brody has spent 31 years helping people cope with growing old. *Philadelphia Inquirer*.

Hessel, D. T., & Kuhn, M. E. (1977). *Maggie Kuhn on aging: A dialogue*. Philadelphia, PA: Westminster Press.

Horowitz, D. (1970). *Empire and revolution: A radical interpretation of contemporary history*. New York, NY: Vintage Books.

Jackson, H. C. (1971a). National goals and priorities in the social welfare of the aging. *The Gerontologist, 11*(1), 88–94.

Jackson, J. J. (1971b). The Blacklands of gerontology. *The International Journal of Aging and Human Development, 2*, 156–171.

Jackson, J. J. (1971c). Negro aged: Toward needed research in social gerontology. *The Gerontologist, 11*(1), Suppl:52–Suppl:57.

Jackson, J. J. (1980). *Minorities and aging*. Belmont, CA: Wadsworth Publishing Company.

King, M. L. (1968). *Chaos or community?* London, UK: Hodder and Stoughton.

Kuhn, M. (1978). Open letter. *The Gerontologist, 18*(5), 422–424.

Kuhn, T. S. (1962). *The structure of scientific revolutions*. Chicago, IL: University of Chicago Press.

Lowi, T. J. (1969). *The end of liberalism: Ideology, policy, and the crisis of public authority*. New York, NY: W. W. Norton.

Lowy, L. (1972). *The function of social work in a changing society: A continuum of practice*. n.p.

Lowy, L., & Miller, L. (1974). Toward greater movement for gerontology in social work education. *The Gerontologist, 14*, 466–467.

McEwen, B. E., & Stellar, E. (1993). Stress and the individual: Mechanisms leading to disease. *Archive of Internal Medicine, 18*, 2093–2101.

Mills, C. W. (1959). *The sociological imagination*. New York, NY: Oxford University Press.

Morris, R., Binstock, R. H., & Rein, M. (1966). *Feasible planning for social change.* New York, NY: Columbia University Press.

Neugarten, B. L. (1974). Age groups in American society and the rise of the young-old. *Annals of the American Academy of Political and Social Science, 415,* 187–198.

Neugarten, B. L. (1979). Policy for the 1980s: Age or need entitlement? In J. P. Hubbard (Ed.), *Aging: Agenda for the eighties, a national journal issues book* (pp. 48–52). Washington, DC: Government Research Corporation.

Neugarten, B. L., & Hagestad, G. O. (1976). Age and the life course. In R. H. Binstock & E. Shanas (Eds.), *Handbook of aging and the social sciences* (pp. 35–55). New York, NY: Van Nostrand Reinhold.

Neugarten, B. L., Moore, J. W., & Lowe, J. C. (1965). Age norms, age constraints, and adult socialization. *American Journal of Sociology, 70,* 710–717.

Piven, F. F., & Cloward, R. A. (1979). *Poor people's movements: Why they succeed, how they fail.* New York, NY: Vintage Books.

Randall, O. A. (1951). Sociological aspects of aging. *Journal of the American Medical Association, 147*(14), 1325–1326.

Randall, O. A. (1965). Some historical developments of social welfare aspects of aging. *The Gerontologist, 5,* Suppl:40–Suppl:49.

Rose, A. M. (1962). The subculture of the aging: A topic for sociological research. *The Gerontologist, 2,* 123–127.

Rose, A. M., & Peterson, W. A. (1965). *Older people and their social world: The sub-culture of the aging.* Philadelphia, PA: F. A. Davis.

Sassoon, A. S. (2000). *Gramsci and contemporary politics: Beyond pessimism of the intellect.* New York, NY: Routledge.

Shanas, E. (1979a). The family as a social support system in old age. *The Gerontologist, 19*(2), 169–174.

Shanas, E. (1979b). Social myth as hypothesis: The case of the family relations of old people. *The Gerontologist, 19,* 3–9.

Tibbitts, C. (Ed.). (1960). *Handbook of social gerontology: Societal aspects of aging.* Chicago, IL: University of Chicago Press.

U.S. Senate Special Committee. (1978). *The graying of nations: Implications.* Hearing before the Special Committee on Aging, United States Senate, Ninety-fifth Congress, first session, Washington, DC, November 10, 1977. Washington: U.S. Govt. Print. Off.

Williams, R. H., Tibbitts, C., & Donahue, W. (Eds.). (1963). *Processes of aging.* New York, NY: Atherton Press.

PART II

Biological Theories and Concepts

ADVANCES IN BIOLOGICAL THEORIES OF AGING
Brian K. Kennedy

Research into the biology of aging has undergone a robust maturation process over the last three decades. The field has evolved from largely studying correlative changes that happen during the aging process to trying to characterize the hundreds of genes and myriad environmental interventions linked to enhanced longevity. Driving this rapid discovery process has been the widespread use of nonvertebrate aging models—such as yeast, worms, and flies—which are cheap to study, age quickly, and have well-characterized biology. Studies of these organisms have led to the identification of candidate molecular pathways that may impact the rate of human aging. Many of these, such as the target of rapamycin (TOR) and insulin/insulin-like growth factor (IGF) pathways, are conserved in mammals. Modulating their activity appears to extend both life span and health span, the functional and disease-free period of life (Junnila, List, Berryman, Murrey, & Kopchick, 2013; Lamming, Ye, Sabatini, & Baur, 2013). Recent research has extended this evidence to humans (Mannick et al., 2014; Tazearslan, Huang, Barzilai, & Suh, 2011). Together, the identification of conserved aging pathways has both generated hypotheses and placed constraints on the way researchers think about molecular events that drive aging.

The flood of genetic and biochemical information on aging has also refined biological theories about *why* and *how* we age. This section of the handbook, "Advances in Biological Theories of Aging," explores new and emerging theories in this area. That so many new ideas have developed recently is a testament to how quickly experimental insights have arisen. Perhaps the biggest recent change is that many researchers in the field now believe that it will be possible in our lifetime to slow aging (Kennedy & Pennypacker, 2014; Longo et al., 2015). Drugs that delay aging are already emerging in mice, and tests are ongoing to delay specific pathologies of aging in humans. The chapters in this section integrate theory and practice, describing interventional strategies that might be employed to prevent disease and slow aging. Aging research has placed us at the brink of a medical revolution, whereby it might be possible to do what was thought to be impossible: delay human aging.

■ AN EVOLVING VIEW OF AGING

Evolution-based hypotheses to explain aging, such as mutation accumulation and antagonistic pleiotropy, are not new (Medawar, 1952; Williams, 1957). In fact, aging has been a source of puzzlement in the context of evolutionary theory since its conception. In the 19th century, August Weisman proposed that aging and senescence remove older individuals from the population so that they do not compete for resources with the young (Weismann, 1889). Although this model is not well supported by empirical data, it is the start of a rich vein of thought about why we age. Evolutionary theories of aging continue to become refined in informative ways. Moreover, an exciting element in recent years involves attempts to test evolutionary concepts in the context of known molecular aging pathways. For instance, there is a trade-off between reproduction and aging: Long-lived organisms often have low fecundity rates. In genetic studies, this model has often been supported, with long-lived mutants in model organisms having reduced fecundity. However, as the number of longevity mutants has grown, this trade-off does not always hold with many mutants dissociating the two phenotypes (Partridge et al., 2005; Walker, McColl, Jenkins, Harris, & Lithgow, 2000). The interface between theory and experiment will continue to refine and shape our perspectives about aging. In Chapter 7, Devin Arbuthnott, Daniel Promislow, and Jacob Moorad cover the history, current viewpoints, and recent advances concerning why we age, as well as anticipate what insights future research might yield.

■ INTERTWINED CAUSES OF AGING

Aging is the biggest risk factor (and one likely cause) for a wide range of chronic diseases that the majority of global disease burden. Given the dramatic increase in the elder population, the concept of targeting aging to prevent or treat these diseases is growing in popularity. This approach has gained momentum in the National Institutes of Health, in part because of the Geroscience initiative under the direction of the National Institute of Aging, which seeks to gain support for research to understand the links between aging and disease (Burch et al., 2014). As a part of this initiative, a meeting was held in 2014 culminating in a review that identified seven molecular events linked to aging (Kennedy et al., 2014). Similar reviews have identified a limited number of overlapping pathways (López-Otín, Blasco, Partridge, Serrano, & Kroemer, 2013). The processes identified in the Geroscience meeting were: (a) adaptation to stress, (b) epigenetics, (c) inflammation, (d) macromolecular damage, (e) metabolism, (f) proteostasis, and (g) stem cells and regeneration (Kennedy et al., 2014). The striking aspect to meeting participants was their interrelatedness: Do epigenetic changes during the aging process lead to enhanced DNA damage, or vice versa? Is inflammation a precursor to the decline of adult stem cells? Gone are the days of scientists working on one model for aging or one hypothesis about what causes aging. Instead, we are in a new research world that is at once exciting and a bit scary, in which the complexity of the aging process is becoming appreciated and a system-level view of aging in an entire organism at least seems theoretically attainable, albeit not in the short term.

Three chapters are targeted at the processes thought to drive aging, focusing on those that have come to the forefront recently. In Chapter 8, Ming Xu and Jim Kirkland address the role of inflammation in aging. This process has become so intimately linked to aging that it has been coined as "inflammaging" (Franceschi et al., 2007). Induction of inflammatory processes are critical to the organism, for instance leading to orchestrated responses to foreign invaders and the repair of damaged tissue. However, chronic inflammation is also a hallmark of aging that clearly promotes a subset of age-associated diseases and likely aging itself. Interestingly, this process has recently been connected to cellular senescence, as cells in this terminal, nonproliferative state are now known to secrete a set of cytokines that can promote localized inflammation, adversely affecting the tissues in which they reside (Coppé et al., 2008; Kuilman et al., 2008). This finding could explain how senescent cells in the body may drive aging processes, even though they never accumulate to high percentages of the population. In support, recent studies suggest that ablation of senescent cells slow the onset of pathology in models of accelerated aging.

In Chapter 9, Pedro Sousa-Victor, Joana Neves, and Heinrich Jasper describe mechanisms that drive the decline of adult stem cell function with age, as well as the consequences of this decline for aging pathologies. Most tissues of the body have resident stem cell populations that are tasked with replacing those that are damaged, thus maintaining tissue function. The mechanisms underlying stem cell decline with age are coming into focus. Although there are unique features with respect to each stem cell population, it is now clear that there are cell-intrinsic changes in stem cells with age as well as noncell autonomous changes that include a loss of factors in young blood that positively affect stem cell function and a rise in deleterious factors in aging blood. These noncell autonomous factors are potential points of intervention to restore stem cell function in aged organisms and further studies to define the specific molecules are of high importance.

Finally, in Chapter 10, Matt Kaeberlein describes the role of protein homeostasis, proteostasis, in driving age-related processes (Balch, Morimoto, Dillin, & Kelly, 2008). All macromolecules in the cell display increasing damage with aging. Recently the cellular proteome has become a point of focus. The proteostatic state of the cell is defined by protein synthesis and turnover. A large number of mutants that lead to life-span extension in model organisms affect both protein synthesis and turnover. It is clear that organisms have evolved elaborate mechanisms to ensure that (a) a functional repertoire of proteins are maintained in cells; (b) many of these processes become dysfunctional with age; and (c) maintaining their function delays at least some aspects of aging.

■ CONCLUSION

For thousands of years, scientists, philosophers, and everyone in between have been puzzled over *why* and *how* we age. Aging and mortality define the human condition and more people than ever are experiencing it firsthand. In the near future, more than 20% of the population will be older than 60 years and the costs to society are manifest. We are living in the "Age" age and how we manage this health crisis will define a lot about global quality of life in the 21st century.

We now know that aging is modifiable. Interventions ranging from genetic to behavioral to pharmacologic extend life span in mammals and delay aging pathologies. The next decade is likely to see increasingly elaborate theories to (a) define the molecular events that drive aging and (b) explain the existence of aging in species shaped by evolution. Moreover, interventional strategies will begin to be tested on humans. Former U.S. Secretary of Defense Donald Rumsfeld once said that there are "known knowns," "known unknowns," and "unknown unknowns," emphasizing that the latter class is often the recipe for disaster. In aging, we may not have enough known knowns, but major progress has been made converting unknown unknowns to known unknowns, and the rate of progress in research into the biology of aging is likely to accelerate as we strive to offset the myriad costs of rapidly aging global societies.

REFERENCES

Balch, W. E., Morimoto, R. I., Dillin, A., & Kelly, J. W. (2008). Adapting proteostasis for disease intervention. *Science, 319*(5865), 916–919.

Burch, J. B., Augustine, A. D., Frieden, L. A., Hadley, E., Howcroft, T. K., Johnson, R., . . . Wise, B. C. (2014). Advances in geroscience: Impact on healthspan and chronic disease. *The Journals of Gerontology, Series A, 69*(Suppl. 1), S1–S3.

Coppé, J. P., Patil, C. K., Rodier, F., Sun, Y., Muñoz, D. P., Goldstein, J., . . . Campisi, J. (2008). Senescence-associated secretory phenotypes reveal cell-nonautonomous functions of oncogenic RAS and the p53 tumor suppressor. *PLoS Biology, 6*(12), 2853–2868.

Franceschi, C., Capri, M., Monti, D., Giunta, S., Olivieri, F., Sevini, F., . . . Salvioli, S. (2007). Inflammaging and anti-inflammaging: A systemic perspective on aging and longevity emerged from studies in humans. *Mechanisms of Ageing and Development, 128*(1), 92–105.

Junnila, R. K., List, E. O., Berryman, D. E., Murrey, J. W., & Kopchick, J. J. (2013). The GH/IGF-1 axis in ageing and longevity. *Nature Reviews: Endocrinology, 9*(6), 366–376.

Kennedy, B. K., Berger, S. L., Brunet, A., Campisi, J., Cuervo, A. M., Epel, E. S., . . . Sierra, F. (2014). Geroscience: Linking aging to chronic disease. *Cell, 159*(4), 709–713.

Kennedy, B. K., & Pennypacker, J. K. (2014). Drugs that modulate aging: The promising yet difficult path ahead. *Translational Research: The Journal of Laboratory and Clinical Medicine, 163*(5), 456–465.

Kuilman, T., Michaloglou, C., Vredeveld, L. C., Douma, S., van Doorn, R., Desmet, C. J., . . . Peeper, D. S. (2008). Oncogene-induced senescence relayed by an interleukin-dependent inflammatory network. *Cell, 133*(6), 1019–1031.

Lamming, D. W., Ye, L., Sabatini, D. M., & Baur, J. A. (2013). Rapalogs and mTOR inhibitors as anti-aging therapeutics. *The Journal of Clinical Investigation, 123*(3), 980–989.

Longo, V. D., Antebi, A., Bartke, A., Barzilai, N., Brown-Borg, H. M., Caruso, C., . . . Fontana, L. (2015). Interventions to slow aging in humans: Are we ready? *Aging Cell, 14*(4), 497–510.

López-Otín, C., Blasco, M. A., Partridge, L., Serrano, M., & Kroemer, G. (2013). The hallmarks of aging. *Cell, 153*(6), 1194–1217.

Mannick, J. B., Del Giudice, G., Lattanzi, M., Valiante, N. M., Praestgaard, J., Huang, B., . . . Klickstein, L. B. (2014). mTOR inhibition improves immune function in the elderly. *Science Translational Medicine, 6*(268), 268–279.

Medawar, P. (1952). *An unsolved problem in biology.* London, UK: H. K. Lewis.

Partridge, L., Gems, D., & Withers, D. J. (2005). Sex and death: What is the connection? *Cell, 120*(4), 461–472.

Tazearslan, C., Huang, J., Barzilai, N., & Suh, Y. (2011). Impaired IGF1R signaling in cells expressing longevity-associated human IGF1R alleles. *Aging Cell, 10*(3), 551–554.

Walker, D. W., McColl, G., Jenkins, N. L., Harris, J., & Lithgow, G. J. (2000). Evolution of lifespan in C. elegans. *Nature, 405*(6784), 296–297.

Weismann, A. (1889). *Essays on hereditary and kindred biological problems.* Oxford, UK: Clarendon Press.

Williams, G. C. (1957). Pleiotropy, natural selection and the evolution of senescence. *Evolution, 11,* 398–411.

CHAPTER 7

Evolutionary Theory and Aging
Devin Arbuthnott, Daniel E. L. Promislow, and Jacob A. Moorad

There is clear value in investigating the genetic, metabolic, and environmental mechanisms underlying processes of aging to understand *how* we age. However, to understand *why* we age, we must turn to evolutionary theories. In exploring the evolutionary mechanisms that may explain why aging arose or changed through time, empirical and theoretical biologists also gain an understanding of why different populations and species show such dramatic diversity in age-related processes. Therefore, evolutionary theories are fundamental to understanding the origin and diversity of aging processes in nature.

In this chapter, we first describe the fundamental evolutionary theories that seek to explain the presence of aging despite its apparent detrimental effects on individual *fitness* (see Box 7.1 for definitions of key terms) and explore key evidence and shortcomings of these theories. We then focus on the observed trade-offs between life span and reproduction, highlighting potential molecular mechanisms by which *selection* can fail to eliminate, or even promote, patterns of senescence. An underexplored avenue by which selection can act on aging, mate choice, and *sexual selection* will then be discussed leading to the development of a verbal model whereby mate choice could promote senescence as a by-product of honest sexual signaling. We finish this chapter by exploring how the described evolutionary theories pertain to human diseases, and identify the critical absence of some important evolutionary processes in the evolutionary theory of aging and disease. Together, these sections will provide an in-depth understanding of why species age, and implications on human aging.

■ EVOLUTIONARY THEORIES OF AGING

Although none would dispute the presence of aging in humans, a consensus regarding aging in natural populations of plants and animals has emerged only over the past few decades. From numerous field studies, it appears that the age-related declines in survival (actuarial senescence) and reproduction (fertility senescence) are common but not ubiquitous (Jones et al., 2014; Promislow, 1991). Moreover, there is tremendous variation in these patterns of demographic senescence across species. A major challenge to evolutionary theory is to explain both the genesis and the diversity of aging in the natural world.

More specifically, a fundamental goal for aging theory is to explain why, if natural selection favors optimal organismal function, aging does not simply evolve away? In fact, numerous models have been proposed to explain why aging has evolved. These

---

BOX 7.1 Definitions of Key Terms

Adaptation: The process by which populations increase mean fitness over time. An adaptive trait (or an adaptation) increases individual fitness in a particular environment or set of environments and may therefore become more prevalent in a population over evolutionary time.

Condition: The pool of available resources available to an individual. The efficiency with which individuals accumulate resources depends on the environment, genetics, and the fit of the individual in the environment (gene × environment interactions). The individual then allocates these limited resources to separate processes (e.g., somatic maintenance, resource acquisition, reproduction).

Condition dependence: A condition-dependent trait is any trait whose expression (presence or size) depends on the extent to which resources are allocated to it. Biologists often assess the condition dependence of a trait by measuring the expression of the trait when resources are readily available versus when resources are scarce.

Constraint: An evolutionary constraint alters the direction or tempo of evolutionary change away from that expected from the action of natural selection alone. A lack of heritable variation for a trait under selection would qualify as a constraint because the trait would not be free to evolve. Antagonistic pleiotropy represents another important form of constraint because negative genetic correlations between two traits under directional selection do not allow these traits to evolve independently of one another.

Fitness: The contribution of an individual or gene to future generations. A simple measure of individual fitness is the number of offspring it produces.

Natural selection: The association between properties, such as traits or gene frequencies, and fitness. When these properties are heritable, natural selection can lead to evolutionary changes. The evolutionary theory of aging shows that the strength of selection for age-specific characters declines. This means that at later ages, fitness is less influenced by variation in age-specific phenotypes.

Sexual selection: The component of natural selection that pertains to competition for reproductive opportunities. This includes competing with individuals of the same sex for potential mates and attracting potential mates.

---

can be classified broadly into three categories with differing perspectives on the adaptive role of aging (Figure 7.1):

1. Aging is an *adaptation*. Fitness is *increased* directly by senescence, and the association between aging and fitness is causal.
2. Aging is a *maladaption*. Aging is detrimental to fitness, but the selection is of insufficient strength to eliminate the spread of aging-related genes.
3. Aging is the result of *constraint*. The relationship between fitness and aging is not causal, but aging emerges as a by-product of selection.

Each evolutionary perspective has a long history, each with its supporters and critics.

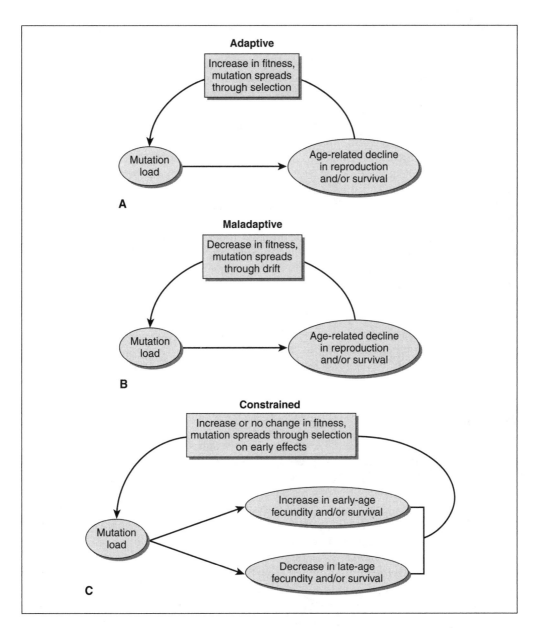

FIGURE 7.1   Conceptual models of three evolutionary theories of aging. (A) Under an adaptive model, mutations that increase rates of aging are favored by selection because they increase fitness. (B) Under a maladaptive model (Medawar's mutation accumulation), mutations that increase aging have spread through genetic drift, because late-acting mutations have little or no effect on fitness. (C) The constrained model (Williams's antagonistic pleiotropy) refers to genes that decrease or have no fitness effects late in life, but spread owing to their beneficial effects early in life.

Adaptation

An adaptive model of aging was perhaps the first articulated evolutionary perspective advocated in the post-Darwin 19th century. August Weismann (1889) suggested that because old individuals consume resources that might be put to better use by the young, natural selection will favor the death of the old. Fundamental to this perspective is the belief that selection works by maximizing the fitness of the group, not the individual. Weismann did not shy away from this viewpoint, arguing that "in regulating duration of life, the advantage of the species, and not the individual, is alone of any importance. This must be obvious to anyone who has once thoroughly thought out the process of natural selection" (Weismann, 1889, p. 10). In fact, the past half century has seen a great deal of thorough thinking on the subject of group selection in general (Okasha, 2006; Queller, 1992; Williams, 1966; Wilson, 1983), and while there is some disagreement on the relative importance of individual- and group-level selection to adaptive evolution, no serious evolutionary biologists would agree with Weismann that individual-level selection is unimportant.

A second problem is that under Weismann's model, the evolution of aging requires the preexistence of aging. Without this, the old are just as valuable to the fitness of the group as the young (and perhaps even more so if selection within cohorts weeds out the frail young before they can become the frail old), and there is no group benefit to be had by removing the old in favor of the young via aging. Although this model cannot explain the origin of senescence, there are situations in which competition and social dynamics can, in principle, shape aging patterns by modifying selection patterns. Competition for resources, for example, can increase aging rates in populations where competing individuals are related to one another (e.g., in families; e.g., Ronce & Promislow, 2010). In contrast, when care or resources are transferred from the old to the young in such populations, selection may favor the evolution of slower aging (e.g., Lee, 2003).

Maladaptation

Although aging cannot evolve de novo directly from adaptation, it can arise from maladaptation. The first influential suggestion of this mechanism is usually attributed to Peter Medawar (1948, 1952), who recognized that the strength of selection for traits that are expressed at specific ages must decrease with increasing age. According to Medawar, provided that a "genetic disaster" (what we might now call a "mutation," specifically a "heritable germ-line mutation") had an effect that became manifest at some late age, selection would be unable to act efficaciously to remove the mutation from the population because late age survival and fertility have little effect on fitness. On the other hand, an early acting deleterious mutation can have a devastating effect on fitness, and selection will act strongly to eliminate it. This is because older individuals have relatively little potential to contribute to the next generation. So long as mutational effects on survival and fertility have some age specificity and the frequencies with which early- and late-acting mutations arise are not too different, over time, the relatively weak selection at late age leads to a situation in which there are more deleterious effects expressed at late age than at early age. In this way, relaxed selection leads to the evolution of aging. Because the buildup of deleterious mutations plays a key role in this mechanism, this is often called the "mutation accumulation" model, or simply MA. Unlike adaptive theories of aging, MA simply hypothesizes that selection is unable to remove aging, rather than selecting directly for it.

Another important distinction between MA and adaptive aging is that the former does not invoke any form of group selection, thereby releasing the evolution of aging from any sort of requirement of kinship or social dynamics. This makes it capable of explaining aging under more general conditions. Another difference is that MA is capable of explaining the evolution of aging from nonaging, meaning that it is sufficient to account for the evolutionary origins of aging. The MA model requires that selection decline with age; Medawar asserts that this is true, but this remained unproven until Hamilton (1966) showed it to be fact. Finally, a key assumption of the MA model is that the effects of at least some mutations are age specific. This last assumption is an empirical issue that has been addressed by a variety of experimental approaches. For example, studies have maintained separate lineages of flies in a regime that eliminates selection, allowing deleterious germ-line mutations with age-specific effects to accumulate (Houle et al., 1994; Pletcher, Houle, & Curtsinger, 1998; Yampolsky, Pearse, & Promislow, 2001). Other studies have estimated age-related changes in genetic variance in natural and laboratory populations (e.g., Charmantier, Perrins, McCleery, & Sheldon, 2006; Promislow, Tatar, Khazaeli, & Curtsinger et al., 1996). In general, these studies present strong evidence for age specificity of mutational effects.

Constraint

Although MA views aging as the result of purely maladaptive processes, the *antagonistic pleiotropy*, or AP, model imagines that senescence is an unfortunate by-product of adaptive processes. Williams introduced such a model in 1957 (Williams, 1957), agreeing with Medawar's assertion that the force of natural selection is attenuated with age, but using this point to argue that genes with early benefit, such as might be delivered by increased reproduction early in life, could spread through a population even if these genes had deleterious late-life effects. Conversely, genes with late-life benefit and early-life costs would be under strong purifying selection to be purged from populations. Williams suggested from this selective asymmetry that the existence of genes characterized by among-age trade-offs will lead to the evolution of aging. The disposable soma theory (Kirkwood, 1977, 1990) is a well-known application of the AP model that emphasizes resource trade-offs between investment in early performance and maintenance. It is an AP model because the nature of the fitness trade-off is separated in time: early reproduction and late survival. However, the disposable soma theory adds to AP by specifying mechanisms underlying the trade-off that are absent in Williams's development of AP.

AP is often characterized as exemplifying an adaptive theory of aging, but this is not correct, as it is not aging per se that increases fitness. In this model, aging is seen as a maladaptive late-life by-product that is associated with a more powerful adaptive change manifested early in life. Aging is indirectly selected for, but only for as long as the constraint remains. The AP gene will be eliminated by natural selection if an alternate allele becomes available that causes the early benefit without the later cost. Like the MA model, AP requires that selection becomes weaker with age, but the difference between models lies in their genetic requirements. AP assumes that genes exist that increase fitness in the young and decrease it in the old. MA requires that genes exist that are more deleterious at old age than at young age. Clearly, it is possible that a mutation can exhibit both qualities, and its contribution to aging could be reasonably assigned to either mechanism. Consider, for example, a gene that contributes to a trade-off that increases early fertility at the cost of late survival, but the late cost is so devastating compared to its weak effect on early fertility that the gene is under negative selection. This gene contributes to senescence, but it persists only through mutational pressure.

■ MODELS MEET THEORY

Early models of MA and AP argued, largely through intuition, that the force of selection should decrease with age, but a formal proof of this assertion had to wait until the mid-1960s. In 1957, Williams suggested that the strength of age-specific selection was proportional to the cumulative probability of survival to that age (Williams, 1957). This led him to suggest that age-independent sources of mortality, or more specifically, *extrinsic mortality*, was a major force in determining the patterns of age-related selection that would shape how aging evolved. However, although it is obvious that less mortality means longer life, it is not true that less age-independent mortality means more *selection* for longer life. It has been understood by theoreticians for more than 20 years that Williams's conjecture is a fallacy (see further discussion). Nevertheless, it has been hugely influential among those who study the evolution of aging even to the present day.

In 1966, Hamilton derived the first formal description of the strength of selection acting to increase age-specific survival and fertility (Hamilton, 1966). In doing so, he provided a sound foundation for the evolutionary theory of aging by showing that selection for vital rates (age-specific survival and fertility) *must* decline with age. Specifically, he showed that age-specific fertility selection was proportional to the product of cumulative survival and a population growth factor; this quantity begins to decline from birth and reaches zero at the last possible age represented in the population. Selection for age-specific survival (or more accurately, selection *against* age-specific mortality) is proportional to the product of cumulative survival and the expected fitness benefit associated with survival at that age. The strength of this selection is at a constant maximum at all preadult ages up to the first age of reproduction, when it begins an irreversible decline and disappears entirely at the last age of reproduction.

Hamilton's derivations can be interpreted in two ways. The first is an axiomatic description of the strength of selection acting to increase vital rates. Although it is important to remember that natural selection is only one component of evolution, this interpretation is remarkably profound and useful. For example, Abrams (1993) and Caswell (2007) demonstrated that the addition of age-independent extrinsic mortality has the effect of decreasing cumulative survival by the same fraction as it increases reproductive value, and for this reason Hamilton's derivations prove that, counter to Williams's conjecture, age-independent mortality cannot alter selection against longevity.

The second way to interpret Hamilton's contribution is to make certain simplifying assumptions about the nature of gene effects and to then project these onto his descriptions of selection in order to model evolutionary end points. In perhaps the best-known population genetic model of senescence, Charlesworth (1994, 2001) assumes linear relationships between the load of deleterious, age-specific mutations, and age-specific mortality to predict that, at an evolutionary equilibrium between the generation of new mutations and selection, the following characteristics of mortality trajectories should evolve: (a) minimal and constant mortality rates at ages up to the first age of reproduction, at which point senescence is first manifested; (b) an increase in mortality rates throughout the reproductive ages; and (c) a "wall-of-death" at the last age of reproduction as mortality mutations are free to accumulate without removal by natural selection. Although such models provide us with valuable confirmation that senescence can evolve by an age-related decline in natural selection, real mortality trajectories can look quite different. Observed patterns of mortality suggest the need for more elaborate models. Three specific departures of mortality trajectories from Charlesworth's models that are occasionally observed are: (a) elevated juvenile mortality; (b) postreproductive survival in some species, including humans; and (c) a late-life deceleration of mortality rates. These features have been explained by relaxing Charlesworth's genetic assumptions in numerous ways. These modifications include nonlinear relationships between mutational load and mortality (Baudisch, 2005), positive phenotypic (Vaupel & Yashin, 1985) and genetic (Charlesworth, 2001) correlations among survival at different ages; age-specific distributions of de novo mutational effects (Moorad & Promislow, 2008); and positive genetic correlations between parental or grandparental care and offspring survival (Lee, 2003).

■ REPRODUCTION AND AGING

Researchers have long recognized that there is an apparent trade-off between reproduction and longevity. In both birds and mammals, long-lived species generally have low fecundity (Holmes et al., 2001; Read & Harvey, 1989). Furthermore, many mutations that increase longevity are accompanied by a decrease in reproductive potential (fecundity and/or fertility) in the nematode *Caenorhabditis elegans* (e.g., insulin-signaling mutations), the fruit fly *Drosophila melanogaster* (e.g., *chico* and mutations in insulin receptor [InR]), and mice (e.g., Snell dwarf mice and little, reviewed in Partridge, Gems, & Withers, 2005a). But what is it about reproduction that decreases life span, or vice versa? Theoretical and empirical work has attempted to disentangle the relationship between these two essential life history components, and whether they trade off directly, or if the two can act independently. Many past researchers have suggested direct links between reproduction and aging, such as resource allocation and gamete production. However, recent work has suggested that the two may be independently affected by common pathways, or that it may not be reproduction at all that decreases life span, but rather the perception of the potential for future reproduction.

The most discussed and accepted model regarding the trade-off between reproduction and life span is the so-called Y-model (de Jong & van Noordwijk, 1992; Roff & Fairbairn, 2007; van Noordwijk & Jong, 1986), in which individuals have limited resources to partition between different life-history traits. Individuals can dedicate some of their limited resources toward energetically costly components of reproduction (e.g., searching and/or competing for mates, mating, gamete production, offspring provisioning), but these resources are then lost to processes of somatic maintenance and repair. As a result, the more the resources are directed toward reproduction, the fewer are available for somatic maintenance and repair, and life span is reduced as a consequence. As such, the Y-model can illustrate the disposable soma theory. The Y-model has often been used to explain patterns of increased life span under diet restriction, with the assumption that resource partitioning is dynamic and plastic. Specifically, many have suggested that when resources are scarce, individuals dedicate their few resources toward somatic maintenance in the hopes that they will survive to reproduce later, while in times of plenty individuals dedicate more of their resources to the short-term gain of reproduction (de Jong & van Noordwijk, 1992; Zera & Harshman, 2001).

However, as pointed out by Reznick, Nunney, and Tessier (2000), such life-history trade-offs are expected under the Y-model only if the genetic variance for resource allocation is greater than the genetic variance for resource acquisition. If there is a great deal of variance among individuals in the ability to acquire resources, then those individuals with the most resources will have more to allocate toward both reproduction and somatic maintenance. Therefore, under this scenario, there would be a positive correlation between reproduction and life span reflecting resource acquisition ability. However, if all individuals were approximately equal in their ability to gain resources, but vary in their partitioning of these resources between reproductive versus nonreproductive processes, then the widespread trade-off between reproduction and life span would be observed. Natural selection may favor resource acquisition ability to a greater extent than particular resource partitioning strategies, which over time would decrease genetic variance for resource acquisition below the variance for resource partitioning, in turn leading to a transition from a positive to a negative correlation between reproduction and life span (Figure 7.2).

What are the energetically costly components of reproduction that directly take resources away from somatic maintenance? Van Voorhies (1992) suggested that it was gamete production, as mating decreased male life span in *C. elegans*, but this mating-induced decrease disappeared in mutants with defective sperm production. However, Gems and Riddle (1996) were unable to repeat this result, and found that mating to either wildtype or spermless males decreased hermaphrodite longevity, suggesting that it is mating, rather than gamete production, that is costly. This could be inferred because hermaphroditic worms can produce offspring directly or by mating males. In fact, costly sexual interactions leading to decreases in longevity have been found in numerous species. In the fruit fly, males use harmful courtship and harassment to induce females to mate (Long, Pischedda, Stewart, & Rice, 2009) and also transfer manipulative sperm proteins (Chapman, 2001), which work together to accelerate aging in mated females (Edward, Fricke, Gerrard, & Chapman, 2011; Fowler

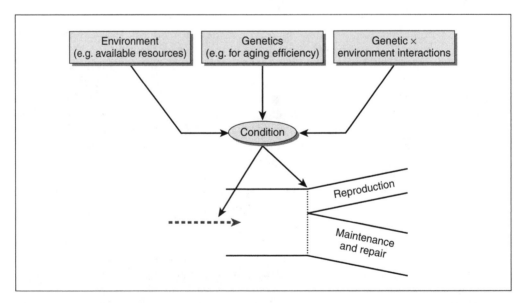

FIGURE 7.2 Y-model of condition dependence. Individuals acquire resources at a rate based on the environment and each individual's genotype-dependent fitness in that environment. The total pool of available resources determines an individual's condition. Condition, in turn, will influence the ability of an individual to acquire resources (dashed arrow) and the way in which that individual will choose to allocate limited resources to activities relating to reproduction or somatic maintenance and repair (dotted line). Using resources for reproduction depletes the resources available for somatic maintenance (and vice versa), which may speed senescence.

and Partridge, 1989; Partridge & Fowler, 1990). In the worm *C. elegans*, mating causes hermaphrodites to shrivel and die sooner, while unmated hermaphrodites continue to grow (Shi & Murphy, 2014).

However, although there is a general trend for longevity to trade-off with reproductive potential, several pieces of evidence suggest that the two life history components might not be directly linked. First, a number of mutations that affect longevity do not influence fecundity, such as the age-1 and daf-2 mutations in *C. elegans* (but see Jenkins, McColl, & Lithgow, 2004; Walker, McColl, Jenkins, Harris, & Lithgow, 2000), and overexpression of Forkhead box type O (dFOXO) in head fat in *D. melanogaster* (Partridge et al., 2005a). Second, although experimental selection for late-life reproduction in *D. melanogaster* initially led to a simultaneous increase in longevity and decrease in early-life reproduction, this trade-off disappeared after 10 years of selection (Leroi, Chippindale, & Rose, 1994). Lastly, Dillin, Crawford, and Kenyon (2002) manipulated insulin signaling in *C. elegans* at different life stages and found that decreasing insulin-signaling activity increased longevity regardless of the time of manipulation, while decreasing insulin-signaling activity only decreased reproduction if it was manipulated at hatching and not later in life. These three lines of evidence suggest that, though longevity and reproduction may be influenced by similar molecular pathways, the effects of these pathways on these two distinct life history components may be separate.

Recent work has also suggested that it may not be reproduction per se that trades off with longevity but instead the perception of reproductive opportunities. Gendron et al. (2013) exposed fruit flies to the scent of either same sex or different sex flies while preventing mating and interactions with different-sex individuals. Surprisingly, those individuals exposed to the smell of opposite-sex individuals showed decreased life span and decreased starvation resistance, even though these individuals did not actually mate or reproduce. Therefore, at least in this species, it does not appear to simply be reproduction that leads directly to a decrease in life span but an investment in reproductive products and activities brought on by the perception of reproduction that decreased longevity.

Sexual Selection and the Evolution of Senescence

In addition to the proximate trade-offs between reproduction and somatic maintenance, there are also potential evolutionary connections between reproduction and aging that may contribute to the origin and diversity of senescence. These evolutionary connections relate to an often-overlooked component of reproduction with respect to aging: sexual selection (Bonduriansky, Maklakov, Zajitschek, & Brooks, 2008). When originally formulating the concept of natural selection, Darwin (1859, 1871) already recognized the important difference between traits that affect survival and those that affect individuals' ability to mate and produce offspring. Today, sexual selection is seen as a subcategory of natural selection pertaining only to traits that influence individuals' ability to compete with same-sex competitors (e.g., male–male competitions over limited females) and/or attract potential mates in sexual species (Andersson, 1994). It has long been recognized that traits that increase sexual fitness (e.g., colorful plumage, large antlers, elaborate courtship behaviors) can decrease nonsexual fitness through energetic costs or by increasing mortality risks, for example by making individuals easier targets for predators (Andersson, 1994).

Because reproductive opportunities and the intensity of competition for mates often differ between males and females, mating systems and sexual selection can lead to divergent life-history strategies between the sexes (Bonduriansky et al., 2008). This often manifests as sexual dimorphism in longevity, with active but short-lived males and longer lived females in most sexual species. The theoretical underpinnings between sexual selection and sexual dimorphism in patterns of aging are explored in the evolutionary literature (Bonduriansky et al., 2008; Maklakov, Fricke, & Arnqvist, 2007; Maklakov & Lummaa, 2013; Promislow, 2003), so we instead focus on the less-discussed mechanisms by which sexual selection might alter patterns of aging in general as well as generate species-level divergence in aging. We focus on two ways in which sexual selection and associated exaggerated traits could affect patterns of aging. First, such traits can influence age-specific adult mortality rates directly, altering the age-distribution of the population and thus affecting the strength of selection against late-acting deleterious mutations. Second, the evolution of mate choice could indirectly select for aging by favoring traits that divert resources away from somatic maintenance and toward traits that enhance mating success (condition-dependent sexual selection).

Sexual Selection and Mortality

Traits used for sexual competition and attraction are famously conspicuous and include many of the most striking traits that we observe in nature, such as bird song, colorful plumage, and elaborate mating dances. However, these traits also attract the attention of predators and competitors; those individuals with the most conspicuous displays are at a greater risk of being seen by predators or challenged by same-sex competitors. For example, female Trinidadian guppies (*Poecilia reticulata*) are attracted to males with large orange spots (Endler & Houde, 1995 ; Houde, 1987). However, such coloration also makes sexually mature males more visible to predators and therefore increases mortality risk among adults (Endler, 1980).

Similarly, males with large weapons (e.g., antlers) or badges of status are challenged more often than lower status males by intraspecific males, and these challenges can lead to injury as well as great energy expenditure. For example, in red-winged blackbirds (*Agelaius phoeniceus*), males possess red "epaulets" on their wings that males use in territorial displays (Searcy & Yasukawa, 1983). When Hansen and Rohwer (1986) experimentally made these red marking larger or smaller in bird dummies, they found that competitor males were more likely to attack males with larger markings than control males or males with reduced markings. Therefore, conspicuous sexual traits can lead to injury from competitors or death via predators and subsequently increase adult mortality risk, which sets the stage for the evolutionary mechanisms of aging described earlier. If possessing elaborate sexual traits decreases the probability of surviving to old age, this decreases the effectiveness of selection against late-acting deleterious mutations. Thus, elaborate sexually dimorphic traits can increase rates of aging both through mutation accumulation and antagonistic pleiotropy.

Such increases in mortality risk raise the question as to why individuals have exaggerated sexual traits at all, rather than staying inconspicuous and surviving longer. It is important to remember that the ultimate measure of an individual's fitness is its contributions to future generations. If an individual can attract more or better mates, this represents an evolutionary advantage, even if it comes at the cost of greater mortality risk and an earlier death. Under this scenario, more offspring inherit both the attractive individuals' exaggerated traits and their increased mortality risk. These traits coevolve with decreased longevity when the fitness dividends associated with more reproductive opportunities outweigh the fitness costs associated with the additional mortality.

Condition Dependence

The majority of evolutionary models of aging assume that all individuals are equally susceptible to mortality within a population. However, as pointed out by Williams and Day (2003), the physiological *condition* of an individual greatly influences his or her susceptibility to mortality. Using mathematical models, Williams and Day showed that including condition-dependent mortality risk can increase overall susceptibility to extrinsic mortality and weaken selection against senescence. However, the particular interactions between condition and fitness gains and mortality can have a great impact on the evolution of aging.

Many of the elaborate traits that individuals use to attract mates and face sexual competitors are costly to produce, making sexual selection a potential mechanism generating condition-dependent traits that affect the evolution of aging. Bright plumage can require individuals to gather excess pigment molecules, and large weapons and courtship behavior often require large amounts of energy to produce (Andersson, 1994). Because these traits often require significant resources, only individuals who are able to gather and efficiently use sufficient resources are able to effectively compete for potential mates. Therefore, these traits often signal an individual's genetic or developmental condition (i.e., are condition dependent).

The preponderance of such costly sexual traits led Zahavi (1975) to propose that individuals found these traits attractive precisely because they are costly to produce; individuals who are able to overcome the handicap of producing and surviving with large and conspicuous traits must have the genes necessary to overcome such obstacles (i.e., are of high genetic quality). Therefore, if females choose to mate with males with exaggerated traits, then their offspring would inherit these "good genes," and increase not only their offspring's survival, but also their offspring's ability to attract mates. Though Zahavi initially framed this handicap hypothesis in terms of surviving with large conspicuous traits, it can be extended to overcoming the costs of producing such traits, allowing individuals to choose mates based on genetic quality (Iwasa, Pomiankowski, & Nee, 1991; Rowe & Houle, 1996). Subsequently, mathematical models and simulations demonstrated that mate preferences might evolve specifically to target condition-dependent display traits, even when such preferences are costly (Pomiankowski, Iwasa, & Nee, 1991; Price, Schluter, & Heckman, 1993; Schluter & Price, 1993). If mating with individuals in good condition confers even slight genetic benefits to offspring, then preferences should consistently evolve to target those traits that most honestly signal condition (Schluter & Price, 1993). For example, in dung beetles, females prefer to mate with males with high courtship rates, and well-fed males are better able to maintain high courtship rates than starved males (Kotiaho, 2001). Furthermore, both courtship rate and condition (mass divided by physical size) are heritable, showing that females choosing to mate with high-condition males are passing on advantageous genes to their offspring.

Therefore, given that preference for condition-dependent traits can evolve in many sexual species, target sexual traits can become more exaggerated through time as preference for these exaggerated traits increases. As discussed in the previous section, however, there are often antagonistic relationships between reproduction and somatic maintenance, and this is the case with the exaggeration of many condition-dependent sexual traits. For example, male field crickets fed excess protein increase their mate-calling effort, but show decreases in longevity (Hunt et al., 2004). Furthermore, the well-fed males lost a greater percentage of their weight after each calling bout than protein-limited males, which suggests that under good conditions, males invest so heavily in reproduction that they die sooner than low condition males (Hunt et al., 2004). In fact, decreasing protein alone often leads to decreases in fertility and increases in longevity (see previous section; Ja et al., 2009; Mair, Piper, & Partridge, 2005; Simpson & Raubenheimer, 2009). It may be that being in good condition generally leads to a higher proportional investment in mate attraction and reproduction, potentially explaining an important component of the extension of life span via dietary restriction. If mate preferences for costly traits demand that individuals invest proportionally more in mate signaling, which in turn leads to shorter life span, it is possible that individuals that are attractive and die young will outcompete any long-lived individuals with low mating and reproductive rates.

■ A MOLECULAR LINK BETWEEN CONDITION-DEPENDENT TRAITS AND AGING

Theoreticians have raised the issue that cheating could undermine the potential of condition dependence as a mechanism for sexual selection (Schluter & Price, 1993; Warren, Gotoh, Dworkin, Emlen, & Lavine, 2013). If a previously honest indicator becomes dishonest ("cheaters" are present), then females gain nothing from mating with elaborate signalers, and selection for such a preference would disappear. One general mechanism to keep traits honest is for preferences to target traits that are directly linked to metabolic pathways integral to other physiological functions (Hill, 2011; Warren, Gotoh, Dworkin, Emlen, & Lavine, 2013). Under this scenario, when individuals are in good condition (e.g., when resources are plentiful), they direct available resources to the physiological processes that are antagonistic with somatic maintenance. Such a trade-off under favorable conditions could potentially contribute to the increases in longevity seen in several species that are kept under diet restriction versus *ad libidum* conditions (e.g., Colman et al., 2009; Partridge, Piper, & Mair, 2005b; Schulz et al., 2007; Weindruch & Walford, 1982).

A series of recent studies propose a general molecular mechanism that directly links sexual selection with aging via the insulin and insulin-like signaling (IIS) pathway. The IIS pathway is highly conserved across animals and controls cell growth and division. IIS levels have been shown to affect such sexual traits as antler size in deer, the tail of swordtail fish, and horns in several beetle species (reviewed in Warren et al., 2013), and can also have large impacts on longevity and senescence, such that downregulation of insulin signaling extends life span and slows aging in a wide range of species, although such changes are often accompanied by decreases in fertility or reproductive rate (Tatar, Bartke, & Antebi, 2003; Toivonen & Partridge, 2009).

Work in two insect examples have suggested that sexual selection and IIS are directly connected. First, in *D. melanogaster* and other insect species, individuals use chemical signals called "cuticular hydrocarbons" (CHCs) to signal to and assess potential mates (Ferveur, 2005; Jallon, 1984). *D. melanogaster*'s CHCs change with age and become less attractive as individuals grow older (Kuo et al., 2012a). Kuo et al. (2012b) also showed that females with a less active mutant Insulin Receptor (InR) live longer, but have CHCs that resemble those of old females. Furthermore, the downregulation of InR in wild-type females made these females "smell" old and decreased their attractiveness, whereas upregulation made females more attractive to males. Therefore, downregulation of insulin gives females a "young" phenotype with respect to survival and longevity, but an "old" phenotype with respect to attractiveness and low fecundity. Second, in the rhinoceros beetle, males use large horns to compete with other males over mates (Emlen,

2000). These horns have been shown to be exceptionally condition dependent (relative to other traits), such that horn size could range from small bumps up to two thirds of the male's body length, depending on developmental nutrition (Emlen, Warren, Johns, Dworkin, & Lavine, 2012). Emlen et al. (2012) hypothesized that the mechanism by which these horns evolved condition dependence was by evolving a highly trait-specific insulin sensitivity. To test this idea, the authors disrupted the InR in different body parts, and found that InR disruption decreased horn size 16% overall, while genitalia and wing size changed only 0% and 2% (respectively) under this treatment. Both of these insect examples confirm a link between IIS and sexual signals, demonstrating the maintenance of honest and unfakeable signals by pairing these signals with essential developmental pathways.

Warren et al. (2013) reviewed these ideas and other relevant data, and proposed that the insulin-signaling pathway acts as a general molecular link between condition and mate choice across the animal kingdom, as IIS plays a role in the development of sexual traits in a wide range of organisms. Also, because insulin signaling acts as a direct link between resource use and attractiveness, mate choice for exaggerated traits can indirectly select for increased insulin signaling and allow mates to directly assess attractiveness based on genetic and environmental "quality" via the resources available to the individual.

Testosterone

Another potentially important system linking sexual traits and somatic condition in vertebrates is that of testosterone. Testosterone often increases sexual competitiveness in males of many species, such as through increasing aggression or dominance signaling, but it impairs immune function (Folstad & Karter, 1992). Therefore, sexual traits may trade-off with immunity in vertebrates. Because of this trade-off (through testosterone or other mechanisms), Hamilton and Zuk (1982) proposed that only males without parasites or disease should be able to display exaggerated traits and outcompete other males. Therefore, females, by choosing the males with the most elaborate displays or defenses, may be choosing to mate with males that are in good health and without parasites. In their "immunocompetence handicap" theory, Folstad and Karter (1992) more generally suggested that those males with elaborate displays are in better health or genetically better equipped to fight infections and parasites. Therefore, by favoring traits that trade-off with immune function, females may be choosing to mate with healthier or genetically superior males, increasing their own fitness or that of their offspring.

In line with the immunocompetence handicap, several recent studies in dogs suggest that sterilized pet dogs live longer and have reduced levels of death due to infectious disease (Hoffman, Creevy, & Promislow, 2013). Interestingly, a similar pattern was described in 19th-century Korean eunuchs (Min, Lee, & Park, 2012).

Sexual Antagonistic Pleiotropy and Aging

Overall, to increase reproductive success, selection may favor changes in pathways that shunt resources away from somatic maintenance and toward reproductive signaling. Similarly, selection may act to favor individuals with mate preferences that target traits that are condition dependent and trade off with somatic maintenance. As a result, there would be direct selection for the exaggeration of such traits in order to increase attractiveness and competitiveness, which may indirectly select for senescence. This represents a form of antagonistic pleiotropy, and because the antagonism is between sexual function and somatic maintenance, it is similar to the disposable soma theory (Kirkwood, 1977; Kirkwood & Holliday, 1979). The strength of sexual selection and competition may therefore determine the indirect selection on senescence and contribute to the variation and patterns of aging among populations and species.

Although consistent with current data, the hypothesis that condition-dependent mate choice has indirectly selected for increased aging has yet to be tested directly. Estimates of the genetic covariance between insulin signaling, condition-dependent attractiveness, mate choice, and rates of senescence would bolster this hypothesis, and one way to assess this possibility directly is through experimental evolution. For example, one could alter the strength of sexual selection in a system (such as by reducing male–female interactions) in species with known connections between insulin sensitivity and sexual signaling, such as rhinoceros beetles or *D. melanogaster*. Over time, if costly traits do not offer reproductive advantages (as would be the case under reduced sexual interactions), then the insulin sensitivity of sexual traits should decrease. If this is observed, then evolutionary connections between insulin sensitivity and patterns of senescence could be measured. Such experiments and data would contribute greatly to our understanding of the selective forces that have shaped variation in patterns of aging both within and among species.

■ GENETIC TESTS OF EVOLUTIONARY THEORIES OF AGING IN HUMAN POPULATIONS

It has been well over 60 years since Medawar's (1946, 1952) and Williams's (1957) groundbreaking insights into the evolutionary forces that can give rise to senescence. The veracity of these models is axiomatic—given an age-structured population and alleles with late-acting deleterious effects, senescence will evolve. Laboratory studies have established the existence of novel deleterious mutations with effects limited to later ages (Pletcher et al., 1998; Yampolsky et al., 2001), and have identified large numbers of genes with major effects on longevity (discussed throughout this book), some of which are conserved over evolutionary timescales (Fontana, Partridge, & Longo, 2010). Our goal here is to review evidence for genes that account for natural variation in mortality risk in human populations, and place these in the context of existing evolutionary theories of aging.

Recent conceptual and technological advances—the sequencing of the human genome and next generation sequencing in particular—now make it possible to identify individual genes associated with age-related morbidity and mortality and potentially to determine whether MA or AP have shaped their evolution. Until now, most discussions of genetic evidence for MA versus AP have focused on quantitative genetic studies of aging. Rather than trying to identify individual genes that affect longevity, quantitative genetic studies provide statistical measures of the degree to which patterns of variation and covariation within and among traits can be explained by heritable genetic factors. Theoreticians have pointed to specific quantitative genetic predictions generated by MA versus AP, and empirical researchers have applied these predictions to lab and field populations. However, as Moorad and Promislow (2009) have pointed out, the theoretical predictions are not straightforward, and in some cases, one cannot distinguish MA from AP based on age-specific patterns of genetic variances and covariances or genetic inbreeding depression. In this light, we focus on traits with single-locus, Mendelian effects, where the predictions are clearer.

Mutation Accumulation

The first and perhaps most famous example in the literature of a "mutation accumulation" gene predates Medawar's papers, and likely stimulated Medawar to develop his theory in the first place. In the early 1930s, Julia Bell established that Huntington's disease (HD) was caused by a single dominant mutation. J. B. S. Haldane, being familiar with Bell's groundbreaking work on the inheritance and etiology of neurological disorders, noted that "the age of onset is a valuable index of the selective disadvantage of the gene" (Haldane, 1941, p. 149). A few years later, citing Bell and Haldane, Medawar pointed directly to HD as a clear example of a gene associated with aging, whose natural frequency rose due to the forces of MA (i.e., the age-related relaxation of selection; Medawar, 1957, pp. 66–67). Although several authors have suggested that the HD allele might be associated with a benefit of high early fecundity, the evidence in support of this hypothesis is decidedly mixed (Albin, 1994).

Whether there are other possible benefits to HD carriers is a topic we come back to in the following section. But the challenge we face in defining an allele as being shaped by MA is that the absence of evidence (for AP effects) is not evidence of absence (as shown, e.g., by Jenkins et al.'s [2004] refutation of the *daf-2* gene in worms having no trade-off). Given the multifaceted ways in which a gene might act, we might consider late-acting deleterious genes as MA genes only insofar as they have not yet been shown to have pleiotropic trade-offs with any early-life traits.

In our search for aging-related genes that are truly shaped by MA, we could consider mitochondrial mutations as particularly good candidates. As we explained in the opening section of this chapter, all loci are subject to the age-related decline in the force of natural selection. However, the rate of decline and efficiency of selection to remove deleterious mutations can vary from gene to gene. Neiman and Taylor (2009) argue that mitochondria should be enriched for age-related mutations. As haploid, uniparentally inherited organelles, they have lower effective population size (N_e) than nuclear-encoded genes. As N_e declines, so too does the ability of selection to purge deleterious alleles. Given the very small number of protein-coding genes in the mitochondria compared to nuclear genes, the low N_e of mitochondria could explain the high number of mitochondrial DNA (mtDNA) mutations known to be associated with human diseases (Taylor & Turnbull, 2005), including aging-related diseases (Wallace, 2005). However, here too, there is a growing literature pointing to AP selecting for high frequency of disease-associated mitochondrial haplotypes (Ballard & Pichaud, 2014). Further studies—both theoretical and empirical—are needed to determine whether mitochondria are truly hotspots for aging-related mutations.

Antagonistic Pleiotropy

Williams's (1957) landmark paper on the evolution of senescence made no reference to specific disease-associated genes, other than a few visible markers in *Drosophila*. With few exceptions, evolutionary studies of Williams's theory have focused either on phenotypic correlations, quantitative genetic studies (including artificial selection), or tests of the effect of extrinsic mortality on aging (but see our earlier critique of this latter hypothesis). Negative phenotypic correlations between early-age and late-age traits or longevity, not only within but even between species (Promislow, 1995), have often been put forward as evidence of AP.

Among the evidence for antagonistic pleiotropy in human populations, we can distinguish three general categories—correlations between traits measured in the absence of genetic information, quantitative genetic correlations without knowledge of specific genes, and identification of specific pleiotropic genes. In the first case, the fact that two traits are correlated at the phenotypic level does not prove that the correlation is due to an underlying gene with AP effects. For example, the human demographic transition (Borgerhoff Mulder, 1998) that occurred following the Industrial Revolution led to a dramatic decrease in fecundity coupled with an equally dramatic and simultaneous increase in longevity. However, these changes are clearly a result of environmental rather than genetic changes. One recent intriguing study found that high birth weight— putatively associated with high fitness—is associated with an increased risk of various cancers (Thomas et al., 2004, 2012). However, this relationship was based on correlations across countries. Wealthy countries tend to have relatively high birth weight and relatively high cancer rates, but whether the correlation has any causal link is unproven. Clearly, environmental factors are among the most important determinants of health span and life span in human populations, but without evidence of an underlying genetic basis, these correlations tell us little about the role of AP in the evolution of aging (Reznick, 1985).

With that in mind, many studies have turned to quantitative genetic studies of age-specific fitness traits. For example, pedigree studies of preindustrial Finnish populations found no evidence for genetic trade-offs between early-age and late-age fecundity (Pettay, Charmantier, Wilson, & Lummaa, 2008), and it found *positive* genetic correlations between age at first reproduction and longevity (Pettay et al., 2008). Whether we can use these genetic correlations to distinguish MA from AP is somewhat controversial. Starting with Michael Rose's groundbreaking work (Rose & Charlesworth, 1980), selection experiments have offered generally strong evidence for negative genetic correlations between early-age and late-age fitness components. At the same time, theoretical treatments have pointed to other quantitative genetic predictions that distinguish MA from AP (Charlesworth & Hughes, 1996; Hughes & Charlesworth, 1994)—predictions that have been tested in both lab and field. However, our own theoretical efforts suggest that these various predictions might not distinguish MA from AP after all (Moorad & Promislow, 2009).

In this light, we turn to molecular genetic tests of the AP theory. Setting age aside, the strongest examples of AP come from studies of congenital diseases and their association with infectious disease. Carriers of the sickle cell allele are resistant to malaria, and more recently it has been shown that those with a single copy of the cystic fibrosis mutation (CFTR) are resistant to typhoid fever (van de Vosse et al., 2005).

Studies of pleiotropy in age-related disease are less clear at this point, but no less intriguing. For example, the BRCA1 mutation is associated with very high rates of breast and ovarian cancer (Friedman et al., 1994). Whereas some have argued that BRCA1 is under positive selection (Huttley et al., 2000), others have argued that it is under negative selection (Pavard & Metcalf, 2007). One recent study from women in the Utah Population Database suggests that carriers of BRCA1 tend to have higher fertility (Smith, Hanson, Mineau, & Buys, 2012).

The molecular basis of such relationships is unknown. However, work by Campisi (2005, 2013) suggests a possible mechanism for a negative relationship between risks of cancer and cellular senescence, mediated at least in part by p53. Campisi argues that cellular senescence, which has evolved at least in part as an anticancer mechanism, can at the same time give rise to age-related pathologies unrelated to cancer. Thus, the very mechanism that has evolved to fight cancer might do so at the expense of increased aging.

Among the most intriguing examples of AP are recent findings of alleles that increase the risk of various neurodegenerative diseases, including those that occur later in life (HD, Parkinson's disease [PD], and Alzheimer's disease [AD]), but confer some fitness benefits. We previously mentioned the case of HD, which Medawar considered a canonical example of a trait that arose due to MA. Subsequent studies suggested that HD might actually be an AP gene, conferring increased fertility, though the data in support of this hypothesis are questionable (reviewed in Albin, 1994). Interestingly, genes associated with HD, PD, and AD (Ou et al., 2013; Plun-Favreau, Lewis, Hardy, Martins, & Wood, 2010; Sorensen, Fenger, & Olsen, 1999) as well as some rarer polyglutamine neurodegenerative diseases (Ji, Sundquist, & Sundquist, 2012) are now being found to have putative anticancer effects.

The primary focus of studies on AP genes has been on age-related reproduction and survival—traits directly related to evolutionary fitness (Fisher, 1930). At least some of the trade-offs shaped by AP might involve traits only indirectly related to fitness, but of great interest nonetheless. The case of AD is particularly interesting. Consider the ApoE ε4 allele, which increases the risk of AD and mortality, and is found at frequencies of up to 30% (Genin et al., 2011). In contrast, the HD allele is typically found at a frequency of less than 0.01% (less than 1 in 10,000). Given very late age at onset in most cases of AD, the evolutionary fitness consequences are likely to be minimal, and one possible explanation for its high frequency is that it confers early-age fitness benefits. We mentioned its association with cancer previously. Although the allele is not known to be associated with any increase in fertility, at least one study has found carriers to have an increase in hormone levels associated with fertility (Jasienska et al., 2015). And in addition to its potentially protective effects on cancer, carriers of the ApoE ε4 allele appear to have improved cognitive function early on (Jochemsen, Muller, van der Graaf, & Geerlings, 2012; Rusted et al., 2013).

These findings illustrate an important point. In the search for AP effects in humans, we should not confine ourselves to looking for alleles that improve early age fertility, fecundity, or survival in the face of late-age deleterious effects. These alleles might have what appear to be very minor effects, on the order of a 1% difference or less in fertility, for example. But from an evolutionary perspective, a 1% difference in mean fecundity early in life would be more than sufficient to maintain a relatively high frequency of an allele with very deleterious effects at middle or late ages. Given that environmental factors and stochasticity are both significant determinants of variation in fitness traits, we are likely able to detect these subtle demographic effects only in very large studies. Although effects on fitness of "secondary" phenotypes—size, hormone levels, behavior, and the like—might not immediately be known, these correlations can give us some important clues into the AP forces that might maintain particular alleles in human populations.

Beyond Medawar and Williams

Starting with Rose's selection experiments in the early 1980s (Rose, 1984; Rose & Charlesworth, 1980), the literature on the evolutionary genetics of aging has focused almost exclusively on two concepts, MA and AP, and on quantitative genetic tests of these ideas. At the same time, evolutionary genetic studies—both theoretical and empirical—have illustrated the central forces that shape genome structure and genetic variation in complex traits. These forces go well beyond the forces of mutation-selection balance and balancing selection typically applied to models of MA and AP. They include such key concepts as drift, positive and negative selection, background selection and hitchhiking, frequency-dependent selection, epigenetics, epistasis, sexually antagonistic coevolution, parental imprinting, and more. These important concepts are typically missing from the literature on the quantitative genetics and population genetics of aging.

We are now seeing these ideas put forward as important forces shaping natural variation for diseases as diverse as cancer (Vasseur & Quintana-Murci, 2013), infectious disease (Karlsson, Kwiatkowski, & Sabeti, 2014), and mental illness (Gratten, Wray, Keller, & Visscher, 2014). An exploration of the roles that these various forces might play in the evolution of aging is beyond the scope of this chapter. We hope, however, that in pointing readers to this interesting existing literature, we will stimulate a broader and more inclusive perspective on the evolutionary genetics of aging. The ideas of Fisher, Haldane, Medawar, Williams, and Hamilton set the stage for the evolutionary genetics of aging. The time is ripe to combine new theory with recent advances in high-throughput molecular biology to identify the pathways that underlie natural variation in age-related morbidity and mortality.

REFERENCES

Abrams, P. A. (1993). Does increased mortality favor the evolution of more rapid senescence? *Evolution, 47,* 877–887.

Albin, R. L. (1994). Antagonistic pleiotropy, mutation accumulation, and human genetic disease. In R. Rose & C. E. Finch (Eds.), *Genetic and evolution of aging* (pp. 307–314). Dordrecht, the Netherlands: Kluwer Academic Publishers.

Andersson, M. (1994). *Sexual selection.* Princeton, NJ: Princeton University Press.

Ballard, J. W. O., & Pichaud, N. (2014). Mitochondrial DNA: More than an evolutionary bystander. *Functional Ecology, 28,* 218–231.

Baudisch, A. (2005). Hamilton's indicators of the force of selection. *Proceedings of the National Academy of Sciences of the United States of America, 102,* 8263–8268.

Bonduriansky, R., Maklakov, A., Zajitschek, F., & Brooks, R. (2008). Sexual selection, sexual conflict and the evolution of ageing and life span. *Functional Ecology, 22,* 443–453.

Borgerhoff Mulder, M. (1998). The demographic transition: Are we any closer to an evolutionary explanation? *Trends Ecology & Evolution, 13,* 266–270.

Campisi, J. (2005). Aging, tumor suppression and cancer: High wire-act! *Mechanisms of Ageing and Development, 126,* 51–58.

Campisi, J. (2013). Aging, cellular senescence, and cancer. *Annual Review of Physiology, 75,* 685–705.

Caswell, H. (2007). Extrinsic mortality and the evolution of senescence. *Trends Ecology & Evolution, 22,* 173–174.

Chapman, T. (2001). Seminal fluid-mediated fitness traits in Drosophila. *Heredity, 87,* 511–521.

Charlesworth, B. (1994). *Evolution in age-structured populations.* Cambridge, UK: Cambridge University Press.

Charlesworth, B. (2001). Patterns of age-specific means and genetic variances of mortality rates predicted by the mutation accumulation theory of aging. *Journal of Theoretical Biology, 210,* 47–65.

Charlesworth, B., & Hughes, K. A. (1996). Age-specific inbreeding depression and components of genetic variance in relation to the evolution of senescence. *Proceedings of the National Academy of Sciences of the United States of America, 93*, 6140–6145.

Charmantier, A., Perrins, C., McCleery, R. H., & Sheldon, B. C. (2006). Quantitative genetics of age at reproduction in wild swans: Support for antagonistic pleiotropy models of senescence. *Proceedings of the National Academy of Sciences of the United States of America, 103*, 6587–6592.

Colman, R. J., Anderson, R. M., Johnson, S. C., Kastman, E. K., Kosmatka, K. J., Beasley, T. M., … Weindruch, R. (2009). Caloric restriction delays disease onset and mortality in rhesus monkeys. *Science, 325*, 201–204.

Darwin, C. (1859). *On the origin of species by means of natural selection or the preservation of favored races in the struggle for life*. London, UK: John Murray.

Darwin, C. (1871). *The descent of man, and selection in relation to sex*. London, UK: John Murray.

de Jong, G., & van Noordwijk, A. J. (1992). Acquisition and allocation of resources: Genetic (co)variances, selection, and life histories. *American Naturalist, 139*, 749–770.

Dillin, A., Crawford, D. K., & Kenyon, C. (2002). Timing requirements for insulin/IGF-1 signaling in *C. elegans*. *Science, 298*, 830–834.

Edward, D. A., Fricke, C., Gerrard, D. T., & Chapman, T. (2011). Quantifying the life-history response to increased male exposure in female *Drosophila melanogaster*. *Evolution, 65*, 564–573.

Emlen, D. J. (2000). Integrating development with evolution: A case study with beetle horns. *Bioscience, 50*, 403–418.

Emlen, D. J., Warren, I. A., Johns, A., Dworkin, I., & Lavine, L. C. (2012). A mechanism of extreme growth and reliable signaling in sexually selected ornaments and weapons. *Science, 337*, 860–864.

Endler, J. A. (1980). Natural selection on color patterns in *Poecilia reticulata*. *Evolution, 34*, 76–91.

Endler, J. A., & Houde, A. E. (1995). Geographic variation in female preferences for male traits in *Poecilia reticulata*. *Evolution, 49*, 456–468.

Ferveur, J. F. (2005). Cuticular hydrocarbons: Their evolution and roles in Drosophila pheromonal communication. *Behavior Genetics, 35*, 279–295.

Fisher, R. A. (1930). *The genetical theory of natural selection*. Oxford, UK: Clarendon Press.

Folstad, I., & Karter, A. J. (1992). Parasites, bright males and the immunocompetence handicap. *The American Naturalist, 139*, 603–622.

Fontana, L., Partridge, L., & Longo, V. D. (2010). Extending healthy life span—From yeast to humans. *Science, 328*, 321–326.

Fowler, K., & Partridge, L. (1989). A cost of mating in female fruitflies. *Nature, 338*, 760–761.

Friedman, L. S., Ostermeyer, E. A., Szabo, C. I., Dowd, P., Lynch, E. D., Rowell, S. E., & King, M. C. (1994). Confirmation of BRCA1 by analysis of germline mutations linked to breast and ovarian cancer in ten families. *Nature Genetics, 8*, 399–404.

Gems, D., & Riddle, D. L. (1996). Longevity in *Caenorhabditis elegans* reduced by mating but not gamete production. *Nature, 379*, 723–725.

Gendron, C. M., Kuo, T. H., Harvanek, Z. M., Chung, B. Y., Yew, J. Y., Dierick, H. A., & Pletcher, S. D. (2013). Drosophila life span and physiology are modulated by sexual perception and reward. *Science, 31*, 544–548.

Genin, E., Hannequin, D., Wallon, D., Sleegers, K., Hiltunen, M., Combarros, O., … Campion, D. (2011). APOE and Alzheimer disease: A major gene with semi-dominant inheritance. *Molecular Psychiatry, 16*, 903–907.

Gratten, J., Wray, N. R., Keller, M. C., & Visscher, P. M. (2014). Large-scale genomics unveils the genetic architecture of psychiatric disorders. *Nature Neuroscience, 17*, 782–790.

Haldane, J. B. S. (1941). *New paths in genetics*. London, UK: Allen and Unwin.

Hamilton, W. D. (1966). The moulding of senescence by natural selection. *Journal of Theoretical Biology, 12*, 12–45.

Hamilton, W. D., & Zuk, M. (1982). Heritable true fitness and bright birds: A role for parasites? *Science, 218*, 384–387.

Hansen, A. J., & Rohwer, S. (1986). Coverable badges and resource defence in birds. *Animal Behaviour, 34*, 69–76.

Hill, G. E. (2011). Condition-dependent traits as signals of the functionality of vital cellular processes. *Ecology Letters, 14*, 625–634.

Hoffman, J. M., Creevy, K. E., & Promislow, D. E. (2013). Reproductive capability is associated with lifespan and cause of death in companion dogs. *PLoS One, 8*, e61082.

Holmes, D. J., Fluckiger, R., & Austad, S. N. (2001). Comparative biology of aging in birds: An update. *Experimental Gerontology, 36*, 869–883.

Houde, A. E. (1987). Mate choice based upon naturally occurring color pattern variation in a guppy population. *Evolution, 41*, 1–10.

Houle, D., Hughes, K. A., Hoffmaster, D. K., Ihara, J., Assimacopoulos, S., Canada, D., & Charlesworth, B. (1994). The effects of spontaneous mutation on quantitative traits. I. Variances and covariances of life history traits. *Genetics, 138*, 773–785.

Hughes, K. A., & Charlesworth, B. (1994). A genetic analysis of senescence in Drosophila. *Nature, 367*, 64–66.

Hunt, J., Brooks, R., Jennions, M. D., Smith, M. J., Bentsen, C. L., & Bussiere, L. F. (2004). High-quality male field crickets invest heavily in sexual display but die young. *Nature, 432*, 1024–1027.

Huttley, G. A., Easteal, S., Southey, M. C., Tesoriero, A., Giles, G. G., McCredie, M. R., … Venter, D. J. (2000). Adaptive evolution of the tumour suppressor BRCA1 in humans and chimpanzees. Australian Breast Cancer Family Study. *Nature Genetics, 25*, 410–413.

Iwasa, Y., Pomiankowski, A., & Nee, S. (1991). The evolution of costly mate preferences II. The "handicap" principle. *Evolution, 45*, 1431–1442.

Ja, W. W., Carvalho, G. B., Zid, B. M., Mak, E. M., Brummel, T., & Benzer, S. (2009). Water- and nutrient-dependent effects of dietary restriction on *Drosophila* lifespan. *Proceedings of the National Academy of Sciences of the United States of America, 106*, 18633–18637.

Jallon, J. M. (1984). A few chemical words exchanged by Drosophila during courtship and mating. *Behavior Genetics, 14*, 441–478.

Jasienska, G., Ellison, P. T., Galbarczyk, A., Jasienski, M., Kalemba-Drozdz, M., Kapiszewska, M.,…Ziomkiewicz, A. (2015). Apolipoprotein E (ApoE) polymorphism is related to differences in potential fertility in women: A case of antagonistic pleiotropy? *Proceedings of the Royal Society B: Biological Sciences, 282*, 20142395.

Jenkins, N. L., McColl, G., & Lithgow, G. J. (2004). Fitness cost of extended lifespan in *Caenorhabditis elegans*. *Proceedings of the Royal Society of London, 271*, 2523–2526.

Ji, J., Sundquist, K., & Sundquist, J. (2012). Cancer incidence in patients with polyglutamine diseases: A population-based study in Sweden. *The Lancet Oncology, 13*, 642–648.

Jochemsen, H. M., Muller, M., van der Graaf, Y., & Geerlings, M. I. (2012). APOE epsilon4 differentially influences change in memory performance depending on age. The SMART-MR study. *Neurobiology of Aging, 33*, e815–e822.

Jones, O. R., Scheuerlein, A., Salguero-Gomez, R., Camarda, C. G., Schaible, R., Casper, B. B.,...Vaupel, J. W. (2014). Diversity of ageing across the tree of life. *Nature, 505*, 169–173.

Karlsson, E. K., Kwiatkowski, D. P., & Sabeti, P. C. (2014). Natural selection and infectious disease in human populations. *Nature Reviews Genetics, 15*, 379–393.

Kirkwood, T. B. L. (1977). Evolution and ageing. *Nature, 270*, 301–304.

Kirkwood, T. B. L. (1990). The disposable soma theory of aging. In D. E. Harrison (Ed.), *Genetic effects on aging III* (pp. 9–19). Caldwell, NJ: Telford Press.

Kotiaho, J. S. (2001). Costs of sexual traits: A mismatch between theoretical considerations and empirical evidence. *Biological Reviews of the Cambridge Philosophical Society, 76*, 365–376.

Kuo, T. H., Fedina, T. Y., Hansen, I., Dreisewerd, K., Dierick, H. A., Yew, J. Y., & Pletcher, S. D. (2012a). Insulin signaling mediates sexual attractiveness in Drosophila. *PLoS Genetics, 8*, e1002684.

Kuo, T. H., Yew, J. Y., Fedina, T. Y., Dreisewerd, K., Dierick, H. A., & Pletcher, S. D. (2012b). Aging modulates cuticular hydrocarbons and sexual attractiveness in *Drosophila melanogaster*. *Journal of Experimental Biology, 215*, 814–821.

Lee, R. D. (2003). Rethinking the evolutionary theory of aging: Transfers, not births, shape senescence in social species. *Proceedings of the National Academy of Sciences of the United States of America, 100*, 9637–9642.

Leroi, A. M., Chippindale, A. K., & Rose, M. R. (1994). Long-term laboratory evolution of a genetic life history trade-off in *Drosophila melanogaster*. 1. The role of genotype-by-environment interaction. *Evolution, 48*, 1244–1257.

Long, T. A., Pischedda, A., Stewart, A. D., & Rice, W. R. (2009). A cost of sexual attractiveness to high-fitness females. *PLoS Biology, 7*, e1000254.

Mair, W., Piper, M. D., & Partridge, L. (2005). Calories do not explain extension of life span by dietary restriction in Drosophila. *PLoS Biology, 3*, e223.

Maklakov, A. A., Fricke, C., & Arnqvist, G. (2007). Sexual selection affects lifespan and aging in the seed beetle. *Aging Cell, 6*, 739–744.

Maklakov, A. A., & Lummaa, V. (2013). Evolution of sex differences in lifespan and aging: Causes and constraints. *Bioessays, 35*, 717–724.

Medawar, P. B. (1946). Old age and natural death. *Modern Quart, 2*, 30–49.

Medawar, P. B. (1952). *An unsolved problem in biology*. London, UK: H.K. Lewis.

Medawar, P. B. (1957). *The uniqueness of the individual*. New York, NY: Basic Books.

Min, K. J., Lee, C. K., & Park, H. N. (2012). The lifespan of Korean eunuchs. *Current Biology, 22*, R792–R793.

Moorad, J. A., & Promislow, D. E. L. (2008). A theory of age-dependent mutation and senescence. *Genetics, 179*, 2061–2073.

Moorad, J. A., & Promislow, D. E. L. (2009). What can genetic variation tell us about the evolution of senescence? *Proceedings of the Royal Society B: Biological Sciences, 276*, 2271–2278.

Neiman, M., & Taylor, D. R. (2009). The causes of mutation accumulation in mitochondrial genomes. *Proceedings of the Royal Society B: Biological Sciences, 276*, 1201–1209.

Okasha, S. (2006). *Evolution and the levels of selection.* New York, NY: Clarendon Press.

Ou, S. M., Lee, Y. J., Hu, Y. W., Liu, C. J., Chen, T. J., Fuh, J. L., & Wang, S. J. (2013). Does Alzheimer's disease protect against cancers? A nationwide population-based study. *Neuroepidemiology, 40*, 42–49.

Partridge, L., & Fowler, K. (1990). Non-mating costs of exposure to males in female *Drosophila melanogaster. Journal of Insect Physiology, 36*, 419–425.

Partridge, L., Gems, D., & Withers, D. J. (2005a). Sex and death: What is the connection? *Cell, 120*, 461–472.

Partridge, L., Piper, M. D., & Mair, W. (2005b). Dietary restriction in Drosophila. *Mechanisms of Ageing and Development, 126*, 938–950.

Pavard, S., & Metcalf, C. J. E. (2007). Negative selection on BRCA1 susceptibility alleles sheds light on the population genetics of late-onset diseases and aging theory. *PLoS One, 2*, e1206.

Pettay, J. E., Charmantier, A., Wilson, A. J., & Lummaa, V. (2008). Age-specific genetic and maternal effects in fecundity of preindustrial Finnish women. *Evolution, 62*, 2297–2304.

Pletcher, S. D., Houle, D., & Curtsinger, J. W. (1998). Age-specific properties of spontaneous mutations affecting mortality in *Drosophila melanogaster. Genetics, 148*, 287–303.

Plun-Favreau, H., Lewis, P. A., Hardy, J., Martins, L. M., & Wood, N. W. (2010). Cancer and neurodegeneration: Between the devil and the deep blue sea. *PLoS Genetics, 6*, e1001257.

Pomiankowski, A., Iwasa, Y., & Nee, S. (1991). The evolution of costly mate preferences. I. Fisher and biased mutation. *Evolution, 45*, 1422–1430.

Price, T., Schluter, D., & Heckman, N. E. (1993). Sexual selection when the female directly benefits. *The Biological Journal of the Linnean Society, 48*, 187–211.

Promislow, D. E. L. (1991). Senescence in natural populations of mammals: A comparative study. *Evolution, 45*, 1869–1887.

Promislow, D. E. L. (1995). New perspectives on comparative tests of antagonistic pleiotropy using Drosophila. *Evolution, 49*, 394–397.

Promislow, D. E. L. (2003). Mate choice, sexual conflict, and evolution of senescence. *Behavior Genetics, 33*, 191–201.

Promislow, D. E. L., Tatar, M., Khazaeli, A., & Curtsinger, J. W. (1996). Age-specific patterns of genetic variance in *Drosophila melanogaster.* I. Mortality. *Genetics, 143*, 839–848.

Queller, D. C. (1992). Quantitative genetics, inclusive fitness, and group selection. *American Naturalist, 139*, 540–558.

Read, A. R., & Harvey, P. H. (1989). Life history differences among the eutherian radiations. *Journal of Zoology, 219*, 329–353.

Reznick, D. (1985). Costs of reproduction: An evaluation of the empirical evidence. *Oikos,44*, 257–267.

Reznick, D., Nunney, L., & Tessier, A. (2000). Big houses, big cars, superfleas and the costs of reproduction. *Trends in Ecology & Evolution, 15*, 421–425.

Roff, D. A., & Fairbairn, D. J. (2007). The evolution of trade-offs: Where are we? *Journal of Evolutionary Biology, 20*, 433–447.

Ronce, O., & Promislow, D. (2010). Kin competition, natal dispersal and the moulding of senescence by natural selection. *Proceedings of the Royal Society of London Series B-Biological Sciences, 277*, 3659–67

Rose, M. (1984). Laboratory evolution of postponed senescence in *Drosophila melanogaster*. *Evolution, 38*, 1004–1010.

Rose, M. R., & Charlesworth, B. (1980). A test of evolutionary theories of senescence. *Nature, 287*, 141–142.

Rowe, L., & Houle, D. (1996). The lek paradox and the capture of genetic variance by condition dependent traits. *Proceedings of the Royal Society of London Series B-Biological Sciences, 263*, 1415–1421.

Rusted, J. M., Evans, S. L., King, S. L., Dowell, N., Tabet, N., & Tofts, P. S. (2013). APOE e4 polymorphism in young adults is associated with improved attention and indexed by distinct neural signatures. *NeuroImage, 65*, 364–373.

Schluter, D., & Price, T. (1993). Honesty, perception and population divergence in sexually selected traits. *Proceedings of the Royal Society of London Series B-Biological Sciences, 253*, 117–122.

Schulz, T. J., Zarse, K., Voigt, A., Urban, N., Birringer, M., & Ristow, M. (2007). Glucose restriction extends *Caenorhabditis elegans* life span by inducing mitochondrial respiration and increasing oxidative stress. *Cell Metabolism, 6*, 280–293.

Searcy, W. A., & Yasukawa, K. (1983). Sexual selection and red-winged blackbirds. *American Scientist, 71*, 166–174.

Shi, C., & Murphy, C. T. (2014). Mating induces shrinking and death in Caenorhabditis mothers. *Science, 343*, 536–540.

Simpson, S. J., & Raubenheimer, D. (2009). Macronutrient balance and lifespan. *Aging, 1*, 875–880.

Smith, K. R., Hanson, H. A., Mineau, G. P., & Buys, S. S. (2012). Effects of BRCA1 and BRCA2 mutations on female fertility. *Proceedings of the Royal Society of London Series B-Biological Sciences, 279*, 1389–1395.

Sorensen, S. A., Fenger, K., & Olsen, J. H. (1999). Significantly lower incidence of cancer among patients with Huntington disease: An apoptotic effect of an expanded polyglutamine tract? *Cancer, 86*, 1342–1346.

Tatar, M., Bartke, A., & Antebi, A. (2003). The endocrine regulation of aging by insulin-like signals. *Science, 299*, 1346–1351.

Taylor, R. W., & Turnbull, D. M. (2005). Mitochondrial DNA mutations in human disease. *Nature Reviews Genetics, 6*, 389–402.

Thomas, F., Elguero, E., Brodeur, J., Roche, B., Missee, D., & Raymond, M. (2012). Malignancies and high birth weight in human: Which cancers could result from antagonistic pleiotropy? *Journal of Evolutionary Medicine, 1*, 1–5.

Thomas, F., Teriokhin, A. T., Budilova, E. V., Brown, S. P., Renaud, F., & Guegan, J. F. (2004). Human birthweight evolution across contrasting environments. *Journal of Evolutionary Biology, 17*, 542–553.

Toivonen, J. M., & Partridge, L. (2009). Endocrine regulation of aging and reproduction in Drosophila. *Molecular and Cellular Endocrinology, 299*, 39–50.

van de Vosse, E., Ali, S., de Visser, A. W., Surjadi, C., Widjaja, S., Vollaard, A. M., & van Dissel, J. T. (2005). Susceptibility to typhoid fever is associated with a polymorphism in the cystic fibrosis transmembrane conductance regulator (CFTR). *Human Genetics, 118*, 138–140.

van Noordwijk, A. J., & Jong, G. D. (1986). Acquisition and allocation of resources: Their influence on variation in life history tactics. *American Naturalist, 128*, 137–142.

Van Voorhies, W. A. (1992). Production of sperm reduces nematode lifespan. *Nature, 360*, 456–458.

Vasseur, E., & Quintana-Murci, L. (2013). The impact of natural selection on health and disease: Uses of the population genetics approach in humans. *Evolutionary Applications, 6*, 596–607.

Vaupel, J. W., & Yashin, A. I. (1985). Heterogeneity's ruses: Some surprising effects of selection on population dynamics. *American Statistician, 39*, 176–195.

Walker, D. W., McColl, G., Jenkins, N. L., Harris, J., & Lithgow, G. J. (2000). Evolution of lifespan in *C. elegans*. *Nature, 405*, 296–297.

Wallace, D. C. (2005). A mitochondrial paradigm of metabolic and degenerative diseases, aging, and cancer: A dawn for evolutionary medicine. *Annual Review of Genetics, 39*, 359–407.

Warren, I. A., Gotoh, H., Dworkin, I. M., Emlen, D. J., & Lavine, L. C. (2013). A general mechanism for conditional expression of exaggerated sexually-selected traits. *Bioessays, 35*, 889–899.

Weindruch, R., & Walford, R. L. (1982). Dietary restriction in mice beginning at 1 year of age: Effect on life-span and spontaneous cancer incidence. *Science, 215*, 1415–1418.

Weismann, A. (1889). *Essay upon heredity and kindred biological problems, Vol. 1*. Oxford, UK: Clarendon Press.

Williams, G. C. (1957). Pleiotropy, natural selection, and the evolution of senescence. *Evolution, 11*, 398–411.

Williams, G. C. (1966). *Adaptation and natural selection*. Princeton, NJ: Princeton University Press.

Wilson, D. S. (1983). The group selection controversy: History and current status. *Annual Review of Ecology and Systematics, 14*, 159–187.

Yampolsky, L. Y., Pearse, L., & Promislow, D. E. L. (2001). Age-specific effects of novel mutations in Drosophila: I. Mortality rates. *Genetica, 110*, 11–29.

Zahavi, A. (1975). Mate selection—A selection for a handicap. *Journal of Theoretical Biology, 53*, 205–214.

Zera, A. J., & Harshman, L. G. (2001). The physiology of life history trade-offs in animals. *Annual Review of Ecology and Systematics, 32*, 95–126.

CHAPTER 8

Inflammation and Aging

Ming Xu and James L. Kirkland

A hallmark of aging is chronic, low-grade inflammation that is "sterile" or not associated with infection (López-Otín, Blasco, Partridge, Serrano, & Kroemer, 2013; Tchkonia, Zhu, van Deursen, Campisi, & Kirkland, 2013). Mounting evidence has shown that an array of proinflammatory cytokines and mediators is frequently elevated in aging populations, including interleukin (IL)-6, tumor necrosis factor (TNF)-α, and C-reactive protein (CRP) (Michaud et al., 2013; Singh & Newman, 2011). It should be noted that, although these mediators are frequently increased in older human subjects, this is not universally the case. The extent of overall elevation, as well as increase in particular mediators, varies among subjects.

In addition to chronological aging, sterile inflammation can be associated with a number of age-related disorders and diseases, including cardiovascular diseases, cancers, type 2 diabetes mellitus (T2DM), bone diseases, neurodegenerative diseases, chronic obstructive pulmonary disease (COPD), and frailty, as considered later (Figure 8.1). Overall, these findings suggest that loss of control of the inflammatory process during aging is a key driver promoting functional decline and chronic disease onset. Here, we describe links between inflammations and chronic disease states, discuss the role of cellular senescence, and outline research on the development of interventions designed to reduce the impact of chronic inflammation in human aging.

■ DOWNSTREAM EFFECTS OF CHRONIC INFLAMMATION

Cardiovascular Diseases

Inflammation is a major contributor to the development and consequences of cardiovascular diseases (Tracy, 2003). Atherosclerosis is perhaps the most frequent form of cardiovascular disease in the elderly, with arterial wall thickening and accumulation of plaques. These predispose to reduced blood flow, clots, and distal ischemia. Atherosclerosis is related to accumulation of low-density lipoprotein (LDL) in the inner layers of blood vessels. Oxidized LDL appears to induce infiltration of immune cells, mainly macrophages and T cells, which then release a range of proinflammatory cytokines, including TNF-α and IL-6 (Ross, 1999). These cytokines activate endothelial cells, causing an increase in procoagulant effects by promoting production of platelet activation factors and inhibiting release of anticoagulant cofactors such as thrombomodulin (Stern, Kaiser, & Nawroth, 1988). These cytokines also directly activate the intrinsic coagulation pathways (Schouten, Wiersinga, Levi, & van der Poll, 2008). Several cytokines, including TNF-α and IL-6, act on endothelial cells to induce arterial contraction and vasoconstriction (Iversen, Nicolaysen, Kvernebo, Benestad, & Nicolaysen, 1999), which further

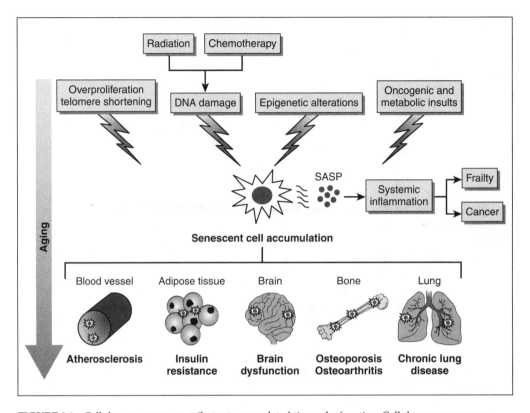

FIGURE 8.1 Cellular senescence contributes to age-related tissue dysfunction. Cellular senescence can be induced by a variety of stimuli and stresses. After senescence becomes established, some senescent cells acquire a senescence-associated secretory phenotype (SASP) that entails secretion of a number of proinflammatory cytokines. The SASP potentially contributes to local and systemic inflammation, frailty, and predisposition to cancer and many other age-related diseases. In addition, the SASP may induce innate immune responses and senescence in adjacent or distant cells.

exacerbates the problem. Thus, age-related chronic inflammation would be expected to increase the incidence or severity of cardiovascular diseases. Consistent with this, high circulating levels of several proinflammatory indicators, including IL-6, TNF-α-related factors, and CRP, are associated with an elevated risk of cardiovascular dysfunction in elderly individuals (Bruunsgaard, Skinhøj, Pedersen, Schroll, & Pedersen, 2000; Cesari et al., 2003; Michaud et al., 2013; Tracy et al., 1997; Volpato et al., 2001).

Cancer

The incidence of cancer rises sharply after people reach middle age (Campisi, 2013). Inflammation and cancer seem to be tightly connected (Balkwill & Mantovani, 2001). Approximately 15% to 20% of deaths from cancer are related to inflammatory responses (Balkwill & Mantovani, 2001). Many types of cancer are also related to or are preceded by chronic inflammation at sites of tumor development (Mantovani, Allavena, Sica, & Balkwill, 2008). Conversely, some anti-inflammatory agents, such as cyclooxygenase (COX)-1 inhibitors and aspirin, seem to decrease the risk of certain types of cancer (Chan, Ogino, & Fuchs, 2007; Flossmann & Rothwell, 2007; Koehne & Dubois, 2004).

Several key inflammatory cytokines, such as TNF-α (Szlosarek & Balkwill, 2003), IL-1β (Voronov et al., 2003), IL-6 (Grivennikov & Karin, 2008), and IL-23 (Langowski et al., 2006), have been found to play important roles in tumorigenesis. These cytokines activate transcription factors, including nuclear factor-κB (NF-κB) and signal transducer and activator of transcription 3 (STAT3), in both tumor and immune cells, leading to production of more inflammatory cytokines and mediators, which in turn contribute to the generation of the tumor inflammatory microenvironment (Mantovani et al., 2008). In addition, inflammatory cytokines, including IL-1β, IL-6, and TNF-α, together with inflammation-induced production of extracellular matrix (ECM) modifiers, such as matrix metalloproteinases (MMP), promote invasion and metastasis of tumor cells (Balkwill, Charles, & Mantovani, 2005). A potential mechanism contributing to tumor invasion involves induction of chemokine receptor expression in cancer cells (Balkwill, 2004; Kulbe et al., 2007). As an increased level of inflammatory cytokines is an important risk factor for cancer (Schetter, Heegaard, & Harris, 2010; Srikrishna & Freeze, 2009), age-related chronic inflammation could be a mechanism that contributes to an increased incidence of cancer in the elderly.

Type 2 Diabetes

Emerging evidence suggests that the inflammation contributes to the pathogenesis of type 2 diabetes (T2D; Donath & Shoelson, 2011). Several studies have suggested that patients with T2D have increased circulating proinflammatory markers, including CRP and IL-6, as well as hemostatic factors such as plasminogen activator inhibitor-1 (PAI-1) (Herder et al., 2005; Pickup, Mattock, Chusney, & Burt, 1997; Spranger et al., 2003). Inflammatory cytokines can activate the c-Jun amino-terminal kinase (JNK; Ip & Davis, 1998) and the IκB kinase-β (IKKβ) pathways (Arkan et al., 2005). After activation, these two pathways phosphorylate serine sites on insulin receptor substrate-1 (IRS-1), which leads to the inhibition of insulin signaling (Aguirre, Uchida, Yenush, Davis, & White, 2000; Gao et al., 2002). Activation of IKKβ also stimulates the NF-κB pathway, leading to increased production of a number of cytokines (Shoelson, Lee, & Yuan, 2003), causing inflammation. Moreover, multiple cytokines induce expression of suppressors of cytokine signaling (SOCS; Rui, Yuan, Frantz, Shoelson, & White, 2002). Several SOCS family members have been implicated in impaired insulin signaling either by interrupting tyrosine phosphorylation or by initiating proteasomal degradation of IRS-1 and IRS-2 (Emanuelli et al., 2001; Mooney et al., 2001; Rui et al., 2002). Thus, the risk of T2D is significantly associated with increased levels of circulating inflammatory mediators, including CRP and IL-6, and in turn both T2DM and increased circulating inflammatory mediators are associated with aging (Pradhan, Manson, Rifai, Buring, & Ridker, 2001; Spranger et al., 2003).

Bone Diseases

Inflammatory cytokines are involved in bone homeostasis (Manolagas & Jilka, 1995). IL-6 plays an essential role in bone remodeling. It promotes osteoporosis both by inhibiting differentiation of osteoblasts into osteocytes, decreasing bone formation (Kaneshiro et al., 2014; Peruzzi et al., 2012) and stimulating osteoclast development, resulting in increased bone resorption (Ishimi et al., 1990; Manolagas, 2000). In addition to IL-6, high levels of CRP and TNF-α–related markers are also associated with fracture risk and bone loss (Cauley et al., 2007; Khosla, Peterson, Egan, Jones, & Riggs, 1994; Koh et al.,

2005; Zheng et al., 1997). IL-6, along with several MMPs whose production is related to inflammation, also plays roles in the pathogenesis of osteoarthritis (Philipot et al., 2014; So et al., 2013).

Brain Dysfunction

Local and circulating inflammatory cytokines can have an impact on the central nervous system (Rosano, Marsland, & Gianaros, 2012). Cytokines can be produced by astrocytes and activated microglia that reside in the brain (Bhat et al., 2012; Hanisch, 2002). Circulating cytokines can induce endothelial cells along the blood–brain barrier to locally secrete cytokines that, in turn, affect brain function (Serrats et al., 2010). Inflammation appears to be a major contributor to the pathogenesis of Alzheimer's disease (AD) (Griffin, 2013). High plasma levels of IL-6, CRP, and TNF-α-related factors have been reported to be predictive of cognitive decline in older populations (Dik et al., 2005; Schram et al., 2007; Yaffe et al., 2003). Elevated levels of IL-6 and TNF-α in the blood are also significantly associated with the risk of AD development (Licastro et al., 2000; Tan et al., 2007).

Frailty

Frailty increases in prevalence with old age and occurs frequently in association with age-related chronic diseases. Phenotypic characteristics of frailty include heightened vulnerability to stresses (e.g., surgery, infection, or trauma), unexplained weight loss, reduced strength, muscle wasting (sarcopenia), poor stamina, low physical activity, slowed moving speed, cachexia, and adipose tissue loss (Bandeen-Roche et al., 2006; Bandeen-Roche, Walston, Huang, Semba, & Ferrucci, 2009; Fried et al., 2001; Kanapuru & Ershler, 2009; Leng, Xue, Tian, Walston, & Fried, 2007; Lucicesare, Hubbard, Searle, & Rockwood, 2010; Qu et al., 2009; Rockwood & Mitnitski, 2011; Rockwood, Mitnitski, Song, Steen, & Skoog, 2006; Walston et al., 2002, 2006, 2009). Frailty is also associated with an increased risk of chronic disease, loss of independence, mortality, and increased health care use (Fried et al., 2001; Rockwood et al., 2006). Sterile, low-grade inflammation is perhaps the most prominent physiologic correlate of the age-related frailty syndrome (Ferrucci et al., 1999; Kanapuru & Ershler, 2009; Leng et al., 2007; Walston et al., 2002). Several key inflammatory mediators including IL-6, CRP, and TNF-α are tightly linked to the incidence of disability, decreased muscle strength, and reduced physical activity in elderly subjects (Cesari et al., 2004; Ferrucci et al., 1999, 2002; Visser et al., 2002).

■ MECHANISMS INITIATING AGE-RELATED INFLAMMATION

The initiating cause(s) of age-related chronic inflammation has not been identified conclusively. Candidate sources include immune system dysregulation, chronic antigenic stimulation (e.g., by latent viruses, such as cytomegalovirus or herpes viruses, neo- or auto-antigen exposure, altered microbiome, or increased gut permeability), oxidative stress, reactive lipids, other metabolites, dysfunctional macromolecules (e.g., unfolded or aggregated proteins, advanced glycation end products [AGEs]), and inflammatory mediators produced by senescent or pre-neoplastic cells (Franceschi et al., 2007; Tchkonia et al., 2013). Chronic inflammation can provoke tissue dysregulation through at least two mechanisms. First, infiltrating immune cells can degrade tissues because of their release of reactive or toxic molecules such as reactive oxygen species (ROS). Second, inflammatory cytokines can induce changes in nearby cells that are independent of the immune system. For example, IL-6 and IL-8 can impede macrophage function, induce innate immune responses, stimulate angiogenesis, promote epithelial and endothelial cell migration and invasion, and disrupt cell–cell communication (Ancrile et al., 2007; Badache & Hynes, 2001; Nagabhushanam et al., 2003; Sebastian, Lloberas, & Celada, 2009; Sparmann & Bar-Sagi, 2004). Additionally, chronic tissue inflammation can contribute to susceptibility to autoimmune diseases and lead to restricted capacity to increase inflammation further when needed in response to infection or other insults. Importantly, this restricted dynamic range of inflammatory and cellular stress responses in older individuals may constrain capacity to respond effectively to infection, cancer, immunization, or injury.

■ AGE-RELATED CHANGES IN THE IMMUNE SYSTEM AND INFLAMMATION

Potentially, changes in immune system function associated with aging contribute to age-related chronic inflammation (Poland, Ovsyannikova, Kennedy, Lambert, & Kirkland, 2014). A general decline in immune system function occurs in old age that entails increased susceptibility to infections, cancers, and autoimmune disorders associated with increased mortality. Particular immune cell types undergo alterations in function with aging. For example, macrophage function is decreased and the activation potential of T cells is impaired in older individuals (Jackola, Ruger, & Miller, 1994; Nikolich-Žugich, 2014; Poland et al., 2014; Sebastian et al., 2009). Furthermore, the ability of anti-inflammatory pathways to keep inflammation in check might also decline with aging, contributing to the chronic, low-grade sterile inflammatory state and tissue damage, a possibility that merits investigation. This imbalance between pro- and anti-inflammatory processes in old age has been termed as "inflammaging" (Franceschi et al., 2007). Immune system dysfunction, combined with lifelong or prolonged antigen exposures, may play an important role in the genesis of the chronic inflammatory state (Franceschi, Bonafè, & Valensin, 2000). Accumulation or prolonged exposure to ROS or other metabolites, such as ceramides or reducing sugars, with aging can alter the structure of proteins, DNA, or membrane lipids, thereby creating neo- or autoantigens. Immune cells can be persistently activated to clear these damaged molecules, which may contribute to age-related chronic inflammation (Cannizzo, Clement, Sahu, Follo, & Santambrogio, 2011). Latent viruses, including cytomegalovirus or herpes viruses, can become reactivated in old age or, by inducing low-level immune activation throughout life, deplete or alter components of the immune system, contributing to chronic inflammation and dysfunction of the immune system (Nikolich-Žugich, 2014).

■ THE CONTRIBUTION OF CELLULAR SENESCENCE TO CHRONIC INFLAMMATION WITH AGING

Recently, mounting evidence suggests that the cellular senescence could play an important role in inducing age-related chronic inflammation. Cellular senescence refers to the irreversible arrest of cell proliferation of progenitor cells without cell death. Although they can appear at any point during life (Meuter et al., 2014), senescent cells accumulate with aging in a number of tissues, including the cardiovascular system, skin, liver, kidney, lung, gastrointestinal system, bone marrow, and adipose tissue (Tchkonia et al., 2013). A variety of stimuli and stresses can induce cellular senescence, including telomere shortening, genomic mutation, epigenetic alterations, drugs, radiation, and oncogenic and metabolic insults (Campisi & d'Adda di Fagagna, 2007; Zhu, Armstrong, Tchkonia, & Kirkland, 2014). Senescent cells can secrete a range of proinflammatory cytokines and chemokines, termed the "senescence-associated secretory phenotype" (SASP; Coppé et al., 2008, 2010; Herbig, Ferreira, Condel, Carey, & Sedivy, 2006; Kuilman et al., 2008). Notably, IL-6, IL-8, and other SASP components are associated with many of the age-related dysfunctions and diseases discussed earlier.

Increasing evidence suggests that the senescent cell accumulation contributes to pathology in multiple diseases (Tchkonia et al., 2013; Xu, Palmer, et al., 2015; Zhu et al., 2014). For example, in cardiovascular disease, senescent smooth muscle and endothelial cells accumulate in atherosclerotic plaques and likely play a key role in atherosclerosis (Sikora, Bielak-Zmijewska, & Mosieniak, 2014). Telomere shortening, an inducer of cellular senescence, is a risk factor for major cardiovascular diseases, including heart failure, atherosclerosis, and hypertension (Fyhrquist, Saijonmaa, & Strandberg, 2013). Senolytic agents—drugs that selectively eliminate senescent cells—enhance cardiovascular function of old mice, leading to increases in cardiac ejection fraction (the proportion of blood pumped during each contraction of the heart) and carotid smooth muscle vascular reactivity (Zhu et al., 2015).

In diabetes, senescent preadipocytes and endothelial cells accumulate in the adipose tissue of obese experimental animals as well as human subjects (Minamino et al., 2009; Tchkonia et al., 2010). Telomere shortening has been found to be associated with the risk of diabetes in South Asian populations (Harte et al., 2012). Several key SASP components, including IL-6 and monocyte chemoattractant protein-1 (MCP-1), appear to contribute to insulin resistance as indicated by in vitro and in vivo studies (Daniele et al., 2014; Handa et al., 2013; Sarvas, Khaper, & Lees, 2013). Diabetes, especially when associated with obesity, is associated with chronic inflammation of adipose tissue (Palmer et al., 2015).

Regarding osteoporosis, cellular senescence is linked to osteoblast dysfunction and bone loss (Kassem & Marie, 2011). In mice with an accelerated aging-like syndrome that leads to osteoporosis, senolytic agents increased vertebral bone mineral content and density (Zhu et al., 2015). Senescent chondrocytes are found in the joints of patients with osteoarthritis (Rose et al., 2012) and have been shown to be part of the pathogenesis of osteoarthritis (Philipot et al., 2014).

In neurodegenerative diseases, more senescent astrocytes were found in brains from subjects with Alzheimer's disease than in subjects without dementia (Bhat et al., 2012). Senescent glial cells have been implicated in Parkinson's disease (Chinta et al., 2013). We found that senolytic drugs delayed age-related neurological dysfunction in progeroid mice (Zhu et al., 2015).

Senescent cells also accumulate in the lungs in smokers, COPD, and idiopathic pulmonary fibrosis. These age-related conditions are also associated with chronic lung inflammation. COPD and idiopathic pulmonary fibrosis are attractive as potential indications for senolytic drugs, perhaps as aerosols (Kirkland & Tchkonia, 2015). In addition to being associated with chronological aging and cellular senescence, each of the aforementioned conditions is also associated with local or systemic inflammation. The same holds true for a number of other age-related disorders (Kirkland & Tchkonia, 2015). Thus, cellular senescence and chronic inflammation appear to be interrelated processes that reinforce each other and contribute to age-related dysfunction and risk for multiple chronic diseases.

Potential Interventions

Anti-inflammatory agents include: (a) aspirin, which inhibits both COX-1 and -2; (b) nonsteroidal anti-inflammatory drugs (NSAIDS), which more specifically inhibit COX-2; (c) certain steroids, such as glucocorticoids, which also inhibit the SASP (Laberge et al., 2012); (d) neutralizing antibodies to block activity of key cytokines such as IL-6 or TNF-α; and (e) inhibitors of key kinases in the inflammatory response such as p38 mitogen-activated protein kinase (MAPK) (Dinarello, 2010). Some of these agents may turn out to reduce low-grade inflammation in older subjects and alleviate age-related tissue dysfunction. However, many of these drugs have side effects that can be severe. In addition, as this is an emerging field and the number of studies are limited, further investigation of the hypothesis that targeting low inflammation could alleviate age-related dysfunction using both animal and human models is required. Additional, safe therapeutic options are needed.

Several emerging approaches for alleviating age-related, chronic, sterile inflammation are on the horizon using agents that target fundamental aging mechanisms. Cellular senescence appears to be a new and promising target for combating age-related dysfunction and diseases as a group, instead of one at a time (Kirkland & Tchkonia, 2015). Elimination of senescent cells in a progeroid mouse model, *BubR1$^{H/H}$* mice, delayed the onset of age-related dysfunction and improved health span (Baker et al., 2011). Senolytic drugs, which can selectively kill senescent cells, restored function of several tissues in chronologically aged, radiation-treated, and progeroid mice (Zhu et al., 2015). The target of rapamycin (TOR) signaling pathway plays an important role in cellular senescence (Anisimov, 2013). Inhibition of this pathway was found to extend life span and improve health span in mammals (Harrison et al., 2009) and reduce immunosenescence in elderly subjects (Mannick et al., 2014). Like rapamycin, metformin extends life span in mice (Anisimov et al., 2008, 2010, 2011; Smith et al., 2010) and inhibits the SASP (Moiseeva et al., 2013). Inhibitors of the Janus kinase (JAK) pathway blunt the SASP in cultured mouse and human cells as well as systemic inflammation in aged mice, leading to reductions in frailty phenotypes (Xu, Tchkonia, et al., 2015). In a placebo-controlled clinical trial, treatment with a JAK1/2 pathway inhibitor led to increased physical activity, reduced frailty, and weight regain in elderly subjects with myelofibrosis (Tefferi, Litzow, & Pardanani, 2011; Verstovsek et al., 2012). Thus, promising new clinical interventions appear to be on the horizon.

■ CONCLUSION

Although more studies are required, evidence to date suggests that drugs that target age-related chronic inflammation and related fundamental aging processes, including cellular senescence or the age-related increase in mammalian target of rapamycin (mTOR) activity, might play an important role in reducing age-related disability, frailty, and multiple chronic diseases as a group. If this is correct, the concept of targeting mechanisms driving aging to prevent or treat associated chronic disease states will be greatly accelerated and medicine as we know it would be transformed.

■ ACKNOWLEDGMENTS

The authors are grateful for the administrative assistance of J. Armstrong. This work was supported by National Institutes of Health grants AG13925, AG041122, AG31736 (Project 4), AG044396, and DK50456, and the Glenn, Ted Nash Long Life, and Noaber Foundations (J.L.K.).

REFERENCES

Aguirre, V., Uchida, T., Yenush, L., Davis, R., & White, M. F. (2000). The c-Jun NH(2)-terminal kinase promotes insulin resistance during association with insulin receptor substrate-1 and phosphorylation of Ser(307). *The Journal of Biological Chemistry, 275*(12), 9047–9054.

Ancrile, B., Lim, K. H., & Counter, C. M. (2007). Oncogenic Ras-induced secretion of IL6 is required for tumorigenesis. *Genes & Development, 21*(14), 1714–1719.

Anisimov, V. N. (2013). Metformin and rapamycin are master-keys for understanding the relationship between cell senescent, aging and cancer. *Aging, 5*(5), 337–338.

Anisimov, V. N., Berstein, L. M., Egormin, P. A., Piskunova, T. S., Popovich, I. G., Zabezhinski, M. A.,…Semenchenko, A. V. (2008). Metformin slows down aging and extends life span of female SHR mice. *Cell Cycle, 7*(17), 2769–2773.

Anisimov, V. N., Berstein, L. M., Popovich, I. G., Zabezhinski, M. A., Egormin, P. A., Piskunova, T. S.,…Poroshina, T. E. (2011). If started early in life, metformin treatment increases life span and postpones tumors in female SHR mice. *Aging, 3*(2), 148–157.

Anisimov, V. N., Egormin, P. A., Piskunova, T. S., Popovich, I. G., Tyndyk, M. L., Yurova, M. N.,…Romanyukha, A. A. (2010). Metformin extends life span of HER-2/neu transgenic mice and in combination with melatonin inhibits growth of transplantable tumors in vivo. *Cell Cycle, 9*(1), 188–197.

Arkan, M. C., Hevener, A. L., Greten, F. R., Maeda, S., Li, Z. W., Long, J. M.,…Karin, M. (2005). IKK-beta links inflammation to obesity-induced insulin resistance. *Nature Medicine, 11*(2), 191–198.

Badache, A., & Hynes, N. E. (2001). Interleukin 6 inhibits proliferation and, in cooperation with an epidermal growth factor receptor autocrine loop, increases migration of T47D breast cancer cells. *Cancer Research, 61*(1), 383–391.

Baker, D. J., Wijshake, T., Tchkonia, T., LeBrasseur, N. K., Childs, B. G., van de Sluis, B.,…van Deursen, J. M. (2011). Clearance of p16Ink4a-positive senescent cells delays ageing-associated disorders. *Nature, 479*(7372), 232–236.

Balkwill, F. (2004). Cancer and the chemokine network. *Nature Reviews. Cancer, 4*(7), 540–550.

Balkwill, F., Charles, K. A., & Mantovani, A. (2005). Smoldering and polarized inflammation in the initiation and promotion of malignant disease. *Cancer Cell, 7*(3), 211–217.

Balkwill, F., & Mantovani, A. (2001). Inflammation and cancer: Back to Virchow? *The Lancet, 357*(9255), 539–545.

Bandeen-Roche, K., Walston, J. D., Huang, Y., Semba, R. D., & Ferrucci, L. (2009). Measuring systemic inflammatory regulation in older adults: Evidence and utility. *Rejuvenation Research, 12*(6), 403–410.

Bandeen-Roche, K., Xue, Q. L., Ferrucci, L., Walston, J., Guralnik, J. M.,…Fried, L. P. (2006). Phenotype of frailty: Characterization in the women's health and aging studies. *The Journals of Gerontology, Series A, 61*(3), 262–266.

Bhat, R., Crowe, E. P., Bitto, A., Moh, M., Katsetos, C. D., Garcia, F. U.,…Torres, C. (2012). Astrocyte senescence as a component of Alzheimer's disease. *PloS One, 7*(9), e45069.

Bruunsgaard, H., Skinhøj, P., Pedersen, A. N., Schroll, M., & Pedersen, B. K. (2000). Ageing, tumour necrosis factor-alpha (TNF-alpha) and atherosclerosis. *Clinical and Experimental Immunology, 121*(2), 255–260.

Campisi, J. (2013). Aging, cellular senescence, and cancer. *Annual Review of Physiology, 75*, 685–705.

Campisi, J., & d'Adda di Fagagna, F. (2007). Cellular senescence: When bad things happen to good cells. *Nature Reviews. Molecular Cell Biology, 8*(9), 729–740.

Cannizzo, E. S., Clement, C. C., Sahu, R., Follo, C., & Santambrogio, L. (2011). Oxidative stress, inflamm-aging and immunosenescence. *Journal of Proteomics, 74*(11), 2313–2323.

Cauley, J. A., Danielson, M. E., Boudreau, R. M., Forrest, K. Y., Zmuda, J. M., Pahor, M.,…Newman, A. B.; Health ABC Study. (2007). Inflammatory markers and incident fracture risk in older men and women: The Health Aging and Body Composition Study. *Journal of Bone and Mineral Research, 22*(7), 1088–1095.

Cesari, M., Penninx, B. W., Newman, A. B., Kritchevsky, S. B., Nicklas, B. J., Sutton-Tyrrell, K.,…Pahor, M. (2003). Inflammatory markers and cardiovascular disease (The Health, Aging and Body Composition [Health ABC] Study). *The American Journal of Cardiology, 92*(5), 522–528.

Cesari, M., Penninx, B. W., Pahor, M., Lauretani, F., Corsi, A. M., Rhys Williams, G.,…Ferrucci, L. (2004). Inflammatory markers and physical performance in older persons: The InCHIANTI study. *The Journals of Gerontology, Series A, 59*(3), 242–248.

Chan, A. T., Ogino, S., & Fuchs, C. S. (2007). Aspirin and the risk of colorectal cancer in relation to the expression of COX-2. *The New England Journal of Medicine, 356*(21), 2131–2142.

Chinta, S. J., Lieu, C. A., Demaria, M., Laberge, R. M., Campisi, J., & Andersen, J. K. (2013). Environmental stress, ageing and glial cell senescence: A novel mechanistic link to Parkinson's disease? *Journal of Internal Medicine, 273*(5), 429–436.

Coppé, J. P., Patil, C. K., Rodier, F., Krtolica, A., Beauséjour, C. M., Parrinello, S.,…Campisi, J. (2010). A human-like senescence-associated secretory phenotype is conserved in mouse cells dependent on physiological oxygen. *PloS One, 5*(2), e9188.

Coppé, J. P., Patil, C. K., Rodier, F., Sun, Y., Muñoz, D. P., Goldstein, J.,…Campisi, J. (2008). Senescence-associated secretory phenotypes reveal cell-nonautonomous functions of oncogenic RAS and the p53 tumor suppressor. *PLoS Biology, 6*(12), 2853–2868.

Daniele, G., Guardado Mendoza, R., Winnier, D., Fiorentino, T. V., Pengou, Z., Cornell, J.,…Folli, F. (2014). The inflammatory status score including IL-6, TNF-a, osteopontin, fractalkine, MCP-1 and adiponectin underlies whole-body insulin resistance and hyperglycemia in type 2 diabetes mellitus. *Acta Diabetologica, 51*(1), 123–131.

Dik, M. G., Jonker, C., Hack, C. E., Smit, J. H., Comijs, H. C., & Eikelenboom, P. (2005). Serum inflammatory proteins and cognitive decline in older persons. *Neurology, 64*(8), 1371–1377.

Dinarello, C. A. (2010). Anti-inflammatory agents: Present and future. *Cell, 140*(6), 935–950.

Donath, M. Y., & Shoelson, S. E. (2011). Type 2 diabetes as an inflammatory disease. *Nature Reviews. Immunology, 11*(2), 98–107.

Emanuelli, B., Peraldi, P., Filloux, C., Chavey, C., Freidinger, K., Hilton, D. J.,...Van Obberghen, E. (2001). SOCS-3 inhibits insulin signaling and is up-regulated in response to tumor necrosis factor-alpha in the adipose tissue of obese mice. *The Journal of Biological Chemistry, 276*(51), 47944–47949.

Ferrucci, L., Harris, T. B., Guralnik, J. M., Tracy, R. P., Corti, M. C., Cohen, H. J.,...Havlik, R. J. (1999). Serum IL-6 level and the development of disability in older persons. *Journal of the American Geriatrics Society, 47*(6), 639–646.

Ferrucci, L., Penninx, B. W., Volpato, S., Harris, T. B., Bandeen-Roche, K., Balfour, J.,...Md, J. M. (2002). Change in muscle strength explains accelerated decline of physical function in older women with high interleukin-6 serum levels. *Journal of the American Geriatrics Society, 50*(12), 1947–1954.

Flossmann, E., & Rothwell, P. M.; British Doctors Aspirin Trial and the UK-TIA Aspirin Trial. (2007). Effect of aspirin on long-term risk of colorectal cancer: Consistent evidence from randomised and observational studies. *The Lancet, 369*(9573), 1603–1613.

Franceschi, C., Bonafè, M., & Valensin, S. (2000). Human immunosenescence: The prevailing of innate immunity, the failing of clonotypic immunity, and the filling of immunological space. *Vaccine, 18*(16), 1717–1720.

Franceschi, C., Capri, M., Monti, D., Giunta, S., Olivieri, F., Sevini, F.,...Salvioli, S. (2007). Inflammaging and anti-inflammaging: A systemic perspective on aging and longevity emerged from studies in humans. *Mechanisms of Ageing and Development, 128*(1), 92–105.

Fried, L. P., Tangen, C. M., Walston, J., Newman, A. B., Hirsch, C., Gottdiener, J.,...McBurnie, M. A.; Cardiovascular Health Study Collaborative Research Group. (2001). Frailty in older adults: Evidence for a phenotype. *The Journals of Gerontology, Series A, 56*(3), M146–M156.

Fyhrquist, F., Saijonmaa, O., & Strandberg, T. (2013). The roles of senescence and telomere shortening in cardiovascular disease. *Nature Reviews. Cardiology, 10*(5), 274–283.

Gao, Z., Hwang, D., Bataille, F., Lefevre, M., York, D., Quon, M. J., & Ye, J. (2002). Serine phosphorylation of insulin receptor substrate 1 by inhibitor kappa B kinase complex. *The Journal of Biological Chemistry, 277*(50), 48115–48121.

Griffin, W. S. (2013). Neuroinflammatory cytokine signaling and Alzheimer's disease. *The New England Journal of Medicine, 368*(8), 770–771.

Grivennikov, S., & Karin, M. (2008). Autocrine IL-6 signaling: A key event in tumorigenesis? *Cancer Cell, 13*(1), 7–9.

Handa, M., Vanegas, S., Maddux, B. A., Mendoza, N., Zhu, S., Goldfine, I. D., & Mirza, A. M. (2013). XOMA 052, an anti-IL-1β monoclonal antibody, prevents IL-1β-mediated insulin resistance in 3T3-L1 adipocytes. *Obesity, 21*(2), 306–309.

Hanisch, U. K. (2002). Microglia as a source and target of cytokines. *Glia, 40*(2), 140–155.

Harrison, D. E., Strong, R., Sharp, Z. D., Nelson, J. F., Astle, C. M., Flurkey, K.,...Miller, R. A. (2009). Rapamycin fed late in life extends lifespan in genetically heterogeneous mice. *Nature, 460*(7253), 392–395.

Harte, A. L., da Silva, N. F., Miller, M. A., Cappuccio, F. P., Kelly, A., O'Hare, J. P.,...McTernan, P. G. (2012). Telomere length attrition, a marker of biological senescence, is inversely correlated with triglycerides and cholesterol in South Asian males with type 2 diabetes mellitus. *Experimental Diabetes Research, 2012*, 895185.

Herbig, U., Ferreira, M., Condel, L., Carey, D., & Sedivy, J. M. (2006). Cellular senescence in aging primates. *Science, 311*(5765), 1257.

Herder, C., Illig, T., Rathmann, W., Martin, S., Haastert, B., Müller-Scholze, S.,...Kolb, H.; KORA Study Group. (2005). Inflammation and type 2 diabetes: Results from KORA Augsburg. *Gesundheitswesen, 67*(Suppl. 1), S115–S121.

Ip, Y. T., & Davis, R. J. (1998). Signal transduction by the c-Jun N-terminal kinase (JNK)– from inflammation to development. *Current Opinion in Cell Biology, 10*(2), 205–219.

Ishimi, Y., Miyaura, C., Jin, C. H., Akatsu, T., Abe, E., Nakamura, Y.,...Hirano, T. (1990). IL-6 is produced by osteoblasts and induces bone resorption. *Journal of Immunology, 145*(10), 3297–3303.

Iversen, P. O., Nicolaysen, A., Kvernebo, K., Benestad, H. B., & Nicolaysen, G. (1999). Human cytokines modulate arterial vascular tone via endothelial receptors. *Pflügers Archiv: European Journal of Physiology, 439*(1–2), 93–100.

Jackola, D. R., Ruger, J. K., & Miller, R. A. (1994). Age-associated changes in human T cell phenotype and function. *Aging, 6*(1), 25–34.

Kanapuru, B., & Ershler, W. B. (2009). Inflammation, coagulation, and the pathway to frailty. *The American Journal of Medicine, 122*(7), 605–613.

Kaneshiro, S., Ebina, K., Shi, K., Higuchi, C., Hirao, M., Okamoto, M.,...Hashimoto, J. (2014). IL-6 negatively regulates osteoblast differentiation through the SHP2/ MEK2 and SHP2/Akt2 pathways in vitro. *Journal of Bone and Mineral Metabolism, 32*(4), 378–392.

Kassem, M., & Marie, P. J. (2011). Senescence-associated intrinsic mechanisms of osteoblast dysfunctions. *Aging Cell, 10*(2), 191–197.

Khosla, S., Peterson, J. M., Egan, K., Jones, J. D., & Riggs, B. L. (1994). Circulating cytokine levels in osteoporotic and normal women. *The Journal of Clinical Endocrinology and Metabolism, 79*(3), 707–711.

Kirkland, J. L., & Tchkonia, T. (2015). Clinical strategies and animal models for developing senolytic agents. *Experimental Gerontology, 68*, 19–25.

Koehne, C. H., & Dubois, R. N. (2004). COX-2 inhibition and colorectal cancer. *Seminars in Oncology, 31*(2, Suppl. 7), 12–21.

Koh, J. M., Khang, Y. H., Jung, C. H., Bae, S., Kim, D. J., Chung, Y. E., & Kim, G. S. (2005). Higher circulating hsCRP levels are associated with lower bone mineral density in healthy pre- and postmenopausal women: Evidence for a link between systemic inflammation and osteoporosis. *Osteoporosis International, 16*(10), 1263–1271.

Kuilman, T., Michaloglou, C., Vredeveld, L. C., Douma, S., van Doorn, R., Desmet, C. J.,...Peeper, D. S. (2008). Oncogene-induced senescence relayed by an interleukin-dependent inflammatory network. *Cell, 133*(6), 1019–1031.

Kulbe, H., Thompson, R., Wilson, J. L., Robinson, S., Hagemann, T., Fatah, R.,...Balkwill, F. (2007). The inflammatory cytokine tumor necrosis factor-alpha generates an autocrine tumor-promoting network in epithelial ovarian cancer cells. *Cancer Research, 67*(2), 585–592.

Laberge, R. M., Zhou, L., Sarantos, M. R., Rodier, F., Freund, A., de Keizer, P. L.,...Campisi, J. (2012). Glucocorticoids suppress selected components of the senescence-associated secretory phenotype. *Aging Cell, 11*(4), 569–578.

Langowski, J. L., Zhang, X., Wu, L., Mattson, J. D., Chen, T., Smith, K.,...Oft, M. (2006). IL-23 promotes tumour incidence and growth. *Nature, 442*(7101), 461–465.

Leng, S. X., Xue, Q. L., Tian, J., Walston, J. D., & Fried, L. P. (2007). Inflammation and frailty in older women. *Journal of the American Geriatrics Society, 55*(6), 864–871.

Licastro, F., Pedrini, S., Caputo, L., Annoni, G., Davis, L. J., Ferri, C.,...Grimaldi, L. M. (2000). Increased plasma levels of interleukin-1, interleukin-6 and alpha-1-antichymotrypsin in patients with Alzheimer's disease: Peripheral inflammation or signals from the brain? *Journal of Neuroimmunology, 103*(1), 97–102.

López-Otín, C., Blasco, M. A., Partridge, L., Serrano, M., & Kroemer, G. (2013). The hallmarks of aging. *Cell, 153*(6), 1194–1217.

Lucicesare, A., Hubbard, R. E., Searle, S. D., & Rockwood, K. (2010). An index of self-rated health deficits in relation to frailty and adverse outcomes in older adults. *Aging Clinical and Experimental Research, 22*(3), 255–260.

Mannick, J. B., Del Giudice, G., Lattanzi, M., Valiante, N. M., Praestgaard, J., Huang, B.,...Klickstein, L. B. (2014). mTOR inhibition improves immune function in the elderly. *Science Translational Medicine, 6*(268), 268ra179.

Manolagas, S. C. (2000). Birth and death of bone cells: Basic regulatory mechanisms and implications for the pathogenesis and treatment of osteoporosis. *Endocrine Reviews, 21*(2), 115–137.

Manolagas, S. C., & Jilka, R. L. (1995). Bone marrow, cytokines, and bone remodeling. Emerging insights into the pathophysiology of osteoporosis. *The New England Journal of Medicine, 332*(5), 305–311.

Mantovani, A., Allavena, P., Sica, A., & Balkwill, F. (2008). Cancer-related inflammation. *Nature, 454*(7203), 436–444.

Meuter, A., Rogmann, L. M., Winterhoff, B. J., Tchkonia, T., Kirkland, J. L., & Morbeck, D. E. (2014). Markers of cellular senescence are elevated in murine blastocysts cultured in vitro: Molecular consequences of culture in atmospheric oxygen. *Journal of Assisted Reproduction and Genetics, 31*(10), 1259–1267.

Michaud, M., Balardy, L., Moulis, G., Gaudin, C., Peyrot, C., Vellas, B.,...Nourhashemi, F. (2013). Proinflammatory cytokines, aging, and age-related diseases. *Journal of the American Medical Directors Association, 14*(12), 877–882.

Minamino, T., Orimo, M., Shimizu, I., Kunieda, T., Yokoyama, M., Ito, T.,...Komuro, I. (2009). A crucial role for adipose tissue p53 in the regulation of insulin resistance. *Nature Medicine, 15*(9), 1082–1087.

Moiseeva, O., Deschênes-Simard, X., St-Germain, E., Igelmann, S., Huot, G., Cadar, A. E.,...Ferbeyre, G. (2013). Metformin inhibits the senescence-associated secretory phenotype by interfering with IKK/NF-κB activation. *Aging Cell, 12*(3), 489–498.

Mooney, R. A., Senn, J., Cameron, S., Inamdar, N., Boivin, L. M., Shang, Y., & Furlanetto, R. W. (2001). Suppressors of cytokine signaling-1 and -6 associate with

0826129420

and inhibit the insulin receptor. A potential mechanism for cytokine-mediated insulin resistance. *The Journal of Biological Chemistry, 276*(28), 25889–25893.

Nagabhushanam, V., Solache, A., Ting, L. M., Escaron, C. J., Zhang, J. Y., & Ernst, J. D. (2003). Innate inhibition of adaptive immunity: Mycobacterium tuberculosis-induced IL-6 inhibits macrophage responses to IFN-gamma. *Journal of Immunology, 171*(9), 4750–4757.

Nikolich-Žugich, J. (2014). Aging of the T cell compartment in mice and humans: From no naive expectations to foggy memories. *Journal of Immunology, 193*(6), 2622–2629.

Palmer, A. K., Tchkonia, T., LeBrasseur, N. K., Chini, E. N., Xu, M., & Kirkland, J. L. (2015). Cellular senescence in type 2 diabetes: A therapeutic opportunity. *Diabetes, 64*(7), 2289–2298.

Peruzzi, B., Cappariello, A., Del Fattore, A., Rucci, N., De Benedetti, F., & Teti, A. (2012). c-Src and IL-6 inhibit osteoblast differentiation and integrate IGFBP5 signalling. *Nature Communications, 3*, 630.

Philipot, D., Guérit, D., Platano, D., Chuchana, P., Olivotto, E., Espinoza, F.,...Brondello, J. M. (2014). p16INK4a and its regulator miR-24 link senescence and chondrocyte terminal differentiation-associated matrix remodeling in osteoarthritis. *Arthritis Research and Therapy, 16*(1), R58.

Pickup, J. C., Mattock, M. B., Chusney, G. D., & Burt, D. (1997). NIDDM as a disease of the innate immune system: Association of acute-phase reactants and interleukin-6 with metabolic syndrome X. *Diabetologia, 40*(11), 1286–1292.

Poland, G. A., Ovsyannikova, I. G., Kennedy, R. B., Lambert, N. D., & Kirkland, J. L. (2014). A systems biology approach to the effect of aging, immunosenescence and vaccine response. *Current Opinion in Immunology, 29*, 62–68.

Pradhan, A. D., Manson, J. E., Rifai, N., Buring, J. E., & Ridker, P. M. (2001). C-reactive protein, interleukin 6, and risk of developing type 2 diabetes mellitus. *Journal of the American Medical Association, 286*(3), 327–334.

Qu, T., Walston, J. D., Yang, H., Fedarko, N. S., Xue, Q. L., Beamer, B. A.,...Leng, S. X. (2009). Upregulated ex vivo expression of stress-responsive inflammatory pathway genes by LPS-challenged CD14(+) monocytes in frail older adults. *Mechanisms of Ageing and Development, 130*(3), 161–166.

Rockwood, K., & Mitnitski, A. (2011). Frailty defined by deficit accumulation and geriatric medicine defined by frailty. *Clinics in Geriatric Medicine, 27*(1), 17–26.

Rockwood, K., Mitnitski, A., Song, X., Steen, B., & Skoog, I. (2006). Long-term risks of death and institutionalization of elderly people in relation to deficit accumulation at age 70. *Journal of the American Geriatrics Society, 54*(6), 975–979.

Rosano, C., Marsland, A. L., & Gianaros, P. J. (2012). Maintaining brain health by monitoring inflammatory processes: A mechanism to promote successful aging. *Aging and Disease, 3*(1), 16–33.

Rose, J., Söder, S., Skhirtladze, C., Schmitz, N., Gebhard, P. M., Sesselmann, S., & Aigner, T. (2012). DNA damage, discoordinated gene expression and cellular senescence in osteoarthritic chondrocytes. *Osteoarthritis and Cartilage/OARS, Osteoarthritis Research Society, 20*(9), 1020–1028.

Ross, R. (1999). Atherosclerosis—An inflammatory disease. *The New England Journal of Medicine, 340*(2), 115–126.

Rui, L., Yuan, M., Frantz, D., Shoelson, S., & White, M. F. (2002). SOCS-1 and SOCS-3 block insulin signaling by ubiquitin-mediated degradation of IRS1 and IRS2. *The Journal of Biological Chemistry, 277*(44), 42394–42398.

Sarvas, J. L., Khaper, N., & Lees, S. J. (2013). The IL-6 paradox: Context dependent interplay of SOCS3 and AMPK. *Journal of Diabetes & Metabolism*, Suppl. 13. doi: 10.4172/2155-6156.S13-003

Schetter, A. J., Heegaard, N. H., & Harris, C. C. (2010). Inflammation and cancer: Interweaving microRNA, free radical, cytokine and p53 pathways. *Carcinogenesis, 31*(1), 37–49.

Schouten, M., Wiersinga, W. J., Levi, M., & van der Poll, T. (2008). Inflammation, endothelium, and coagulation in sepsis. *Journal of Leukocyte Biology, 83*(3), 536–545.

Schram, M. T., Euser, S. M., de Craen, A. J., Witteman, J. C., Frölich, M., Hofman, A.,…Westendorp, R. G. (2007). Systemic markers of inflammation and cognitive decline in old age. *Journal of the American Geriatrics Society, 55*(5), 708–716.

Sebastian, C., Lloberas, J., & Celada, A. (2009). Molecular and cellular aspects of macrophage aging. In T. Fulop (Ed.), *Handbook on immunosenescence* (pp. 919–945). Dordrecht, the Netherlands: Springer Science + Business Media B.V.

Serrats, J., Schiltz, J. C., García-Bueno, B., van Rooijen, N., Reyes, T. M., & Sawchenko, P. E. (2010). Dual roles for perivascular macrophages in immune-to-brain signaling. *Neuron, 65*(1), 94–106.

Shoelson, S. E., Lee, J., & Yuan, M. (2003). Inflammation and the IKK beta/I kappa B/NF-kappa B axis in obesity- and diet-induced insulin resistance. *International Journal of Obesity and Related Metabolic Disorders, 27*(Suppl. 3), S49–S52.

Sikora, E., Bielak-Zmijewska, A., & Mosieniak, G. (2014). Cellular senescence in ageing, age-related disease and longevity. *Current Vascular Pharmacology, 12*(5), 698–706.

Singh, T., & Newman, A. B. (2011). Inflammatory markers in population studies of aging. *Ageing Research Reviews, 10*(3), 319–329.

Smith, D. L., Elam, C. F., Mattison, J. A., Lane, M. A., Roth, G. S., Ingram, D. K., & Allison, D. B. (2010). Metformin supplementation and life span in Fischer-344 rats. *The Journals of Gerontology, Series A, 65*(5), 468–474.

So, M. W., Lee, E. J., Lee, H. S., Koo, B. S., Kim, Y. G., Lee, C. K., & Yoo, B. (2013). Protective effects of ginsenoside Rg3 on human osteoarthritic chondrocytes. *Modern Rheumatology/The Japan Rheumatism Association, 23*(1), 104–111.

Sparmann, A., & Bar-Sagi, D. (2004). Ras-induced interleukin-8 expression plays a critical role in tumor growth and angiogenesis. *Cancer Cell, 6*(5), 447–458.

Spranger, J., Kroke, A., Möhlig, M., Hoffmann, K., Bergmann, M. M., Ristow, M.,…Pfeiffer, A. F. (2003). Inflammatory cytokines and the risk to develop type 2 diabetes: Results of the prospective population-based European Prospective Investigation into Cancer and Nutrition (EPIC)-Potsdam Study. *Diabetes, 52*(3), 812–817.

Srikrishna, G., & Freeze, H. H. (2009). Endogenous damage-associated molecular pattern molecules at the crossroads of inflammation and cancer. *Neoplasia, 11*(7), 615–628.

Stern, D. M., Kaiser, E., & Nawroth, P. P. (1988). Regulation of the coagulation system by vascular endothelial cells. *Haemostasis, 18*(4–6), 202–214.

Szlosarek, P. W., & Balkwill, F. R. (2003). Tumour necrosis factor alpha: A potential target for the therapy of solid tumours. *The Lancet. Oncology, 4*(9), 565–573.

Tan, Z. S., Beiser, A. S., Vasan, R. S., Roubenoff, R., Dinarello, C. A., Harris, T. B.,…Seshadri, S. (2007). Inflammatory markers and the risk of Alzheimer disease: The Framingham Study. *Neurology, 68*(22), 1902–1908.

Tchkonia, T., Morbeck, D. E., Von Zglinicki, T., Van Deursen, J., Lustgarten, J., Scrable, H.,…Kirkland, J. L. (2010). Fat tissue, aging, and cellular senescence. *Aging Cell, 9*(5), 667–684.

Tchkonia, T., Zhu, Y., van Deursen, J., Campisi, J., & Kirkland, J. L. (2013). Cellular senescence and the senescent secretory phenotype: Therapeutic opportunities. *The Journal of Clinical Investigation, 123*(3), 966–972.

Tefferi, A., Litzow, M. R., & Pardanani, A. (2011). Long-term outcome of treatment with ruxolitinib in myelofibrosis. *The New England Journal of Medicine, 365*(15), 1455–1457.

Tracy, R. P. (2003). Emerging relationships of inflammation, cardiovascular disease and chronic diseases of aging. *International Journal of Obesity and Related Metabolic Disorders, 27*(Suppl. 3), S29–S34.

Tracy, R. P., Lemaitre, R. N., Psaty, B. M., Ives, D. G., Evans, R. W., Cushman, M.,…Kuller, L. H. (1997). Relationship of C-reactive protein to risk of cardiovascular disease in the elderly. Results from the Cardiovascular Health Study and the Rural Health Promotion Project. *Arteriosclerosis, Thrombosis, and Vascular Biology, 17*(6), 1121–1127.

Verstovsek, S., Mesa, R. A., Gotlib, J., Levy, R. S., Gupta, V., DiPersio, J. F.,…Kantarjian, H. M. (2012). A double-blind, placebo-controlled trial of ruxolitinib for myelofibrosis. *The New England Journal of Medicine, 366*(9), 799–807.

Visser, M., Pahor, M., Taaffe, D. R., Goodpaster, B. H., Simonsick, E. M., Newman, A. B.,…Harris, T. B. (2002). Relationship of interleukin-6 and tumor necrosis factor-alpha with muscle mass and muscle strength in elderly men and women: The Health ABC Study. *The Journals of Gerontology, Series A, 57*(5), M326–M332.

Volpato, S., Guralnik, J. M., Ferrucci, L., Balfour, J., Chaves, P., Fried, L. P., & Harris, T. B. (2001). Cardiovascular disease, interleukin-6, and risk of mortality in older women: The women's health and aging study. *Circulation, 103*(7), 947–953.

Voronov, E., Shouval, D. S., Krelin, Y., Cagnano, E., Benharroch, D., Iwakura, Y.,…Apte, R. N. (2003). IL-1 is required for tumor invasiveness and angiogenesis. *Proceedings of the National Academy of Sciences of the United States of America, 100*(5), 2645–2650.

Walston, J., Hadley, E. C., Ferrucci, L., Guralnik, J. M., Newman, A. B., Studenski, S. A.,…Fried, L. P. (2006). Research agenda for frailty in older adults: Toward a better understanding of physiology and etiology: Summary from the American Geriatrics Society/National Institute on Aging Research Conference on Frailty in Older Adults. *Journal of the American Geriatrics Society, 54*(6), 991–1001.

Walston, J., McBurnie, M. A., Newman, A., Tracy, R. P., Kop, W. J., Hirsch, C. H.,…Fried, L. P.; Cardiovascular Health Study. (2002). Frailty and activation of the inflammation and coagulation systems with and without clinical comorbidities: Results from the Cardiovascular Health Study. *Archives of Internal Medicine, 162*(20), 2333–2341.

Walston, J. D., Matteini, A. M., Nievergelt, C., Lange, L. A., Fallin, D. M., Barzilai, N.,...Reiner, A. P. (2009). Inflammation and stress-related candidate genes, plasma interleukin-6 levels, and longevity in older adults. *Experimental Gerontology, 44*(5), 350–355.

Xu, M., Palmer, A. K., Ding, H., Weivoda, M. M., Pirtskhalava, T., White, T. A., ... Kirkland, J. L. (2015). Targeting senescent cells enhances adipogenesis and metabolic function in old age. *eLife, 4*, e12997.

Xu, M., Tchkonia, T., Ding, H., Ogrodnik, M., Lubbers, E. R., Pirtskhalava, T.,... Kirkland, J. L. (2015). JAK inhibition alleviates the cellular senescence-associated secretory phenotype and frailty in old age. *Proceedings of the National Academy of Sciences of the United States of America, 112*(46), e6301–6310.

Yaffe, K., Lindquist, K., Penninx, B. W., Simonsick, E. M., Pahor, M., Kritchevsky, S.,...Harris, T. (2003). Inflammatory markers and cognition in well-functioning African-American and white elders. *Neurology, 61*(1), 76–80.

Zheng, S. X., Vrindts, Y., Lopez, M., De Groote, D., Zangerle, P. F., Collette, J.,...Reginster, J. Y. (1997). Increase in cytokine production (IL-1 beta, IL-6, TNF-alpha but not IFN-gamma, GM-CSF or LIF) by stimulated whole blood cells in postmenopausal osteoporosis. *Maturitas, 26*(1), 63–71.

Zhu, Y., Armstrong, J. L., Tchkonia, T., & Kirkland, J. L. (2014). Cellular senescence and the senescent secretory phenotype in age-related chronic diseases. *Current opinion in Clinical Nutrition and Metabolic Care, 17*(4), 324–328.

Zhu, Y., Tchkonia, T., Pirtskhalava, T., Gower, A. C., Ding, H., Giorgadze, N.,...Kirkland, J. L. (2015). The Achilles' heel of senescent cells: From transcriptome to senolytic drugs. *Aging Cell, 14*(4), 644–658.

CHAPTER 9

Theories of Stem Cell Aging

Pedro Sousa-Victor, Joana Neves, and Heinrich Jasper

Adult stem cells are undifferentiated, multipotent progenitor cells residing within a fully differentiated tissue that are required to replace damaged or lost cells. Adult stem cells are also referred to as "somatic" stem cells, and they are defined by two basic properties: self-renewal and multipotency. Self-renewal refers to the capacity to produce a daughter cell with similar stem cell properties. Multipotency refers to the capacity to engage differentiation programs leading to the generation of a limited number of mature cell types that constitute their corresponding adult host tissue. Upon homeostatic pressure, imposed by homeostatic demand (normal turnover of differentiated tissues) or tissue damage (an injury), some stem cells are activated, after which both fundamental functions need to be coordinated. Failure to self-renew will result in a depletion of the stem cell pool, while failure to engage the appropriate differentiation programs will compromise tissue maintenance and regeneration.

Adult stem cells are not sheltered from the aging process, and the molecular and cellular mechanisms underlying stem cell aging are now beginning to be understood. The consequences of aging on stem cell function vary greatly among tissues, involving defects in activation, self-renewal, and differentiation. Despite these differences, the outcome of these defects will ultimately be a loss of homeostatic capacity, tissue dysfunction, and degenerative or hyperplastic pathologies (Liu & Rando, 2011; Oh, Lee, & Wagers, 2014).

Intercellular communication between the stem cell and its surrounding milieu is critical for normal stem cell function. This includes communication between stem cells and the local microenvironment (the niche), as well as between stem cells and the systemic environment. Accordingly, age-associated alterations in the stem cell environment have significant impact on stem cell function and are important determinants of stem cell aging (Jasper & Kennedy, 2012; Jones & Rando, 2011). Yet, accumulating evidence suggests that stem cell–specific alterations that impair their capacity to respond to niche-derived and systemic stimuli also contribute to the age-associated loss of regenerative capacity in many tissues. Recent studies further suggest that stem cells can provide signals that modulate immune function in their environment, but the impact of this latter activity on the aging organism remains largely unexplored (Martino, Pluchino, Bonfanti, & Schwartz, 2011; Pluchino et al., 2005; Wang, Chen, Cao, & Shi, 2014b).

In this chapter, we discuss current theories of stem cells aging, focusing on the molecular and cellular determinants leading to loss of stem cell function with age and on the consequences for tissue regeneration and homeostasis. Furthermore, we discuss the emerging concept of stem cells as immune modulators. Finally, we elaborate the theory that declining adult stem cell function precipitates normal aging.

■ MODELS OF STEM CELL AGING

The last decade has seen significant advances in the understanding of the biology of aging along with important discoveries in the field of regenerative biology in vertebrate and invertebrate model systems. This combination of factors yielded an optimal environment for advances in the biology of stem cell aging.

Although invertebrate model systems have long been used in aging studies, somatic stem cell aging research (as opposed to research on aging of germline stem cells) in nonvertebrate models was possible only after the identification of a population of stem cells in the midgut of the intestinal tract of the fruit fly, *Drosophila melanogaster* (Micchelli & Perrimon, 2006; Ohlstein & Spradling, 2006). The intestinal stem cell (ISC) resides on the basal side of the epithelium and is the only proliferating cell type in the *Drosophila* midgut. Upon homeostatic (normal turnover of intestinal tissue) or regenerative pressure (e.g., after an injury caused by an external agent), the ISC is activated and divides to give rise to another stem cell and an intermediate, nonproliferating progenitor, the enteroblast (EB), which can further differentiate into two specialized cell types— the enterocyte (EC) and the enteroendocrine cell (EE). The simple architecture of the *Drosophila* intestinal epithelium, the availability of tools for genetic manipulation, and the short life span of *Drosophila* have allowed rapid progress in our understanding of somatic stem cell aging, and have helped to characterize mechanisms of stem cell aging conserved in vertebrates (Biteau, Hochmuth, & Jasper, 2011; Jones & Rando, 2011).

In vertebrates, murine model systems have taken the lead, but other organisms are being utilized. Despite their remarkable regenerative capacity, teleost vertebrate model organisms, such as zebrafish, have not been used in the aging biology field, mostly because of the long life spans (3.5 years on average for zebrafish). To overcome this limitation, the short-lived teleost fish African killifish *Nothobranchius furzeri*, with an average life span of 10 weeks, is emerging as a model for aging studies, including stem cell aging, with tools for genetic manipulation currently being developed (Harel et al., 2015; Valenzano, Sharp, & Brunet, 2011).

In mammals, somatic stem cells have been identified in several adult tissues and most aging studies have focused primarily in six systems (Figure 9.1): the skeletal muscle stem cell (also known as "satellite cell"); the hematopoietic stem cell (HSC); the neural stem cell (NSC), the mesenchymal stem cell (MSC), the ISC, and the skin stem cell. Mammalian models used in biomedical research exhibit relatively long life spans (e.g., 2–3 years for mice), which slows the pace of discovery in aging research. As a means to overcome this problem, mouse models of progeria syndromes have often been used to uncover key regulators of stem cell aging. Progeroid syndromes are genetic disorders that mimic premature aging, leading to the development of aging features at younger age. Because these are usually monogenic diseases, mouse models carrying mutations in the relevant genes can be used as progeria models and thus accelerate aging research, although caution in the interpretation of results is necessary, as progerias may represent only certain, and not all, aspects of the normal aging process.

Although the different stem cell populations accomplish the same basic function, their activity throughout the life of an organism is extremely variable and depends on the specific demands of the tissues in which they reside. Low turnover tissues, such as the skeletal muscle or the nervous system, do not routinely replace their differentiated cells—the muscle fibers and the neurons, respectively. In these tissues, the stem cell remains in a dormant state throughout most of the organism life. This dormant state is referred to as quiescence and is characterized by a reversible exit from the cell

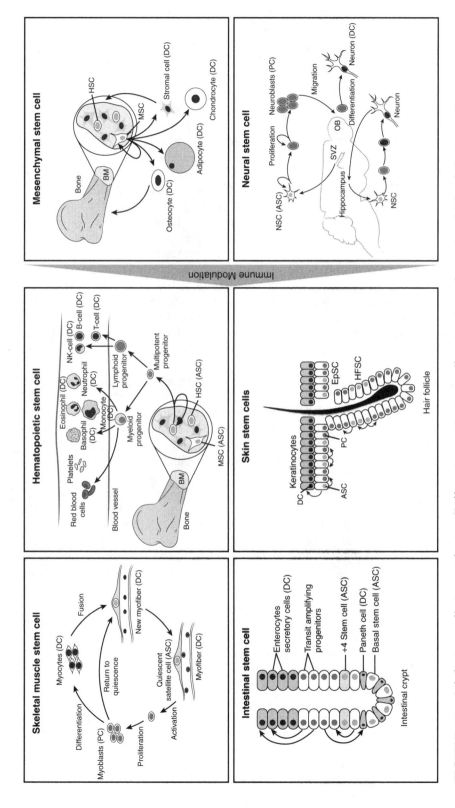

FIGURE 9.1 Adult stem cells in vertebrates. Different somatic stem cell systems are shown in which adult stem cells are represented by the letters ASC, progenitor cells by the word "progenitor" or the letters PC, and differentiated cells by the letters DC. All renderings in this figure are simplified versions of the activation and differentiation process of the stem cell in each system.

BM = bone marrow; EpSC, epidermal stem cell; HFSC, hair follicle stem cell; HSC, hematopoietic stem cell; MSC, mesenchymal stem cell; NSC = neural stem cell; OB, olfactory bulb; SVZ, subventricular zone.

155

cycle and low metabolic activity. Although quiescent, the satellite cells and NSCs can be readily activated in response to specific cues. Under such conditions, they will reenter cell cycle and proliferate (a process known as "activation") to give rise to a population of transient-activated progenitors, the myoblasts and neuroblasts, which will further differentiate into mature cell types—myofibers and neurons (Gage, 2002; Zhang et al., 2013). A subpopulation of these activated progenitors has to reinstate the quiescent state so that the stem cell pool can be maintained. In both compartments, a decrease of the proliferative activity of stem cells with aging is observed. In the skeletal muscle, this loss of proliferative capacity results in defective self-renewal and ultimately depletion of the stem cell population, and is also accompanied by a deficiency in differentiation, resulting in increased fibrotic scars after an injury in old mice. The decline in satellite cell function has been attributed to systemic factors; yet it is also a consequence of the failure to regulate the reversible quiescent state, ultimately leading to a transition to a senescent state (Sousa-Victor, Garcia-Prat, Serrano, Perdiguero, & Munoz-Canoves, 2015). This senescent state is a characteristic of many aged cell populations, which is defined by irreversible cell cycle arrest. It has evolved as a cancer-protective mechanism, but it is also believed to be the driving force behind many age-related pathologies.

In contrast, the diminished proliferative capacity of neural progenitors with age is proposed to be associated with an increase in the quiescent population of NSCs (Hattiangady & Shetty, 2008; Lugert et al., 2010; Miron et al., 2013). However, it still remains controversial whether this results or not in a depletion of the stem cell pool with contradictory data supporting opposing views (Hattiangady & Shetty, 2008; Miron et al., 2013; Molofsky et al., 2006). However, these reports refer to stem cells found in different regions of the brain, and it is likely that they correspond to functionally different populations with distinct aging phenotypes.

High turnover tissues are those that replace their differentiated cell types on a regular basis. This is the case of the blood, the intestine, or the skin. In these tissues, homeostatic renewal requires high stem cell activity throughout life, although recent studies have identified and characterized also quiescent stem cell populations that serve as "reserve" stem cell populations in these tissues (Tian et al., 2011).

HSCs sustain hematopoiesis, that is, the generation of the entire blood system. This includes cells of two main lineages: the lymphoid lineage comprising the B and T white blood cells that play central roles in cell-mediated immunity; and the myeloid lineage that comprises the red blood cells, the platelets, and a different set of white blood cells, involved in the first line of defense of the body, also referred to as "innate immunity." In aging mice, the hematopoietic lineage skews toward myeloid differentiation at the expense of lymphoid differentiation, compromising immune function. Moreover, myeloid progenitors overproliferate leading to unlimited self-renewal, resulting in myeloid hyperplasia. Because hematopoiesis is a frequent process, its deregulation during aging leads to a wide range of pathological conditions and associated impairments in blood cell composition, particularly myeloid leukemias and deficiencies in immune competence. In contrast, under stress-induced regenerative pressure, old HSCs show impaired self-renewal and proliferative potential, which results in defective blood reconstitution and diminished regenerative capacity (Flach et al., 2014; Rossi, Jamieson, & Weissman, 2008).

Similarly, the intestine and the skin, which function as barrier epithelia, frequently replenish their differentiated cell types and the function of their stem cells is central to this process. ISCs display a remarkable capacity to maintain their proliferative potential throughout life, a function that has been attributed to high levels of telomerase activity

(Schepers, Vries, van den Born, van de Wetering, & Clevers, 2011). Telomerase is an enzyme responsible for maintaining the telomeres—a repetitive DNA sequence at the ends of chromosomes, which protects them from deterioration and fusion—over rounds of cell division. Consistently, telomerase-deficient mice display an age-related decrease in ISCs in the small intestine, and exhibit a deficient response to stresses that challenge the regenerative potential of the gastrointestinal system (Rudolph et al., 1999). Skin stem cells are also affected by aging. In particular, hair follicle stem cells, which are responsible for the renewal of hair, hyperproliferate with aging while decreasing their function and stress tolerance. This has been, at least in part, attributed to the increase in pro-inflammatory signals that negatively impact stem cell function (Doles, Storer, Cozzuto, Roma, & Keyes, 2012).

MSCs have the ability to differentiate into bone, cartilage, and fat; however, their main physiological function seems to be independent from the traditional stem cell–like activity. In fact, both native and transplanted MSCs play important immune modulatory functions: They secrete molecules that can influence the state of immune cells, which in turn can influence stem cell function through the secretion of pro-inflammatory and anti-inflammatory molecules. This immune modulatory function supports tissue repair after damage and there is evidence that their depletion can lead to tissue dysfunctions (Roberts et al., 2013). Therefore, MSCs seem to be important mediators of tissue homeostasis and their loss of function with age may have important consequences for organismal aging (Fukada, Ma, & Uezumi, 2014). MSC aging is characterized by a decline in cell number and function, regulated by most of the same molecular mechanisms underlying the aging process of other somatic stem cell populations (Yu & Kang, 2013). However, how this age-associated decline affects their immune modulatory and supportive function and what the consequences for organismal aging are remain largely unexplored questions (Fukada et al., 2014; Sepulveda et al., 2014; Yu et al., 2014).

Despite the differences in their function and plasticity, current studies suggest that the molecular and cellular mechanisms that determine adult stem cell aging are conserved mostly among these different systems. In the next section, we discuss the common hallmarks of adult stem cell aging and how they influence stem cell function in different tissues.

▪ DETERMINANTS OF STEM CELL AGING

Adult stem cell aging is the result of a combination of factors, including extrinsic cues from the local and systemic environment as well as cell-intrinsic alterations of the stem cell. The stem cell is surrounded by other cells that include the differentiated cell types that constitute their host tissues, the blood vessels, and resident and circulating immune cells. This complex environment surrounding the stem cell is referred to as "the niche" and it is a source of signaling cues that modulate stem cell activation, self-renewal, and differentiation. Alterations in cell composition and secreted molecules in the niche are known to be a source of age-related stem cell decline. In addition, secreted molecules found in the blood can also modulate stem cell function and age-associated changes of the systemic environment have detrimental consequences for stem cell function. This was first demonstrated by studies using heterochronic parabiosis, in which the circulatory systems of two animals of different ages were surgically combined. These studies demonstrated that old stem cell function could be rejuvenated when exposed to young blood, while the function of stem cells from the younger animal in the heterochronic pair would decline in the presence of old serum. These studies indicate that there are factors present in the old circulatory system that can drive loss of stem cell function, while the young blood may potentially contain factors, otherwise depleted in the old serum, that promote stem cell activity (Conboy et al., 2005). These findings spawned a large number of studies to identify such factors, with interesting leads that are subject of intense investigation and debate (Oh et al., 2014).

Stem cell intrinsic aging refers to biological phenomena that will occur intracellularly in the stem cell that will irreversibly compromise its ability to perform its functions. These include accumulation of protein, DNA, and organelle damage as well as metabolic changes that deregulate cell function.

Although often looked at as two independent mechanisms of stem cell aging, it is becoming evident that extrinsic and intrinsic aging are in fact interconnected processes. First, because aging is a progressive process, it is likely that environmental dysregulation may cause several defects that accumulate intrinsically, while secreted signals from the aging environment likely impair intracellular signaling in the adult stem cell, exacerbating the environmental effects. Second, because some stem cell populations have themselves the ability to influence the surrounding environment, it is also likely that a feed-forward loop acts cooperatively to drive stem cell aging at the organism level, accounting for the progressive nature of the aging process (Jung & Brack, 2014; Oh et al., 2014).

Stem Cell Intrinsic Changes

OXIDATIVE STRESS

The concept of stem cell aging resulting from accumulation of cellular and mitochondrial oxidative damage is directly linked with the decades-old "free radical theory of aging." Given that aging is a universal process affecting all organs and tissues, Dr. Harman assumed a common underlying basic mechanism driving aging and proposed free radicals as its determinant (Harman, 1956). Reactive oxygen species (ROS) are formed as a by-product of cellular respiration. The accumulation of ROS in the aged cell can lead to macromolecular damage and disruption of proper mitochondria function, which drives a higher production of ROS in a cycle that eventually results in a cellular breakdown (Harman, 1956).

The causal relation between oxidative cellular damage and the aging process is controversial and recent studies indicate that the age-associated accumulation of cellular ROS might not be sufficient to explain the phenomenon of aging. In the nematode *Caenorhabditis elegans*, increased oxidative stress caused by deletion of superoxide dismutase genes does not result in altered life span (Van Raamsdonk & Hekimi, 2012) and inappropriately elevated ROS generation is compatible with extended longevity of nematodes (Van Raamsdonk & Hekimi, 2009; Yee, Yang, & Hekimi, 2014). ROS are also fundamental signaling molecules, and dysregulation of the redox state might have an impact on stem cell function independently of macromolecular damage. Indeed, Nrf2, a master regulator of the cellular redox state, specifically controls the proliferative activity of progenitor cells in the *Drosophila* intestine and mouse trachea (Biteau et al., 2011; Paul et al., 2014; Smith, Ladi, Mayer-Proschel, & Noble, 2000). Loss of Nrf2 activity causes accumulation of ROS in ISCs, a condition that is required for stem cell proliferation during regeneration, but accelerates age-associated dysplasia of the intestinal epithelium (Biteau et al., 2011). A low intracellular concentration of ROS is now considered a critical condition for proper stem cell function and excessive cellular ROS levels are associated with loss of self-renewal capacity, abnormal proliferation, and malignancy in different tissues (Holmstrom & Finkel, 2014).

MITOCHONDRIAL FUNCTION AND METABOLISM

The importance of oxidative stress in stem cell aging is also supported by work done with the Sirtuin (Sirt) family of proteins. After initial reports showing that Sir2 could extend life span of *Saccharomyces cerevisiae* (Kaeberlein, McVey, & Guarente, 1999), extensive research efforts were dedicated to exploring the potential role of Sirtuins in the biology of aging (Longo & Kennedy, 2006). One example is the study of the role of SIRT3 in HSCs. SIRT3 is highly expressed in HSCs, where it regulates stress responses (Brown et al., 2013). Although SIRT3 is dispensable for HSC maintenance in young mice under homeostatic conditions, it seems essential under stress or at an advanced age. Re-establishment of the levels and activity of SIRT3 in aged HSCs reduced the age-associated increase in ROS levels and improved their regenerative capacity (Brown et al., 2013). Sirtuins are also emerging as important modulators of metabolic end epigenetic states, and it can be expected that these functions contribute to their positive effects on SC maintenance.

Mitochondrial dysfunction has long been considered an important factor in aging (Bratic & Larsson, 2013; Jensen & Jasper, 2014). The association between mitochondrial integrity and aging has been reinforced by the observation that different tissues display an age-dependent accumulation of mitochondrial DNA (mtDNA) mutations. MtDNA, unlike nuclear DNA, is located in the mitochondria and, although it codes for a very small proportion of genes, it is essential for organismal function. Mouse models that accumulate somatic mtDNA mutations exhibit reduced life span and premature onset of aging-related phenotypes, suggesting a causative link between mtDNA mutations and aging phenotypes in mammals (Kujoth et al., 2005; Trifunovic et al., 2004). Interestingly, the accumulation of mtDNA mutations in HSCs can cause differentiation blockage and the disappearance of downstream progenitors. However, this impairment seems to be molecularly distinct from what is observed in physiological HSC aging, arguing against the idea that mtDNA mutations are primary drivers of HSC aging (Norddahl et al., 2011). Nevertheless, the progeroid phenotypes that result from increased mtDNA mutagenesis impact different populations of somatic stem cells and can be attenuated through the supplementation with antioxidants, supporting a link between mitochondrial dysfunction, ROS accumulation, and the decline of stem cell function in aging organisms (Ahlqvist et al., 2012).

Recent studies are going beyond the traditional role of mitochondria in the context of the free radical theory of aging and are exploring specific changes in metabolic pathways as consequences of mitochondrial dysfunction that contribute to the aging process (Bratic & Larsson, 2013). Caloric restriction (CR), known to enhance longevity, results in improved stem cell function and is also associated with increased mitochondrial content. Consistently, in vitro manipulations of nutrients to enhance mitochondrial energy production recapitulate the beneficial effects of CR on muscle stem cells (Cerletti, Jang, Finley, Haigis, & Wagers, 2012).

Among the molecular mediators of these responses are likely common nutrient sensing signaling pathways, including the insulin/Foxo and the Tor signaling pathways. FoxO subfamily proteins promote the long-term maintenance of several stem cell populations in flies and mice. In the *Drosophila* midgut, insulin signaling and Foxo regulate proliferation of ISCs and the regenerative response to tissue damage (Biteau et al., 2010;

Biteau, Hochmuth, & Jasper, 2008). A dysregulated ISC response leads to intestinal dysplasia, a phenotype that is observed in aging animals and is characterized by improper growth and differentiation of the epithelia. Limiting insulin signaling or overexpression of Foxo target genes in the progenitor cells is sufficient to limit ISC proliferation, thus extending life span (Biteau et al., 2010). In mouse HSCs, Foxo proteins are critical to prevent age-related oxidative stress and to prevent dysfunction and loss of stem cells (Tothova et al., 2007).

The mTOR pathway, also widely linked to organismal aging, is one of the main effectors of the organism's response to CR (Kapahi et al., 2010; Laplante & Sabatini, 2012). The activity of the mTOR pathway is increased in HSCs from aged mice, and increasing mTOR signaling through conditional deletion of Tsc1 is sufficient to cause premature aging of HSCs in young mice (Chen, Liu, & Zheng, 2009). Consistently, the persistent activation of mTOR signaling leads to the depletion of epidermal stem cells and accelerated age-dependent hair loss in mice, a phenotype that can be reversed through rapamycin supplementation (Castilho, Squarize, Chodosh, Williams, & Gutkind, 2009).

GENOMIC INSTABILITY AND EPIGENETIC ALTERATIONS

The quiescent state of stem cells is associated with a low ROS-producing metabolic state, which prevents damage to cells (Shyh-Chang, Daley, & Cantley, 2013). Nevertheless, the long-term exposure of stem cells to genotoxic agents during their lifetimes does seem to have an impact on DNA integrity, and signs of DNA damage can be detected in aged stem cells from different tissues (Burkhalter, Rudolph, & Sperka, 2015). This accumulation of DNA damage might arise from a reduced capacity of the aged stem cell to repair DNA, or from defects in faithfully replicating DNA (Flach et al., 2014). The fact that different progeroid syndromes, including Hutchinson–Gliford, Werner, and Cockayne's, are linked to mutations affecting DNA repair factors (Burtner & Kennedy, 2010) supports an important role for DNA repair pathways in physiological aging. Replicative stress, that is, potential sources of cellular damage that can occur during DNA replication, and the associated DNA damage response were also directly linked with the premature exhaustion of the HSC pool in Fanconi anemia (FA), an inherited DNA repair deficiency syndrome (Ceccaldi et al., 2012).

A possible consequence of the age-associated accumulation of genome-wide mutations and DNA damage in aging stem cells is change in chromatin that leads to widespread deregulation in gene expression. Chromatin refers to the complex formed between DNA and proteins that allows the compaction of the genetic material into the nucleus. It can exist in two forms: Euchromatin, a less condensed form that allows gene expression, and heterochromatin, a highly compacted form usually associated with transcriptional repression. These forms are generated and maintained by epigenetic marks, which involve alterations to histone proteins (the proteins around which DNA is wrapped) or to the DNA molecule itself. Changes in the maintenance and organization of these epigenetic states likely contribute to global heterochromatin loss and resulting cellular alterations in aged organisms (Tsurumi & Li, 2012; Villeponteau, 1997). Age-dependent changes in the epigenome, including histone modifications such as methylation, acetylation, and ubiquitination, can also affect chromatin structure in stem cells (Rando & Chang, 2012). Global transcriptome and epigenome analysis comparing young and aged HSCs revealed that the expression of key epigenetic regulators decreases with age (Sun et al., 2014). In satellite cells, a genome-wide study indicated that the global epigenetic landscape is altered in aged quiescent cells compared to young quiescent cells (Liu et al., 2013).

A deeper understanding of the causes and consequences of epigenetic changes, as well as insight into how these changes influence stem cell function in aging organisms is needed and will be subject to investigation in the years to come.

Inflammaging and the Stem Cell Niche

Adult stem cells reside within a niche and are in close proximity to blood vessels; therefore, they are constantly exposed to signaling cues derived from soluble proteins that reach the stem cell niche via the bloodstream or other cells that compose their local environment. Aging is accompanied by a generic dysregulation of intercellular signaling often linked with the development of a pro-inflammatory condition, referred to as "inflammaging." This is thought to be, at least in part, a driving force for aging phenotypes, including those of stem cells (Franceschi & Campisi, 2014; Neves, Demaria, Campisi, & Jasper, 2015). Because the cross talk between immune cells and stem cells is an important determinant of regenerative capacity (Aurora & Olson, 2014; Kokaia, Martino, Schwartz, & Lindvall, 2012), it is likely that aging-driven inflammation is itself an important determinant of stem cell aging.

INFLAMMATORY SIGNALS

The impact of the systemic environment on stem cell aging was demonstrated in heterochronic parabiosis experiments, in which the blood systems of old and young mice were connected. These experiments showed that the aged systemic environment has an important contribution to stem and progenitor cell loss of function in the skeletal muscle, central nervous system (CNS), liver, and heart (Brack et al., 2007; Conboy et al., 2005; Loffredo et al., 2013; Ruckh et al., 2012; Villeda et al., 2011). The molecular and cellular cues responsible for these effects, however, are only beginning to be understood. Villeda et al. (2011) identified the chemokine eotaxin (CCL11) as a mediator of the effects of old serum on the decline in hippocampal neurogenesis, learning, and memory. Eotaxin is elevated in old serum and exogenous administration of the chemokine in young animals can reproduce the adverse effects of old blood on hippocampal neurogenesis, although the mechanism behind this function is still unknown (Villeda et al., 2011).

Although some studies point to a lack of anti-inflammatory signals as a driver of stem cell loss of function with age, there is also substantial evidence supporting the negative impact of pro-inflammatory signals on stem cell function (Mirantes, Passegue, & Pietras, 2014). Interleukin-6 (IL-6), for example, a pro-inflammatory molecule whose expression substantially increases with age, can reprogram multipotent progenitors derived from HSCs to promote differentiation into the myeloid lineage at the expense of the lymphoid lineage (Ishihara & Hirano, 2002; Maeda et al., 2005; Reynaud et al., 2011). Although the immune modulatory actions described previously seem to be beneficial in the context of acute inflammation in response to infection (Schurch, Riether, & Ochsenbein, 2014; Zhao et al., 2014), in the context of chronic inflammation, they have deleterious effects leading to cancer phenotypes, such as chronic myelogenous leukemia (Reynaud et al., 2011).

SYSTEMIC AND NICHE FACTORS

In addition to inflammatory signals, signaling cues from growth factors classically involved in the regulation of proliferation and differentiation during development are known to also regulate adult stem cell function. Moreover, dysregulation of these signaling pathways during aging contributes to the age-associated decline in stem cell function. An important emerging concept in this context is how the integration of these different inputs regulates the ability of the stem cell to maintain reversible quiescence while also maintaining the capacity to activate and generate the appropriate progeny. Fibroblast growth factor (FGF) and epidermal growth factor receptor (EGFR) signaling are important mitogenic cues—signals that promote cell proliferation—during development, acting through the activation of the mitogen-activated protein kinase (MAPK) pathway. These pathways also control stem cell function and their dysregulation has been linked to adult stem cell aging in different systems. In mammalian skeletal muscle, FGF2 expression is increased in the aging myofiber, leading to a disruption of satellite cell quiescence because of spontaneous mitogenic activity, which can be rescued by inhibition of FGF signaling (Chakkalakal, Jones, Basson, & Brack, 2012). It is important to note that satellite cells are equipped with a safeguard mechanism to protect them from this spontaneous mitogenic activity during aging. Sprouty1, a negative regulator of FGF signaling, is expressed in satellite cells, and its genetic ablation in aged SCs causes a depletion of the satellite cell pool and diminished regenerative capacity (Chakkalakal et al., 2012). This is likely the result of an inability to reinstate the quiescent state, leading to apoptosis at the expense of self-renewal (Shea et al., 2010). Therefore, during aging, only cells that can maintain robust Sprouty1 activity are protected from the effects of spontaneous and persistent activation of MAPK signaling. In the *Drosophila* midgut, different safeguard systems have been described: EE cells secrete the neuroendocrine hormone Bursicon to inhibit expression of the visceral muscle–derived epidermal growth factor (EGF)-like ligand vein, reinstating the quiescent state of ISCs (Scopelliti et al., 2014). Similarly, the visceral muscle expresses the bone morphogenetic protein (BMP) homolog decapentaplegic (Dpp), negatively regulating ISC proliferation and thus promoting tissue homeostasis after damage has been repaired (Guo, Driver, & Ohlstein, 2013).

Regulatory pathways such as Notch, transforming growth factor (TGF)-β, and Wnt signaling pathways control a range of cellular processes, including adult stem cell function. A disturbance in the balance of Notch signaling between stem cells and the intermediate progenitors is observed in the aging brain, skeletal muscle, and hematopoietic system, with important consequences for the decline in regenerative capacity of these tissues (Bjornson et al., 2012; Conboy, Conboy, Smythe, & Rando, 2003; Duncan et al., 2005; Lugert et al., 2010; Mizutani, Yoon, Dang, Tokunaga, & Gaiano, 2007; Mourikis et al., 2012). Also, in the aging ISC compartment of the *Drosophila* midgut, impaired Notch signaling is associated with misdifferentiation of the stem cell population, rather than with stem cell maintenance (Biteau et al., 2008). Importantly, Notch signaling synergizes with Wnt and TGF-β signaling and a dysregulation in the balance of these pathways can contribute to stem cell loss of function in different stem cell compartments (Brack, Conboy, Conboy, Shen, & Rando, 2008; Carlson, Hsu, & Conboy, 2008; Duncan et al., 2005).

The discoveries described previously highlight that deregulation of common signaling pathways affects stem cell aging in different compartments. Therefore, there is hope that common approaches directed toward attenuation of the age-associated systemic alterations may indeed result in a rejuvenation of different stem cell pools simultaneously. Evidence supporting this idea is provided by parabiosis studies, as well as by more recent studies in which systemic delivery of specific factors can rejuvenate several stem cell compartments simultaneously. Growth differentiation factor 11 (GDF11) was shown to rejuvenate neurogenic and skeletal muscle stem cell compartments and reestablish skeletal muscle regenerative capacity and neurogenesis in aged animals (Katsimpardi et al., 2014; Sinha et al., 2014). A recent contradictory report claims, however, that GDF11 increases in the old serum and has a negative impact on muscle regeneration (Egerman et al., 2015).

In the same line of thinking, interventions such as dietary restriction and exercise have been shown to positively modulate stem cell function in the different compartments and attenuate aging-associated dysfunction (Cerletti et al., 2012; Shefer, Rauner, Yablonka-Reuveni, & Benayahu, 2010; van Praag, Shubert, Zhao, & Gage, 2005; Yilmaz et al., 2012).

■ CONSEQUENCES OF STEM CELL AGING AND REJUVENATION STRATEGIES

Stem Cell Exhaustion and Senescence Versus Hyperplasia

The stem cell dysfunction that accompanies organismal aging results in many cases in the exhaustion of the available stem cell pools. By contrast, age-related perturbed cell-cycle activity can also result in hyperplastic phenotypes where stem cells acquire new functions and proliferative potential. In both circumstances, stem cell dysfunction contributes to the loss of somatic homeostasis and organ failure (Loffredo et al., 2013).

Self-renewal is an essential property of stem cells often impaired in aged organisms. This process is fundamental for replenishment of stem cell populations and can be impaired by premature/inadequate terminal differentiation or by the engagement of stress response processes such as senescence and apoptosis. Age-related stem cell depletion can be observed in different tissues such as the brain (Molofsky et al., 2006) and skeletal muscle (Sousa-Victor et al., 2014). In response to aging determinants described previously, the stem cell can irreversibly exit the cell cycle and become senescent, a state generally associated with the upregulation of cell cycle inhibitors like p53/p21 and p16INK4a (Sharpless & DePinho, 2007). Senescence markers can be found in resident stem cell populations of the skeletal muscle and fat tissue of the BubR1 progeroid mice (Baker, Weaver, & van Deursen, 2013). In physiologically aged mice, quiescent satellite cells enter a pre-senescent state associated with the upregulation of p16INK4a. On proliferative pressure, these cells are unable to perform regenerative functions and undergo accelerated senescence. Silencing of p16INK4a restores the stem cell self-renewal capacity and improves the muscle regenerative potential (Sousa-Victor et al., 2014). A similar quiescence-to-senescence transition on cell cycle entry was reported in aged HSCs with elevated levels of DNA damage and p16INK4a expression (Wang, Lu, Sakk, Klein, & Rudolph, 2014a). Silencing of p16INK4a reestablishes the repopulating capacity of aged HSCs (Janzen et al., 2006). Increased expression of p16INK4a is also associated with a decline in self-renewal capacity of the aged progenitor population of the subventricular zone (SVZ) of the brain. Consistently, p16INK4a-deficient mice displayed improved olfactory bulb neurogenesis and increased self-renewal potential of SVZ multipotent progenitors (Molofsky et al., 2006).

Loss of Homeostatic Capacity and Reduced Life Span

One critical question in the stem cell aging field is to what extent stem cell aging contributes to organismal aging and life span. Evidence from *Drosophila* studies suggests that preservation of ISC proliferative homeostasis can extend life span (Biteau et al., 2010, 2011; Guo, Karpac, Tran, & Jasper, 2014). This can be achieved through the attenuation, without complete blockade, of insulin/insulin-like growth factor (IGF) and Jun-N-terminal kinase (JNK) signaling so that regenerative capacity is maintained, but hyperplastic phenotypes are prevented (Biteau et al., 2010). Overexpression of stress protective genes (Biteau et al., 2010) or of the transcriptional regulator of energy metabolism—proliferator-activated receptor-gamma coactivator-1 (PGC-1) (Rera et al., 2011), specifically in ISCs and EBs, yields similar results. Although these experiments determine that life span depends on proficient stem cell function in *Drosophila*, it remains to be tested whether: (a) delaying stem cell aging in one compartment prevents aging of other tissues; and (b) preventing stem cell function in mammals also extends organismal life span.

Unlike *Drosophila*, mammals have several adult stem cell compartments that vary in their contribution to tissue homeostasis. Stem cells from high turnover tissues, such as blood or the intestine, have important homeostatic functions to sustain tissue renewal in basal conditions. In other compartments, such as the skeletal muscle, stem cell function is dedicated mostly to repair of injuries. In addition, other stem cell types, such as MSCs or NSCs, are proposed to have important regulatory functions that expand their "traditional" stem cell function. It is likely that aging of stem cell populations that contribute to tissue homeostasis or produce immune modulatory cues has more impact on overall tissue and organismal aging than aging of stem cells whose function is solely dedicated to repair in response to injury. Consistent with this view, conditional ablation of satellite cells from young skeletal muscles may not contribute to the development of sarcopenic phenotypes (Fry et al., 2015), while depletion of skeletal muscle-associated MSCs results in loss of muscle mass (Roberts et al., 2013). Similarly, depletion of MSCs from the bone marrow results in aging-like phenotypes of the hematopoietic system. Supporting the hypothesis that loss of homeostatic capacity may have consequences for organismal life span, aging of stem cells in the hematopoietic and intestinal compartments results in pathologies that increase mortality rate, such as myeloid leukemias and intestinal cancers (Rossi et al., 2008), and preservation of ISC activity can prolong life span of mice with telomere dysfunction (Sperka et al., 2012). Finally, because inflammaging is thought to be a major driving force for organismal aging (Franceschi & Campisi, 2014) and the immune modulatory properties of MSCs exhibit dynamic plasticity (Wang et al., 2014b), it is tempting to suggest that MSC aging may be an important contributor for organismal aging (Fukada et al., 2014) and that modulation of their activity can improve health span and life span. The capability of endogenous and transplanted NSCs to deliver immune modulatory cues is also increasingly recognized (Kokaia et al., 2012; Moyon et al., 2015; Pluchino et al., 2005) in the context of injury models and it would be interesting to explore whether this capacity can be harnessed to ameliorate age-associated pathological conditions in the CNS, such as Parkinson's or Alzheimer's, diseases classically associated with pro-inflammatory environments (Hirsch & Hunot, 2009; Latta, Brothers, & Wilcock, 2014).

Stem Cell Rejuvenation Strategies

A better understanding of the underlying mechanisms of aging is now opening new avenues of research that explore rejuvenation strategies based on counteracting the determinants of stem cell aging. Common aging determinants across stem cell pools raise hope that universal rejuvenation strategies can be applied, while tissue-specific consequences of stem cell aging will help to select local interventions to reestablish organ function.

In addition to systemic factors described previously, stem cell–specific interventions in pathways dysregulated in aging have already resulted in successful rejuvenation in the skeletal muscle compartment. Transient inhibition of MAPKs in isolated aged satellite cells increased self-renewal and improved their regenerative potential when transplanted into old muscles (Bernet et al., 2014; Cosgrove et al., 2014). These effects were reported in association with a repression of p16INK4a. Consistently, genetic rejuvenation of old satellite cells is also possible through p16INK4a silencing (Sousa-Victor et al., 2014). Because p16INK4a upregulation is a common hallmark of stem cell aging across tissues, these strategies may have a broader application. Consistently, an inducible genetic model for senescent cell clearance based on the ablation of p16INK4a-expressing cells was shown to delay the onset of age-related pathologies in progeroid mice (Baker et al., 2011). Because senescent cells are a source of pro-inflammatory signals, which negatively impact stem cell function, it is likely that strategies aimed at attenuating inflammation in aging will have similar rejuvenation potential.

REFERENCES

Ahlqvist, K. J., Hamalainen, R. H., Yatsuga, S., Uutela, M., Terzioglu, M., Gotz, A., . . . Suomalainen, A. (2012). Somatic progenitor cell vulnerability to mitochondrial DNA mutagenesis underlies progeroid phenotypes in Polg mutator mice. *Cell Metabolism, 15*, 100–109.

Aurora, A. B., & Olson, E. N. (2014). Immune modulation of stem cells and regeneration. *Cell Stem Cell, 15*, 14–25.

Baker, D. J., Weaver, R. L., & van Deursen, J. M. (2013). p21 both attenuates and drives senescence and aging in BubR1 progeroid mice. *Cell Reports, 3*, 1164–1174.

Baker, D. J., Wijshake, T., Tchkonia, T., LeBrasseur, N. K., Childs, B. G., van de Sluis, B., . . . van Deursen, J. M. (2011). Clearance of p16Ink4a-positive senescent cells delays ageing-associated disorders. *Nature, 479*, 232–236.

Bernet, J. D., Doles, J. D., Hall, J. K., Kelly Tanaka, K., Carter, T. A., & Olwin, B. B. (2014). p38 MAPK signaling underlies a cell-autonomous loss of stem cell self-renewal in skeletal muscle of aged mice. *Nature Medicine, 20*, 265–271.

Biteau, B., Hochmuth, C. E., & Jasper, H. (2008). JNK activity in somatic stem cells causes loss of tissue homeostasis in the aging Drosophila gut. *Cell Stem Cell, 3*, 442–455.

Biteau, B., Hochmuth, C. E., & Jasper, H. (2011). Maintaining tissue homeostasis: Dynamic control of somatic stem cell activity. *Cell Stem Cell, 9*, 402–411.

Biteau, B., Karpac, J., Supoyo, S., Degennaro, M., Lehmann, R., & Jasper, H. (2010). Lifespan extension by preserving proliferative homeostasis in Drosophila. *PLoS Genetics, 6*, e1001159.

Bjornson, C. R., Cheung, T. H., Liu, L., Tripathi, P. V., Steeper, K. M., & Rando, T. A. (2012). Notch signaling is necessary to maintain quiescence in adult muscle stem cells. *Stem Cells, 30*, 232–242.

Brack, A. S., Conboy, I. M., Conboy, M. J., Shen, J., & Rando, T. A. (2008). A temporal switch from notch to Wnt signaling in muscle stem cells is necessary for normal adult myogenesis. *Cell Stem Cell, 2,* 50–59.

Brack, A. S., Conboy, M. J., Roy, S., Lee, M., Kuo, C. J., Keller, C., & Rando, T. A. (2007). Increased Wnt signaling during aging alters muscle stem cell fate and increases fibrosis. *Science, 317,* 807–810.

Bratic, A., & Larsson, N. G. (2013). The role of mitochondria in aging. *The Journal of Clinical Investigation, 123,* 951–957.

Brown, K., Xie, S., Qiu, X., Mohrin, M., Shin, J., Liu, Y., . . . Chen, D. (2013). SIRT3 reverses aging-associated degeneration. *Cell Reports, 3,* 319–327.

Burkhalter, M. D., Rudolph, K. L., & Sperka, T. (2015). Genome instability of ageing stem cells—Induction and defence mechanisms. *Ageing Research Reviews, 23*(Pt. A), 29–36.

Burtner, C. R., & Kennedy, B. K. (2010). Progeria syndromes and ageing: What is the connection? *Nature Reviews Molecular Cell Biology, 11,* 567–578.

Carlson, M. E., Hsu, M., & Conboy, I. M. (2008). Imbalance between pSmad3 and Notch induces CDK inhibitors in old muscle stem cells. *Nature, 454,* 528–532.

Castilho, R. M., Squarize, C. H., Chodosh, L. A., Williams, B. O., & Gutkind, J. S. (2009). mTOR mediates Wnt-induced epidermal stem cell exhaustion and aging. *Cell Stem Cell, 5,* 279–289.

Ceccaldi, R., Parmar, K., Mouly, E., Delord, M., Kim, J. M., Regairaz, M., . . . Soulier, J. (2012). Bone marrow failure in Fanconi anemia is triggered by an exacerbated p53/ p21 DNA damage response that impairs hematopoietic stem and progenitor cells. *Cell Stem Cell, 11,* 36–49.

Cerletti, M., Jang, Y. C., Finley, L. W., Haigis, M. C., & Wagers, A. J. (2012). Short-term calorie restriction enhances skeletal muscle stem cell function. *Cell Stem Cell, 10,* 515–519.

Chakkalakal, J. V., Jones, K. M., Basson, M. A., & Brack, A. S. (2012). The aged niche disrupts muscle stem cell quiescence. *Nature, 490,* 355–360.

Chen, C., Liu, Y., & Zheng, P. (2009). mTOR regulation and therapeutic rejuvenation of aging hematopoietic stem cells. *Science Signaling, 2,* ra75.

Conboy, I. M., Conboy, M. J., Smythe, G. M., & Rando, T. A. (2003). Notch-mediated restoration of regenerative potential to aged muscle. *Science, 302,* 1575–1577.

Conboy, I. M., Conboy, M. J., Wagers, A. J., Girma, E. R., Weissman, I. L., & Rando, T. A. (2005). Rejuvenation of aged progenitor cells by exposure to a young systemic environment. *Nature, 433,* 760–764.

Cosgrove, B. D., Gilbert, P. M., Porpiglia, E., Mourkioti, F., Lee, S. P., Corbel, . . . Blau, H. M. (2014). Rejuvenation of the muscle stem cell population restores strength to injured aged muscles. *Nature Medicine, 20,* 255–264.

Doles, J., Storer, M., Cozzuto, L., Roma, G., & Keyes, W. M. (2012). Age-associated inflammation inhibits epidermal stem cell function. *Genes & Development, 26,* 2144–2153.

Duncan, A. W., Rattis, F. M., DiMascio, L. N., Congdon, K. L., Pazianos, G., Zhao, C., . . . Reya, T. (2005). Integration of Notch and Wnt signaling in hematopoietic stem cell maintenance. *Nature Immunology, 6,* 314–322.

Egerman, M. A., Cadena, S. M., Gilbert, J. A., Meyer, A., Nelson, H. N., Swalley, S. E.,... Glass, D. J. (2015). GDF11 Increases with age and inhibits skeletal muscle regeneration. *Cell Metabolism, 22*, 54–56.

Flach, J., Bakker, S. T., Mohrin, M., Conroy, P. C., Pietras, E. M., Reynaud, D.,... Passegué, E. (2014). Replication stress is a potent driver of functional decline in ageing haematopoietic stem cells. *Nature, 512*, 198–202.

Franceschi, C., & Campisi, J. (2014). Chronic inflammation (inflammaging) and its potential contribution to age-associated diseases. *The Journals of Gerontology, Series A, 69*(Suppl. 1), S4–S9.

Fry, C. S., Lee, J. D., Mula, J., Kirby, T. J., Jackson, J. R., Liu, F.,... Peterson, C. A. (2015). Inducible depletion of satellite cells in adult, sedentary mice impairs muscle regenerative capacity without affecting sarcopenia. *Nature Medicine, 21*, 76–80.

Fukada, S., Ma, Y., & Uezumi, A. (2014). Adult stem cell and mesenchymal progenitor theories of aging. *Frontiers in Cell and Developmental Biology, 2*, 10.

Gage, F. H. (2002). Neurogenesis in the adult brain. *The Journal of Neuroscience, 22*, 612–613.

Guo, L., Karpac, J., Tran, S. L., & Jasper, H. (2014). PGRP-SC2 promotes gut immune homeostasis to limit commensal dysbiosis and extend lifespan. *Cell, 156*, 109–122.

Guo, Z., Driver, I., & Ohlstein, B. (2013). Injury-induced BMP signaling negatively regulates Drosophila midgut homeostasis. *The Journal of Cell Biology, 201*, 945–961.

Harel, I., Benayoun, B. A., Machado, B., Singh, P. P., Hu, C. K., Pech, M. F.,... Brunet, A. (2015). A platform for rapid exploration of aging and diseases in a naturally short-lived vertebrate. *Cell, 160*, 1013–1026.

Harman, D. (1956). Aging: A theory based on free radical and radiation chemistry. *Journal of Gerontology, 11*, 298–300.

Hattiangady, B., & Shetty, A. K. (2008). Aging does not alter the number or phenotype of putative stem/progenitor cells in the neurogenic region of the hippocampus. *Neurobiology of Aging, 29*, 129–147.

Hirsch, E. C., & Hunot, S. (2009). Neuroinflammation in Parkinson's disease: A target for neuroprotection? *The Lancet Neurology, 8*, 382–397.

Holmstrom, K. M., & Finkel, T. (2014). Cellular mechanisms and physiological consequences of redox-dependent signalling. *Nature Reviews Molecular Cell Biology, 15*, 411–421.

Ishihara, K., & Hirano, T. (2002). IL-6 in autoimmune disease and chronic inflammatory proliferative disease. *Cytokine & Growth Factor Reviews, 13*, 357–368.

Janzen, V., Forkert, R., Fleming, H. E., Saito, Y., Waring, M. T., Dombkowski, D. M.,... Scadden, D. T. (2006). Stem-cell ageing modified by the cyclin-dependent kinase inhibitor p16INK4a. *Nature, 443*, 421–426.

Jasper, H., & Kennedy, B. K. (2012). Niche science: The aging stem cell. *Cell Cycle, 11*, 2959–2960.

Jensen, M. B., & Jasper, H. (2014). Mitochondrial proteostasis in the control of aging and longevity. *Cell Metabolism, 20*, 214–225.

Jones, D. L., & Rando, T. A. (2011). Emerging models and paradigms for stem cell ageing. *Nature Cell Biology, 13*, 506–512.

Jung, Y., & Brack, A. S. (2014). Cellular mechanisms of somatic stem cell aging. *Current Topics in Developmental Biology, 107*, 405–438.

Kaeberlein, M., McVey, M., & Guarente, L. (1999). The SIR2/3/4 complex and SIR2 alone promote longevity in *Saccharomyces cerevisiae* by two different mechanisms. *Genes & Development, 13*, 2570–2580.

Kapahi, P., Chen, D., Rogers, A. N., Katewa, S. D., Li, P. W., Thomas, E. L., & Kockel, L. (2010). With TOR, less is more: A key role for the conserved nutrient-sensing TOR pathway in aging. *Cell Metabolism, 11*, 453–465.

Katsimpardi, L., Litterman, N. K., Schein, P. A., Miller, C. M., Loffredo, F. S., Wojtkiewicz, G. R.,…Rubin, L. L. (2014). Vascular and neurogenic rejuvenation of the aging mouse brain by young systemic factors. *Science, 344*, 630–634.

Kokaia, Z., Martino, G., Schwartz, M., & Lindvall, O. (2012). Cross-talk between neural stem cells and immune cells: The key to better brain repair? *Nature Neuroscience, 15*, 1078–1087.

Kujoth, G. C., Hiona, A., Pugh, T. D., Someya, S., Panzer, K., Wohlgemuth, S. E.,…Prolla, T. A. (2005). Mitochondrial DNA mutations, oxidative stress, and apoptosis in mammalian aging. *Science, 309*, 481–484.

Laplante, M., & Sabatini, D. M. (2012). mTOR signaling in growth control and disease. *Cell, 149*, 274–293.

Latta, C. H., Brothers, H. M., & Wilcock, D. M. (2014). Neuroinflammation in Alzheimer's disease; a source of heterogeneity and target for personalized therapy. *Neuroscience, 302*, 103–111.

Liu, L., Cheung, T. H., Charville, G. W., Hurgo, B. M., Leavitt, T., Shih, J.,…Rando, T. A. (2013). Chromatin modifications as determinants of muscle stem cell quiescence and chronological aging. *Cell Reports, 4*, 189–204.

Liu, L., & Rando, T. A. (2011). Manifestations and mechanisms of stem cell aging. *The Journal of Cell Biology, 193*, 257–266.

Loffredo, F. S., Steinhauser, M. L., Jay, S. M., Gannon, J., Pancoast, J. R., Yalamanchi, P.,…Lee, R. T. (2013). Growth differentiation factor 11 is a circulating factor that reverses age-related cardiac hypertrophy. *Cell, 153*, 828–839.

Longo, V. D., & Kennedy, B. K. (2006). Sirtuins in aging and age-related disease. *Cell, 126*, 257–268.

Lugert, S., Basak, O., Knuckles, P., Haussler, U., Fabel, K., Gotz, M.,…Giachino, C. (2010). Quiescent and active hippocampal neural stem cells with distinct morphologies respond selectively to physiological and pathological stimuli and aging. *Cell Stem Cell, 6*, 445–456.

Maeda, K., Baba, Y., Nagai, Y., Miyazaki, K., Malykhin, A., Nakamura, K.,… Coggeshall, K. M. (2005). IL-6 blocks a discrete early step in lymphopoiesis. *Blood, 106*, 879–885.

Martino, G., Pluchino, S., Bonfanti, L., & Schwartz, M. (2011). Brain regeneration in physiology and pathology: The immune signature driving therapeutic plasticity of neural stem cells. *Physiological Reviews, 91*, 1281–1304.

Micchelli, C. A., & Perrimon, N. (2006). Evidence that stem cells reside in the adult Drosophila midgut epithelium. *Nature, 439*, 475–479.

Mirantes, C., Passegue, E., & Pietras, E. M. (2014). Pro-inflammatory cytokines: Emerging players regulating HSC function in normal and diseased hematopoiesis. *Experimental Cell Research, 329*, 248–254.

Miron, V. E., Boyd, A., Zhao, J. W., Yuen, T. J., Ruckh, J. M., Shadrach, J. L., ... ffrench-Constant, C. (2013). M2 microglia and macrophages drive oligodendrocyte differentiation during CNS remyelination. *Nature Neuroscience, 16*, 1211–1218.

Mizutani, K., Yoon, K., Dang, L., Tokunaga, A., & Gaiano, N. (2007). Differential Notch signalling distinguishes neural stem cells from intermediate progenitors. *Nature, 449*, 351–355.

Molofsky, A. V., Slutsky, S. G., Joseph, N. M., He, S., Pardal, R., Krishnamurthy, J., ... Morrison, S. J. (2006). Increasing p16INK4a expression decreases forebrain progenitors and neurogenesis during ageing. *Nature, 443*, 448–452.

Mourikis, P., Sambasivan, R., Castel, D., Rocheteau, P., Bizzarro, V., & Tajbakhsh, S. (2012). A critical requirement for notch signaling in maintenance of the quiescent skeletal muscle stem cell state. *Stem Cells, 30*, 243–252.

Moyon, S., Dubessy, A. L., Aigrot, M. S., Trotter, M., Huang, J. K., Dauphinot, L., ... Lubetzki, C. (2015). Demyelination causes adult CNS progenitors to revert to an immature state and express immune cues that support their migration. *The Journal of Neuroscience, 35*, 4–20.

Neves, J., Demaria, M., Campisi, J., & Jasper, H. (2015). Of flies, mice, and men: Evolutionarily conserved tissue damage responses and aging. *Developmental Cell, 32*, 9–18.

Norddahl, G. L., Pronk, C. J., Wahlestedt, M., Sten, G., Nygren, J. M., Ugale, A., ... Bryder, D. (2011). Accumulating mitochondrial DNA mutations drive premature hematopoietic aging phenotypes distinct from physiological stem cell aging. *Cell Stem Cell, 8*, 499–510.

Oh, J., Lee, Y. D., & Wagers, A. J. (2014). Stem cell aging: Mechanisms, regulators and therapeutic opportunities. *Nature Medicine, 20*, 870–880.

Ohlstein, B., & Spradling, A. (2006). The adult Drosophila posterior midgut is maintained by pluripotent stem cells. *Nature, 439*, 470–474.

Paul, M. K., Bisht, B., Darmawan, D. O., Chiou, R., Ha, V. L., Wallace, W. D. C., ... Gomperts, B. N. (2014). Dynamic changes in intracellular ROS levels regulate airway basal stem cell homeostasis through Nrf2-dependent Notch signaling. *Cell Stem Cell, 15*, 199–214.

Pluchino, S., Zanotti, L., Rossi, B., Brambilla, E., Ottoboni, L., Salani, G., ... Martino, G. (2005). Neurosphere-derived multipotent precursors promote neuroprotection by an immunomodulatory mechanism. *Nature, 436*, 266–271.

Rando, T. A., & Chang, H. Y. (2012). Aging, rejuvenation, and epigenetic reprogramming: Resetting the aging clock. *Cell, 148*, 46–57.

Rera, M., Bahadorani, S., Cho, J., Koehler, C. L., Ulgherait, M., Hur, J. H., ... Walker, D. W. (2011). Modulation of longevity and tissue homeostasis by the Drosophila PGC-1 homolog. *Cell Metabolism, 14*, 623–634.

Reynaud, D., Pietras, E., Barry-Holson, K., Mir, A., Binnewies, M., Jeanne, M.,…Passegue, E. (2011). IL-6 controls leukemic multipotent progenitor cell fate and contributes to chronic myelogenous leukemia development. *Cancer Cell, 20,* 661–673.

Roberts, E. W., Deonarine, A., Jones, J. O., Denton, A. E., Feig, C., Lyons, S. K.,…Fearon, D. T. (2013). Depletion of stromal cells expressing fibroblast activation protein-alpha from skeletal muscle and bone marrow results in cachexia and anemia. *The Journal of Experimental Medicine, 210,* 1137–1151.

Rossi, D. J., Jamieson, C. H., & Weissman, I. L. (2008). Stems cells and the pathways to aging and cancer. *Cell, 132,* 681–696.

Ruckh, J. M., Zhao, J. W., Shadrach, J. L., van Wijngaarden, P., Rao, T. N., Wagers, A. J., & Franklin, R. J. (2012). Rejuvenation of regeneration in the aging central nervous system. *Cell Stem Cell, 10,* 96–103.

Rudolph, K. L., Chang, S., Lee, H. W., Blasco, M., Gottlieb, G. J., Greider, C., & DePinho, R. A. (1999). Longevity, stress response, and cancer in aging telomerase-deficient mice. *Cell, 96,* 701–712.

Schepers, A. G., Vries, R., van den Born, M., van de Wetering, M., & Clevers, H. (2011). Lgr5 intestinal stem cells have high telomerase activity and randomly segregate their chromosomes. *The EMBO Journal, 30,* 1104–1109.

Schurch, C. M., Riether, C., & Ochsenbein, A. F. (2014). Cytotoxic CD8+ T cells stimulate hematopoietic progenitors by promoting cytokine release from bone marrow mesenchymal stromal cells. *Cell Stem Cell, 14,* 460–472.

Scopelliti, A., Cordero, J. B., Diao, F., Strathdee, K., White, B. H., Sansom, O. J., & Vidal, M. (2014). Local control of intestinal stem cell homeostasis by enteroendocrine cells in the adult Drosophila midgut. *Current Biology, 24,* 1199–1211.

Sepulveda, J. C., Tome, M., Fernandez, M. E., Delgado, M., Campisi, J., Bernad, A., & Gonzalez, M. A. (2014). Cell senescence abrogates the therapeutic potential of human mesenchymal stem cells in the lethal endotoxemia model. *Stem Cells, 32,* 1865–1877.

Sharpless, N. E., & DePinho, R. A. (2007). How stem cells age and why this makes us grow old. *Nature Reviews Molecular Cell Biology, 8,* 703–713.

Shea, K. L., Xiang, W., LaPorta, V. S., Licht, J. D., Keller, C., Basson, M. A., & Brack, A. S. (2010). Sprouty1 regulates reversible quiescence of a self-renewing adult muscle stem cell pool during regeneration. *Cell Stem Cell, 6,* 117–129.

Shefer, G., Rauner, G., Yablonka-Reuveni, Z., & Benayahu, D. (2010). Reduced satellite cell numbers and myogenic capacity in aging can be alleviated by endurance exercise. *PloS One, 5,* e13307.

Shyh-Chang, N., Daley, G. Q., & Cantley, L. C. (2013). Stem cell metabolism in tissue development and aging. *Development, 140,* 2535–2547.

Sinha, M., Jang, Y. C., Oh, J., Khong, D., Wu, E. Y., Manohar, R.,…Wagers, A. J. (2014). Restoring systemic GDF11 levels reverses age-related dysfunction in mouse skeletal muscle. *Science, 344,* 649–652.

Smith, J., Ladi, E., Mayer-Proschel, M., & Noble, M. (2000). Redox state is a central modulator of the balance between self-renewal and differentiation in a dividing glial precursor cell. *Proceedings of the National Academy of Sciences of the United States of America, 97,* 10032–10037.

Sousa-Victor, P., Garcia-Prat, L., Serrano, A. L., Perdiguero, E., & Munoz-Canoves, P. (2015). Muscle stem cell aging: Regulation and rejuvenation. *Trends in Endocrinology and Metabolism, 26*(6), 287–296.

Sousa-Victor, P., Gutarra, S., Garcia-Prat, L., Rodriguez-Ubreva, J., Ortet, L., Ruiz-Bonilla, V.,...Munoz-Canoves, P. (2014). Geriatric muscle stem cells switch reversible quiescence into senescence. *Nature, 506,* 316–321.

Sperka, T., Song, Z., Morita, Y., Nalapareddy, K., Guachalla, L. M., Lechel, A.,...Rudolph, K. L. (2012). Puma and p21 represent cooperating checkpoints limiting self-renewal and chromosomal instability of somatic stem cells in response to telomere dysfunction. *Nature Cell Biology, 14,* 73–79.

Sun, D., Luo, M., Jeong, M., Rodriguez, B., Xia, Z., Hannah, R.,...Goodell, M. A. (2014). Epigenomic profiling of young and aged HSCs reveals concerted changes during aging that reinforce self-renewal. *Cell Stem Cell, 14,* 673–688.

Tian, H., Biehs, B., Warming, S., Leong, K. G., Rangell, L., Klein, O. D., & de Sauvage, F. J. (2011). A reserve stem cell population in small intestine renders Lgr5-positive cells dispensable. *Nature, 478,* 255–259.

Tothova, Z., Kollipara, R., Huntly, B. J., Lee, B. H., Castrillon, D. H., Cullen, D. E.,...Gilliand, D. G. (2007). FoxOs are critical mediators of hematopoietic stem cell resistance to physiologic oxidative stress. *Cell, 128,* 325–339.

Trifunovic, A., Wredenberg, A., Falkenberg, M., Spelbrink, J. N., Rovio, A. T., Bruder, C. E.,...Larsson, N. G. (2004). Premature ageing in mice expressing defective mitochondrial DNA polymerase. *Nature, 429,* 417–423.

Tsurumi, A., & Li, W. X. (2012). Global heterochromatin loss: A unifying theory of aging? *Epigenetics, 7,* 680–688.

Valenzano, D. R., Sharp, S., & Brunet, A. (2011). Transposon-mediated transgenesis in the short-lived African Killifish *Nothobranchius furzeri,* a vertebrate model for aging. *G3 (Bethesda, Md.), 1,* 531–538.

van Praag, H., Shubert, T., Zhao, C., & Gage, F. H. (2005). Exercise enhances learning and hippocampal neurogenesis in aged mice. *The Journal of Neuroscience, 25,* 8680–8685.

Van Raamsdonk, J. M., & Hekimi, S. (2009). Deletion of the mitochondrial superoxide dismutase sod-2 extends lifespan in *Caenorhabditis elegans. PLoS Genetics, 5,* e1000361.

Van Raamsdonk, J. M., & Hekimi, S. (2012). Superoxide dismutase is dispensable for normal animal lifespan. *Proceedings of the National Academy of Sciences of the United States of America, 109,* 5785–5790.

Villeda, S. A., Luo, J., Mosher, K. I., Zou, B., Britschgi, M., Bieri, G.,...Wyss-Coray, T. (2011). The ageing systemic milieu negatively regulates neurogenesis and cognitive function. *Nature, 477,* 90–94.

Villeponteau, B. (1997). The heterochromatin loss model of aging. *Experimental Gerontology, 32,* 383–394.

Wang, J., Lu, X., Sakk, V., Klein, C. A., & Rudolph, K. L. (2014a). Senescence and apoptosis block hematopoietic activation of quiescent hematopoietic stem cells with short telomeres. *Blood, 124,* 3237–3240.

Wang, Y., Chen, X., Cao, W., & Shi, Y. (2014b). Plasticity of mesenchymal stem cells in immunomodulation: Pathological and therapeutic implications. *Nature Immunology, 15,* 1009–1016.

Yee, C., Yang, W., & Hekimi, S. (2014). The intrinsic apoptosis pathway mediates the pro-longevity response to mitochondrial ROS in *C. elegans. Cell, 157,* 897–909.

Yilmaz, O. H., Katajisto, P., Lamming, D. W., Gultekin, Y., Bauer-Rowe, K. E., Sengupta, S., . . . Sabatini, D. M. (2012). mTORC1 in the Paneth cell niche couples intestinal stem-cell function to calorie intake. *Nature, 486,* 490–495.

Yu, K. R., & Kang, K. S. (2013). Aging-related genes in mesenchymal stem cells: A mini-review. *Gerontology, 59,* 557–563.

Yu, K. R., Lee, J. Y., Kim, H. S., Hong, I. S., Choi, S. W., Seo, Y., . . . Kang, K. S. (2014). A p38 MAPK-mediated alteration of COX-2/PGE2 regulates immunomodulatory properties in human mesenchymal stem cell aging. *PloS One, 9,* e102426.

Zhang, G., Li, J., Purkayastha, S., Tang, Y., Zhang, H., Yin, Y., . . . Cai, D. (2013). Hypothalamic programming of systemic ageing involving IKK-beta, NF-kappaB and GnRH. *Nature, 497,* 211–216.

Zhao, J. L., Ma, C., O'Connell, R. M., Mehta, A., DiLoreto, R., Heath, J. R., & Baltimore, D. (2014). Conversion of danger signals into cytokine signals by hematopoietic stem and progenitor cells for regulation of stress-induced hematopoiesis. *Cell Stem Cell, 14,* 445–459.

CHAPTER 10

Proteostasis and Aging

Matt Kaeberlein

In order to maintain proper function, cells have evolved several mechanisms to ensure that the proteome is protected and protein homeostasis (proteostasis) is preserved. These mechanisms include regulation of mRNA translation and protein synthesis, expression of chaperones that assist with protein folding, and machinery to repair or degrade damaged proteins. There is abundant evidence that loss of protein homeostasis contributes to a variety of age-associated diseases in people, particularly neurodegenerative disorders such as Alzheimer's disease (AD) and Parkinson's disease (PD). Studies in model organisms strongly support the idea that proteostasis is critical for healthy longevity and that enhanced proteostasis is associated with longevity both across species and within species. This chapter provides an overview of the evidence supporting the theory that loss of protein homeostasis is a conserved mechanism of aging.

The past two decades have seen rapid advances in our understanding of the molecular processes that underlie aging. Numerous factors have been implicated as casually contributing to age-related declines in function at the cellular and organismal levels. Among these, nine "hallmarks of aging" have been recently suggested to be particularly important. These include genomic instability, telomere attrition, epigenetic alterations, deregulated nutrient sensing, mitochondrial dysfunction, cellular senescence, stem cell exhaustion, altered intercellular communication, and loss of proteostasis (Lopez-Otin, Blasco, Partridge, Serrano, & Kroemer, 2013).

Some of these hallmarks of aging are likely to be relevant only in complex organisms like mammals; for example, telomere attrition and cellular senescence probably are not significant drivers of aging in primarily post-mitotic organisms like *Caenorhabditis elegans*. Others, however, appear to be highly evolutionarily conserved with respect to their role in aging and longevity. Among these, failure to maintain proteostasis appears to play a central role in aging at subcellular, cellular, tissue, and organismal levels.

The term proteostasis is derived from the words "protein" and "homeostasis," and can be defined as the process by which the cell maintains homeostasis of the cellular protein content or proteome (Balch, Morimoto, Dillin, & Kelly, 2008). Cells have evolved a rich and complex network of mechanisms by which they continuously monitor the state of the proteome and adapt the proteome to changing external and internal stimuli. These mechanisms include general protein quality control systems such as the ubiquitin proteasome system (UPS) and autophagy, as well as compartment-specific stress responses such as the endoplasmic reticulum unfolded protein response (ER-UPR), the mitochondrial (MT)-UPR, and the cytosolic heat shock response (HSR). During aging, these protein quality control mechanisms appear to either degrade or become overwhelmed, leading to an increasing burden of proteotoxic stress, primarily in the form of misfolded, chemically modified, or aggregated proteins. This chapter provides an overview of current evidence that loss of proteostasis is a central driver of aging and age-related disease, based on studies from a variety of model systems and clinical data.

■ PROTEIN HOMEOSTASIS AND AGE-ASSOCIATED DISEASE

It has been recognized for many decades that several age-associated neurodegenerative diseases are associated with protein aggregation. This is best characterized in the case of AD, PD, and Huntington's disease (HD; Kikis, Gidalevitz, & Morimoto, 2010). All of these diseases are age associated, with AD and PD occurring with relatively late onset, and HD occurring at variable ages depending on the severity of the causal genetic defect (discussed further subsequently).

Prevalence of AD is strongly age associated and accounts for 60% to 70% of dementia cases (Burns & Iliffe, 2009; Querfurth & LaFerla, 2010). It has long been recognized that AD is closely associated with the presence of senile plaques and neurofibrillary tangles in the brain, which are extracellular deposits largely composed of amyloid beta and hyperphosphorylated tau, respectively (Bancher et al., 1989; Cras et al., 1991). It remains unclear whether the extracellular protein aggregates themselves are pathogenic in AD or represent a response to an intracellular toxic species of misfolded protein such as amyloid beta oligomers (Viola & Klein, 2015).

The primary pathological feature of PD is loss of dopaminergic neurons in the substantia nigra (Davie, 2008). This cell loss is associated with aggregation of alpha synuclein and ubiquitin in neuronal inclusions called "Lewy bodies" (Schulz-Schaeffer, 2010). As with AD, it remains unclear whether the formation of Lewy bodies in PD is toxic in and of itself or represents a protective mechanism to remove toxic oligomeric protein species from solution (Obeso et al., 2010).

HD is caused by an expanded cytosine–adenine–guanine (CAG) repeat in the Huntingtin gene, which leads to a form of the protein with an expanded polyglutamine region (Walker, 2007). This expanded polyglutamine repeat induces protein misfolding and aggregation of the Huntingtin protein, with the severity of the defect and age of onset of disease symptoms proportional to the length of the CAG repeat. Although the precise mechanisms of disease progression in HD remain unknown, as does the normal role of the Huntingtin protein, several other diseases are associated with polyglutamine expansions in other proteins. These include several forms of spinocerebellar ataxia, Machado–Joseph disease, and spinal bulbar muscular atrophy X-linked type 1. These findings suggest that polyglutamine toxicity caused by loss of proteostasis contributes HD and other polyglutamine diseases (Fan et al., 2014; Shao & Diamond, 2007).

Although the link between loss of proteostasis and disease is strongest in age-associated neurodegenerative disorders, there is growing evidence that misfolding and aggregation of proteins also contribute to other age-related diseases, as well as functional decline in numerous tissues and organ systems accompanying the aging process. For example, loss of proteostasis has been implicated in diabetes (Jaisson & Gillery, 2014), heart disease (Christians, Mustafi, & Benjamin, 2014; Martins-Marques, Ribeiro-Rodrigues, Pereira, Codogno, & Girao, 2015; Sandri & Robbins, 2014), and kidney disease (Inagi, Ishimoto, & Nangaku, 2014; Kitamura, 2008), among others.

■ EVIDENCE THAT PROTEIN QUALITY CONTROL CAN MODULATE LIFE SPAN

There are numerous mechanisms that have evolved to allow cells to maintain proteostasis in the face of internal and external challenges. These include controls over the production of proteins at the level of transcription and translation; systems to facilitate the proper folding and localization of proteins; and processes to degrade misfolded, damaged, or otherwise extraneous proteins (Figure 10.1).

As discussed previously, the failure of these systems is associated with reduced survival and increased disease burden in humans; however, compelling evidence for a direct role of proteostasis in aging is derived from studies in model systems where enhanced protein quality control is associated with increased longevity and healthy aging. In this section, we present evidence that each of the major protein quality control mechanisms can impact life span in model systems.

mRNA Translation and Aging

Synthesis of new proteins places perhaps the largest burden on protein homeostasis within cells. Just the production of a ribosome involves transcription and translation of numerous individual protein subunits and mRNAs, processing and assembly of these factors, and import and export between the nucleus and the cytoplasm (Fromont-Racine,

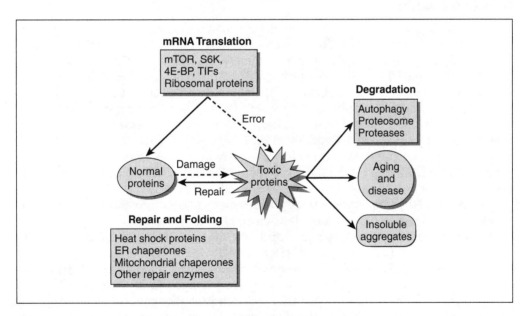

FIGURE 10.1. Model for the role of protein homeostasis in aging. Several mechanisms act to ensure proper protein folding and function that also impact aging and disease. These include control of protein synthesis through regulation of mRNA translation, chaperones to assist in proper folding and refolding of denatured proteins, and degradation pathways to break down damaged proteins. The role of insoluble aggregates in aging and disease is less clear and there is evidence that this may represent an additional mechanism for removing toxic soluble proteins from solution.

mTOR, mechanistic target of rapamycin; S6K, ribosomal S6 kinase; 4E-BP, eukaryotic translation initiation factor 4E binding protein 1; TIFs, translation initiation factors.

Figure modified from Kaeberlein and Kennedy (2007).

Senger, Saveanu, & Fasiolo, 2003; Nissan, Bassler, Petfalski, Tollervey, & Hurt, 2002; Woolford & Baserga, 2013; Zemp & Kutay, 2007). As proteins are synthesized on the ribosome, they are often engaged immediately by chaperones that assist in proper folding and, in some cases, import and targeting to specific cellular compartments such as the ER or mitochondria (Preissler & Deuerling, 2012). It is therefore not surprising that a common response to proteotoxic and other forms of stress is a rapid reduction in global mRNA translation (Liu & Qian, 2014; Sherman & Qian, 2013).

Several studies have identified signaling pathways that regulate mRNA translation, as well as the mRNA translation machinery itself, as important modulators of aging in model systems (Kaeberlein & Kennedy, 2007, 2008, 2011; Kennedy & Kaeberlein, 2009). This includes components of the mechanistic target of rapamycin (mTOR) pathway, translation initiation factors, ribosome biogenesis factors, and subunits of the ribosome itself. In nearly every case, life-span extension is associated with a reduction in global mRNA translation, although there is some evidence that differential translation of specific mRNAs may contribute to enhanced longevity (Steffen et al., 2008; Zid et al., 2009), perhaps in combination with less overall protein synthesis. In both yeast and worms, there is evidence that a reduction in global mRNA translation is associated with enhanced proteostasis (Charmpilas, Daskalaki, Papandreou, & Tavernarakis, 2014; Steffen et al., 2012), although whether this is causally related to the life-span extension is unknown.

Hsf1 and the HSR

Protein homeostasis is highly dependent on the action of chaperones and co-chaperones that assist in the proper folding or refolding of proteins into stable, functional conformations. Chaperones can be grouped into families including HSP70, HSP90, DNAJ/HSP40, HSP60, and small heat shock proteins (HSPs), and are found in all major cellular compartments (Labbadia & Morimoto, 2015). Chaperone defects have been implicated in a variety of diseases, including early-onset cataracts, spastic paraplegia and ataxia, cardiomyopathy and cardiac disease, Charcot–Marie–Tooth disease, and PD (Davey et al., 2006; Engert et al., 2000; Evgrafov et al., 2004; Hansen et al., 2002; Litt et al., 1998; Tang et al., 2005). Chaperone expression is greatly altered in neurodegenerative diseases, including AD, PD, and HD, and it is thought that the chaperones generally function to delay the progression of these diseases (Leak, 2014).

In response to different types of stress, chaperones and co-chaperones can be induced to assist with an elevated proteotoxic burden and restore proteostasis. These responses are largely compartment specific and include the ER-UPR, the MT-UPR, and the cytosolic/nuclear HSR. Chaperones of the HSR are greatly induced by thermal stress (hence the name "heat shock response"), but are also induced by other forms of stress that induce protein misfolding, such as oxidative stress and hypoxia (Leak, 2014).

The HSR has been strongly implicated in aging in several organisms, including yeast, worms, and flies. The HSR is mediated by activation of heat shock transcription factors (HSFs), most notably Hsf1. Activation of Hsf1 is sufficient to extend life span in *C. elegans* (Hsu, Murphy, & Kenyon, 2003; Morley & Morimoto, 2004) and is important for life-span extension and enhanced resistance to proteotoxic stress downstream of the insulin-like signaling pathway, reduced mTOR signaling, and dietary restriction (Cohen, Bieschke, Perciavalle, Kelly, & Dillin, 2006; Seo et al., 2013; Steinkraus et al., 2008). Increased expression of Hsf1 also extends chronological life span in the fission yeast *Schizosaccharomyces pombe* (Ohtsuka, Azuma, Murakami, & Aiba, 2011). The effects of Hsf1 overexpression on life span in mice have not yet been reported; however, one recent study showed amelioration of deficits from Hsf1 overexpression in a mouse model of AD (Pierce et al., 2013).

The UPS

The UPS functions, along with autophagy, as one of two primary mechanisms for degradation of proteins. Proteins in both the nucleus and the cytoplasm are targeted for degradation by the proteasome through covalent polyubiquitination of lysine residues by a complex and highly conserved series of three distinct enzymes (reviewed in Glickman & Ciechanover, 2002): an ubiquitin activase (or E1), an ubiquitin conjugase (or E2), and an ubiquitin ligase (or E3). The proteasome itself is a highly conserved multicatalytic enzyme consisting of more than 30 subunits (Finley, 2009). Several studies have documented a decline in proteasome activity with age (Carrard, Bulteau, Petropoulos, & Friguet, 2002; Vernace, Schmidt-Glenewinkel, & Figueiredo-Pereira, 2007), although at least one study failed to detect such a decline in mice (Cook et al., 2009), and proteasome defects are associated with several diseases including amyotrophic lateral sclerosis (ALS), PD, HD, and spinocerebellar ataxia (Atkin & Paulson, 2014; Guo et al., 2014; Zheng, Geetha, & Babu, 2014).

A direct role for the proteasome as a longevity-promoting complex was first established in yeast, in which it was found that deletion of *UBR2*, which encodes a negative regulator of proteasome activity, resulted in extended life span (Kruegel et al., 2011). A more recent study addressed the downstream targets of the proteasome relevant to yeast aging (Yao et al., 2015). Interestingly, while enhanced proteasome function may lead to life-span extension through turnover of damaged proteins, another mechanism was uncovered, in which proteasome-mediated turnover of a transcription factor, Mig1, leads to enhanced respiratory metabolism and benefits to longevity. This finding highlights the complex interactions between different pathways affecting longevity. Subsequent to the initial yeast study, this observation has been extended to both *C. elegans* and *Drosophila melanogaster* with reports that overexpression of specific proteasomal subunits can extend life span. In fruit flies, overexpression of the non-ATPase subunit of the 19S proteasome particle extends life span and enhances resistance to polyglutamine toxicity (Tonoki et al., 2009), while in *C. elegans*, overexpression of RPN-6, which stabilizes the interaction between the 19S and 20S proteasome, similarly increases life span (Vilchez et al., 2012).

Autophagy and Mitophagy

Autophagy is the other major cellular mechanism for degradation of proteins and involves targeting of substrates for degradation in the lysosome (Mizushima, Levine, Cuervo, & Klionsky, 2008; Yorimitsu & Klionsky, 2005). Unlike the proteasome, however, autophagy can be more general and encompass not just degradation of proteins, but also other cellular macromolecules and even entire organelles, such as mitochondrial degradation via mitophagy. At least three distinct types of autophagy have been described: chaperone-mediated autophagy, microautophagy, and macroautophagy. For the purposes of this chapter, we group all forms of autophagy together when considering evidence for their roles in aging; however, we refer interested readers to several excellent reviews for more depth on this topic (Feng, Yao, & Klionsky, 2015; Kon & Cuervo, 2010; Li, Li, & Bao, 2012; Wang & Mao, 2014).

As with other proteostatic mechanisms, defects in autophagy have been linked with several diseases, and particularly strongly linked with neurodegenerative disorders including AD, PD, and ALS (Frake, Ricketts, Menzies, & Rubinsztein, 2015; Martinez-Vicente, 2015). Tau, alpha synuclein, amyloid beta, and polyglutamine proteins are all known to be substrates for autophagy, and accumulation of autophagic vesicles has been reported in animal models of these diseases and clinical brain samples. One study also indicated that autophagy can specifically degrade progerin, the toxic protein expressed in the premature aging disease Hutchinson–Gilford progeria syndrome (Cao et al., 2011; Graziotto, Cao, Collins, & Krainc, 2012).

Like the proteasome, autophagy has been found to decline during aging in multiple studies and model systems (Cuervo & Dice, 2000), and several longevity-promoting pathways are known to regulate autophagy. This is best characterized in *C. elegans* where reduced insulin-like signaling, dietary restriction, and inhibition of mTOR have all been shown to activate autophagy and to require autophagy for life span extension (Hansen et al., 2008; Jia & Levine, 2007; Melendez et al., 2003). Recently, a transcription factor homologous to mammalian TFEB, HLH-30, was shown to be an important regulator of autophagy in *C. elegans* whose overexpression is sufficient to increase life span in that organism (Lapierre et al., 2013). Although it remains possible that functions of HLH-30 in addition to autophagy regulation underlie its effects on life span, this observation supports the idea that activation of autophagy is sufficient to enhance longevity in *C. elegans*.

The ER-UPR

The ER is a critical cellular system for protein folding and proteostasis. Nearly one third of all cellular proteins are estimated to utilize the ER for folding, posttranslational modification, and trafficking to their ultimate functional location (Schroder & Kaufman, 2005a, 2005b). The primary mechanism by which the ER responds to protein stress is through the ER-UPR, which results in the activation of a variety of chaperones and other factors involved in restoring proteostasis within the ER (Schroder & Kaufman, 2005a, 2005b). Several studies have indicated that the ER-UPR is induced in a variety of disease states, including age-related neurodegeneration, metabolic disease, and cancer, and prolonged ER-UPR activation can result in cell death (Stutzbach et al., 2013; Wang & Kaufman, 2012).

A direct role for the ER-UPR in aging is best supported from studies in yeast and worms indicating that induction of the ER-UPR is associated with life span extension in some cases. In worms, aging is associated with increased ER stress, and expression of a constitutively active form of the ER-UPR transcription factor XBP-1 is sufficient to extend life span (Taylor & Dillin, 2013). The ER-UPR has also been implicated as an important downstream target involved in life-span extension, resulting from reduced signaling through the insulin-like signaling pathway and overexpression of the worm sirtuin SIR-2.1 (Henis-Korenblit et al., 2010; Viswanathan, Kim, Berdichevsky, & Guarente, 2005). In yeast, activation of the ER-UPR is similarly associated with longer replicative life span and is required for replicative life-span extension from several mutations that impair ER secretory function (Labunskyy et al., 2014).

The MT-UPR

Similar to the ER-UPR, mitochondria have a compartment-specific stress response referred to as the "MT-UPR." The MT-UPR is induced in response to a variety of forms of mitochondrial stress including depletion of mitochondrial DNA, expression of a misfolding-prone protein in the mitochondrial membrane, deficiency for electron transport chain components, and exposure of cells to reactive oxygen species generating compounds such as paraquat (Benedetti, Haynes, Yang, Harding, & Ron, 2006; Martinus et al., 1996; Runkel, Liu, Baumeister, & Schulze, 2013; Zhao et al., 2002). Activation of the MT-UPR leads to a transcriptional response in the nucleus that increases expression of several nuclear encoded mitochondrial genes, including mitochondrial chaperonins 10 (Hsp10) and 60 (Hsp60), mitochondrial DnaJ, and the mitochondrial ClpP protease (Zhao et al., 2002). The MT-UPR has been studied most extensively in *C. elegans* using a transcriptional green fluorescent protein (GFP) reporter for mitochondrial Hsp70 (HSP-6; Bennett, Choi, & Kaeberlein, 2014). Numerous genes have been identified that induce expression of this reporter when knocked down, including several components of the electron transport chain, mitochondrial import machinery, and mitochondrial proteases (Haynes & Ron, 2010).

It has been documented that several gene knockdowns in *C. elegans* that induce the HSP-6 reporter also increase life span. These cases are primarily restricted to genes encoding components of the electron transport chain or mitochondrial ribosomal proteins (Bennett & Kaeberlein, 2014). Based on these observations, it was proposed that activation of the MT-UPR plays a direct, causal role in life-span extension in *C. elegans* (Durieux, Wolff, & Dillin, 2011) and, perhaps, in mice (Houtkooper et al., 2013). Subsequent studies have weakened this model, however, by showing that induction of the MT-UPR in several cases is neither necessary nor sufficient to increase life span (Bennett et al., 2014). The situation is further complicated by the fact that most of the studies indicating a role for the MT-UPR in aging have restricted their analysis to the HSP-6 reporter, which is problematic considering that the HSP-6 ortholog is not induced as part of the MT-UPR in mammalian cells (Zhao et al., 2002). Further studies are therefore needed to better understand the MT-UPR, its role, if any, in aging and disease, and additional mitochondrial stress response mechanisms that may be involved in healthy aging.

■ COMPARATIVE BIOLOGY OF AGING AND PROTEOSTASIS

Along with the data from the commonly used laboratory models and clinical studies described previously, there is growing evidence from comparative biological approaches that maintenance of proteostasis is a key attribute underlying healthy longevity. One example of this is a series of studies carried out on the naked mole rat, an exceptionally long-lived rodent species that lives about 10-fold longer than laboratory mice or rats (Buffenstein, 2005). Naked mole rat proteins are remarkably resistant to denaturation and are able to retain enzymatic function despite much higher levels of protein carbonylation in vivo (De Waal et al., 2013). Naked mole rate tissues also show elevated proteasome activity and, recently, a cytosolic factor was detected from naked mole rat cells that is able to protect proteasomes of other species, including yeast, mice, and humans, from proteasome inhibition (Rodriguez, Edrey, Osmulski, Gaczynska, & Buffenstein, 2012; Rodriguez et al., 2014).

Comparative approaches have also identified a striking correlation between proteostasis and longevity in diverse species. In one study, levels of insoluble protein carbonyls were examined in mice, rats, bats, marmosets, and naked mole rats, with lower levels of these insoluble carbonyls correlating with species longevity (Rodriguez et al., 2014). In another study, it was shown that extracts from clams with exceptional longevity were far more resistant to protein unfolding than extracts from shorter-lived clams (Treaster et al., 2014). Of particular interest in this latter report was evidence that a soluble factor from the extremely long-lived clam could confer enhanced resistance to denaturing conditions on proteins from shorter-lived species. Recently, immunoproteasome activity and expression were also found to be correlated with species longevity in fibroblasts derived from mice and primates. Immunoproteasomes can act as replacements for the three catalytic subunits of the proteasome and can be induced by immune and inflammatory signaling (Ferrington & Gregerson, 2012). Interestingly, in this study, interventions shown to increase life span in mice, including treatment with the mTOR inhibitor rapamycin, also induced immunoproteasome expression (Pickering, Lehr, & Miller, 2015). Another recent report showed a similar correlation between species longevity and other proteostasis pathways including autophagy and HSPs in fibroblasts derived from rodents, marsupials, and bats (Pride et al., 2015).

Although it is difficult to draw causal inferences from these types of comparative approaches, these observations make a compelling case that mechanisms for maintaining proteostasis are strongly associated with longevity across a broad evolutionary range. When taken in combination with the more direct evidence from short-lived model organisms, they also suggest that such mechanisms are likely necessary for extreme longevity and may play a direct role in promoting such longevity.

■ LOOKING FORWARD

Protein homeostasis appears to be of central importance during aging in a variety of different species; loss of protein homeostasis clearly contributes to age-related disease and declines in function in people. Because multiple, at least partially redundant, mechanisms are in place to ensure maintenance of protein homeostasis and the appropriate response to proteotoxic stress, it is perhaps not surprising that evidence can be found supporting a role for several of these mechanisms in aging and disease. Such studies have generally looked at each of these mechanisms individually, however, and defining the interactions between these various proteostatic pathways is likely to be important for understanding the role of proteostasis in normal cellular function and healthy organismal longevity. A few attempts have been made to better define the "proteostatic network," which can be thought of as an integrated collection of machinery that acts to maintain proteome integrity within cells and between tissues (Labbadia & Morimoto, 2015; Matus, Nassif, Glimcher, & Hetz, 2009). As described previously, the proteostasis network includes mechanisms for regulating mRNA translation and protein synthesis, molecular chaperones, and machinery for degradation of damaged or misfolded proteins. The interaction and interrelationships between these various components of the network are still only poorly understood and studies aimed at defining these interactions should be an area of emphasis going forward.

A second area of interest and active research is the development of pharmacological approaches to enhance proteostasis. Such drugs have the potential to be used as therapies for a swath neurodegenerative and other diseases associated with proteotoxicity, as well as interventions to promote healthy aging. One example of this kind of compound would be drugs that target known longevity pathways that also impact proteostasis. A good illustration of this idea is rapamycin, a specific inhibitor of mTOR. Rapamycin or genetic inhibition of mTOR has been shown to delay aging and increase life span in yeast, worms, flies, and several strains of mice (Kaeberlein, 2013, 2014). It is important to note that rapamycin has also been shown to enhance proteostasis in each of these species (Johnson, Rabinovitch, & Kaeberlein, 2013; Johnson, Sangesland, Kaeberlein, & Rabinovitch, 2015), and several studies have documented dramatic improvements from rapamycin treatment in mouse models of AD (Caccamo et al., 2009; Lin et al., 2013; Majumder, Richardson, Strong, & Oddo, 2011; Orr, Salinas, Buffenstein, & Oddo, 2014; Spilman et al., 2010). Pharmacological modifiers of other aging-related pathways, including sirtuins and insulin/insulin-like growth factor (IGF)-1-like signaling, may also prove to be potent enhancers of proteostasis.

In addition to targeting aging-related pathways, it may be possible to enhance proteostasis by targeting the proteostasis machinery itself (i.e., chaperones, proteasome, autophagy) or through the use of molecular chaperones that can directly aid in preventing denaturation or promoting protein refolding. For example, purification of the cytosolic factor from naked mole rats that enhances proteasome function (described previously) could allow for the development of a drug that can be used to enhance proteasome function in vivo. Likewise, the development of pharmacological chaperones has been described. Such molecules can function like a molecular scaffold to allow specific proteins prone to misfolding to fold properly within the cell (Parenti, Andria, & Valenzano, 2015) or they can act in a general manner to enhance proteostasis (Alavez & Lithgow, 2012). Going forward, these approaches have great potential to allow development of interventions that can attenuate disease and enhance healthy aging.

REFERENCES

Alavez, S., & Lithgow, G. J. (2012). Pharmacological maintenance of protein homeostasis could postpone age-related disease. *Aging cell, 11*(2), 187–191.

Atkin, G., & Paulson, H. (2014). Ubiquitin pathways in neurodegenerative disease. *Frontiers in Molecular Neuroscience, 7*, 63.

Balch, W. E., Morimoto, R. I., Dillin, A., & Kelly, J. W. (2008). Adapting proteostasis for disease intervention. *Science, 319*(5865), 916–919.

Bancher, C., Brunner, C., Lassmann, H., Budka, H., Jellinger, K., Wiche, G.,...Wisniewski, H. M. (1989). Accumulation of abnormally phosphorylated tau precedes the formation of neurofibrillary tangles in Alzheimer's disease. *Brain Research, 477*(1–2), 90–99.

Benedetti, C., Haynes, C. M., Yang, Y., Harding, H. P., & Ron, D. (2006). Ubiquitin-like protein 5 positively regulates chaperone gene expression in the mitochondrial unfolded protein response. *Genetics, 174*(1), 229–239.

Bennett, C. F., Choi, H., & Kaeberlein, M. (2014). Searching for the elusive mitochondrial longevity signal in *C. elegans. Worm, 30*, e959404.

Bennett, C. F., & Kaeberlein, M. (2014). The mitochondrial unfolded protein response and increased longevity: Cause, consequence, or correlation? *Experimental Gerontology, 56C*, 142–146.

Bennett, C. F., Vander Wende, H., Simko, M., Klum, S., Barfield, S., Choi, H.,...Kaeberlein, M. (2014). Activation of the mitochondrial unfolded protein response does not predict longevity in *Caenorhabditis elegans. Nature Communications, 5*, 3483.

Buffenstein, R. (2005). The naked mole-rat: A new long-living model for human aging research. *The Journals of Gerontology, Series A, 60*(11), 1369–1377.

Burns, A., & Iliffe, S. (2009). Alzheimer's disease. *British Medical Journal, 338*, b158.

Caccamo, A., Majumder, S., Deng, J. J., Bai, Y., Thornton, F. B., & Oddo, S. (2009). Rapamycin rescues TDP-43 mislocalization and the associated low molecular mass neurofilament instability. *The Journal of Biological Chemistry, 284*(40), 27416–27424.

Cao, K., Graziotto, J. J., Blair, C. D., Mazzulli, J. R., Erdos, M. R., Krainc, D., & Collins, F. S. (2011). Rapamycin reverses cellular phenotypes and enhances mutant protein clearance in Hutchinson-Gilford progeria syndrome cells. *Science Translational Medicine, 3*(89), 89ra58.

Carrard, G., Bulteau, A. L., Petropoulos, I., & Friguet, B. (2002). Impairment of proteasome structure and function in aging. *International Journal of Biochemistry & Cell Biology, 34*(11), 1461–1474.

Charmpilas, N., Daskalaki, I., Papandreou, M. E., & Tavernarakis, N. (2014). Protein synthesis as an integral quality control mechanism during ageing. *Ageing Research Reviews, 23*(Pt. A), 75–89.

Christians, E. S., Mustafi, S. B., & Benjamin, I. J. (2014). Chaperones and cardiac misfolding protein diseases. *Current Protein & Peptide Science, 15*(3), 189–204.

Cohen, E., Bieschke, J., Perciavalle, R. M., Kelly, J. W., & Dillin, A. (2006). Opposing activities protect against age-onset proteotoxicity. *Science, 313*(5793), 1604–1610.

Cook, C., Gass, J., Dunmore, J., Tong, J., Taylor, J., Eriksen, J.,...Petrucelli, L. (2009). Aging is not associated with proteasome impairment in UPS reporter mice. *PloS One, 4*(6), e5888.

Cras, P., Kawai, M., Lowery, D., Gonzalez-DeWhitt, P., Greenberg, B., & Perry, G. (1991). Senile plaque neurites in Alzheimer disease accumulate amyloid precursor protein. *Proceedings of the National Academy of Sciences of the United States of America, 88*(17), 7552–7556.

Cuervo, A. M., & Dice, J. F. (2000). Age-related decline in chaperone-mediated autophagy. *The Journal of Biological Chemistry, 275*(40), 31505–31513.

Davey, K. M., Parboosingh, J. S., McLeod, D. R., Chan, A., Casey, R., Ferreira, P.,...Bernier, F. P. (2006). Mutation of DNAJC19, a human homologue of yeast inner mitochondrial membrane co-chaperones, causes DCMA syndrome, a novel autosomal recessive Barth syndrome-like condition. *Journal of Medical Genetics, 43*(5), 385–393.

Davie, C. A. (2008). A review of Parkinson's disease. *British Medical Bulletin, 86*, 109–127.

De Waal, E. M., Liang, H., Pierce, A., Hamilton, R. T., Buffenstein, R., & Chaudhuri, A. R. (2013). Elevated protein carbonylation and oxidative stress do not affect protein structure and function in the long-living naked-mole rat: A proteomic approach. *Biochemical and Biophysical Research Communications, 434*(4), 815–819.

Durieux, J., Wolff, S., & Dillin, A. (2011). The cell-non-autonomous nature of electron transport chain-mediated longevity. *Cell, 144*(1), 79–91.

Engert, J. C., Berube, P., Mercier, J., Dore, C., Lepage, P., Ge, B.,...Richter, A. (2000). ARSACS, a spastic ataxia common in northeastern Quebec, is caused by mutations in a new gene encoding an 11.5-kb ORF. *Nature Genetics, 24*(2), 120–125.

Evgrafov, O. V., Mersiyanova, I., Irobi, J., Van Den Bosch, L., Dierick, I., Leung, C. L.,...Timmerman, V. (2004). Mutant small heat-shock protein 27 causes axonal

Charcot-Marie-Tooth disease and distal hereditary motor neuropathy. *Nature Genetics, 36*(6), 602–606.

Fan, H. C., Ho, L. I., Chi, C. S., Chen, S. J., Peng, G. S., Chan, T. M.,...Harn, H. J. (2014). Polyglutamine (PolyQ) diseases: Genetics to treatments. *Cell Transplant, 23*(4–5), 441–458.

Feng, Y., Yao, Z., & Klionsky, D. J. (2015). How to control self-digestion: Transcriptional, post-transcriptional, and post-translational regulation of autophagy. *Trends in Cell Biology, 25*(6), 354–363.

Ferrington, D. A., & Gregerson, D. S. (2012). Immunoproteasomes: Structure, function, and antigen presentation. *Progress in Molecular Biology and Translational Science, 109*, 75–112.

Finley, D. (2009). Recognition and processing of ubiquitin-protein conjugates by the proteasome. *Annual Review of Biochemistry, 78*, 477–513.

Frake, R. A., Ricketts, T., Menzies, F. M., & Rubinsztein, D. C. (2015). Autophagy and neurodegeneration. *Journal of Clinical Investigation, 125*(1), 65–74.

Fromont-Racine, M., Senger, B., Saveanu, C., & Fasiolo, F. (2003). Ribosome assembly in eukaryotes. *Gene, 313*, 17–42.

Glickman, M. H., & Ciechanover, A. (2002). The ubiquitin-proteasome proteolytic pathway: Destruction for the sake of construction. *Physiological Reviews, 82*(2), 373–428.

Graziotto, J. J., Cao, K., Collins, F. S., & Krainc, D. (2012). Rapamycin activates autophagy in Hutchinson-Gilford progeria syndrome: Implications for normal aging and age-dependent neurodegenerative disorders. *Autophagy, 8*(1), 147–151.

Guo, L., Giasson, B. I., Glavis-Bloom, A., Brewer, M. D., Shorter, J., Gitler, A. D., & Yang, X. (2014). A cellular system that degrades misfolded proteins and protects against neurodegeneration. *Molecular Cell, 55*(1), 15–30.

Hansen, J. J., Durr, A., Cournu-Rebeix, I., Georgopoulos, C., Ang, D., Nielsen, M. N.,...Bross, P. (2002). Hereditary spastic paraplegia SPG13 is associated with a mutation in the gene encoding the mitochondrial chaperonin Hsp60. *American Journal of Human Genetics, 70*(5), 1328–1332.

Hansen, M., Chandra, A., Mitic, L. L., Onken, B., Driscoll, M., & Kenyon, C. (2008). A role for autophagy in the extension of lifespan by dietary restriction in *C. elegans*. *PLoS Genetics, 4*(2), e24.

Haynes, C. M., & Ron, D. (2010). The mitochondrial UPR—Protecting organelle protein homeostasis. *Journal of Cell Science, 123*(Pt. 22), 3849–3855.

Henis-Korenblit, S., Zhang, P., Hansen, M., McCormick, M., Lee, S. J., Cary, M., & Kenyon, C. (2010). Insulin/IGF-1 signaling mutants reprogram ER stress response regulators to promote longevity. *Proceedings of the National Academy of Sciences of the United States of America, 107*(21), 9730–9735.

Houtkooper, R. H., Mouchiroud, L., Ryu, D., Moullan, N., Katsyuba, E., Knott, G.,...Auwerx, J. (2013). Mitonuclear protein imbalance as a conserved longevity mechanism. *Nature, 497*(7450), 451–457.

Hsu, A. L., Murphy, C. T., & Kenyon, C. (2003). Regulation of aging and age-related disease by DAF-16 and heat-shock factor. *Science, 300*(5622), 1142–1145.

Inagi, R., Ishimoto, Y., & Nangaku, M. (2014). Proteostasis in endoplasmic reticulum—New mechanisms in kidney disease. *Nature Reviews Nephrology, 10*(7), 369–378.

Jaisson, S., & Gillery, P. (2014). Impaired proteostasis: Role in the pathogenesis of diabetes mellitus. *Diabetologia, 57*(8), 1517–1527.

Jia, K., & Levine, B. (2007). Autophagy is required for dietary restriction-mediated life span extension in *C. elegans. Autophagy, 3*(6), 597–599.

Johnson, S. C., Rabinovitch, P. S., & Kaeberlein, M. (2013). mTOR is a key modulator of ageing and age-related disease. *Nature, 493*(7432), 338–345.

Johnson, S. C., Sangesland, M., Kaeberlein, M., & Rabinovitch, P. S. (2015). Modulating mTOR in aging and health. *Interdisciplinary Topics in Gerontology and Geriatrics, 40*, 107–127.

Kaeberlein, M. (2013). mTOR inhibition: From aging to autism and beyond. *Scientifica (Cairo), 2013*, 849186.

Kaeberlein, M. (2014). Rapamycin and ageing: When, for how long, and how much? *Journal of Genetics and Genomics, 41*(9), 459–463.

Kaeberlein, M., & Kennedy, B. K. (2007). Protein translation. *Aging Cell, 6*(6), 731–734.

Kaeberlein, M., & Kennedy, B. K. (2008). Protein translation. *Aging Cell, 7*(6), 777–782.

Kaeberlein, M., & Kennedy, B. K. (2011). Hot topics in aging research: Protein translation and TOR signaling. *Aging Cell, 10*(2), 185–190.

Kennedy, B. K., & Kaeberlein, M. (2009). Hot topics in aging research: Protein translation. *Aging Cell, 8*(6), 617–623.

Kikis, E. A., Gidalevitz, T., & Morimoto, R. I. (2010). Protein homeostasis in models of aging and age-related conformational disease. *Advances in Experimental Medicine and Biology, 694*, 138–159.

Kitamura, M. (2008). Endoplasmic reticulum stress and unfolded protein response in renal pathophysiology: Janus faces. *American Journal of Physiology: Renal Physiology, 295*(2), F323–F334.

Kon, M., & Cuervo, A. M. (2010). Chaperone-mediated autophagy in health and disease. *FEBS Letters, 584*(7), 1399–1404.

Kruegel, U., Robison, B., Dange, T., Kahlert, G., Delaney, J. R., Kotireddy, S., . . . Schmidt, M. (2011). Elevated proteasome capacity extends replicative lifespan in *Saccharomyces cerevisiae. PLoS Genetics, 7*(9), e1002253.

Labbadia, J., & Morimoto, R. I. (2015). The biology of proteostasis in aging and disease. *Annual Review of Biochemistry, 84*, 435–464.

Labunskyy, V. M., Gerashchenko, M. V., Delaney, J. R., Kaya, A., Kennedy, B. K., Kaeberlein, M., & Gladyshev, V. N. (2014). Lifespan extension conferred by endoplasmic reticulum secretory pathway deficiency requires induction of the unfolded protein response. *PLoS Genetics, 10*(1), e1004019.

Lapierre, L. R., De Magalhaes Filho, C. D., McQuary, P. R., Chu, C. C., Visvikis, O., Chang, J. T., . . . Hansen, M. (2013). The TFEB orthologue HLH-30 regulates autophagy and modulates longevity in *Caenorhabditis elegans. Nature Communications, 4*, 2267.

Leak, R. K. (2014). Heat shock proteins in neurodegenerative disorders and aging. *Journal of Cell Communication and Signaling, 8*(4), 293–310.

Lin, A. L., Zheng, W., Halloran, J. J., Burbank, R. R., Hussong, S. A., Hart, M. J.,…Galvan, V. (2013). Chronic rapamycin restores brain vascular integrity and function through NO synthase activation and improves memory in symptomatic mice modeling Alzheimer's disease. *Journal of Cerebral Blood Flow & Metabolism, 33*(9), 1412–1421.

Litt, M., Kramer, P., LaMorticella, D. M., Murphey, W., Lovrien, E. W., & Weleber, R. G. (1998). Autosomal dominant congenital cataract associated with a missense mutation in the human alpha crystallin gene CRYAA. *Human Molecular Genetics, 7*(3), 471–474.

Li, W. W., Li, J., & Bao, J. K. (2012). Microautophagy: Lesser-known self-eating. *Cellular and Molecular Life Sciences: CMLS, 69*(7), 1125–1136.

Liu, B., & Qian, S. B. (2014). Translational reprogramming in cellular stress response. *Wiley Interdisciplinary Reviews: RNA, 5*(3), 301–315.

Lopez-Otin, C., Blasco, M. A., Partridge, L., Serrano, M., & Kroemer, G. (2013). The hallmarks of aging. *Cell, 153*(6), 1194–1217.

Majumder, S., Richardson, A., Strong, R., & Oddo, S. (2011). Inducing autophagy by rapamycin before, but not after, the formation of plaques and tangles ameliorates cognitive deficits. *PloS One, 6*(9), e25416.

Martinez-Vicente, M. (2015). Autophagy in neurodegenerative diseases: From pathogenic dysfunction to therapeutic modulation. *Seminars in Cell & Developmental Biology, 40*, 115–126.

Martins-Marques, T., Ribeiro-Rodrigues, T., Pereira, P., Codogno, P., & Girao, H. (2015). Autophagy and ubiquitination in cardiovascular diseases. *DNA and Cell Biology, 34*(4), 243–251.

Martinus, R. D., Garth, G. P., Webster, T. L., Cartwright, P., Naylor, D. J., Hoj, P. B., & Hoogenraad, N. J. (1996). Selective induction of mitochondrial chaperones in response to loss of the mitochondrial genome. *European Journal of Biochemistry/ FEBS, 240*(1), 98–103.

Matus, S., Nassif, M., Glimcher, L. H., & Hetz, C. (2009). XBP-1 deficiency in the nervous system reveals a homeostatic switch to activate autophagy. *Autophagy, 5*(8), 1226–1228.

Melendez, A., Talloczy, Z., Seaman, M., Eskelinen, E. L., Hall, D. H., & Levine, B. (2003). Autophagy genes are essential for dauer development and life-span extension in *C. elegans. Science, 301*(5638), 1387–1391.

Mizushima, N., Levine, B., Cuervo, A. M., & Klionsky, D. J. (2008). Autophagy fights disease through cellular self-digestion. *Nature, 451*(7182), 1069–1075.

Morley, J. F., & Morimoto, R. I. (2004). Regulation of longevity in *Caenorhabditis elegans* by heat shock factor and molecular chaperones. *Molecular Biology of the Cell, 15*(2), 657–664.

Nissan, T. A., Bassler, J., Petfalski, E., Tollervey, D., & Hurt, E. (2002). 60S pre-ribosome formation viewed from assembly in the nucleolus until export to the cytoplasm. *The EMBO Journal, 21*(20), 5539–5547.

Obeso, J. A., Rodriguez-Oroz, M. C., Goetz, C. G., Marin, C., Kordower, J. H., Rodriguez, M.,…Halliday, G. (2010). Missing pieces in the Parkinson's disease puzzle. *Nature Medicine, 16*(6), 653–661.

Ohtsuka, H., Azuma, K., Murakami, H., & Aiba, H. (2011). hsf1 (+) extends chronological lifespan through Ecl1 family genes in fission yeast. *Molecular Genetics and Genomics, 285*(1), 67–77.

Orr, M. E., Salinas, A., Buffenstein, R., & Oddo, S. (2014). Mammalian target of rapamycin hyperactivity mediates the detrimental effects of a high sucrose diet on Alzheimer's disease pathology. *Neurobiology of Aging, 35*(6), 1233–1242.

Parenti, G., Andria, G., & Valenzano, K. J. (2015). Pharmacological chaperone therapy: Preclinical development, clinical translation, and prospects for the treatment of lysosomal storage disorders. *Molecular Therapy, 23*(7), 1138–1148.

Pickering, A. M., Lehr, M., & Miller, R. A. (2015). Lifespan of mice and primates correlates with immunoproteasome expression. *Journal of Clinical Investigation, 125*(5), 2059–2068.

Pierce, A., Podlutskaya, N., Halloran, J. J., Hussong, S. A., Lin, P. Y., Burbank, R.,…Galvan, V. (2013). Over-expression of heat shock factor 1 phenocopies the effect of chronic inhibition of TOR by rapamycin and is sufficient to ameliorate Alzheimer's-like deficits in mice modeling the disease. *Journal of Neurochemistry, 124*(6), 880–893.

Preissler, S., & Deuerling, E. (2012). Ribosome-associated chaperones as key players in proteostasis. *Trends in Biochemical Sciences, 37*(7), 274–283.

Pride, H., Yu, Z., Sunchu, B., Mochnick, J., Coles, A., Zhang, Y.,…Perez, V. I. (2015). Long-lived species have improved proteostasis compared to phylogenetically-related shorter-lived species. *Biochemical and Biophysical Research Communications, 457*(4), 669–675.

Querfurth, H. W., & LaFerla, F. M. (2010). Alzheimer's disease. *The New England Journal of Medicine, 362*(4), 329–344.

Rodriguez, K. A., Edrey, Y. H., Osmulski, P., Gaczynska, M., & Buffenstein, R. (2012). Altered composition of liver proteasome assemblies contributes to enhanced proteasome activity in the exceptionally long-lived naked mole-rat. *PloS One, 7*(5), e35890.

Rodriguez, K. A., Osmulski, P. A., Pierce, A., Weintraub, S. T., Gaczynska, M., & Buffenstein, R. (2014). A cytosolic protein factor from the naked mole-rat activates proteasomes of other species and protects these from inhibition. *Biochimica et Biophysica Acta, 1842*(11), 2060–2072.

Runkel, E. D., Liu, S., Baumeister, R., & Schulze, E. (2013). Surveillance-activated defenses block the ROS-induced mitochondrial unfolded protein response. *PLoS Genetics, 9*(3), e1003346.

Sandri, M., & Robbins, J. (2014). Proteotoxicity: An underappreciated pathology in cardiac disease. *Journal of Molecular and Cellular Cardiology, 71*, 3–10.

Schroder, M., & Kaufman, R. J. (2005a). ER stress and the unfolded protein response. *Mutation Research, 569*(1–2), 29–63.

Schroder, M., & Kaufman, R. J. (2005b). The mammalian unfolded protein response. *Annual Review of Biochemistry, 74*, 739–789.

Schulz-Schaeffer, W. J. (2010). The synaptic pathology of alpha-synuclein aggregation in dementia with Lewy bodies, Parkinson's disease and Parkinson's disease dementia. *Acta Neuropathologica, 120*(2), 131–143.

Seo, K., Choi, E., Lee, D., Jeong, D. E., Jang, S. K., & Lee, S. J. (2013). Heat shock factor 1 mediates the longevity conferred by inhibition of TOR and insulin/IGF-1 signaling pathways in *C. elegans. Aging Cell, 12*(6), 1073–1081.

Shao, J., & Diamond, M. I. (2007). Polyglutamine diseases: Emerging concepts in pathogenesis and therapy. *Human Molecular Genetics, 16 Spec No. 2*, R115–R123.

Sherman, M. Y., & Qian, S. B. (2013). Less is more: Improving proteostasis by translation slow down. *Trends in Biochemical Sciences, 38*(12), 585–591.

Spilman, P., Podlutskaya, N., Hart, M. J., Debnath, J., Gorostiza, O., Bredesen, D.,...Galvan, V. (2010). Inhibition of mTOR by rapamycin abolishes cognitive deficits and reduces amyloid-beta levels in a mouse model of Alzheimer's disease. *PloS One, 5*(4), e9979.

Steffen, K. K., MacKay, V. L., Kerr, E. O., Tsuchiya, M., Hu, D., Fox, L. A.,...Kaeberlein, M. (2008). Yeast life span extension by depletion of 60s ribosomal subunits is mediated by Gcn4. *Cell, 133*(2), 292–302.

Steffen, K. K., McCormick, M. A., Pham, K. M., MacKay, V. L., Delaney, J. R., Murakami, C. J.,...Kennedy, B. K. (2012). Ribosome deficiency protects against ER stress in *Saccharomyces cerevisiae. Genetics, 191*(1), 107–118.

Steinkraus, K. A., Smith, E. D., Davis, C., Carr, D., Pendergrass, W. R., Sutphin, G. L.,...Kaeberlein, M. (2008). Dietary restriction suppresses proteotoxicity and enhances longevity by an hsf-1-dependent mechanism in *Caenorhabditis elegans. Aging Cell, 7*(3), 394–404.

Stutzbach, L. D., Xie, S. X., Naj, A. C., Albin, R., Gilman, S., Group, P. S. P. G. S.,...Schellenberg, G. D. (2013). The unfolded protein response is activated in disease-affected brain regions in progressive supranuclear palsy and Alzheimer's disease. *Acta Neuropathologica Communications, 1*(1), 31.

Tang, B. S., Zhao, G. H., Luo, W., Xia, K., Cai, F., Pan, Q.,...Dai, H. P. (2005). Small heat-shock protein 22 mutated in autosomal dominant Charcot-Marie-Tooth disease type 2L. *Human Genetics, 116*(3), 222–224.

Taylor, R. C., & Dillin, A. (2013). XBP-1 is a cell-nonautonomous regulator of stress resistance and longevity. *Cell, 153*(7), 1435–1447.

Tonoki, A., Kuranaga, E., Tomioka, T., Hamazaki, J., Murata, S., Tanaka, K., & Miura, M. (2009). Genetic evidence linking age-dependent attenuation of the 26S proteasome with the aging process. *Molecular and Cellular Biology, 29*(4), 1095–1106.

Treaster, S. B., Ridgway, I. D., Richardson, C. A., Gaspar, M. B., Chaudhuri, A. R., & Austad, S. N. (2014). Superior proteome stability in the longest lived animal. *Age (Dordr), 36*(3), 9597.

Vernace, V. A., Schmidt-Glenewinkel, T., & Figueiredo-Pereira, M. E. (2007). Aging and regulated protein degradation: Who has the UPPer hand? *Aging Cell, 6*(5), 599–606.

Vilchez, D., Morantte, I., Liu, Z., Douglas, P. M., Merkwirth, C., Rodrigues, A. P.,...Dillin, A. (2012). RPN-6 determines *C. elegans* longevity under proteotoxic stress conditions. *Nature, 489*(7415), 263–268.

Viola, K. L., & Klein, W. L. (2015). Amyloid beta oligomers in Alzheimer's disease pathogenesis, treatment, and diagnosis. *Acta Neuropathologica, 129*(2), 183–206.

Viswanathan, M., Kim, S. K., Berdichevsky, A., & Guarente, L. (2005). A role for SIR-2.1 regulation of ER stress response genes in determining *C. elegans* life span. *Developmental Cell, 9*(5), 605–615.

Walker, F. O. (2007). Huntington's disease. *The Lancet, 369*(9557), 218–228.

Wang, G., & Mao, Z. (2014). Chaperone-mediated autophagy: Roles in neurodegeneration. *Translational Neurodegeneration, 3*, 20.

Wang, S., & Kaufman, R. J. (2012). The impact of the unfolded protein response on human disease. *The Journal of Cell Biology, 197*(7), 857–867.

Woolford, J. L., Jr., & Baserga, S. J. (2013). Ribosome biogenesis in the yeast *Saccharomyces cerevisiae*. *Genetics, 195*(3), 643–681.

Yao, Y., Tsuchiyama, S., Yang, C., Bulteau, A. L., He, C., Robison, B., ... Schmidt, M. (2015). Proteasomes, Sir2, and Hxk2 form an interconnected aging network that impinges on the AMPK/Snf1-regulated transcriptional repressor Mig1. *PLoS Genetics, 11*(1), e1004968.

Yorimitsu, T., & Klionsky, D. J. (2005). Autophagy: Molecular machinery for self-eating. *Cell Death & Differentiation, 12*(Suppl. 2), 1542–1552.

Zemp, I., & Kutay, U. (2007). Nuclear export and cytoplasmic maturation of ribosomal subunits. *FEBS Letters, 581*(15), 2783–2793.

Zhao, Q., Wang, J., Levichkin, I. V., Stasinopoulos, S., Ryan, M. T., & Hoogenraad, N. J. (2002). A mitochondrial specific stress response in mammalian cells. *The EMBO Journal, 21*(17), 4411–4419.

Zheng, C., Geetha, T., & Babu, J. R. (2014). Failure of ubiquitin proteasome system: Risk for neurodegenerative diseases. *Neurodegenerative Diseases, 14*(4), 161–175.

Zid, B. M., Rogers, A. N., Katewa, S. D., Vargas, M. A., Kolipinski, M. C., Lu, T. A., ... Kapahi, P. (2009). 4E-BP extends lifespan upon dietary restriction by enhancing mitochondrial activity in Drosophila. *Cell, 139*(1), 149–160.

PART III

Psychological Theories and Concepts

ADVANCES IN PSYCHOLOGICAL THEORIES OF AGING
Jacqui Smith

What are the definitive processes and trajectories of psychological aging? What progress have we made in answering this question in any domain of psychological functioning? As I looked back at previous efforts to summarize the state of psychological theories of aging and asked colleagues for their ideas about the emergence of *new* theories in the past decade, I realized that, with some exceptions, psychologists remain entrenched in long-standing concepts, metaphors, and unsolved issues. Among others, these include mechanisms such as reserve, selection, and compensation, and concepts such as differential aging, multidirectional change trajectories, differentiation/dedifferentiation, plasticity, and the potential and limits of modifiability (see also Dixon, 2011).

There are, however, signs of change. Increasingly, for example, long-standing psychological theories are being recast in a new generation of efforts to understand and model the complexities, dynamics, and interdependencies of change over time. Traditionally, psychological theories have employed one of the mechanisms or concepts mentioned earlier, and have focused on only one area of psychological functioning (e.g., memory, sensorimotor integration, emotion-regulation, self-perceptions, social relationships, and personality). In some respects, this approach is similar to the medical sciences, which continue to be dominated by disease-specific theories and models. However, some contemporary theories are beginning to develop explanations for associations *across* areas of psychological functioning as exemplified in Chapter 12 by Ngo, Sands, and Isaacowitz, which probes the linkages between trajectories of cognitive and emotional age-related change.

With contemporary advances in the collection of multidimensional and multilevel data, and Big Data tools to analyze and model the synchronization and interdependencies of functioning over time (e.g., at neural, biological, and behavioral levels), we might expect more of these integrative theories to evolve in the next decades. Indeed, there are already signs of movement in this direction. As Birren (1999) and Baltes (1997) noted previously, the processes of psychological aging are inherently intertwined not only with each other, but also with changes in physical health, social and historical context, and biological aging. In the future, as new theories of *biopsychosocial change over time* emerge, it will indeed become more difficult to categorize contemporary theories as being distinctly about *psychological* aging. This is not a critique of the discipline. Rather, it points to the fact that most psychologists in the field of aging have acknowledged the complexities inherent in aging and have taken up the challenge to outline age-related processes that generalize across functional domains and operate as a multivariate system.

Another sign of change lies in new efforts to integrate concepts of psychological aging. Regardless of the specificity or generality of the theory, it is important that theories of psychological aging address questions about the patterning and timing of age-related change as well as the causal determinants, underlying mechanisms, and contexts of age-related change (see also Salthouse, 2006). Questions about the patterning of psychological change have long been prominent in life-span theories of development and aging. Early theories of cognitive aging, for example, described different directions (growth, stability, and decline), metrics (quantity and quality), and different rates of change across various dimensions of functioning (e.g., episodic vs. long-term memory; fluid vs. crystallized intelligence). Theories in other areas of psychological functioning (e.g., personality) typically dealt with variance in the capacity of individuals to adapt and change at different ages.

Over the past decade, new theories have integrated concepts of capacity and patterning of age-related change. One is the Scaffolding Theory of Aging and Cognition (STAC), which outlines the operation of protective lifelong experiences and biological processes associated with the enrichment of brain capacity (reserve) and the buildup of compensatory neural pathways (or scaffolds; Park & Reuter-Lorenz, 2009; Reuter-Lorenz & Park, 2014). This theory proposes ways in which these processes, together, serve to buffer the deleterious effects of functional and structural brain changes in later life. In addition, it encompasses trajectories of both normal and pathological cognitive aging.

Four chapters (Chapters 11–14) in this part also address questions about efficacy or capacity of psychological reserves (e.g., cognitive, social, and self-related beliefs) to buffer physical health and biological challenges. In Chapter 15, Hülür, Ram, and Gerstorf consider the multiple sources of psychological reserve (sometimes called "resilience"). On one hand, these reserves may contribute to a longer life and be maintained at relatively high levels over many years. On the other hand, they may eventually be challenged by biological multimorbidity in the final years of life. Charles and Hong in Chapter 11 review theories about stability and change in emotional experience throughout adulthood and into old age, and the important role of positive emotional experience in adapting to age-related changes in social context and health. They point out, however, that even the strength of this highly protective mechanism may be vulnerable to frailty in the oldest old. In Chapter 13, Uchino, Ong, Queen, and Kent de Grey consider the role of changes in building up and utilizing reserves of social support across the life span for health outcomes. Meisner and Levy in Chapter 14 discuss the psychological, behavioral, and physiological pathways through which societal age stereotypes are internalized as self-stereotypes.

There are still relatively few theories that address the timing of critical changes in patterns of psychological aging. Why do these changes occur earlier in life for some people and domains but later for others? What are the predictors or precursors of the onset of qualitative differences in change (e.g., pathological cognitive aging)? Certainly many theories account for potential sources of differential trajectories of change in early life (e.g., Uchino and colleagues, and Meisner and Levy) and others attempt to estimate the onset of terminal change in very old age (e.g., Hülür et al.). These issues along with other vexing questions may take some time to come to the fore in theoretical work.

Future theories might entertain new questions such as: Why should humans invest in years of acquiring knowledge if this does not result in well-functioning brains that are built to last? Does "building a smart child" pay psychological dividends at the end of life? (E.g., does it improve happiness, health, social activity and integration, and the ability to live independently until the end of life?) When in the life course are "booster shots" needed to sustain psychological functioning—how many and how often? How many protective personal psychological resources are required to deal with all of the potential threats to integrity and to benefit from the *longevity dividend* (Goldman et al., 2013; Smith & Ryan, 2016; Vaupel, 2010)?

Recent years have brought the rapid expansion of publicly available data from large representative surveys that include psychological, physical, cellular, and genetic data. These data provide a rich platform for all researchers to engage in theory-guided research and contribute new insights. Increasingly, these studies are also being linked to geographic and administrative data. The retrospective collection of life histories from participants in ongoing studies of aging will further extend current possibilities to trace antecedents to change during midlife and old age. Smaller experimental studies will, of course, continue to be especially important contexts to complement findings from Big Data and to test and derive theories about specific mechanisms. In effect, there remains much to be learned about psychological aging. New analytical methods, measurement tools, and Big Data will spur new theories in the upcoming years.

REFERENCES

Baltes, P. B. (1997). On the incomplete architecture of human ontogeny. Selection, optimization, and compensation as foundation of developmental theory. *American Psychologist, 52*(4), 366–380.

Birren, J. E. (1999). Theories of aging: A personal perspective. In V. L. Bengtson & K. W. Schaie (Eds.), *Handbook of theories of aging* (pp. 459–471). New York, NY: Springer Publishing Company.

Dixon, R. A. (2011). Enduring theoretical themes in psychological aging: Derivation, functions, perspectives, and opportunities. In K. W. Schaie & S. L. Willis (Eds.). *Handbook of the psychology of aging* (7th ed., pp. 3–23). San Diego, CA: Elsevier.

Goldman, D. P., Cutler, D., Rowe, J. W., Michaud, P. C., Sullivan, J., Peneva, D., & Olshansky, S. J. (2013). Substantial health and economic returns from delayed aging may warrant a new focus for medical research. *Health Affairs (Project Hope), 32*(10), 1698–1705.

Park, D. C., & Reuter-Lorenz, P. (2009). The adaptive brain: Aging and neurocognitive scaffolding. *Annual Review of Psychology, 60*, 173–196.

Reuter-Lorenz, P. A., & Park, D. C. (2014). How does it STAC up? Revisiting the scaffolding theory of aging and cognition. *Neuropsychology Review, 24*(3), 355–370.

Salthouse, T. A. (2006). Theoretical issues in the psychology of aging. In K. W. Schaie & S. L. Willis (Eds.), *Handbook of the psychology of aging* (6th ed., pp. 3–13). San Diego, CA: Elsevier.

Smith, J., & Ryan, L. H. (2016). Psychological vitality in the oldest old. In K. W. Schaie & S. L. Willis (Eds.), *Handbook of the psychology of aging* (8th ed., pp. 303–319). San Diego, CA: Elsevier. doi:http://dx.doi.org/10.1016/B978-0-12-411469-2.00016-9

Vaupel, J. W. (2010). Biodemography of human ageing. *Nature, 464*(7288), 536–542.

CHAPTER 11

Theories of Emotional Well-Being and Aging

Susan T. Charles and Joanna Hong

Psychological science is grounded in empiricism, with the understood goal of gathering objective data on which to base our conclusions. Yet, we are not objective in our observations. Existing beliefs and assumptions shape our approach to science, influencing the questions we ask and the interpretation of our results. In so doing, we are bound to view our research topic not as unbiased agents, but instead as researchers directed, consciously or not, by current theory.

The study of emotion and aging is no exception, and findings are inherently viewed through the lens of current theory. A comparison between two studies published almost 50 years apart illustrates this point. The first investigation, with results published in the *Journal of Gerontology* in 1962, examined four types of emotional experience (feelings of boredom, irritation, anger, and being lonely) among people ranging in age from 50 to older than 80 years (Dean, 1962). Findings revealed that the frequencies of feeling irritated and angry decreased with each successively older age group. Boredom were similar across all age groups, as were feelings of loneliness with the exception of the oldest group, aged greater than 80 years. These oldest adults reported higher frequencies of loneliness relative to the younger groups. The results, summarized in an article titled "Aging and the Decline of Affect," supported the hypothesis that emotions would follow the same deteriorating pattern as visual and tactual acuity, with the eventual loss in the ability to experience them. The author further concluded that the findings were consistent with the then-popular disengagement theory, which described how people gradually and willingly withdraw from social interactions with others as they grow older.

Nearly 50 years later, another study examined a similar question (Stone, Schwartz, Broderick, & Deaton, 2010). People of different ages were asked about their reports of emotional experience. Similar to the study nearly 50 years prior, results revealed that the levels of reported anger declined with age. Other negative emotions, including stress and worry, were also reported less frequently among the oldest adults in the study. From these findings, the authors concluded that well-being increases with age, with older adults being happier and less stressed. They interpreted these findings as indicative of possible increase in wisdom and a greater ability of older adults to regulate their emotions compared to younger adults, consistent with current theories in life-span developmental psychology (Stone et al., 2010).

Both studies yielded nearly identical results. The interpretations, however, could not have been more different: one study showed evidence of decline and deterioration, and the other of increased well-being and greater regulation abilities. Admittedly, the more recent study also benefited from additional questions about happiness that were not included in the older study. Yet, the choice of emotions under investigation for each study was also guided by current theory. Given the focus on deterioration and decline

193

with aging, asking questions about happiness 50 years ago was probably not even a consideration.

The earlier example underscores the need to understand our current theories of emotion and aging that shape existing work. To place research into its proper perspective, we begin this chapter by outlining findings and theories generated in the early years of gerontology, when the formal study of emotions and aging had just begun. We then focus on the past 20 years of research, with an emphasis on current theories that are being tested in the field. We end by discussing how our current emphases are shaping present research programs, and we offer directions for future studies of how emotional experience and emotion regulation vary across the adult life span.

■ HISTORICAL CONTEXT

The first theories of emotion and aging began simply, following assumptions established in biological and cognitive aging research. Early in the 20th century, physiologists such as Pavlov studied aging in animal models, adding objective findings from their laboratories to bolster the adage that old dogs had difficulties learning tricks (see review by Birren, 1961). A popular term to describe life-span development in these early years was deterioration; researchers described visual, cognitive, and tactual deterioration with age. Within this context, abilities were thought to peak at age 28 or 30 years and slowly decline thereafter. In this view and based on their observations at the time, scientists maintained that older adults had emotional experiences similar to those of "neurotic individuals irrespective of aging," which were characterized with words such as negativism, apathy, anxiety, guilt feelings, depression, and self-pity (Banham, 1951, p. 175). In addition, findings showing decline in the frequency of affect—including decrease in anger and irritation—were evidence of deterioration in the ability to experience emotions (e.g., Dean, 1962). The reason for this decrease in emotional experience was largely explained by the disengagement theory. This theory described how older adults, nearing the end of life, begin to disengage from the world, emotionally distancing themselves from others in a symbolic preparation for death (Cumming & Henry, 1961; see historical review by Achenbaum & Bengtson, 1994).

Traditional View Questioned

The belief of ubiquitous deterioration had its critics even in these early years (see review by Achenbaum & Bengtson, 1994), yet the common assumption of aging and socioemotional decline remained largely unchecked until the late 1980s and early 1990s. At that time, researchers began to examine both the frequency and intensity of negative and positive emotional states, with results that refuted earlier assumptions (e.g., Lawton, Kleban, Rajagopal, & Dean, 1992; Malatesta & Kalnok, 1984). Findings indicated that age differences in emotional experience were characterized by "more similarities than dissimilarities" (Malatesta & Kalnok, 1984, p. 308). Emotions were sometimes reported less frequently among older than younger adults, but older adults reported similar levels of intensity when emotions were experienced. In addition, older age was not related to lower levels of positive emotional experiences. These early cross-sectional results were the beginning of a series of cross-sectional studies finding age-related decrease in negative emotions and similar and sometimes higher levels of positive emotions (Carstensen, Pasupathi, Mayr, & Nesselroade, 2000; Carstensen et al., 2011; Mroczek & Kolarz, 1998).

Furthermore, the majority of older adults were reporting high levels of affective well-being and highly satisfying interpersonal relationships (see review by Charles & Carstensen, 2010). Rates of anger and stress were lower than those of younger adults (as had been noted in early studies but replicated across the decades when comparing age differences in later-born cohorts as well), and sadness levels were similar across age groups (e.g., Dean, 1962; Stone et al., 2010). When asked about satisfaction with close friends and family members, reports increased over time in one longitudinal study (Carstensen, 1992). When asked about their ability to control their emotional experiences, older adults reported more success than did younger adults (Gross et al., 1997). Similarly, in studies in the 1990s examining coping strategies, older age was related to positive outcomes (Diehl, Coyle, & Labouvie-Vief, 1996). For example, a study examining reported coping strategies among adults ranging from 10 years to older than 70 years found that more efficacious strategies, such as seeing problems as life lessons (i.e., principalization) and downplaying the negative aspects of the situation (i.e., reversal), were highest among people in their 60s; likewise, the use of strategies including expressing aggression toward others (turning against object) or toward the self declined across all the age groups (Diehl et al., 1996). These studies, from laboratories predominantly in North America and Europe, found consistent support for similar if not higher rates of well-being among older adults compared to younger adults and positive trajectories of coping styles and reported emotional control.

Throughout the late 20th and early 21st centuries, longitudinal studies have emerged showing that negative affect decreases and overall positive experience is similar, if not sometimes higher, with age (Carstensen et al., 2011; Charles, Reynolds, & Gatz, 2001). Large cross-sectional studies have also observed this general pattern of age-related declines in levels of negative affect and similar, if not higher, levels of positive affect (Kunzmann, Little, & Smith, 2000; Mroczek & Kolarz, 1998; Stone et al., 2010). As a result, researchers coined the phrase the "paradox of aging" to describe the relatively high rates of emotional well-being despite age-related declines in other physical and cognitive processes.

■ ADAPTING AND RESPONDING TO LOSS

Even before research emerged showing similar and sometimes higher levels of well-being among older adults, scientists were already discussing how older adults could maintain high levels of well-being in later life. According to activity theory, older adults would maintain high levels of well-being if they continued to engage in the activities they had during middle age, and find substitute activities when maintenance was no longer possible (e.g., volunteering after retirement; Havighurst, 1951). Similarly, continuity theory posited that older adults who stayed active and engaged in activities that allowed them to maintain their previous activity level would maintain high levels of well-being (Atchley, 1989). The goal, then, was to adapt to aging in a way that made it possible to continue engaging in the same activities as one did in midlife.

Baltes and Baltes (1990) recognized the importance of staying active and engaged in late life, yet they also maintained that age-related losses would make the same lifestyle enjoyed in one's midlife impossible to sustain in later years. They formulated a meta-model called "selective optimization with compensation" (SOC) to describe how older adults maintain functioning despite age-related declines. The SOC model acknowledges the reduced reserve capacities that often accompany aging and that lead to fewer domains of functioning (Baltes & Baltes, 1990). To adapt successfully in response to an increasing number of losses, people need to select areas of functioning in their lives that are important for them to maintain and that are possible given environmental, biological, and personal considerations. Sometimes, this selection involves altering goals or selecting new domains in their lives. After selecting a domain, older adults then strive to work to maintain or enhance their reserves to maintain the quantity and quality of their chosen life work. Finally, when plasticity or adaptive potential prevents them from successfully achieving their goals, SOC posits that people will compensate by using psychological strategies or technological aids. For example, worse memory may be compensated by using more mnemonic aids, just as a cane can be used to help with gait instability (Baltes & Baltes, 1990).

The SOC serves as a general model of development, specifically for later life, which states how people maintain active, engaged lifestyles at the same time that they are faced with an increasing number of losses in their lives. The model was not specific to the domains selected or the resources necessary, but many researchers have examined the processes by which people adapt to losses in many areas of their lives to optimize functioning (see review by Ouwehand, de Ridder, & Bensing, 2007). Researchers have used SOC, for example, to describe how older adults who use selection, optimization, and compensatory behaviors report higher levels of positive emotions and lower levels of loneliness (Freund & Baltes, 1998) as well as other socioemotional experiences (Baltes & Carstensen, 1996; Urry & Gross, 2010).

■ LOSS AS GAIN: EXTENDING THE PARADOX OF AGING

The aforementioned models discuss adaptations by older adults in response to decreasing cognitive and physiological capacities (e.g., Baltes & Baltes, 1990). Other researchers have pointed to serendipitous benefits in light of these declining resources. They posit the "paradox of aging" is a concept that not only describes relatively high levels of well-being reported by older adults despite facing losses in their lives, but also describes the phenomenon whereby age-related losses are themselves associated with emotion-related gains.

Fewer Social Roles, Fewer Stressors

As a growing number of studies suggested, older adults did not seem to be emotionally disengaged from others, and they were not reporting lower-intensity emotional experiences (e.g., Lawton et al., 1992). Their lives, however, were undeniably different than those of younger adults, and psychologists began examining life circumstances to explain age-related differences in social and emotional well-being (Folkman, Lazarus, Pimley, & Novacek, 1987). For years, sociologists have studied the association between older age and loss in social roles, and psychologists discussed how these losses may threaten a person's self-esteem and identity (e.g., Havighurst, 1961). At the same time, freedom from these social roles could also release people from potentially unpleasant experiences. For example, researchers explained the relatively high emotional well-being among older adults as freedom from often-stressful work-related and child-rearing responsibilities (e.g., Lawton, 2001). In addition, older adults reported more leisure time than younger adults did, and their freedom to select their own activities also potentially explained the high levels of well-being reported by older adults (e.g., Ginn & Fast, 2006). Consistent with this view, research indicates that older adults experience fewer negative major life events as well as minor daily stressors compared to younger adults (e.g., Brose, Scheibe, & Schmiedek, 2013). Moreover, age differences in emotional well-being are often no longer present once researchers adjust for the number of daily stressors in people's lives (e.g., Brose et al., 2013; Charles et al., 2010).

Lower Cognitive Functioning, Less Processing

Other theories described how cognitive declines may be related to enhanced emotion regulation (Labouvie-Vief & Medler, 2002). For example, dynamic integration theory stated that emotion regulation and emotional reasoning are related to cognitive development (Labouvie-Vief, 2003; Labouvie-Vief & Medler, 2002). According to this theory, the ability to understand complex information increases throughout adolescence and into adulthood. As a result, adults are able to evaluate complicated emotional information better and analyze both positive and negative aspects of the situation to integrate differing and often seemingly contradictory aspects of the situation. As people age and their cognitive abilities decline, however, their ability to evaluate cognitively complex information decreases. According to this theory, older adults will thus focus away from negative information, which is often more complex than positive information, and engage in more positive and simplified views of their world.

Physiological Decline as an Advantage

Still other theories focused on the serendipitous benefits of physiological decline. For years, researchers had studied how age-related declines in physiological regulation influence emotional functioning (e.g., Cannon, 1942). These declines had been well documented; yet newer hypotheses portrayed these declines as benefiting emotion regulation (e.g., Cacioppo, Berntson, Bechara, Tranel, & Hawkley, 2011). These arguments maintained that reductions in physiological arousal result in lower arousal levels that are easier to regulate (Cacioppo, Berntson, Klein, & Poehlmann, 1997; Levenson, 2000).

This stance has expanded to include age-related declines in brain structure and functioning (Cacioppo et al., 2011). The amygdalar aging hypothesis, for example, posits that age-related declines in the amygdala are responsible for age-related reductions in negative emotional experiences. This theory states that even though the amygdala is responsive to both negative and positive information, declines in the structure will have greater influence on negative reactivity than positive reactivity. Other researchers disagree with this stance, but maintain that declines in physiological functioning may motivate older adults to use different types of emotion regulation strategies, and these compensatory strategies may be even more effective for maintaining affective well-being (Urry & Gross, 2010).

■ MOVING AWAY FROM LOSS: SOCIOEMOTIONAL SELECTIVITY THEORY

According to the aforementioned models, age-related declines explain age-related gains in happiness and well-being. Bad news, then, is seen as good news for both cognitive and physical functioning. Before the advent of Carstensen's socioemotional selectivity theory (SST), few researchers focused on areas of gain that may enhance emotion regulation abilities with age. SST is a life-span theory positing that people's motivations are governed largely by the time they perceive is left in their lives (Carstensen, 2006). According to the theory, this temporal perspective shifts the relative importance of two primary motivational goals that govern much of human behavior: those focused on emotional meaningfulness and emotional experience, and those focused on knowledge and information gain (Carstensen, 1995; Carstensen, Isaacowitz, & Charles, 1999).

When people are young, they perceive time left in the life span as seemingly endless, which leads them to prioritize information-related goals even at the risk of potential emotional costs. In other words, to prepare for the expansive and long future, young adults pursue knowledge-acquisition goals despite potential emotional distress. As people grow older, however, their temporal horizon narrows. Recognizing that time left to live is decreasing, older adults prioritize emotion-related goals, which results in behaviors that include engaging in meaningful social interactions and placing greater importance on emotional experience and affective well-being (Carstensen et al., 1999; Carstensen, 2006).

SST, then, explains why older adults prioritize more positively valenced stimuli, and why they are more selective in choosing social environments that afford the greatest emotional reward than younger adults. For example, past research has found that older adults decrease the frequency of their interactions with peripheral relationships while maintaining or increasing the frequency of contact with those whom they are closest to, such as spouses or children (Carstensen, 1992). Although the size of their social network decreases, older adults report high levels of emotional closeness, satisfaction, and intimacy with their close interpersonal relationships (see review by Charles & Carstensen, 2010).

Positivity Effect

SST posits that the greater emphasis on emotionally salient goals leads to a greater focus on, attention to, and memory for positive over negative information (see review by Carstensen & Mikels, 2005; Carstensen, Mikels, & Mather, 2006). This phenomenon, termed the "positivity effect," refers to older adults preferring, attending to, and remembering relatively more positive or less negative stimuli compared to their younger counterparts (Carstensen & Mikels, 2005). For example, when older adults are shown images of positive, negative, and neutral stimuli followed by a distraction task, they recall an increased amount of positive information than negative information (Charles, Mather & Carstensen, 2003). Using eye gaze to examine attention to positive information, researchers find that older adults have a greater attentional bias to positive faces in comparison to neutral and negative faces (e.g., Isaacowitz, Wadlinger, Goren, & Wilson, 2006; Mather & Carstensen, 2003). Positivity effect is also evident in older adults' autobiographical memory. When asked to recall negative and positive memories from the past, older adults indicate higher levels of positive emotions in comparison to negative emotions (Mather & Carstensen, 2005). This finding has been replicated a number of times, with results indicating more pronounced effects in situations where older adults are able to view information without specific instructions or expectations placed on them (Reed, Chan, & Mikels, 2014).

The Importance of Cognitive Control

The cognitive control hypothesis grew from studies examining how cognitive functioning influences the positivity effect (Mather, 2006). This hypothesis states that older adults with the highest cognitive functioning show the greatest bias toward positive stimuli and the best emotion regulation strategies. In a series of studies, Mather and Knight (2005) examined the role of cognitive control in the positivity effect. First, they found that older adults with high executive performance displayed the positivity effect when recalling emotional stimuli. Older adults with lower executive functioning failed to show the positivity effect, instead remembering a greater proportion of negative images. In another study, they manipulated cognitive control by having younger and older adults view positive, negative, and neutral images either in a divided-attention paradigm (where cognitive control would be compromised), or in a control condition without any additional distractions. They found that older adults in the divided-attention task did not display the positivity effect, but older adults in the control condition again replicated other studies showing that older age is related to better memory for positive relative to neutral images (Mather & Knight, 2005).

Other studies revealed that processing emotional information may be less cognitively demanding for older adults relative to younger adults. One study, for example, had older and younger adults downregulate unpleasant emotional experience while they completed a difficult cognitive task (Scheibe & Blanchard-Fields, 2009). Findings indicate that the older adults' performance on the cognitive task was less affected by the emotion regulation task than that of the younger adults. Another study found that older and younger adults showed similar performance for a working memory task comprising emotional stimuli; for nonemotional stimuli, however, older adults showed the normative age-related decrement in performance (Mikels, Larkin, Reuter-Lorenz, & Carstensen, 2005).

■ INTEGRATING THE STRENGTHS AND VULNERABILITIES OF AGING

SST inspired many developmental studies examining thoughts and behaviors that promote positive emotional functioning (see review by Charles & Carstensen, 2010). Older adults were focusing, appraising, and remembering events both from their own lives and those experienced in laboratory studies as more positive, less negative, or both, compared to their younger counterparts. At the same time, researchers were faced with conflicting findings regarding linear increases in well-being with age. First, studies were now moving beyond the focus on average sample means and starting to document the variability in trajectories of well-being across time for positive and negative affect (Griffin, Mroczek, & Spiro, 2006). These findings set the stage for examining how different health-related and psychosocial factors influenced affective experience over time (e.g., Cho et al., 2013). Results showed that the phenomenon of terminal drop—declines in functioning during the 3- to 5-year period before death—also applied to well-being (e.g., Gerstorf, Ram, Röcke, Lindenberger, & Smith, 2008; Gerstorf, Ram, Estabrook, et al., 2008). In addition, researchers examining performance of thoughts and behaviors related to emotion regulation found mixed support for age-related superiority. For example, older and younger adults were equally adept at emotion regulation strategies such as inhibiting or amplifying their facial expressions in response to negative stimuli (e.g., Kunzmann, Kupperbusch, & Levenson, 2005). However, when recognizing emotional facial expressions, older adults often performed worse than younger adults (e.g., Sullivan, Ruffman, & Hutton, 2007).

The Theoretical Model of Strength and Vulnerability Integration

The theoretical model of strength and vulnerability integration (SAVI) was formulated to address these discrepant findings (Charles, 2010; Charles & Piazza, 2009). SAVI recognizes both strengths and vulnerabilities related to age, and posits that by understanding an individual's current circumstances, researchers can integrate information about these strengths and vulnerabilities to make specific predictions about emotion regulation and emotional well-being across the adult life span.

The Strengths of Aging

SAVI posits that the strengths of aging are defined as older adults employing thoughts and behaviors that allow them to avoid or at least reduce their exposure to negative experiences that elicit high levels of emotional distress more often than younger adults. For example, interpersonal tensions are the most common and most upsetting stressor that people experience on a day-to-day basis (Almeida, 2005). Yet, older adults report fewer interpersonal stressors and often even higher levels of satisfaction and happiness with family and close friends than younger adults (Charles & Piazza, 2007; see review by Luong, Charles, & Fingerman, 2010). When older adults cannot avoid tense social situations, they opt to avoid conflict more often than younger adults (e.g., Sorkin & Rook, 2006). When presented with pictures of different emotional valence, older adults will shift their attention to the more positive, or least negative, image to a greater extent than younger adults (e.g., Isaacowitz, Toner, Goren, & Wilson, 2008). When they must focus on negative experiences, older adults are more likely to appraise negative situations as less distressing (e.g., Charles & Carstensen, 2008), and to report less negative emotions in response to unpleasant events than younger adults (Luong & Charles, 2014).

The reason for these strengths lies in changes in perspective with age, a perspective shaped strongly by time left to live as well as time lived. SAVI incorporates SST to explain why older adults have greater strengths in employing emotion regulation strategies compared to younger adults. As described earlier, SST posits that time left to live shifts motivational goals so that older adults increasingly prioritize emotionally meaningful experiences, and maintain high levels of emotional well-being. Many studies illustrating the use of emotion regulation skills by older adults (such as attentional deployment and less negative cognitive appraisals) were based on predictions by SST (see review by Charles & Carstensen, 2010). In addition, SAVI also recognizes the importance of time lived, which provides people with life experiences and self-knowledge that inform emotional well-being (e.g., Blanchard-Fields, 2007). This self-knowledge may also include greater awareness of limitations as well, and avoiding situations eliciting high levels of arousal are particularly beneficial in the face of age-related declines in physiological functioning.

The Vulnerabilities of Aging

SAVI posits that the higher levels of emotional well-being reported by older adults are primarily the result of avoiding the experience of highly distressing events. When they fail to avoid negative distress and experience high levels of physiological arousal, SAVI posits that older adults have less capability to downregulate these experiences than younger adults.

Researchers have focused on age differences in cardiovascular reactivity, given the importance of cardiovascular response for emotional arousal (Cacioppo et al., 1997). Although much heterogeneity exists in the rate and extent of age-related declines, researchers have found that older age is related to stiffer or less flexible vasculature. As indicated by increase in blood pressure levels, capability of the vascular to adjust to perturbations of the system decreases with age (Kaess et al., 2012). In addition, age-related neurological changes lead to reductions in heart-rate variability (Voss et al., 2013). Both these processes result in greater blood pressure reactivity in response to stressors with age (see review by Uchino, Birmingham, & Berg, 2010).

In addition to cardiovascular reactivity, researchers have also studied age-related differences in adrenal functioning in response to stressors (e.g., Selye, 1962). The glucocorticoid hypothesis was formulated to explain why many studies using nonhuman samples showed that age was related to higher levels of cortisol (Sapolsky, Krey & McEwen, 1986). This hypothesis focused on the hypothalamic–pituitary–adrenal (HPA) axis, a term for the pathway activated when someone perceives a threat to his or her well-being. According to the hypothesis, older age is related to a decreasing ability to down-regulate the HPA axis, resulting in delayed recovery from an emotion-eliciting event and resulting higher levels of cortisol.

Despite being a popular model, little evidence suggests that aging is related to delays in cortisol recovery after a stressor among humans. One study supporting this age-related hypothesis found that high levels of trait-like negative affect were unrelated to cortisol levels for people ranging from their mid-30s to early 50s (Piazza, Charles, Stawski, & Almeida, 2013). For people ranging from 50s to mid-80s, however, those with high levels of trait-like negative affect had much higher levels of daily (i.e., area under the curve) levels of cortisol than their less negative counterparts. This same study also found that among people low in negative affect, only older adults had evening cortisol levels that were elevated on days when stressors occurred; people in their mid-50s and younger had cortisol levels that were unrelated to daily stressors (Piazza et al., 2013). The authors interpret these findings as indicating that sustained, high levels of negative affect are related to higher levels of cortisol for older adults, but not their relatively younger counterparts (i.e., those in their mid-50s and younger). Laboratory studies examining age differences in cortisol reactivity to and recovery from a stressor are less consistent, with some finding greater reactivity to a stressor with age (Agrigoroaei et al., 2013) and others finding no difference with age (see review by Kudielka, Hellhammer, & Wüst, 2009). These findings point to levels of sustained, as opposed to acute, emotional distress having worse effects on cortisol levels for older adults—consistent with SAVI—but further studies will have to replicate and further substantiate this claim.

SAVI's tenet that sustained levels of emotional distress are more caustic for older adults with more vulnerable physiological systems is also consistent with findings from a study that examined the association among age, trait-like levels of anger, and metabolic syndrome (Boylan & Ryff, 2013). The metabolic syndrome refers to a constellation of conditions including high blood pressure, high glucose levels, and excess fat around the abdomen and waist that predispose people to life-threatening illnesses such as stroke, diabetes, and cardiovascular disease. Among people who reported experiencing high chronic levels of anger, only those ranging in age from their mid-50s and older had a higher likelihood of having metabolic syndrome compared to their same-aged, less-angry peers (Boylan & Ryff, 2013).

Understanding Context to Integrate Strengths and Weaknesses

SAVI posits that when people are in a position where they can avoid negative situations, or attenuate their exposure to caustic events, they will report higher levels of well-being compared to younger adults (e.g., Charles, Piazza, Luong, & Almeida, 2009).

However, when they cannot avoid situations that elicit distress and accompany physiological arousal, age differences will attenuate if not disappear completely. Consistent with SAVI, older adults often report fewer stressors and daily hassles than younger adults do (e.g., Aldwin, Jeong, Igarashi, & Spiro, 2014; Stawski, Sliwinski, Almeida, & Smyth, 2008). However, when they do experience stressors, they sometimes report even greater reactivity than younger adults (Aldwin et al., 2014; Sliwinski, Almeida, Smyth, & Stawski, 2009).

What, then, determines whether older adults are in a position to avoid a distressing event? Current circumstances—external and internal to the individual—influence the extent to which people are able to avoid or mitigate exposure to negative life events. In negative situations characterized by uncontrollability, older adults cannot plan ahead and select out of the situation. They cannot avoid or appraise away the situation, and they cannot escape so they can later remember the situation more fondly. When they are faced with these situations, SAVI predicts that strengths of aging will be difficult if not impossible to employ, and emotional well-being will suffer as a result. For example, the death of someone who provided a sense of belonging and meaning to life is not a situation that can be avoided by superior emotion regulation strategies. Other situations characterized by a high degree of uncontrollability include caregiving for a spouse with dementia; living with a debilitating disease with a declining yet unpredictable course trajectory; or living with an uncertain financial future with limited job prospects. For example, a recent study found that the paradox of older age associated with high levels of emotional well-being did not apply to countries with lower national wealth (i.e., gross domestic product [GDP]; Swift et al., 2014). In these studies, the association between GDP and well-being was even stronger for older adults relative to younger adults.

Other uncontrollable internal factors can also serve to either enhance or exacerbate the strengths and vulnerabilities of aging. For example, one effective emotion regulation strategy is knowing what situations may be unpleasant, and avoiding them. When people experience cognitive decline, they will have more difficulty in evaluating their current situations and deciding among potential alternative actions. Cognitive performance is also related to attention and appraisal performance, with lower-performing older adults no longer displaying the positivity effects exhibited by their higher-functioning peers (Knight et al., 2007; Mather & Knight, 2005).

Another, more subtle, factor that can affect strengths and weaknesses of emotion regulation is the personality trait neuroticism. Neuroticism was originally conceptualized as a measure of autonomic reactivity, such that high levels of neuroticism represented a more sensitive, reactive neural system that was prone to disruption and instability (Eysenck, 1947). Consistent with this early view, researchers have documented that people with higher levels of neuroticism report greater numbers of negative and uncontrollable major negative life events and daily stressors, and are more reactive to these stressors (e.g., Suls & Martin, 2005). Higher levels of neuroticism, then, are related to greater difficulty in avoiding negative arousal. SAVI posits that experiencing this arousal becomes more costly to well-being with age. Consistent with this prediction, older adults high in neuroticism do not experience lower levels of negative affect with age (Charles, Reynolds, & Gatz, 2001), and they are more—not less—reactive to daily stressors compared to their younger, equally neurotic peers (Mroczek & Almeida, 2004).

Of course, life circumstances can also work in the opposite direction, enhancing emotion regulation efficacy among older adults. For example, better physical conditioning enhances the ability to respond to distressing situations. In one study, men who underwent exercise training showed significant reductions in cardiovascular reactivity and cortisol reactivity to stressors (Klaperski, von Dawans, Heinrichs & Fuchs, 2014). As such, factors that reduce age-related declines in physiological functioning may attenuate these vulnerabilities when modulating high levels of emotional arousal.

Standing on the Shoulders of Giants

SAVI is a new theoretical model in the literature that makes explicit hypotheses about age differences in different contexts. Yet, no single aspect of SAVI is unique on its own. The thoughts and behaviors described as the strengths of aging have been documented by a growing number of studies discussing enhanced emotion regulation strategies among older adults (see review by Charles & Carstensen, 2010). The vast majority of these studies were motivated by SST, a theory that SAVI incorporates to explain these strengths. In addition, the importance of experience gained from time lived is not new for life-span researchers (Blanchard-Fields, 2007; Magai, Consedine, Krivoshekova, Kudadjie-Gyamfi, & McPherson, 2006), nor is the idea that older adults have self-knowledge about their own limitations (Baltes & Baltes, 1990).

The vulnerabilities of aging are also not novel. Greater dysregulation in physiological processes with age were discussed by early pioneers in psychology, such as Cannon (1942), a man who coined the term "homeostasis" and developed one of the first theories explaining emotional functioning (Cannon–Bard theory). As described earlier, SOC discusses the balance between optimizing areas that are maintained or enhanced (strengths) of aging to compensate for the increasing losses, or vulnerabilities, that characterize the aging process.

Finally, SAVI discusses the need to understand the circumstances of life to place the strengths and vulnerabilities within their proper context. Without knowledge of these factors, both internal and external to the individual, researchers will be unable to predict whether older adults are able to use their strengths and avoid high arousal situations. Gerontologists, however, have long recognized circumstances that cause high levels of distress such as bereavement and loneliness; caregiving; and living with the chronic stress or unremitting, uncontrollable pain.

The novelty in SAVI lies in the integration of current circumstances, strengths, and vulnerabilities to make predictions. We cannot focus on strengths without recognizing vulnerabilities. We cannot predict how older adults will select and engage in emotion regulation strategies without an awareness of current circumstances. By this integration, we can make specific predictions. For example, SAVI predicts that age differences will be greatest (i.e., more beneficial for older adults) before and after the negative event is experienced. However, at the time when people experience stressors, SAVI predicts that current circumstances will play a strong role to attenuate age differences, such that they may disappear altogether. Similarly, SAVI posits that age differences will be greatest for questions asking about general levels of well-being, where people rely on appraisal and beliefs about their emotions, as opposed to those asking about emotions over a shorter period of time, when people can use situational cues on which to base their judgments. Indeed, age differences in emotional experience grow stronger across measures of emotions that use increasingly longer time intervals (i.e., comparing daily to monthly reports of well-being; Charles et al., 2015).

■ MOVING THE FIELD FORWARD

Statistical models are becoming more complex, capturing the vast heterogeneity in our data. The multifactorial influences on any predicted outcome point to the fact that, "no one size fits all." It is tempting to sum up any finding by stating that "heterogeneity exists with age, showing that patterns of [insert psychosocial variable of interest here] are complex." We know that human behaviors are complex; since the introduction of the Gaussian curve, we recognize that not everyone falls along the mean of any phenomenon under investigation. We also, however, need to generate findings to help us understand and predict average tendencies for future behaviors. We cannot do so without an understanding of the larger picture; we cannot do so if our findings lack patterns of relationships from which to build our future theory. Theory influences the questions people ask, the methods they select, and the interpretations of their results. SAVI emphasizes both age-related strengths and weaknesses, with a new emphasis on understanding current circumstances to determine the extent to which age-related strengths and weaknesses shape emotion regulation and emotional well-being across the life span.

Attention to Context

Instead of highlighting people who are successfully aging, SAVI provides a theory that will stimulate research identifying the context, or situations, for successful aging. For years, researchers have focused on studying emotional distress among at-risk older adults living in difficult circumstances, such as spousal caregiving or bereaved individuals. More recently, however, researchers have focused on the daily lives of older adults, understanding the environmental context for their emotional experiences (Smith, Ryan, Queen, Becker, & Gonzalez, 2014; Wrzus, Müller, Wagner, Lindenberger, & Riediger, 2013). This important work will enable us to examine the situations where people engage in emotion regulation strategies successfully, and those situations that make regulating emotions difficult for older adults. For example, this new work is showing that in situations in which older adults can minimize their exposure to a negative situation, they report less emotional distress than younger adults (Birditt, 2014). However, when they cannot avoid this exposure and encounter distressing situations, they experience similar, if not higher, levels of negative affect than their younger counterparts (Birditt, 2014; Charles et al., 2009).

Determining the Regulation Strategies That Are Most Important

The study of emotion and aging has burgeoned in recent years, with researchers carefully distinguishing between different types of emotion regulation strategies (e.g., reappraisal vs. facial suppression) and assessing various aspects of emotional well-being (e.g., mean levels, and variability in emotional experience). However, the underlying question to all of this research would be: What thoughts and behaviors regarding emotional experiences are important for regulation in daily life and what aspects of emotional experience itself are most important for the older adult, given differences in social roles and differences in life context?

Even the terms we use may be slightly problematic when studying emotion regulation. For example, we discuss emotion regulation strategies in response to an emotion-eliciting event. The term strategy implies marshalling resources or plans of action. In using this term, are we implying that people are consciously choosing a course of action? When people reported doing nothing, we still refer to this as a strategy (sometimes referred to as "passive emotion regulation"). In a sample of men ranging from

48- to 91-years old, older age was related to endorsing fewer reactions to problems in general (Aldwin, Sutton, Chiara, & Spiro, 1996). The oldest men in this study reported using fewer coping strategies and expending less effort when using these coping strategies than younger adults, yet with similar levels of success in these situations. This research is also consistent with findings showing that older adults generate fewer coping strategies when asked how to respond to hypothetical problems relative to younger adults (Thornton, Paterson, & Yeung, 2013) and more often reported doing nothing in response to negative social interactions (Charles, Carstensen, & McFall, 2001). They not only endorsed this strategy for themselves, but also recommended this strategy to others who find themselves in the same situation (Charles et al., 2001). As a result, the most important aspect of emotion regulation for older adults is the most minimalist, least effortful tactic of all—nothing. The question, then, would be: What environments provide successful outcomes for this behavior? Whereas some situations are suited for doing nothing—such as choosing not to argue with a friend or family member over a trivial point—other situations may have deleterious consequences. For example, ignoring a troubling physical symptom, or ignoring the disapprobation of a boss, may be unwise for multiple reasons, and short-term avoidance of mild to moderate distress may lead to long-term severe emotional distress. Older adults may be more adept at understanding when no action is best (Blanchard-Fields, Mienaltowski, & Seay, 2007), but more research is needed in this area.

The Feasibility of Real World to Laboratory Translation

If older adults do benefit from situations in which they can successfully avoid experiences of negative affect, then several challenges arise in the literature. First, bringing people to the lab, asking them to participate in an emotion regulation strategy, and then waiting to see if they do nothing is problematic practically and statistically. In practical considerations, older adults are aware that you are interested in studying their responses. Even if social desirability played no role, which is doubtful (e.g., Soubelet & Salthouse, 2011), designing a study where emotion regulation was assessed by people refusing to comply or leaving the situation would be difficult.

Studying age differences when people are instructed to engage in different emotion regulation strategies in response to negative events may be helpful to evaluate basic differences between these processes. However, a critical question for this research would be: How often do people of these different age groups engage in each of these emotion regulation strategies in their daily lives? If they rarely use these strategies in daily life, then understanding age differences is less helpful. Finally, research testing the positivity effect has found that age differences favoring older adults were stronger in paradigms where people were given no explicit instructions when viewing the emotional stimuli. The goal in moving the field forward, then, is to understand what older adults are doing when left to their own devices. Understanding how these strategies are specific to the circumstances of their daily lives, such as the types of social partners with whom they interact, the cognitive demands on the situation, and the time pressure they are experiencing, only enhances the complexity of the study. Yet, we need to understand emotion regulation as it appears in the daily lives of older adults if we have goals to translate research into policy recommendations. Often, laboratory studies focus on the number of strategies generated (e.g., Thornton et al., 2013) or instructing people to engage in specific emotion regulation strategies (e.g., Shiota & Levenson, 2009). We need to carefully evaluate how these types of strategies correspond with their current circumstances.

Refine Theory

Criticism is easy. Building theory and understanding how new research fits into existing models, changes aspects of certain models, or redefines them completely are difficult. Yet, existing theory would benefit from people not only testing their boundary conditions, but also offering refinements when new evidence is available. For example, studies have found that perceiving time as diminishing leads to increased priority to emotional goals (see review by Charles & Carstensen, 2010). At the same time, studies of terminal decline document decline in emotional well-being when people are close to death (Gerstorf, Ram, Röcke, Lindenberger, & Smith, 2008). These seemingly conflicting findings may be reconciled if people agree on a definition of time perception. In addition, SAVI predicts that physiological vulnerability associated with age is problematic when people need to modulate physiological arousal generated by emotional events. Yet, understanding what age-related changes are problematic and how these changes relate (or not) to subjective experience are fairly unexplored questions. Finally, refinements to existing theory can help to place new findings into the broader literature. Moreover, if our current theories do not hold up to scrutiny, they must be discarded and replaced by a newer paradigm to explain age differences in emotional experience.

■ SUMMARY AND CONCLUSION

Theories on emotion and aging have varied, with some focused on deterioration and decline, and others on gains. More recently, researchers have acknowledged age-related losses and gains for emotional experience. SAVI offers a model that examines how current circumstances influence the gains (or strengths) and losses (or vulnerabilities) on the emotional well-being of older adults. SAVI is a complex model, taking into account individual differences in external and internal factors that shape the current environment where emotion regulation takes place. Researchers need to refine and understand all aspects of age-related strengths, the vulnerabilities, and the circumstances that determine how they are used to predict well-being. We must do so by studying the context of life for older adults and the emotion regulation strategies used most often (and with more success) in their daily lives. No theory belongs to a specific person or lab, but to the scientific community at large. We must take our theories and constantly question, constantly refine, and eventually move forward in our understanding of how emotional experience varies by age so that we can use this knowledge to enhance the lives of the growing number of older adults in our society.

REFERENCES

Achenbaum, W. A., & Bengtson, V. L. (1994). Re-engaging the disengagement theory of aging: On the history and assessment of theory development in gerontology. *The Gerontologist, 34*(6), 756–763.

Agrigoroaei, S., Polito, M., Lee, A., Kranz-Graham, E., Seeman, T., & Lachman, M. E. (2013). Cortisol response to challenge involving low controllability: The role of control beliefs and age. *Biological Psychology, 93*(1), 138–142.

Aldwin, C. M., Jeong, Y. J., Igarashi, H., & Spiro, A. (2014). Do hassles and uplifts change with age? Longitudinal findings from the VA Normative Aging Study. *Psychology and Aging, 29*(1), 57–71.

Aldwin, C. M., Sutton, K. J., Chiara, G., & Spiro, A. (1996). Age differences in stress, coping, and appraisal: Findings from the Normative Aging Study. *The Journals of Gerontology, Series B, 51*(4), P179–P188.

Almeida, D. M. (2005). Resilience and vulnerability to daily stressors assessed via diary methods. *Current Directions in Psychological Science, 14,* 64–68.

Atchley, R. C. (1989). A continuity theory of normal aging. *The Gerontologist, 29*(2), 183–190.

Baltes, M. M., & Carstensen, L. L. (1996). The process of successful ageing. *Ageing & Society, 16,* 397–422.

Baltes, P. B., & Baltes, M. M. (1990). Psychological perspectives on successful aging: The model of selective optimization with compensation. In P. B. Baltes & M. M. Baltes (Eds.), *Successful aging: Perspectives from the behavioral sciences* (pp. 1–34). New York, NY: Cambridge University Press.

Banham, K. M. (1951). Senescence and the emotions: A genetic theory. *The Journal of Genetic Psychology, 78*(2), 175–183.

Birditt, K. S. (2014). Age differences in emotional reactions to daily negative social encounters. *The Journals of Gerontology, Series B, 69*(4), 557–566.

Birren, F. (1961). *Color psychology and color therapy.* New York, NY: University Books.

Blanchard-Fields, F. (2007). Everyday problem solving and emotion: An adult developmental perspective. *Current Directions in Psychological Science, 16,* 26–31.

Blanchard-Fields, F., Mienaltowski, A., & Seay, R. B. (2007). Age differences in everyday problem-solving effectiveness: Older adults select more effective strategies for interpersonal problems. *The Journals of Gerontology, Series B, 62*(1), P61–P64.

Boylan, J. M., & Ryff, C. D. (2013). Varieties of anger and the inverse link between education and inflammation: Toward an integrative framework. *Psychosomatic Medicine, 75*(6), 566–574.

Brose, A., Scheibe, S., & Schmiedek, F. (2013). Life contexts make a difference: Emotional stability in younger and older adults. *Psychology and Aging, 28*(1), 148–159.

Cacioppo, J. T., Berntson, G. G., Bechara, A., Tranel, D., & Hawkley, L. C. (2011). Could an aging brain contribute to subjective well being? The value added by a social neuroscience perspective. In A. Todorov, S. T. Fiske, & D. Prentice (Eds.), *Social neuroscience: Toward understanding the underpinnings of the social mind.* New York, NY: Oxford University Press.

Cacioppo, J. T., Berntson, G. G., Klein, D. J., & Poehlmann, K. M. (1997). Psychophysiology of emotion across the life span. *Annual Review of Gerontology and Geriatrics, 17,* 27–74.

Cannon, W. B. (1942). *Problems of aging.* Baltimore, MD: Lippincott Williams & Wilkins.

Carstensen, L. L. (1992). Social and emotional patterns in adulthood: Support for socioemotional selectivity theory. *Psychology and Aging, 7*(3), 331–338.

Carstensen, L. L. (1995). Evidence for a life-span theory of socioemotional selectivity. *Current Directions in Psychological Science, 4,* 151–156.

Carstensen, L. L. (2006). The influence of a sense of time on human development. *Science, 312*(5782), 1913–1915.

Carstensen, L. L., Isaacowitz, D. M., & Charles, S. T. (1999). Taking time seriously. A theory of socioemotional selectivity. *The American Psychologist, 54*(3), 165–181.

Carstensen, L. L., & Mikels, J. A. (2005). At the intersection of emotion and cognition: Aging and the positivity effect. *Current Directions in Psychological Science, 14*, 117–121.

Carstensen, L. L., Mikels, J. A., & Mather, M. (2006). Aging and intersection of cognition, motivation and emotion. In J. E. Birren & K. Warner Schaie (Eds.), *Handbook of the psychology of aging* (pp. 343–362). Burlington, MA: Elsevier.

Carstensen, L. L., Pasupathi, M., Mayr, U., & Nesselroade, J. R. (2000). Emotional experience in everyday life across the adult life span. *Journal of Personality and Social Psychology, 79*(4), 644–655.

Carstensen, L. L., Turan, B., Scheibe, S., Ram, N., Ersner-Hershfield, H., Samanez-Larkin, G. R.,...Nesselroade, J. R. (2011). Emotional experience improves with age: Evidence based on over 10 years of experience sampling. *Psychology and Aging, 26*(1), 21–33.

Charles, S. T. (2010). Strength and vulnerability integration: A model of emotional well-being across adulthood. *Psychological Bulletin, 136*(6), 1068–1091.

Charles, S. T., & Carstensen, L. L. (2008). Unpleasant situations elicit different emotional responses in younger and older adults. *Psychology and Aging, 23*(3), 495–504.

Charles, S. T., & Carstensen, L. L. (2010). Social and emotional aging. *Annual Review of Psychology, 61*, 383–409.

Charles, S. T., Carstensen, L. L., & McFall, R. M. (2001). Problem-solving in the nursing home environment: Age and experience differences in emotional reactions and responses. *Journal of Clinical Geropsychology, 7*, 319–330.

Charles, S. T., Luong, G., Almeida, D. M., Ryff, C., Sturm, M., & Love, G. (2010). Fewer ups and downs: Daily stressors mediate age differences in negative affect. *The Journals of Gerontology, Series B, 65*(3), 279–286.

Charles, S. T., Mather, M., & Carstensen, L. L. (2003). Focusing on the positive: Age differences in memory for positive, negative, and neutral stimuli. *Journal of Experimental Psychology, 85*, 163–178.

Charles, S. T., & Piazza, J. R. (2007). Memories of social interactions: Age differences in emotional intensity. *Psychology and Aging, 22*(2), 300–309.

Charles, S. T., & Piazza, J. R. (2009). Age differences in affective well being: Context matters. *Social and Personality Psychology Compass, 3*, 711–724.

Charles, S. T., Piazza, J. R., Luong, G., & Almeida, D. M. (2009). Now you see it, now you don't: Age differences in affective reactivity to social tensions. *Psychology and Aging, 24*(3), 645–653.

Charles, S. T., Piazza, J. R., Mogle, J. A., Urban, E. J., Sliwinski, M. J., & Almeida, D. M. (2015). Age differences in emotional well-being vary by temporal recall. *The Journals of Gerontology, Series B*, gbv011.

Charles, S. T., Reynolds, C. A., & Gatz, M. (2001). Age-related differences and change in positive and negative affect over 23 years. *Journal of Personality and Social Psychology, 80*(1), 136–151.

Cho, J., Martin, P., Poon, L. W., MacDonald, M., Jazwinski, S. M., Green, R. C.,…Davey, A.; Georgia Centenarian Study. (2013). Age group differences in positive and negative affect among oldest-old adults: Findings from the Georgia Centenarian Study. *International Journal of Aging & Human Development, 77*(4), 261–288.

Cumming, E., & Henry, W. E. (1961). *Growing old, the process of disengagement.* New York, NY: Basic Books.

Dean, L. R. (1962). Aging and the decline of affect. *Journal of Gerontology, 17,* 440–446.

Diehl, M., Coyle, N., & Labouvie-Vief, G. (1996). Age and sex differences in strategies of coping and defense across the life span. *Psychology and Aging, 11*(1), 127–139.

Eysenck, H. J. (1947). Screening-out the neurotic. *The Lancet, 1*(6451), 530.

Folkman, S., Lazarus, R. S., Pimley, S., & Novacek, J. (1987). Age differences in stress and coping processes. *Psychology and Aging, 2*(2), 171–184.

Freund, A. M., & Baltes, P. B. (1998). Selection, optimization, and compensation as strategies of life management: Correlations with subjective indicators of successful aging. *Psychology and Aging, 13,* 531–543.

Gerstorf, D., Ram, N., Estabrook, R., Schupp, J., Wagner, G. G., & Lindenberger, U. (2008). Life satisfaction shows terminal decline in old age: Longitudinal evidence from the German Socio-Economic Panel Study (SOEP). *Developmental Psychology, 44*(4), 1148–1159.

Gerstorf, D., Ram, N., Röcke, C., Lindenberger, U., & Smith, J. (2008). Decline in life satisfaction in old age: Longitudinal evidence for links to distance-to-death. *Psychology and Aging, 23*(1), 154–168.

Ginn, J., & Fast, J. (2006). Employment and social integration in midlife: Preferred and actual time use across welfare regime types. *Research on Aging, 28,* 669–690.

Griffin, P. W., Mroczek, D. K., & Spiro, A. III. (2006). Variability in affective change among aging men: Longitudinal findings from the VA Normative Aging Study. *Journal of Research in Personality, 40,* 942–965.

Gross, J. J., Carstensen, L. L., Pasupathi, M., Tsai, J., Skorpen, C. G., & Hsu, A. Y. (1997). Emotion and aging: Experience, expression, and control. *Psychology and Aging, 12*(4), 590–599.

Havighurst, R. J. (1951). *Developmental tasks and education.* New York, NY: Longmans, Green.

Havighurst, R. J. (1961). Successful aging. *The Gerontologist, 1,* 8–13.

Isaacowitz, D. M., Toner, K., Goren, D., & Wilson, H. R. (2008). Looking while unhappy: Mood-congruent gaze in young adults, positive gaze in older adults. *Psychological Science, 19*(9), 848–853.

Isaacowitz, D. M., Wadlinger, H. A., Goren, D., & Wilson, H. R. (2006). Is there an age-related positivity effect in visual attention? A comparison of two methodologies. *Emotion, 6*(3), 511–516.

Kaess, B. M., Rong, J., Larson, M. G., Hamburg, N. M., Vita, J. A., Levy, D., . . . Mitchell, G. F. (2012). Aortic stiffness, blood pressure progression, and incident hypertension. *Journal of the American Medical Association, 308*(9), 875–881.

Klaperski, S., von Dawans, B., Heinrichs, M., & Fuchs, R. (2014). Effects of a 12-week endurance training program on the physiological response to psychosocial stress in men: A randomized controlled trial. *Journal of Behavioral Medicine, 37*(6), 1118–1133.

Knight, M., Seymour, T. L., Gaunt, J. T., Baker, C., Nesmith, K., & Mather, M. (2007). Aging and goal-directed emotional attention: Distraction reverses emotional biases. *Emotion, 7*(4), 705–714.

Kudielka, B. M., Hellhammer, D. H., & Wüst, S. (2009). Why do we respond so differently? Reviewing determinants of human salivary cortisol responses to challenge. *Psychoneuroendocrinology, 34*(1), 2–18.

Kunzmann, U., Kupperbusch, C. S., & Levenson, R. W. (2005). Behavioral inhibition and amplification during emotional arousal: A comparison of two age groups. *Psychology and Aging, 20*(1), 144–158.

Kunzmann, U., Little, T. D., & Smith, J. (2000). Is age-related stability of subjective well-being a paradox? Cross-sectional and longitudinal evidence from the Berlin Aging Study. *Psychology and Aging, 15*(3), 511–526.

Labouvie-Vief, G. (2003). Dynamic integration: Affect, cognition, and the self in adulthood. *Current Directions in Psychological Science, 12,* 201–206.

Labouvie-Vief, G., & Medler, M. (2002). Affect optimization and affect complexity: Modes and styles of regulation in adulthood. *Psychology and Aging, 17*(4), 571–588.

Lawton, M. P. (2001). Emotion in later life. *Current Directions in Psychological Science, 10,* 120–124.

Lawton, M. P., Kleban, M. H., Rajagopal, D., & Dean, J. (1992). Dimensions of affective experience in three age groups. *Psychology and Aging, 7*(2), 171–184.

Levenson, R. W. (2000). Expressive, physiological, and subjective changes in emotion across adulthood. In S. H. Qualls & N. Abeles (Eds.), *Dialogues about aging: Psychology responds to the aging revolution* (pp. 123–140). Washington, DC: American Psychological Association.

Luong, G., & Charles, S. T. (2014). Age differences in affective and cardiovascular responses to a negative social interaction: The role of goals, appraisals, and emotion regulation. *Developmental Psychology, 50*(7), 1919–1930.

Luong, G., Charles, S. T., & Fingerman, K. L. (2010). Better with age: Social relationships across adulthood. *Journal of Social and Personal Relationship, 28,* 9–23.

Magai, C., Consedine, N. S., Krivoshekova, Y. S., Kudadjie-Gyamfi, E., & McPherson, R. (2006). Emotion experience and expression across the adult life span: Insights from a multimodal assessment study. *Psychology and Aging, 21*(2), 303–317.

Malatesta, C. Z., & Kalnok, M. (1984). Emotional experience in younger and older adults. *Journal of Gerontology, 39*(3), 301–308.

Mather, M. (2006). A review of decision-making processes: Weighing the risks and benefits of aging. In L. L. Carstensen & C. R. Hartel (Eds.), *When I'm 64* (pp. 145–173). Washington, DC: National Academies Press.

Mather, M., & Carstensen, L. L. (2003). Aging and attentional biases for emotional faces. *Psychological Science, 14*(5), 409–415.

Mather, M., & Carstensen, L. L. (2005). Aging and motivated cognition: The positivity effect in attention and memory. *Trends in Cognitive Sciences, 9*(10), 496–502.

Mather, M., & Knight, M. (2005). Goal-directed memory: The role of cognitive control in older adults' emotional memory. *Psychology and Aging, 20,* 554–570.

Mikels, J. A., Larkin, G. R., Reuter-Lorenz, P. A., & Carstensen, L. L. (2005). Divergent trajectories in the aging mind: Changes in working memory for affective versus visual information with age. *Psychology and Aging, 20*(4), 542–553.

Mroczek, D. K., & Almeida, D. M. (2004). The effect of daily stress, personality, and age on daily negative affect. *Journal of Personality, 72*(2), 355–378.

Mroczek, D. K., & Kolarz, C. M. (1998). The effect of age on positive and negative affect: A developmental perspective on happiness. *Journal of Personality and Social Psychology, 75*(5), 1333–1349.

Ouwehand, C., de Ridder, D. T., & Bensing, J. M. (2007). A review of successful aging models: Proposing proactive coping as an important additional strategy. *Clinical Psychology Review, 27*(8), 873–884.

Piazza, J. R., Charles, S. T., Stawski, R. S., & Almeida, D. M. (2013). Age and the association between negative affective states and diurnal cortisol. *Psychology and Aging, 28*(1), 47–56.

Reed, A. E., Chan, L., & Mikels, J. A. (2014). Meta-analysis of the age-related positivity effect: Age differences in preferences for positive over negative information. *Psychology and Aging, 29,* 1–15.

Sapolsky, R. M., Krey, L. C., & McEwen, B. S. (1986). The neuroendocrinology of stress and aging: The glucocorticoid cascade hypothesis. *Endocrine Reviews, 7*(3), 284–301.

Scheibe, S., & Blanchard-Fields, F. (2009). Effects of regulating emotions on cognitive performance: What is costly for young adults is not so costly for older adults. *Psychology and Aging, 24*(1), 217–223.

Selye, H. (1962). The dermatologic implications of stress and calciphylaxis. *The Journal of Investigative Dermatology, 39,* 259–275.

Shiota, M. N., & Levenson, R. W. (2009). Effects of aging on experimentally instructed detached reappraisal, positive reappraisal, and emotional behavior suppression. *Psychology and Aging, 24*(4), 890–900.

Sliwinski, M. J., Almeida, D. M., Smyth, J., & Stawski, R. S. (2009). Intraindividual change and variability in daily stress processes: Findings from two measurement-burst diary studies. *Psychology and Aging, 24*(4), 828–840.

Smith, J., Ryan, L. H., Queen, T. L., Becker, S., & Gonzalez, R. (2014). Snapshots of mixtures of affective experiences in a day: Findings from the health and retirement study. *Journal of Population Ageing, 7*(1), 55–79.

Sorkin, D. H., & Rook, K. S. (2006). Dealing with negative social exchanges in later life: Coping responses, goals, and effectiveness. *Psychology and Aging, 21*(4), 715–725.

Soubelet, A., & Salthouse, T. A. (2011). Influence of social desirability on age differences in self-reports of mood and personality. *Journal of Personality, 79*(4), 741–762.

Stawski, R. S., Sliwinski, M. J., Almeida, D. M., & Smyth, J. M. (2008). Reported exposure and emotional reactivity to daily stressors: The roles of adult age and global perceived stress. *Psychology and Aging, 23*(1), 52–61.

Stone, A. A., Schwartz, J. E., Broderick, J. E., & Deaton, A. (2010). A snapshot of the age distribution of psychological well-being in the United States. *Proceedings of the National Academy of Sciences of the United States of America, 107*(22), 9985–9990.

Sullivan, S., Ruffman, T., & Hutton, S. B. (2007). Age differences in emotion recognition skills and the visual scanning of emotion faces. *The Journals of Gerontology, Series B, 62*(1), P53–P60.

Suls, J., & Martin, R. (2005). The daily life of the garden-variety neurotic: Reactivity, stressor exposure, mood spillover, and maladaptive coping. *Journal of Personality, 73*(6), 1485–1509.

Swift, H. J., Vauclair, C. M., Abrams, D., Bratt, C., Marques, S., & Lima, M. L. (2014). Revisiting the paradox of well-being: The importance of national context. *The Journals of Gerontology, Series B, 69*(6), 920–929.

Thornton, W. L., Paterson, T. S., & Yeung, S. E. (2013). Age differences in everyday problem solving: The role of problem context. *International Journal of Behavioral Development, 37*, 13–20.

Uchino, B. N., Birmingham, W., & Berg, C. A. (2010). Are older adults less or more physiologically reactive? A meta-analysis of age-related differences in cardiovascular reactivity to laboratory tasks. *The Journals of Gerontology, Series B, 65*(2), 154–162.

Urry, H. L., & Gross, J. J. (2010). Emotion regulation in older age. *Current Directions in Psychological Science, 19*, 352–357.

Voss, A., Schroeder, R., Fischer, C., Heitmann, A., Peters, A., & Perz, S. (2013). Influence of age and gender on complexity measures for short term heart rate variability analysis in healthy subjects. *Conference Proceedings: Annual International Conference of the IEEE Engineering in Medicine and Biology Society, 2013*, 5574–5577.

Wrzus, C., Müller, V., Wagner, G. G., Lindenberger, U., & Riediger, M. (2013). Affective and cardiovascular responding to unpleasant events from adolescence to old age: Complexity of events matters. *Developmental Psychology, 49*(2), 384–397.

CHAPTER 12

Emotion–Cognition Links in Aging: Theories and Evidence

Nhi Ngo, Molly Sands, and Derek M. Isaacowitz

Throughout adulthood, individuals may experience changes in both cognitive and emotional processes. On the one hand, aging is associated primarily with declines in cognitive function; older adults experience more difficulty with executive function, working memory, and fluid cognitive processing (Craik & Salthouse, 2011). On the other hand, in the domain of emotion, some people actually seem to experience higher levels of affective well-being as they age. Older adults report less frequent experiences of negative emotions and relatively stable levels of positive affect (Charles, Reynolds, & Gatz, 2001). As people age, they also report more satisfying social relationships (Luong, Charles, & Fingerman, 2010), less variable moods (Carstensen et al., 2011), and preserved memory enhancement for emotional information (Kensinger, Allard, & Krendl, 2014). These seemingly contrary findings about the life-span trajectories of cognitive and emotional processes have raised interesting theoretical questions about the developmental trajectories of cognition and emotion across the life span. Is it the case that cognition and emotion have separate development pathways, or that age-related changes in one process lead to changes in the other?

As emotion and cognition are processes integrated in the brain, interacting to produce behaviors (Pessoa, 2008; Phelps, 2006), changes in emotion and cognition in late adulthood may not be independent of each other. In this chapter, we review and evaluate prominent theoretical models that link age-related changes in emotional processes with changes in cognition. These various approaches all highlight the importance of emotion–cognition interactions for explaining age-related changes in emotional experience; however, they diverge in their perspectives of what underlying factors may drive such changes. First, we review the socioemotional selectivity theory (SST; Carstensen, Isaacowitz, & Charles, 1999), which attributes better emotional outcomes with age to changes in motivation that result in cognition becoming more positively oriented. We also introduce neuroscientific perspectives and review how these perspectives interpret age-associated changes in the brain in terms of cognitive–emotional processing. Then we discuss the dynamic integration theory (DIT), which outlines how older adults may optimize emotional experience to compensate for reduced affective complexity resulting from declines in fluid cognitive processing. Finally, we evaluate the current evidence for and the potential contributions of these theories.

■ CHANGES IN EMOTION REGULATION GOALS LEAD TO CHANGES IN COGNITION

Socioemotional Selectivity Theory

SST is arguably the primary theoretical framework currently used to generate hypotheses about how the relationship between emotion and cognition may vary with age across adulthood. SST posits that as people age, they view their future time left in life as more limited, which motivates them to prioritize positive emotional goals. At any point in development, individuals have a certain amount of resources to devote toward goal pursuit, and although younger adults, for whom time seems more expansive, may prioritize knowledge acquisition or novel experiences that are useful for the future, older adults are motivated to prioritize their current hedonic state (Carstensen, Isaacowitz, & Charles, 1999). As emotional goals become more salient throughout adulthood (e.g., Carstensen & Turk-Charles, 1994), older adults are theorized to place increased importance on emotion regulation as a way to achieve positive emotional outcomes. One way to attain these hedonic goals for older adults may be through positively oriented cognitive processing of emotional information (see Mather & Carstensen, 2005 for a review).

Affective information is typically more salient than nonemotional content for both younger and older adults (Charles, Mather, & Carstensen, 2003). However, older adults have been found to remember and attend to a higher ratio of positive compared to negative emotional information as opposed to younger adults for whom negative affective stimuli tend to be the most salient (Mather & Carstensen, 2005). These age-related positivity effects in cognitive processing have been investigated in a number of domains and are often seen as one way for older adults to accomplish positive emotional goals (Reed & Carstensen, 2012).

Initially, positivity effects were found in studies that explored age differences in memory for emotional materials. Despite an age-related decline in overall memory performance, older adults recalled more positive than negative or neutral images (Charles, Mather, & Carstensen, 2003). In a second study, Charles et al. (2003) found that negative mood was positively correlated with negative image recall, but did not fully explain the age by valence effect. Younger adults still had better memory for negative content than older adults regardless of current mood. In this study, the researchers also evaluated how engagement, measured by time spent viewing images, influenced memory and found that, surprisingly, both age groups spent more time viewing negative images than other types of stimuli. These findings have been interpreted to suggest that shifts in cognitive processing reflect emotion regulation goals; however, they also inspired many questions about the mechanisms underlying age differences in memory.

One possible explanation for improved memory for positive emotional content is increased attention to, or engagement with, positive stimuli. In order to gain a more nuanced understanding of age differences in engagement with emotional content, our lab has focused on differences in visual attention. Studies using eye-tracking methods to examine visual attention have also found age-related positivity effects (see Isaacowitz, 2012 for a review). Older adults tend to look away from angry and sad faces, and direct attention toward happy facial expressions, whereas younger adults attend more to fearful faces or do not display an attentional bias (Isaacowitz, Waldinger, Goren, & Wilson, 2006a, 2006b). Older adults' moods also seem to benefit more from positivity-oriented cognition in their emotional experience. Positivity effects in visual attention (i.e., looking away from negative stimuli and toward neutral or positive content) are associated with better moods for older adults in response to facial expressions (Isaacowitz,

Toner, & Neupert, 2009), emotional films (Lohani & Isaacowitz, 2014), and negatively valenced health information (Isaacowitz & Choi, 2012).

Positivity effects that emerge in older adults' memory for and attention to emotional information pose the question of whether positively oriented cognitive processing facilitates emotional well-being (e.g., cognition influences emotion) or whether mood-congruent information is preferentially processed (e.g., emotion influencing cognition). In other words, positivity in cognition may increase positive affect, or older adults' higher levels of positive affect may make mood-congruent positive stimuli more salient. In another study in our lab, older and younger adults' moods were experimentally manipulated and their gaze was tracked while they viewed facial expressions. We found that older adults were more likely to use positivity in cognition as an emotion regulation strategy to improve mood. Older adults allocated their attention toward positive facial expressions when in a negative mood, as opposed to younger adults who tended to exhibit mood congruent rather than regulatory gaze patterns (Gaze et al., 2008). This study suggests that as people age, shifts in attention may in fact serve regulatory purposes, more so than in young adulthood.

If the prioritization of emotion regulation goals in late adulthood is the main cause of positive cognition, manipulating emotional goals in younger adults should lead to similar results. Several studies of attention and memory have found this pattern (Kennedy, Mather, & Carstensen, 2004; Light & Isaacowitz, 2006; Pruzan & Isaacowitz, 2006). Older adults also naturally exhibit a preference and better memory for positive information when making health care decisions but, when instructed to focus on information gathering, age differences were attenuated (Löckenhoff & Carstensen, 2007). As positivity effects can be induced in a broader adult sample by instructing emotion-regulation goals or eliminated in older adult samples by increasing the salience of other types of goals, such as knowledge acquisition, it suggests that positively oriented cognition is a motivated process.

Although there are studies that do not find an age difference in positivity (e.g., Grühn, Smith, & Baltes, 2005; Kensinger, Brierley, Medford, Growdon, & Corkin, 2002; Majerus & D'Argembeau, 2011), Reed, Chan, and Mikels (2014) argued that these studies place constraints on participants' chronically activated hedonic goals, thus preventing the positivity effect from emerging. This argument is supported by their meta-analysis that revealed positivity effects to be strongest for older adults in studies with more naturalistic, unconstrained designs (e.g., no instructions or manipulated resources), suggesting that top-down motivational processes are responsible for changes in cognitive processing. However, questions remain concerning whether age differences result from motivated processes that lead to better encoding of positive emotional content or from a more basic decline in negative emotional memory.

SST provides a valuable framework to explain age differences in attention and memory for emotional materials and to link positive cognition to positive emotional experience in old age. Emotion regulation, however, is a resource-demanding process, and recent discussions of SST (Mather, 2012; Nashiro, Sakaki, & Mather, 2011; Samanez-Larkin & Carstensen, 2011) have focused on behavioral and neural changes in old age that implicate cognitive control in the emotion regulation process, and subsumed these discussions under the Cognitive Control model (CCM).

Cognitive Control Model

CCM extends the SST framework by emphasizing the top-down nature of the positivity effect and positing that chronically activated emotional goals are implemented with the help of cognitive control resources (Mather, 2012; Nashiro, Sakaki, & Mather, 2011). To fulfill their emotional goals, older adults need to engage in emotion regulation, which has been shown in younger adults to require cognitive control (Ochsner & Gross, 2005). In that sense, only older adults with sufficient cognitive resources should be able to successfully orient their attention and memory to positive materials, and consequently achieve better emotional experience. In a series of experiments, Mather & Knight (2005) found that repeated retrieval enhanced older adults' memories for positive but not negative emotional images, suggesting that when asked to retrieve information, older adults process positive emotional information more elaborately. They also found that older adults with better cognitive abilities exhibited stronger positivity effects in memory, indicating that cognitive control resources are important for attaining positive emotional goals. If placed under cognitive load, older adults' memory bias for positive images was reversed and they actually recalled more negative than positive emotional images (Mather & Knight, 2005). Under divided-attention conditions, which reduce the availability of cognitive resources, older adults were also less likely to exhibit positivity effects in their fixation patterns. Interestingly, younger adults' fixation patterns were also altered in the divided-attention condition and their negativity bias was reduced, suggesting cognitive control might also have a role in emotion processing for younger adults (Knight et al., 2007). It seems that, despite age-related declines in cognitive function, older adults allocate more cognitive resources to control the processing of emotional information than younger adults.

However, a study of memory for emotionally valenced words found that a visual discrimination distracter task did not lead to the reversal of positivity effects, raising questions about the role of cognitive control in older adults' memory bias (Thomas & Hasher, 2006). Allard and Isaacowitz (2008) conducted a study using a within-subjects design to gain a more nuanced view of how divided attention, or reduced cognitive control, influences attention to emotional stimuli. They found, as in Thomas and Hasher (2006), that positivity effects can emerge under conditions of divided attention. It is interesting to note that their finding that positivity effects did arise despite other cognitive or attentional demands used distracter tasks that did not compete with the stimuli (e.g., the cognitive load task and the emotion task were not at the same time). In light of these findings, it seems that some level of top-down cognitive control is necessary for positivity effects to emerge, but full allocation of cognitive resources probably is not necessary for older adults to influence their attentional patterns (Allard & Isaacowitz, 2008). There is some automatic saliency of negative information, and it is beneficial for older adults to detect when there are threats in their environment. However, as hedonic goals become more salient with age, attentional biases driven by qualities of the stimuli can be overridden with cognitive control processes when the necessary resources are available.

In sum, SST and frameworks derived from this model attribute differences in the cognitive processing of emotional stimuli to older adults' emotional goals. SST sets itself apart by focusing on motivation, and argues for an account of age-related changes that are not inherently driven by cognitive and biological decline. In fact, cognitive control is theorized to be a central resource used to shift cognitive processing and attain positive emotional goals. However, as we discuss later in the chapter, other theories have proposed alternative approaches to changes in older adults' emotion and cognition links by incorporating changes in cognitive and neural development.

■ CHANGES IN THE BRAIN AND CHANGES IN EMOTION–COGNITION LINKS: CAUSE OR CONSEQUENCE?

Age comes with structural and functional changes in the brain, and several theories have emphasized the role of such changes for age differences in cognitive and emotional processes. Of particular interest is the amygdala, a structure with broad connectivity to areas implicated in cognitive functioning such as the sensory cortices, the hippocampal complex, and the prefrontal cortex. Connectivity between these brain regions enables the amygdala to modulate cognitive and social behaviors in response to emotional cues (Phelps, 2006). With age, there is a linear reduction in gray matter in limbic and paralimbic structures, including the amygdala, although this rate is significantly less than that of the whole brain (Grieve, Clark, Williams, Peduto, & Gordon, 2005). Although it is unclear how reduction in volume directly affects amygdala functioning, older adults appear to experience functional changes in this brain region as well, resulting in lower activation to negative stimuli than younger adults (Mather et al., 2004). Several theories have proposed that changes in the brain and changes in emotion and cognition in older adults are causally linked, although each theory differs in how they conceptualize the direction of this causal link.

Aging Brain Model

SST theorists view the change in amygdala activation as a direct result of chronic emotional regulatory goals. In contrast, Cacioppo, Berntson, Bechara, Tranel, and Hawkley (2011) proposed the Aging Brain model (ABM), in which improvement in subjective well-being in later life is seen as rooted in age-related changes in the amygdala. This model posits that age-related impairments in amygdala functioning result in reduced activation to negative stimuli but preserved activation for positive stimuli (e.g., Gunning-Dixon et al., 2003; Mather et al., 2004). These neural differences are thought to, in turn, lead to age-associated decreases in arousal to negative stimuli, which diminishes the memory advantage of emotionally arousing events and improves subjective well-being.

Although current research in this domain is all correlational and cannot provide direct evidence for this model, a study using patients with amygdala/anterior temporal lesions provided some support for the causal link between amygdala functioning and felt arousal from negative stimuli (Berntson, Bechara, Damasio, Tranel, & Cacioppo, 2007). Six patients aged 22 to 65 years rated affective pictures on positivity, negativity, and arousal. Compared to the control group, which comprised patients with lesions sparing areas involved in emotion processing, the experimental group had lower self-reported arousal for negative pictures, but similar arousal to positive and neutral pictures. There was no group difference in valence rating, indicating the decrease in arousal was not caused by impairment to valence discrimination. This finding is consistent with previous research that also shows that lesions to the amygdala are associated with lower arousal to negative stimuli (Adolphs, Russell, & Tranel, 1999; Winston, Gottfried, Kilner, & Dolan, 2005). Although data from the experimental group came from a wide age range, additional comparisons of arousal rating data from two older patients older than 80 years with lesions outside of the amygdala/anterior temporal regions reveal more similarity with middle-aged amygdala-damaged patients than younger normal controls and middle-aged lesion controls. This result implies that age-related, and not lesion-related, change in the amygdala might have led to diminished felt arousal to negative stimuli.

Fronto-Amygdalar Age-Related Differences in Emotion: For Emotion Regulation, Compensation, or Self-Referential Processing?

The reduced activation within the amygdala noted in ABM is also part of a documented phenomenon termed "fronto-amygdalar age-related differences in emotion" (FADE; Davis, Dennis, Daselaar, Fleck, & Cabeza, 2008). Coupled with a decrease in activation in the amygdala (e.g., Iidaka et al., 2002; Tessitore et al., 2005), older adults also recruit more of the prefrontal cortex (PFC; Gunning-Dixon et al., 2003; Gutchess, Kensinger, & Schacter, 2007; Leclerc & Kensinger, 2008; Tessitore et al., 2005; Williams et al., 2006) compared with younger adults when perceiving negative stimuli. A similar pattern of PFC engagement was found during memory encoding of emotional materials regardless of valence, although there was no age difference in amygdala activation (St. Jacques, Dolcos, & Cabeza, 2009; Kensinger & Schacter, 2008; Murty et al., 2009).

There are a few available interpretations for the FADE phenomenon. The most popular account attributes the fronto-amygdala shift to older adults' prioritizing emotion regulation, with the PFC exerting cognitive control to inhibit amygdala response to negative stimuli (St. Jacques et al., 2009). This account further supports the CCM's proposal that age differences in patterns of brain activity during emotional processing are motivated by differential emotional goals (Mather, 2012). From this perspective, if the amygdala were less responsive with age due to structural or functional changes solely in that brain region, a difference in responding across valences and under all conditions would be anticipated. However, amygdala responses remain intact for older adults in response to positive stimuli (Erk, Walter, & Abler, 2008; Mather et al. 2004; although see Kensinger et al., 2014) and age differences are attenuated under some experimental conditions (Wright, Wedig, Williams, Rauch, & Albert, 2006).

It is interesting to note that age-related declines in limbic system responding are accompanied by an increase, for older adults, in activity in prefrontal brain areas associated with emotion regulation in response to negative emotional content, which may account for diminished amygdala responding (Nashiro, Sakaki, & Mather, 2011). If emotion regulation is driving older adults' reduced responses to negative emotional information, it is likely that areas like the PFC are inhibiting amygdala responses. If older adults are pursuing chronically activated hedonic goals, and thus are continually motivated to regulate their emotions, researchers would expect to observe age-related increases in connectivity between regulatory frontal brain regions and the limbic system in response to negative emotional content.

In a functional MRI (fMRI) study, older adults exhibited diminished amygdala and hippocampus responding coupled with greater dorsolateral PFC activity, compared to younger adults, during memory encoding and recognition of negatively valenced images (Murty et al., 2009). In addition, the links between prefrontal and amygdala responding were stronger for negative than neutral images in older adults, suggesting greater connectivity for aversive stimuli. Another fMRI study found that medial prefrontal cortex (mPFC) activity was greater for older adults in response to fearful facial expressions, but lower than younger adults when viewing happy faces. The authors interpret these findings to indicate increases in older adults' emotion regulation in response to negative stimuli (Williams et al., 2006). Older adults also showed greater functional connectivity than younger adults between the anterior cingulate cortex (ACC), another brain area often involved in emotion regulation, and the amygdala during an emotional image-rating task (Jacques, Dolcos, & Cabeza, 2010). In sum, activation and connectivity between brain areas key to emotion processing seem to differ by valence, which provides support for accounts suggesting negative emotional content motivates differences in cognitive processing of emotional stimuli reflected in neural responding.

Another explanation for FADE is the more general posterior-to-anterior shift with aging (PASA) not exclusive to emotional processing. PASA denotes a pattern of decreased activity in posterior brain regions, particularly the occipital lobe and the medial temporal lobe, but increased activity in anterior regions, particularly the PFC, in older adults. This shift occurs in various cognitive domains, including visual perception (e.g., Grady et al., 1994), attention (e.g., Madden et al., 2002), and recognition memory (e.g., Cabeza et al., 2004). The increase in PFC activity has also been associated with better cognitive performance (Dennis & Cabeza, 2008). Because of the role of the PFC in controlled processes and occipital lobe in more automatic, sensory processes, PASA is viewed as a compensatory mechanism that allows older adults to boost performance by using top-down control to compensate for bottom-up decline (Grady et al., 1994; Dennis & Cabeza, 2008). Evidence of the PASA pattern provides avenues to extend classic cognitive aging theories such as the sensory deficit theory (Lindenberger & Baltes, 1994), the resources deficit theory and the environmental support hypothesis (Craik, 1986), the speed deficit theory (Salthouse, 1996), the inhibition deficit theory, and the recollection deficit theory (Yonelinas, 2002) to include predictions about underlying neural mechanisms. Changes in amygdala activation and therefore emotional processing may be a part of a global change in neural recruitment that affects multiple cognitive domains.

Focusing specifically on the mPFC and its effect on memory encoding, Kensinger and Leclerc (2009) proposed that the increase in frontal activity is indicative of older adults' enhanced self-referential processes. This account does not contradict CCM (Mather, 2012); it posits that age-related change in frontal engagement can be caused by multiple mechanisms. As part of the PASA pattern, mPFC recruitment has been found to increase with age. This area has been associated with interpreting and elaborating on emotional information in a personal or contextual way (Amodio & Frith, 2006; Qin & Northoff, 2011; Salzman & Fusi, 2010). The increased mPFC activity during emotional processing, which implies deeper elaboration, can explain the preserved memory enhancement effect of emotional information, despite cognitive decline in old age (Kensinger et al., 2014). However, there is a valence-dependent age difference in activation of mPFC during encoding: Across a range of stimuli, older adults have more mPFC activation for positive than for negative information, whereas the pattern is reversed for younger adults (Leclerc & Kensinger, 2008, 2010, 2011). This age-related reversal is also present for self-related positive words (Gutchess, Kensinger, & Schacter, 2007). These findings, although different from those that found age-related mPFC engagement for negative valence (e.g., Williams et al., 2006), raise the possibility that the role of mPFC is not simply to regulate emotions (although see Mather, 2012, for evidence that response to each valence is determined by the involvement or lack thereof of the ventromedial PFC, as opposed to lateral or general PFC).

Besides regulating emotion, mPFC has been found to be at the center of a neural network unique to self-referential processing. The mPFC is hypothesized to direct attention inward for self-reflection or to bind self-relevant experiences (Kensinger et al., 2014). However, self-relevant processing is not entirely independent from emotional processing: Affective information directly impacts one's affective experiences and is therefore inherently self-relevant. Inversely, information that is interpreted in a personal way can be meaningful and emotionally important (Kensinger et al., 2014). Future research needs to address these shared characteristics between the two domains and investigate whether older adults' preserved memory enhancement effects for emotional materials and their recruitment of mPFC stem from a common mechanism between emotional and self-relevant processes.

■ CHANGE IN COGNITIVE DEVELOPMENT AFFECTS EMOTIONAL PROCESSING

Unlike other theories that emphasize older adults' ability to apply available cognitive resources to emotional processes, the DIT (Labouvie-Vief, 2003; Labouvie-Vief, Diehl, Jain, & Zhang, 2007; Labouvie-Vief, Gilet, & Mella, 2014) posits that cognitive decline negatively affects older adults' integration of complex affective states, thus causing them to optimize their emotional experience through preferences for positive stimuli. The core tenet of this theory lies in the concept of equilibrium. In biological processes, equilibrium is the ideal state, around which small deviations occur in opposite directions to balance one another. Extreme deviations in either direction can cause damage to the biological system; thus equilibrium processes strive to maintain homeostasis through tension reduction. Tension is associated with negative emotions, and relieving tension to achieve equilibrium can lead to rewarding positive emotions. With each challenge individuals face to reduce tension, they develop a more cognitively complex representation of the situation and attain a higher level of development. Disequilibrium, therefore, is essential to development in promoting cognitive complexity. Through practice and developing cognitive understanding of new and challenging situations, experiences that deviate from the norm will no longer lead to disequilibrium, both cognitively and emotionally. Throughout development from childhood to adulthood, cognitive–emotional development is therefore synchronous with cognitive understanding.

This course of development operates in a similar fashion at a biological level. Over the years, growing connectivity between the prefrontal areas and the limbic system and increasingly automated relevant neural networks allow for a better cognitive–emotional integration and an improved emotion regulation (e.g., findings from Casey et al., 1997 and Luna et al., 2001, on reduced prefrontal activation in adults compared with children during inhibition or directed attention, indicating that adults require less regulation efforts in cognitively demanding tasks). This process of automization, or crystallization, reduces regulation burden that depends on fluid processes, which declines in later life. Although crystallized knowledge is largely intact in late adulthood, fluid processes can affect crystallization when crystallized knowledge needs to be retrieved and implemented. DIT views later adulthood as a period where the decline in fluid processes creates difficulty for maintaining general equilibrium. Cognitive–emotional systems become more likely to be overwhelmed, and older adults are more vulnerable to higher levels of tension. There has been evidence for a positive linear association between valence and arousal in older adults (higher arousal is viewed as negative), whereas the relationship is curvilinear for younger adults (Keil & Freund, 2009). Older adults appear to have greater interdependence of cognitive and emotional processes, and decline in fluid functioning results in difficulties in processing emotional stimuli, which in turn disrupts cognitive performance. In a study by Wurm, Labouvie-Vief, Aycock, Rebucal, and Koch (2004), older adults were more sensitive to high-arousal words, but remembered fewer of the more arousing words. Hess and Ennis (2012) found that older adults had higher reactivity levels, as measured by systolic blood pressure, but worse performance than younger adults. Although older adults are less easily aroused than younger adults, in stressful situations older adults exhibit more reactivity than younger adults in systolic blood pressure (although not in heart rate; see review by Uchino, Birmingham, & Berg, 2010).

As high levels of arousal can impede complex, integrated behaviors (Labouvie-Vief & Marquez, 2004), and older adults are more vulnerable in situations that induce high arousal, they need a mechanism to maintain their affective balance. Labouvie-Vief and colleagues (2007) described two modes of emotional processing that interact dynamically to help older adults compensate for the consequences of their decline in cognitive complexity and preserve well-being. The first one is *affect optimization*, which is the tendency to process information in order to maximize positive and minimize negative affect. The second, *affect complexity*, is the ability to integrate positive and negative states, allowing a focus on objectivity, personal growth, emotional and conceptual complexity. These two modes of processing coordinate so that if one decreases, the other increases. Because affect complexity measures tend to correlate with measures of cognitive functioning, on which older adults have exhibited deficits, it would follow that affect complexity also declines with age, as evidenced by findings that older adults tend to simplify valence in their emotion-related judgment (e.g., Mather & Johnson, 2000). In exchange, affect optimization increases with age, as a compensation strategy to maintain subjective well-being. DIT thus emphasizes the effect of simplified cognition on emotion regulation and affective experience, and predicts that older adults with fewer cognitive resources will be worse at maintaining subjective well-being.

■ HOW DO THESE THEORIES CONTRIBUTE TO OUR UNDERSTANDING OF THE EMOTION–COGNITION INTERFACE ACROSS THE LIFE SPAN?

The theories discussed earlier have all provided useful conceptual frameworks to explain empirical findings in research on age-associated changes in emotion and cognition. Most theories aim to reconcile the seemingly separate developmental pathways of cognition and emotion: as people age, although cognition gets worse, emotion does not. Investigation into preserved emotional functioning has led SST theorists to notice the pattern of positivity in older adults' attention and memory, and to propose that the positivity effect is a way for older adults to accomplish emotional goals. SST was the key reason researchers started investigating potential age-related positivity effects in attention and memory. Other theories have since proposed alternative explanations for the positivity effect, while also accounting for cognitive and neurological decline in old age. Thus, despite their common goal and shared domain of interest, theories on the interaction between cognition and emotion across the life span are distinctive in important aspects.

Motivational Shift or Cognitive and Neurological Decline?

A key difference between the theories discussed earlier is whether they consider motivation as a causal factor for changes in cognition and emotion. SST and CCM conceptualize positive cognition as motivated cognition, in which attention to and memory for positive stimuli serve as emotion regulatory goals to assure subjective well-being in older adults. These goals in turn produce an increase in PFC activity to exert cognitive control to inhibit activity in the amygdala. Older adults' motivation, therefore, shapes their cognition, and age differences in amygdala activation to positive and negative stimuli are a consequence of these motivational and cognitive changes. In contrast, the ABM posits that decreased activity in the amygdala with age, due to structural and functional decline, is the cause of the positivity effect in attention and memory in older adults. Similarly, DIT emphasizes cognitive decline, which has roots in structural and functional decline in the brain, as the main antecedent for preserved subjective well-being in old age. ABM and DIT, therefore, provide more neurologically based explanations for age-related changes in emotional processing, whereas SST postulates motivation as the cause of such changes.

Evidence so far has not fully supported decline-based accounts. Findings that positivity in memory can be successfully manipulated (Kennedy et al., 2004; Löckenhoff & Carstensen, 2007) or how positivity effects disappear under cognitive load (Mather & Knight, 2005; Knight et al., 2007, although see Allard & Isaacowitz, 2008) suggest that better cognitive control, presumably for emotion regulation purposes, leads to positively oriented cognition. Although whether preferred processing of positive stimuli actually results in better mood is often inferred and less often tested (Isaacowitz & Blanchard-Fields, 2012), there is some evidence of older adults with better executive control being able to avoid negative mood by looking less at negative stimuli (Isaacowitz, Toner, Goren, & Wilson, 2008; Isaacowitz, Toner, & Neupert, 2009). This contrasts with predictions from DIT, which posits that negative affect is more cognitively demanding and therefore older adults with less cognitive control would exhibit more processing of positive affect.

However, a recent event-related potential (ERP) study (Foster, Davis, & Kisley, 2013) did find a positive correlation between cognitive functioning and more late positive potentials (LPP) in response to negative images in older adults. This finding supports the perspective of DIT that positivity in older adults' cognition may result from declines in cognitive functioning. Nevertheless, the findings can also be interpreted to speak to the ability of older adults with higher cognitive levels to process negative stimuli at the early stage of perception so as to gain information, and only engage in controlled processing of positive stimuli in a later stage. This interpretation would be consistent with previous research that shows balanced processing of positive and negative information within 1,000 ms, but positivity effects later (Isaacowitz, Allard, Murphy, & Schlangel, 2009; Knight et al., 2007). However, the authors did not directly test for this explanation, thus leaving open venues for future research to examine the time course and relative roles of automatic and controlled processes in positive cognition and affect.

Similarly, evidence for the neurological decline account (ABM) has been scant, and there has been some evidence supporting preserved functioning of the amygdala with age (e.g., Dolcos, Katsumi, & Dixon, 2014; Grieve et al., 2005). The hypothesis that decline in amygdala functioning in older adults reduces amygdala activity to negative stimuli has also been challenged by findings that both younger and older adults have comparable amygdala responses to negative-novel stimuli and neutral stimuli (Wright et al., 2006).

Cognitive and biological changes are part and parcel to aging, but as discussed earlier, evidence seems to support a motivational account when it comes to positivity in cognitive processing. Motivation has been found to be an important factor in older adults' emotional processing, and can provide plausible explanations for age-related differences in emotion regulation and perception (Sands, Ngo, & Isaacowitz, 2016). Throughout the life span, goals might change to suit developmental needs and available resources. Motivation theories such as selection, optimization, and compensation (SOC; Baltes, 1997; Freund & Baltes, 1998); selection, optimization, and compensation with emotion regulation (SOC-ER; Urry & Gross, 2010); or the selective engagement hypothesis (Hess, 2006) have provided conceptual guidance for empirical research in multiple fields such as decision making, social cognition, and emotion regulation. Although more direct testing of the process–outcome link between emotion regulation goals and positive cognition proposed by SST is necessary, motivation, whether considered under SST or other motivation-focused theoretical frameworks, would offer new ways to approach the question of why emotion functioning appears to be preserved despite cognitive decline.

Brain Change: General or Specific?

The role of motivation in age-related changes in positive cognition is often supported by neural evidence of prefrontal activity—regions that have previously been associated with cognitive control in emotion regulation. However, neuroscientific research has also linked the PFC to self and other judgment (see Denny, Kober, Wager, & Ochsner, 2012 for a meta-analysis), and to contextualization of emotional information in a self-relevant manner (Amodio & Frith, 2006; D'Argembeau et al., 2011). If PFC activity indicates only emotion regulation efforts in older adults, their PFC activity should be most evident in response to negative stimuli, which is indeed the case in several studies (Gunning-Dixon et al., 2003; Tessitore et al., 2005; Williams et al., 2006). However, there has also been evidence that older adults show greater mPFC activity (Leclerc & Kensinger, 2008, 2010, 2011) and stronger functional connectivity between the PFC and the amygdala for positive rather than negative stimuli (Addis, Leclerc, Muscatell, & Kensinger, 2010), particularly older adults with higher life satisfaction (Waldinger, Kensinger, & Schulz, 2011).

These findings for PFC response to both negative and positive stimuli might be more complementary than contradictory, and point to more general age-related top-down processing of emotional information. One form of this top-down processing could be emotion regulation, and another form could be self-referential processing of emotional information (Kensinger et al., 2014). Furthermore, age-related increases in PFC activity have been shown in other cognitive domains, characterized by the PASA pattern (Davis et al., 2008), raising the possibility that the prefrontal shift in emotion processing is part of a larger change in the aging brain. A compensation account (increased anterior activity compensates for posterior activity decline) and a dedifferentiation account (brain regions become less specialized and respond more similarly to different cognitive tasks) have been proposed to explain PASA, but more research needs to be conducted to determine the cause of this pattern and further our understanding of the age-related change in PFC-amygdala interaction in processing of emotional stimuli.

The Role of Arousal

Dimensional conceptualizations of affect, which highlight the importance of both the hedonic valence and arousal components of affect, have raised questions about the implications of age differences in arousal for affective experience and regulation. Older adults seem to find highly arousing stimuli increasingly aversive (Keil & Freund, 2009), and since negative stimuli tend to be higher in arousal than positive or neutral stimuli, arousal may play a key role in motivating positivity in cognitive processing. In an image-rating task, younger adults show linear patterns within positive and negative valence categories, with higher arousal being associated with either more pleasant or more unpleasant ratings depending on image valence. However, older adults' valence ratings of emotional images seemed to be driven more so by stimulus arousal rather than valence; they rated low arousal images as more pleasant, and high-arousal images as more unpleasant (Keil & Freund, 2009).

The role of arousal for the interface of emotion and cognition, especially physiological reactivity and flexibility, is one aspect that differentiates between the theoretical models reviewed in this chapter. On the one hand, studies have found that older adults report fewer intense negative emotions (e.g., Charles & Carstensen, 2008; Charles, Reynolds, & Gatz, 2001) and experience lower levels of physiological reactivity in response to negative emotional experiences (e.g., Levenson, Carstensen, Friesen, & Ekman, 1991; Levenson, Carstensen, & Gottman, 1994). The SST framework has attributed these age differences to changes in motivation that lead to positivity in cognitive processing that ultimately enhances emotion regulation. However, on the other hand, in some contexts older adults may also experience higher levels of negative affect (Mroczek & Almeida, 2004) and heightened levels of physiological arousal in emotional situations (Uchino, Holt-Lunstad, Bloor, & Campo, 2005). DIT posits that, in highly arousing situations, age-related cognitive decline may impede the integration of interdependent cognitive and affective processes that facilitate emotion regulation (Labouvie-Vief, Gilet, & Mella, 2014). Recently, there have been some efforts to reconcile the seemingly contradictory findings about the developmental trajectories of cognitive and emotional functioning.

Morgan and Scheibe (2014) propose a series of mechanisms that may explain why declines in cognitive functioning can still be accompanied by maintenance or improvements in affective well-being. First, age-related changes in the autonomic nervous system result in diminished physiological reactivity in emotional situations, which may reduce the difficulty of emotion regulation. Age differences in physiological flexibility also appear to be context dependent. Although reactivity in response to emotional experience is often diminished, older adults simultaneously experience decreases in physiological flexibility, which may make downregulating existing high-arousal states more difficult (see the SAVI model by Charles, 2010, for a review). In addition, they hypothesize that, in line with SST, chronically activated hedonic goals may motivate older adults to allocate more cognitive resources for emotion regulation so that cognitive decline may be compensated for by increased effort. Finally, they propose that emotion regulation may become more efficient, and therefore limited resources may still be used more effectively with age (Morgan & Scheibe, 2014).

The *overpowering hypothesis* also aims to reconcile these contrary findings, and complements findings about differences in physiological responding, by attributing differences to the complexity of the emotional situation (Wrzus, Müller, Wagner, Lindenberger, & Riediger, 2012). According to this framework, older adults have decreased negative responses to low-arousal situations that may elicit small amounts of negative affect (e.g., argument about household chores) but increased emotional reactivity in complex, highly arousing negative situations that place high demands on resources that decline with age. In an experience-sampling study, older age was associated with heightened negative affect and physiological reactivity to complex aversive events. However, in response to minor stressors, there were no apparent age differences in subjective affect and physiological responding was actually diminished for older adults (Wrzus et al., 2012).

Although research has only recently incorporated arousal into the conceptualization of emotional and cognitive changes in old age, because arousal is crucial to emotion regulation efficiency, theories that argue for the role of emotional goals (such as SST and CCM) need to consider not only the effect of stimulus valence, but also the level of arousal that the stimulus elicits in older adults' affective experiences. Arousal is also important to theories that focus on the role of cognitive and neurological development in emotional response (such as DIT, ABM, PASA, self-referential processing), as arousal is seen as impairing older adults' performance (from DIT's perspective), but can also facilitate performance to reduce age differences (e.g., older adults have preserved enhanced memory for emotionally arousing stimuli regardless of valence, which can be caused by preserved functioning of the amygdala). In addition, incorporating arousal into the study of age differences in emotion regulation may shed light on preferences and the effectiveness of various regulatory strategies (see Sands & Isaacowitz, 2016). Future research will benefit from addressing the role of arousal regardless of the perspective from which they operate.

Does Cognition Influence Emotion, or Does Emotion Influence Cognition, or Both?

Most of the theories reviewed earlier in this chapter focus on how cognitive changes support emotional ones. Fewer theories have considered the effects of aging on how emotion influences cognition, though some theories of this nature exist in the broader literature (e.g., the broaden and build theory, Fredrickson, 2001; the somatic marker hypothesis, Damasio, Everitt, & Bishop, 1996; the Affect Infusion model, Forgas, 1995; the affect-as-information hypothesis, Clore & Huntsinger, 2007; and the arousal-biased competition theory, Mather & Sutherland, 2011).

The affect-as-information hypothesis in particular has received much empirical support (Schwarz, 2011). The hypothesis proposes that mood and emotion influence judgment by assigning values to the object of judgment, or providing feedback on one's own thoughts and inclinations. This hypothesis also predicts that positive emotions promote relational processing, which converges with predictions from the Affect Infusion model (positive emotions promoting substantive processing; Forgas, 1995) and the Broaden and Build model (positive emotions broadening the scope of cognition) (Fredrickson, 2001). This conceptual framework, similar to others, makes no developmental predictions, and most of the evidence has been from younger adult samples.

So far, only a few studies with older adults have explored the effect of mood on judgment across the life span. A study on the effect of induced sad mood on recall of word lists and autobiographical events, and performance on a lexical ambiguity task, showed that older adults were more likely to exhibit mood congruency than younger adults (Knight, Maines, & Robinson, 2002). In another study, positive mood eliminated the age differences in correspondence bias present in neutral mood and exacerbated age differences in negative mood (Mienaltowski & Blanchard-Fields, 2005). Older adults might have been more motivated to regulate their negative mood, which comes at a cognitive cost and impairs their performance on the attitude attribution task. Positive mood, in contrast, can broaden attention (Fredrickson, 2001) and promote substantive processing (Clore & Huntsinger, 2007; Forgas, 1995), and might increase younger and older adults' motivation to complete the task, or encourage them to attend to situational rather than dispositional causes. However, in another study, positive and negative mood did not affect product evaluation differently across age groups (Hess, Beale, & Miles, 2010), suggesting that affect-as-information processes remain intact in old age. The effect of mood on judgment in younger and older adults thus seems to vary depending on the type of judgment.

Another theory that might be relevant to the aging literature is the arousal competition biased theory, which posits that the affective state of the perceiver may also play a role in the salience of information. Specifically, this theory proposes that arousal, regardless of the source, enhances memory for objects that dominate in selective attention (Mather & Sutherland, 2011). In other words, arousal creates a favorable bias toward information that is more relevant, or perceptually more salient, and then enhances memory encoding for this information regardless of its inherent level of arousal. Although old age may come with declines in physiological activation and the ability to sense bodily states (Mendes, 2010), arousal may still play a key role in memory salience. For older adults, internal arousal influences memory for neutral stimuli. In a study of memory of alphabet letters, recall was enhanced for nonaffective stimuli that are high in visual salience (e.g., higher contrast letters) if the perceiver was in a high-arousal affective state at the time of stimulus presentation (Sutherland & Mather, 2015). The arousal level of the stimuli also influences salience; highly arousing stimuli in some circumstances have diminished positivity effects in cognitive processing (e.g., Streubel & Kunzmann, 2011; also see Wurm et al., 2004) suggesting that arousal might be the key moderator of emotional effects on cognition in old age.

Given demonstrated complexity in age differences in emotional experience, cognitive functioning, and the effect of emotional goals on cognition, the question of whether emotion influences cognition or cognition influences emotion may be too simplistic. Older adults' chronic goals are to maintain a positive state and reduce negative affect, which results in their preferred processing of positive stimuli. The positivity in cognition in turn leads to either an increase in positive affect or a decrease in negative affect, which again can have downstream effects of task performance, even when the task does not have an affective component. The idea is that older adults constantly try to regulate their emotions—and in fact, there has been evidence that they tend to regulate more rapidly than younger adults (Larcom & Isaacowitz, 2009). The constant and rapid regulation might create an affective feedback loop that makes it challenging to discern causes and consequences in older adults' behaviors.

Furthermore, current neuroimaging evidence points to complex integration of emotion and cognition in the brain: regions that activate during emotion processing have also been involved in other mental processes, such as cognitive control, memory, theory of mind, navigation, among others (Lindquist & Barrett, 2012; Pessoa, 2008). For example, activity in the dorsolateral PFC is modulated by the valence of the stimuli during response inhibition (Goldstein et al., 2007) and working memory tasks (Gray, Braver, & Raichle, 2002; Perlstein, Elbert, & Stenger, 2002). Areas traditionally marked as affective, such as the amygdala, the orbitofrontal cortex, the ventromedial PFC, and the ACC, are highly interconnected with other parts of the brain and function as a connectivity hub (Pessoa, 2008; Phelps, 2006). Along with behavioral evidence, neural findings have encouraged theorists to take up a more network-based and constructionist approach (Barrett, 2006; Barrett, 2013; Lindquist, 2013; Pessoa, 2008) that considers emotion and cognition to be integrated at different levels of processing, and has no clear demarcation of functionality in the brain. Future research in the interaction of emotion and cognition in aging, therefore, can take a more dynamic and psychological construction view to the question of how the link between emotion and cognition changes across the life span.

■ CONCLUSION

Several theories have proposed motivation, neurological changes, and cognitive development as being involved in changes in the developmental trajectory of emotion–cognition links throughout the life span, although there is yet a consensus on which factors are causes and which are consequences of such changes. Most theories in aging have also focused on the effect of cognition on emotion and have yet to explore how emotion can also influence cognition. However, the question of directionality might not be as crucial as understanding how the integration of emotion and cognition, which has been demonstrated with behavioral and neuroimaging evidence, can change with age. Put another way, it seems clear that emotion–cognition links vary as a function of age. Although theories exist regarding which comes first and why, future research that better describes the dynamic interplay of cognitive and emotional processes over time within individuals may provide better tests of existing theories, or may suggest new theoretical directions as well.

REFERENCES

Addis, D. R., Leclerc, C. M., Muscatell, K. A., & Kensinger, E. A. (2010). There are age-related changes in neural connectivity during the encoding of positive, but not negative, information. *Cortex: A Journal Devoted to the Study of the Nervous System and Behavior, 46*(4), 425–433.

Adolphs, R., Russell, J. A., & Tranel, D. (1999). A role for the human amygdala in recognizing emotional arousal from unpleasant stimuli. *Psychological Science, 10,* 167–171.

Allard, E., & Isaacowitz, D. (2008). Are preferences in emotional processing affected by distraction? Examining the age-related positivity effect in visual fixation within a dual-task paradigm. *Aging, Neuropsychology, and Cognition.* Retrieved from http://www.tandfonline.com/doi/abs/10.1080/13825580802348562

Amodio, D. M., & Frith, C. D. (2006). Meeting of minds: The medial frontal cortex and social cognition. *Nature Reviews. Neuroscience, 7*(4), 268–277.

Baltes, P. B. (1997). On the incomplete architecture of human ontogeny. Selection, optimization, and compensation as foundation of developmental theory. *The American Psychologist, 52*(4), 366–380.

Barrett, L. F. (2006). Are emotions natural kinds? *Perspectives on Psychological Science: A Journal of the Association for Psychological Science, 1*(1), 28–58.

Barrett, L. F. (2013). Psychological construction: The Darwinian approach to the science of emotion. *Emotion Review, 5,* 379–389.

Berntson, G. G., Bechara, A., Damasio, H., Tranel, D., & Cacioppo, J. T. (2007). Amygdala contribution to selective dimensions of emotion. *Social Cognitive and Affective Neuroscience, 2*(2), 123–129.

Cabeza, R., Daselaar, S. M., Dolcos, F., Prince, S. E., Budde, M., & Nyberg, L. (2004). Task-independent and task-specific age effects on brain activity during working memory, visual attention and episodic retrieval. *Cerebral Cortex, 14*(4), 364–375.

Cacioppo, J. T., Berntson, G. G., Bechara, A., Tranel, D., & Hawkley, L. C. (2011). Could an aging brain contribute to subjective well-being? The value added by a social neuroscience perspective. *Social Neuroscience: Toward Understanding the Underpinnings of the Social Mind,* 249–262.

Carstensen, L. L., Isaacowitz, D. M., & Charles, S. T. (1999). Taking time seriously: A theory of socioemotional selectivity. *The American Psychologist, 54,* 165. Retrieved from http://onlinelibrary.wiley.com/doi/10.1111/j.1540–5907.2007.00307.x/full

Carstensen, L. L., Turan, B., Scheibe, S., Ram, N., Ersner-Hershfield, H., Samanez-Larkin, G. R.,...Nesselroade, J. R. (2011). Emotional experience improves with age: Evidence based on over 10 years of experience sampling. *Psychology and Aging, 26*(1), 21–33.

Carstensen, L. L., & Turk-Charles, S. (1994). The salience of emotion across the adult life span. *Psychology and Aging, 9*(2), 259–264.

Casey, B. J., Castellanos, F. X., Giedd, J. N., Marsh, W. L., Hamburger, S. D., Schubert, A. B.,...Rapoport, J. L. (1997). Implication of right frontostriatal circuitry in response inhibition and attention-deficit/hyperactivity disorder. *Journal of the American Academy of Child and Adolescent Psychiatry, 36*(3), 374–383.

Charles, S. T. (2010). Strength and vulnerability integration: A model of emotional well-being across adulthood. *Psychological Bulletin, 136*(6), 1068.

Charles, S. T., & Carstensen, L. L. (2008). Unpleasant situations elicit different emotional responses in younger and older adults. *Psychology and Aging, 23*(3), 495–504.

Charles, S. T., Mather, M., & Carstensen, L. L. (2003). Aging and emotional memory: The forgettable nature of negative images for older adults. *Journal of Experimental Psychology. General, 132*(2), 310–324.

Charles, S. T., Reynolds, C. A., & Gatz, M. (2001). Age-related differences and change in positive and negative affect over 23 years. *Journal of Personality and Social Psychology, 80*(1), 136–151.

Clore, G. L., & Huntsinger, J. R. (2007). How emotions inform judgment and regulate thought. *Trends in Cognitive Sciences, 11*(9), 393–399.

Craik, F. I. M. (1986). A functional account of age differences in memory. In F. Klix & H. Hagendorf (Eds.), *Human memory and cognitive capabilities: Mechanisms and performances* (pp. 409–422). Amsterdam, The Netherlands: Elsevier.

Craik, F. I. M., & Salthouse, T. A. (2011). *The handbook of aging and cognition* (3rd ed.). New York, NY: Psychology Press.

D'Argembeau, A., Jedidi, H., Balteau, E., Bahri, M., Phillips, C., & Salmon, E. (2011). Valuing one's self: Medial prefrontal involvement in epistemic and emotive investments in self-views. *Cerebral Cortex, 22*, 659–667.

Damasio, A. R., Everitt, B. J., & Bishop, D. (1996). The somatic marker hypothesis and the possible functions of the prefrontal cortex [and discussion]. *Philosophical Transactions of the Royal Society B: Biological Sciences, 351*, 1413–1420.

Davis, S. W., Dennis, N. A., Daselaar, S. M., Fleck, M. S., & Cabeza, R. (2008). Que PASA? The posterior-anterior shift in aging. *Cerebral Cortex 18*(5), 1201–1209.

Dennis, N. A., & Cabeza, R. (2008). Neuroimaging of healthy cognitive aging. In F. I. M. Craik & T. A. Salthouse (Eds.), *The handbook of aging and cognition* (3rd ed., pp. 1–54). New York, NY: Psychology Press.

Denny, B. T., Kober, H., Wager, T. D., & Ochsner, K. N. (2012). A meta-analysis of functional neuroimaging studies of self and other judgments reveals a spatial gradient for mentalizing in medial prefrontal cortex. *Journal of Cognitive Neuroscience, 24*(8), 1742–1752.

Dolcos, S., Katsumi, Y., & Dixon, R. A. (2014). The role of arousal in the spontaneous regulation of emotions in healthy aging: A fMRI investigation. *Frontiers in Psychology, 5*, 681.

Erk, S., Walter, H., & Abler, B. (2008). Age-related physiological responses to emotion anticipation and exposure. *Neuroreport, 19*(4), 447–452.

Forgas, J. P. (1995). Mood and judgment: The affect infusion model (AIM). *Psychological Bulletin, 117*(1), 39–66.

Foster, S. M., Davis, H. P., & Kisley, M. A. (2013). Brain responses to emotional images related to cognitive ability in older adults. *Psychology and Aging, 28*(1), 179–190.

Fredrickson, B. L. (2001). The role of positive emotions in positive psychology: The broaden-and-build theory of positive emotions. *The American Psychologist, 56*(3), 218–226.

Freund, A. M., & Baltes, P. B. (1998). Selection, optimization, and compensation as strategies of life management: Correlations with subjective indicators of successful aging. *Psychology and Aging, 13*(4), 531–543.

Gaze, M., Adults, Y., Gaze, P., Isaacowitz, D. M., Toner, K., Goren, D., & Wilson, H. R. (2008). Looking while unhappy: Mood-congruent gaze in young adults, positive gaze in older adults. *Psychological Science, 19*, 848–853.

Goldstein, M., Brendel, G., Tuescher, O., Pan, H., Epstein, J., Beutel, M., … Silbersweig, D. (2007). Neural substrates of the interaction of emotional stimulus processing and motor inhibitory control: An emotional linguistic go/no-go fMRI study. *Neuroimage, 36*(3), 1026–1040.

Grady, C. L., Maisog, J. M., Horwitz, B., Ungerleider, L. G., Mentis, M. J., Salerno, J. A., … Haxby, J. V. (1994). Age-related changes in cortical blood flow activation during visual processing of faces and location. *The Journal of Neuroscience, 14*(3, Pt. 2), 1450–1462.

Gray, J. R., Braver, T. S., & Raichle, M. E. (2002). Integration of emotion and cognition in the lateral prefrontal cortex. *Proceedings of the National Academy of Sciences of the United States of America, 99*(6), 4115–4120.

Grieve, S. M., Clark, C. R., Williams, L. M., Peduto, A. J., & Gordon, E. (2005). Preservation of limbic and paralimbic structures in aging. *Human Brain Mapping, 25*(4), 391–401.

Grühn, D., Smith, J., & Baltes, P. B. (2005). No aging bias favoring memory for positive material: Evidence from a heterogeneity-homogeneity list paradigm using emotionally toned words. *Psychology and Aging, 20*(4), 579–588.

Gunning-Dixon, F. M., Gur, R. C., Perkins, A. C., Schroeder, L., Turner, T., Turetsky, B. I., … Gur, R. E. (2003). Age-related differences in brain activation during emotional face processing. *Neurobiology of Aging, 24*(2), 285–295.

Gutchess, A. H., Kensinger, E. A., & Schacter, D. L. (2007). Aging, self-referencing, and medial prefrontal cortex. *Social Neuroscience, 2*(2), 117–133.

Hess, T. M. (2006). Adaptive aspects of social cognitive functioning in adulthood: Age-related goal and knowledge influences. *Social Cognition, 24*, 279–309.

Hess, T. M., Beale, K. S., & Miles, A. (2010). The impact of experienced emotion on evaluative judgments: The effects of age and emotion regulation style. *Neuropsychology, Development, and Cognition. Section B, Aging, Neuropsychology and Cognition, 17*(6), 648–672.

Hess, T. M., & Ennis, G. E. (2012). Age differences in the effort and costs associated with cognitive activity. *The Journals of Gerontology, Series B, 67*(4), 447–455.

Iidaka, T., Okada, T., Murata, T., Omori, M., Kosaka, H., Sadato, N., & Yonekura, Y. (2002). Age-related differences in the medial temporal lobe responses to emotional faces as revealed by fMRI. *Hippocampus, 12*(3), 352–362.

Isaacowitz, D. M. (2012). Mood regulation in real-time: Age differences in the role of looking. *Current Directions in Psychological Science, 21*(4), 237–242.

Isaacowitz, D. M., Allard, E. S., Murphy, N. A., & Schlangel, M. (2009). The time course of age-related preferences toward positive and negative stimuli. *The Journals of Gerontology, Series B, 64*(2), 188–192.

Isaacowitz, D. M., & Blanchard-Fields, F. (2012). Linking process and outcome in the study of emotion and aging. *Perspectives on Psychological Science: A Journal of the Association for Psychological Science, 7*(1), 3–17.

Isaacowitz, D. M., & Choi, Y. (2012). Looking, feeling, and doing: Are there age differences in attention, mood, and behavioral responses to skin cancer information? *Health Psychology: Official Journal of the Division of Health Psychology, American Psychological Association, 31*(5), 650–659.

Isaacowitz, D. M., Toner, K., Goren, D., & Wilson, H. R. (2008). Looking while unhappy mood-congruent gaze in young adults, positive gaze in older adults. *Psychological Science, 19*(9), 848–853.

Isaacowitz, D. M., Toner, K., & Neupert, S. D. (2009). Use of gaze for real-time mood regulation: Effects of age and attentional functioning. *Psychology and Aging, 24*(4), 989–994.

Isaacowitz, D. M., Wadlinger, H. A., Goren, D., & Wilson, H. R. (2006a). Is there an age-related positivity effect in visual attention? A comparison of two methodologies. *Emotion, 6*(3), 511–516.

Isaacowitz, D. M., Wadlinger, H. A., Goren, D., & Wilson, H. R. (2006b). Selective preference in visual fixation away from negative images in old age? An eye-tracking study. *Psychology and Aging, 21*(1), 40–48.

Jacques, P. S., Dolcos, F., & Cabeza, R. (2010). Effects of aging on functional connectivity of the amygdala during negative evaluation: A network analysis of fMRI data. *Neurobiology of Aging, 31*(2), 315–327.

Keil, A., & Freund, A. M. (2009). Changes in the sensitivity to appetitive and aversive arousal across adulthood. *Psychology and Aging, 24*(3), 668–680.

Kennedy, Q., Mather, M., & Carstensen, L. L. (2004). The role of motivation in the age-related positivity effect in autobiographical memory. *Psychological Science, 15*(3), 208–214.

Kensinger, E. A., Allard, E. R., & Krendl, A. C. (2014). The effects of age on memory for socioemotional material: An affective neuroscience perspective. In P. Verhaeghen & C. Hertzog (Eds.), *The Oxford handbook of emotion, social cognition, and problem solving in adulthood* (p. 26). New York, NY: Oxford University Press.

Kensinger, E. A., Brierley, B., Medford, N., Growdon, J. H., & Corkin, S. (2002). Effects of normal aging and Alzheimer's disease on emotional memory. *Emotion, 2*(2), 118–134.

Kensinger, E. A., & Leclerc, C. M. (2009). Age-related changes in the neural mechanisms supporting emotion processing and emotional memory. *European Journal of Cognitive Psychology, 21*, 192–215.

Kensinger, E. A., & Schacter, D. L. (2008). Neural processes supporting young and older adults' emotional memories. *Journal of Cognitive Neuroscience, 20*(7), 1161–1173.

Knight, B. G., Maines, M. L., & Robinson, G. S. (2002). The effects of sad mood on memory in older adults: A test of the mood congruence effect. *Psychology and Aging, 17*(4), 653–661.

Knight, M., Seymour, T. L., Gaunt, J. T., Baker, C., Nesmith, K., & Mather, M. (2007). Aging and goal-directed emotional attention: Distraction reverses emotional biases. *Emotion, 7*(4), 705–714.

Labouvie-Vief, G. (2003). Dynamic integration: Affect, cognition and the self in adulthood. *Current Directions in Psychological Science, 12*, 201–206.

Labouvie-Vief, G., Diehl, M., Jain, E., & Zhang, F. (2007). Six-year change in affect optimization and affect complexity across the adult life span: A further examination. *Psychology and Aging, 22*(4), 738–751.

Labouvie-Vief, G., Gilet, A.-L., & Mella, N. (2014). The dynamics of cognitive–emotional integration: Complexity and hedonics in emotional development. In P. Verhaeghen & C. Hertzog (Eds.), *The Oxford handbook of emotion, social cognition, and problem solving in adulthood* (p. 83). New York, NY: Oxford University Press.

Labouvie-Vief, G., & Marquez, M. G. (2004). Dynamic integration: Affect optimization and differentiation in development. *Motivation, emotion, and cognition: Integrative perspectives on intellectual functioning and development* (pp. 237–272). Mahwah, NJ: Erlbaum.

Larcom, M. J., & Isaacowitz, D. M. (2009). Rapid emotion regulation after mood induction: Age and individual differences. *The Journals of Gerontology, Series B, 64*(6), 733–741.

Leclerc, C. M., & Kensinger, E. A. (2008). Age-related differences in medial prefrontal activation in response to emotional images. *Cognitive, Affective and Behavioral Neuroscience, 8*(2), 153–164.

Leclerc, C. M., & Kensinger, E. A. (2010). Age-related valence-based reversal in recruitment of medial prefrontal cortex on a visual search task. *Social Neuroscience, 5*(5–6), 560–576.

Leclerc, C. M., & Kensinger, E. A. (2011). Neural processing of emotional pictures and words: A comparison of young and older adults. *Developmental Neuropsychology, 36*(4), 519–538.

Levenson, R. W., Carstensen, L. L., Friesen, W. V., & Ekman, P. (1991). Emotion, physiology, and expression in old age. *Psychology and Aging, 6*(1), 28–35.

Levenson, R. W., Carstensen, L. L., & Gottman, J. M. (1994). The influence of age and gender on affect, physiology, and their interrelations: A study of long-term marriages. *Journal of Personality and Social Psychology, 67*(1), 56–68.

Light, J., & Isaacowitz, D. (2006). The effect of developmental regulation on visual attention: The example of the "biological clock." *Cognition and Emotion, 20*, 623–645.

Lindenberger, U., & Baltes, P. B. (1994). Sensory functioning and intelligence in old age: A strong connection. *Psychology and Aging, 9*(3), 339–355.

Lindquist, K. A. (2013). Emotions emerge from more basic psychological ingredients: A modern psychological constructionist model. *Emotion Review, 5*, 356–368.

Lindquist, K. A., & Barrett, L. F. (2012). A functional architecture of the human brain: Emerging insights from the science of emotion. *Trends in Cognitive Sciences, 16*(11), 533–540.

Löckenhoff, C. E., & Carstensen, L. L. (2007). Aging, emotion, and health-related decision strategies: Motivational manipulations can reduce age differences. *Psychology and Aging, 22*(1), 134–146.

Lohani, M., & Isaacowitz, D. M. (2014). Age differences in managing response to sadness elicitors using attentional deployment, positive reappraisal and suppression. *Cognition and Emotion, 28*(4), 678–697.

Luna, B., Thulborn, K. R., Munoz, D. P., Merriam, E. P., Garver, K. E., Minshew, N. J.,...Sweeney, J. A. (2001). Maturation of widely distributed brain function subserves cognitive development. *NeuroImage, 13*(5), 786–793.

Luong, G., Charles, S. T., & Fingerman, K. L. (2010). Better with age: Social relationships across adulthood. *Journal of Social and Personal Relationships, 28,* 9–23.

Madden, D. J., Langley, L. K., Denny, L. L., Turkington, T. G., Provenzale, J. M., Hawk, T. C., & Coleman, R. E. (2002). Adult age differences in visual word identification: Functional neuroanatomy by positron emission tomography. *Brain and Cognition, 49*(3), 297–321.

Majerus, S., & D'Argembeau, A. (2011). *Semantic knowledge supports verbal short-term memory: The case of emotional words.* Symposium presentation invited by P. Hoffman, S. Saito, M. Lambon-Ralph, International Conference on Memory (ICOM) V. York, United Kingdom.

Mather, M. (2012). The emotion paradox in the aging brain. *Annals of the New York Academy of Sciences, 1251,* 33–49.

Mather, M., Canli, T., English, T., Whitfield, S., Wais, P., Ochsner, K.,...Carstensen, L. L. (2004). Amygdala responses to emotionally valenced stimuli in older and younger adults. *Psychological Science, 15*(4), 259–263.

Mather, M., & Carstensen, L. L. (2005). Aging and motivated cognition: The positivity effect in attention and memory. *Trends in Cognitive Sciences, 9*(10), 496–502.

Mather, M., & Johnson, M. K. (2000). Choice-supportive source monitoring: Do our decisions seem better to us as we age? *Psychology and Aging, 15*(4), 596–606.

Mather, M., & Knight, M. (2005). Goal-directed memory: The role of cognitive control in older adults' emotional memory. *Psychology and Aging, 20*(4), 554–570.

Mather, M., & Sutherland, M. R. (2011). Arousal-biased competition in perception and memory. *Perspectives on Psychological Science: A Journal of the Association for Psychological Science, 6*(2), 114–133.

Mendes, W. B. (2010). Weakened links between mind and body in older age: The case for maturational dualism in the experience of emotion. *Emotion Review, 2,* 240–244.

Mienaltowski, A., & Blanchard-Fields, F. (2005). The differential effects of mood on age differences in the correspondence bias. *Psychology and Aging, 20*(4), 589–600.

Morgan, E. S., & Scheibe, S. (2014). Reconciling cognitive decline and increased well-being with age: The role of increased emotion regulation efficiency. In P. Verhaeghen & C. Hertzog (Eds.), *The Oxford handbook of emotion, social cognition, and problem solving in adulthood* (p. 155). New York, NY: Oxford University Press.

Mroczek, D. K., & Almeida, D. M. (2004). The effect of daily stress, personality, and age on daily negative affect. *Journal of Personality, 72*(2), 355–378.

Murty, V. P., Sambataro, F., Das, S., Tan, H. Y., Callicott, J. H., Goldberg, T. E., Meyer-Lindenberg, A., . . . Mattay, V. S. (2009). Age-related alterations in simple declarative memory and the effect of negative stimulus valence. *Journal of Cognitive Neuroscience, 21*(10), 1920–1933.

Nashiro, K., Sakaki, M., & Mather, M. (2011). Age differences in brain activity during emotion processing: Reflections of age-related decline or increased emotion regulation? *Gerontology, 58*, 156–163.

Ochsner, K. N., & Gross, J. J. (2005). The cognitive control of emotion. *Trends in Cognitive Sciences, 9*(5), 242–249.

Perlstein, W. M., Elbert, T., & Stenger, V. A. (2002). Dissociation in human prefrontal cortex of affective influences on working memory-related activity. *Proceedings of the National Academy of Sciences of the United States of America, 99*(3), 1736–1741.

Pessoa, L. (2008). On the relationship between emotion and cognition. *Nature Reviews. Neuroscience, 9*(2), 148–158.

Phelps, E. A. (2006). Emotion and cognition: Insights from studies of the human amygdala. *Annual Review of Psychology, 57*, 27–53.

Pruzan, K., & Isaacowitz, D. M. (2006). An attentional application of socioemotional selectivity theory in college students. *Social Development, 15*, 326–338.

Qin, P., & Northoff, G. (2011). How is our self related to midline regions and the default-mode network? *Neuroimage, 57*(3), 1221–1233.

Reed, A. E., & Carstensen, L. L. (2012). The theory behind the age-related positivity effect. *Frontiers in Psychology, 3*, 339.

Reed, A. E., Chan, L., & Mikels, J. A. (2014). Meta-analysis of the age-related positivity effect: Age differences in preferences for positive over negative information. *Psychology and Aging, 29*(1), 1–15.

Salthouse, T. A. (1996). The processing-speed theory of adult age differences in cognition. *Psychological Review, 103*(3), 403–428.

Salzman, C. D., & Fusi, S. (2010). Emotion, cognition, and mental state representation in amygdala and prefrontal cortex. *Annual Review of Neuroscience, 33*, 173–202.

Samanez-Larkin, G. R., & Carstensen, L. L. (2011). Socioemotional functioning and the aging brain. In J. Decety & J. T. Cacioppo (Eds.) *The Oxford handbook of social neuroscience* (pp. 507–521). New York, NY: Oxford University Press.

Sands, M., & Isaacowitz, D. M. (2016). Situation selection across adulthood: The role of arousal. *Cognition and Emotion*, 1–8.

Sands, M., Ngo, N., & Isaacowitz, D. M. (2016). The interplay of motivation and emotion: View from adulthood and old age. In M. Lewis, J. M. Haviland-Jones, & L. F. Barrett (Eds.), *Handbook of emotions* (pp. 336–349). New York, NY: Guilford Press.

Schwarz, N. (2011). Feelings-as-information theory. In P. A. M. Van Lange, A. Kruglanski, & E. T. Higgins (Eds.), *Handbook of theories of social psychology* (pp. 289–308). Thousand Oaks, CA: Sage.

St. Jacques, P. L., Dolcos, F., & Cabeza, R. (2009). Effects of aging on functional connectivity of the amygdala for subsequent memory of negative pictures: A network analysis of functional magnetic resonance imaging data. *Psychological Science, 20*(1), 74–84.

Streubel, B., & Kunzmann, U. (2011). Age differences in emotional reactions: Arousal and age-relevance count. *Psychology and Aging, 26*(4), 966–978.

Sutherland, M. R., & Mather, M. (2015). Negative arousal increases the effects of stimulus salience in older adults. *Experimental Aging Research, 41*(3), 259–271.

Tessitore, A., Hariri, A. R., Fera, F., Smith, W. G., Das, S., Weinberger, D. R., & Mattay, V. S. (2005). Functional changes in the activity of brain regions underlying emotion processing in the elderly. *Psychiatry Research, 139*(1), 9–18.

Thomas, R. C., & Hasher, L. (2006). The influence of emotional valence on age differences in early processing and memory. *Psychology and Aging, 21*(4), 821–825.

Uchino, B. N., Birmingham, W., & Berg, C. A. (2010). Are older adults less or more physiologically reactive? A meta-analysis of age-related differences in cardiovascular reactivity to laboratory tasks. *The Journals of Gerontology, Series B, 65*(2), 154–162.

Uchino, B. N., Holt-Lunstad, J., Bloor, L. E., & Campo, R. A. (2005). Aging and cardiovascular reactivity to stress: Longitudinal evidence for changes in stress reactivity. *Psychology and Aging, 20*(1), 134–143.

Urry, H. L., & Gross, J. J. (2010). Emotion regulation in older age. *Current Directions in Psychological Science, 19*, 352–357.

Waldinger, R. J., Kensinger, E. A., & Schulz, M. S. (2011). Neural activity, neural connectivity, and the processing of emotionally valenced information in older adults: Links with life satisfaction. *Cognitive, Affective & Behavioral Neuroscience, 11*(3), 426–436.

Williams, L. M., Brown, K. J., Palmer, D., Liddell, B. J., Kemp, A. H., Olivieri, G.,...Gordon, E. (2006). The mellow years?: Neural basis of improving emotional stability over age. *The Journal of Neuroscience, 26*(24), 6422–6430.

Winston, J. S., Gottfried, J. A., Kilner, J. M., & Dolan, R. J. (2005). Integrated neural representations of odor intensity and affective valence in human amygdala. *The Journal of Neuroscience, 25*(39), 8903–8907.

Wright, C. I., Wedig, M. M., Williams, D., Rauch, S. L., & Albert, M. S. (2006). Novel fearful faces activate the amygdala in healthy young and elderly adults. *Neurobiology of Aging, 27*(2), 361–374.

Wrzus, C., Müller, V., Wagner, G. G., Lindenberger, U., & Riediger, M. (2012). Affective and cardiovascular responding to unpleasant events from adolescence to old age: Complexity of events matters. *Developmental Psychology, 49*, 384–397.

Wurm, L. H., Labouvie-Vief, G., Aycock, J., Rebucal, K. A., & Koch, H. E. (2004). Performance in auditory and visual emotional stroop tasks: A comparison of older and younger adults. *Psychology and Aging, 19*(3), 523–535.

Yonelinas, A. P. (2002). The nature of recollection and familiarity: A review of 30 years of research. *Journal of Memory and Language, 46*, 441–517.

CHAPTER 13

Theories of Social Support in Health and Aging
Bert N. Uchino, Anthony D. Ong, Tara L. Queen, and Robert G. Kent de Grey

Social support from close relationships is one of the most well-documented psychosocial predictors of physical health outcomes (Berkman, Glass, Brissette, & Seeman, 2000; Cohen, 2004; Holt-Lunstad, Smith, & Layton, 2010; Uchino, 2004). As a result, the concept of social support has played an important role across disciplines including psychology, sociology, neuroscience, and medicine. It can be defined as the perceived availability (i.e., perceived support) or actual exchange (i.e., received support) of resources from others. These important resources include emotional (e.g., expressions of caring), informational (e.g., information that might be used to deal with stress), tangible (e.g., direct material aid, also referred to as "instrumental," "practical," or "financial" support), and belonging (e.g., others to engage in social activities) support (Cohen, Mermelstein, Kamarck, & Hoberman, 1985; Cutrona & Russell, 1990). Social support is distinguishable from other health-relevant social processes including social integration (i.e., structural characteristics of one's social network; see Chapter 18 by Wong and Waite, this volume) and social negativity (i.e., conflict; see Brooks & Dunkel-Schetter, 2011).

Much of the work on social support and health has been conducted by researchers focused on disease-related outcomes (e.g., physiology, mortality). As a result, we know much less about how social support from close relationships is related to health across the life span and how developmental processes might influence such links. This is an important omission because many chronic conditions develop slowly over time and hence may be influenced by life-span support processes. In addition, chronic conditions in the aging adult present unique developmental challenges that increase the need for quality social support. In the present chapter, epidemiological work on social support and health is reviewed first, followed by major life-span models that have implications for understanding these issues. A life-span model of social support and health that has been informed by these perspectives is reviewed, including critical directions for future work.

■ SOCIAL SUPPORT AND PHYSICAL HEALTH

Research linking social support to disease outcomes has a long and rich history. One of the earliest studies by Blazer (1982) examined a community sample of older adults in Durham County, North Carolina. Even when considering standard control variables such as physical health status and smoking, perceptions of social support from close others predicted lower mortality rates. These results held even when considering structural measures of social integration (e.g., important social roles) thereby showing an independent association with health.

The reliability and strength of the link between social support and health has subsequently been confirmed in recent meta-analyses. Holt-Lunstad et al. (2010) examined 148 studies comprising more than 300,000 participants from around the globe including the United States, Europe, Asia, and Australia. They found that social support was associated with a 46% increased likelihood of survival. Importantly, the link between social support and mortality was consistent across age, sex, geographical region, initial health status, and cause of death (Holt-Lunstad et al., 2010). Indeed, effect sizes for these associations were comparable to standard biomedical risk factors including smoking and physical activity. Shor, Roelfs, and Yogev (2013) further showed that social support from familial sources were especially strong predictors of lower mortality.

Although social support predicts mortality, it is not the case that all indicators are similarly predictive of health outcomes. There is significant variability based on how social support is operationalized (Uchino, 2004). In prior work, the concepts of perceived and received support have been used interchangeably with the assumption that individuals high in perceived support also received more support from others (Barrera, 1986; Dunkel-Schetter & Bennett, 1990; Uchino, 2009). However, measures of perceived and received support are only moderately correlated and hence seem to represent distinct constructs (Haber, Cohen, Lucas, & Baltes, 2007). In one meta-analysis, perceived support was significantly related to increased survival whereas measures of received support did not predict survival (Holt-Lunstad et al., 2010). In fact, several epidemiological studies examining received support (especially tangible support) found it to be associated with *higher* subsequent mortality rates (Forster & Stoller, 1992; Krause, 1997). Thus, one important distinction in this literature is between perceived and received support, which has significant theoretical and applied implications (Uchino, 2009; Wills & Shinar, 2000).

■ THEORETICAL PERSPECTIVES ON SOCIAL SUPPORT IN HEALTH AND AGING

Most of the work on social support and health does not take into account the rich theoretical perspectives in the life-span development literature. One potential reason for this omission is that most life-span theories are about how aging influences sociomotivational processes more generally and are not as specific to social support. Major life-span perspectives and their implications for social support processes are reviewed in the following paragraphs, starting with more general theoretical frameworks followed by those more specific to social interactions.

Life-Span Perspectives on Social Support

Broad perspectives on life-span development and social interactions come from the theory of selection, optimization, and compensation (SOC; Baltes, 1997) and motivational theory (MT; Heckhausen, Wrosch, & Schulz, 2010). These perspectives argue that aging is associated with challenges that can be met with adaptive processes that facilitate adjustment. SOC focuses on how the processes of selection (e.g., goal specification), optimization (e.g., attentional focus, effort), and compensation (e.g., increased attentional focus, effort) can help individuals maintain functioning or regulate age-related losses (Baltes, 1997). Importantly, one way individuals can compensate for age-related losses is via social support (i.e., help by others). MT also postulates that age-related decreases in primary control capacity elicit the need for secondary control strategies such as enhanced self-regulation and/or perceived control. In addition, individuals can compensate for decreases in primary control capacity via compensatory primary control, which includes seeking the help of others. Thus, both SOC and MT postulate that receiving social support from others can play an adaptive role in compensating for the challenges associated with aging.

Socioemotional selectivity theory (SST) and the related strength and vulnerability integration (SAVI) model focus more specifically on the role of social processes in life-span development (Carstensen, Isaacowitz, & Charles, 1999; Charles, 2010). SST highlights the importance of emotional goals as individuals age, which lead older individuals to actively select or prioritize emotionally close social ties to more peripheral ones (Carstensen et al., 1999). Thus, the social networks of older adults should contain more emotionally close relationships that might be rich sources of social support. An added perspective on SST is provided by Fingerman's social input model that highlights the dyadic nature of relationships in that older individuals may also have more positive relationships because others treat them better (Fingerman & Charles, 2010).

The SAVI model is a more general perspective built on SST and explains why older adults often have better well-being and takes into account both perceptions of time left and experience gained over time (Charles, 2010). With experience, individuals have learned to avoid negative situations and/or de-escalate existing negativity with close others by using selective strategies, some of which are activated after the fact (Blanchard-Fields, 2007; Charles, 2010). By incorporating aspects of SST, the predictions of SAVI regarding social support are similar although it also stipulates conditions under which older adults might suffer more from the aging process. One such condition is the loss of social belongingness, which might be more impactful to older adults given age-related vulnerabilities (Charles, 2010).

Finally, the Convoy model is the most specific model in terms of life-span approaches to social support. It argues that the need for different relationships and support resources depends heavily on a variety of personal and situational (e.g., age, socioeconomic status) factors (Antonucci, Ajrouch, & Birditt, 2013; Kahn & Antonucci, 1980). This model is also unique in that it explicitly acknowledges the difference between perceived and received support and the double-edged nature of relationships; that is, their ability to deliver responsive support and upsetting interpersonal conflict. It further predicts that the ability of social support to bolster self-efficacy and reduce stress may be major pathways linking relationships to health (Antonucci et al., 2013).

Limitation of Existing Life-Span Theories for Social Support Processes

The rich literature on life-span development has highlighted a number of important processes that are likely to occur when faced with life challenges (Baltes, 1997; Carstensen et al., 1999). However, these models are more limited when applied directly to understanding links between social support and health across the life span. With the exception of the convoy model (Antonucci et al., 2013), these models typically do not draw the crucial distinction between perceived and received support, which appears to differentially influence health. In addition, all of these models highlight the challenges associated with aging in older adulthood and hence speak less to the development of social support earlier in life. Finally, none of the models highlights the specific biological pathways and their implications on how social support and disease development may unfold together over the life span. This is important because social support processes from a life-span perspective may highlight how relationships influence the long-term development of more chronic conditions, as opposed to the course of already diagnosed chronic conditions. In the next section, a life-span model of support that addresses these challenges is presented along with research on its basic premise.

■ A LIFE-SPAN THEORY OF SOCIAL SUPPORT AND HEALTH

In order to elaborate on the developmental processes over time that might impact social support from close relationships and health, a life-span model of support has been proposed that attempts to integrate prior work and models across disciplines (Uchino, 2009). An important aspect of the model is that it explicitly proposes the separability of perceived and received social support in the context of early and late life-span development processes. Thus, different antecedent and mediating processes are thought to link perceived and received support to health. It also makes predictions about how social support may impact health across the life span, including the specification of more concrete psychological and/or biological mechanisms and disease endpoints.

Overview of Theory

As shown in Figure 13.1, the perceived availability of social support is thought to originate in the early family environment (Sarason, Sarason, & Shearin, 1986). If perceived support develops in the context of early parent–child interactions, an important question becomes what else *codevelops* in the context of such familial environments (Shaw, Krause, Chatters, Connell, & Ingersoll-Dayton, 2004). The model specifies that individuals with nurturing early family environments develop positive psychosocial profiles, including perceived support, certain personality traits/individual differences, social skills, self-esteem, and feelings of personal control (also see Flaherty & Richman, 1986; Shaw et al., 2004). These positive profiles are in turn predicted to be associated with health via distinct mechanisms, especially proactive coping (Aspinwall & Taylor, 1997), healthy behavioral choices, cooperation with medical regimens (DiMatteo, 2004), and disease-specific biological mechanisms. Importantly, it is also postulated that perceived support should be linked to chronic disease development over time due to its early familial influences, stability, and association with other positive profiles.

In contrast to perceived support, received support is more of a situational factor that arises in response to stressful circumstances (see Figure 13.2; Barrera, 2000; Carver, Scheier, & Weintraub, 1989; Thoits, 1986). The health implications of viewing received support as more of a situational factor is that the antecedent conditions and mediators may differ substantially from perceived support. As shown in the top half of Figure 13.2, the stress context will play a focal role in the effectiveness of coping options, only one of which includes receiving support. Based on these contextual processes, potential psychological pathways at different points of the coping process are evident. For instance, depending on at what point support is received, it may then have influences on psychological, behavioral, and biological pathways, such as alterations in one's sense of control, health behaviors, or cardiovascular function, in a positive or negative manner (Bolger & Amarel, 2007; Testa & Collins, 1997). This latter point is important because receiving support is not always beneficial and dependent on its responsiveness to the context (Reis, 2007). Thus, this model incorporates both positive and negative interpersonal transactions, which is important because receiving less responsive support (e.g., insensitivity, criticism) are predictors of negative health

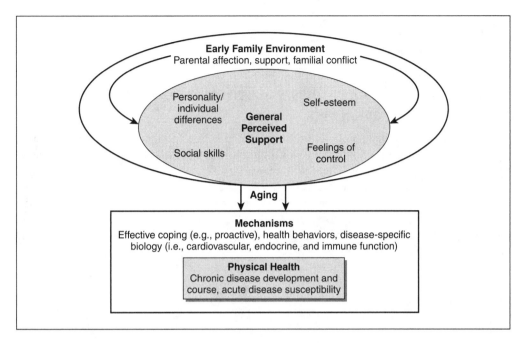

FIGURE 13.1 Life-span model linking perceived support to physical health.

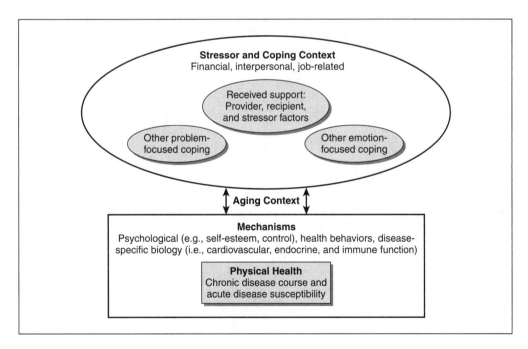

FIGURE 13.2 Life-span model linking received social support to physical health.

outcomes in their own right (De Vogli, Chandola, & Marmot, 2007; Rook, 2015). Because of these processes, it is hypothesized that received support should primarily influence acute disease susceptibility and the course of diagnosed chronic disease in a healthy or unhealthy manner depending on contextual factors. Finally, how an individual copes with health problems also influences their close relationships; hence, the importance of modeling reciprocal influences (Berg & Upchurch, 2007; Bolger, Foster, Vinokur, & Ng, 1996; Coyne & Smith, 1991).

Evidence for the Life-Span Theory of Social Support: Perceived Support and Health

Although more work is needed, there is evidence for this life-span theory of social support and health. Consistent with Figure 13.1, nurturing parent–child transactions including caring, affection, positive involvement, and low conflict appear to set the basis for supportive relational schemas (Flaherty & Richman, 1986). Perceived support is also stable over time (despite changes in social circumstances) and linked to individuals' retrospective perceptions of their early familial experiences whether assessed in adolescence or emerging adulthood (Doucet & Aseltine, 2003; Engels, Dekovic, & Meeus, 2002; Graves, Wang, Mead, Johnson, & Klag, 1998).

Consistent with the theory, these early family processes have also been linked to health at different stages of the life span. Retrospective reports of parental interest and negative behavior have been shown to predict self-reported physical problems experienced during adolescence and young adulthood (e.g., headaches, cough, pain; Mechanic, 1980). In addition, harsh family environments have been linked to an increase in a proinflammatory phenotype over time in adolescents (Miller & Chen, 2010). These associations between perceptions of early parent–child relationships and health during adolescence suggest that these patterns have potential to continue through life, predicting health outcomes throughout adulthood. Consistent with this possibility, longitudinal studies on parental support in young adulthood and midlife health have found that adults who reported higher parental warmth and closeness were less likely to have (a) poor self-rated health (Poon & Knight, 2013), (b) components of the metabolic syndrome (Miller et al., 2011), and (c) diagnosed diseases at midlife (Russek & Schwartz, 1997), including cardiovascular disease (Dong et al., 2004). Finally, Shaw et al. (2004) assessed retrospective reports of early parental relationships in adults (aged 25–75 years). Participants who reported less support from parents during childhood had more chronic conditions in adulthood (Shaw et al., 2004). The relationships between parental support and adult health did not vary by age, suggesting that the effects of parental support persist even into older adulthood.

The model in Figure 13.1 also predicts that strong perceptions of social support codevelop with other positive psychosocial processes to form a profile that is conducive to health. Prior work suggests that perceived support is related to personality factors such as a secure attachment style, higher optimism, and lower hostility (Anders & Tucker, 2000; Gallo & Smith, 1999). Importantly, these personality factors have established links to physical health and appear to have significant interpersonal origins (Gallo & Smith, 1999). The early family environment is also linked to a broad array of psychosocial processes relevant to physical health (Repetti, Robles, & Reynolds, 2011). For instance, low family support has been related to poorer coping strategies in children (Hardy, Power, & Jaedicke, 1993). Such early familial processes also influence the development of basic social skills that are important for the formation of supportive social networks (Sarason, Sarason, Hacker, & Basham, 1985). In fact, links are also evident between perceived support and feelings of control, self-efficacy, and self-esteem in young and older adults (e.g., Shaw et al., 2004; Symister & Friend, 2003). These associations are important because these psychological factors also appear to have influences on physical health in their own right (Shaw et al., 2004).

The downstream consequence of a positive early family environment and psychosocial profile is that such individuals can cope more effectively, flexibly, and proactively with life stressors. That is, they have choices and a broader skill/coping set that can be used to manage and anticipate the challenges in life. Consistent with this view, perceived social support is related to greater proactive coping (Aspinwall & Taylor, 1997) and existing longitudinal studies have found social support to predict lower stress exposure (e.g., Russell & Cutrona, 1991). Thus, individuals high in perceived support appear to live less turbulent lives over the life span, which may translate to better physical health over the years.

This life-span view also addresses the phase of the disease process that should be impacted by perceived support. That is, due to its early family origins, stability, and association with other positive profiles, perceived support should be linked to lower chronic disease development (i.e., incidence) than measures of received support via long-term age-related benefits to cardiovascular, endocrine, and immune function. There is evidence that perceived support is related to a lower risk for the development of cardiovascular disease (Cené et al., 2012; Orth-Gomér, Rosengren, & Wilhelmsen, 1993; Wang, Mittleman, & Orth-Gomer, 2005; but see Ikeda et al., 2008). Given the characteristics of perceived support, the model also predicts that it will have beneficial influences on acute disease risk and the prognosis for diagnosed chronic diseases more generally. Evidence exists linking social support to better infectious diseases outcomes and the course of chronic conditions such as cardiovascular disease (Barth, Schneider, & von Känel, 2010; Uchino, Vaughn, Carlisle, & Birmingham, 2012).

Evidence for the Life-Span Theory of Social Support: Received Support and Health

In contrast to perceived support, received support is less likely to represent early familial processes but a situational factor that is sought or provided in response to stress based on stressor and social–personal resources (Barrera, 2000). This argument, of course, is a relative one but consistent with various models that include support seeking as an increasingly important resource across the life span (Baltes, 1997; Berg & Upchurch, 2007; Carver et al., 1989; Heckhausen, Wrosch, & Schulz, 2010; Thoits, 1986). Consistent with this resource perspective, most studies have found that received support is increased as a function of age (i.e., aged 55–104 years; Lang & Carstensen, 1994; Martire, Schulz, Mittelmark, & Newsom, 1999; van Tilburg, 1998; but see Antonucci & Akiyama, 1987).

As shown in Figure 13.2, an important aspect of this view of received support based on the broader coping literature is that not all forms of coping are beneficial and its effectiveness may depend heavily on the stress and coping context (Berg & Upchurch, 2007; Bolger, Zuckerman, & Kessler, 2000). Of these contextual processes, provider (e.g., relationship quality), recipient (e.g., choice in receiving support), and stressor (e.g., match between stressor and type of support) characteristics appear important (Uchino, 2009). For instance, a key provider characteristic is past conflict that can undermine the effectiveness of received support. A number of studies have shown that perceiving a support provider as a source of "ambivalence" can decrease the efficacy of received support (Holt-Lunstad, Uchino, Smith, & Hicks, 2007; Reblin, Uchino, & Smith, 2010).

These contextual factors influencing the efficacy of received support appear to be shaped by culture and related socialization processes. Flaherty and Richman (1989) found evidence that socialization processes result in women both preferring and bene-fiting more from receiving emotional support. Likewise, it has been found that men may benefit more from receiving instrumental support, especially from other men (Craig & Deichert, 2002). At a broad level, research on cultural differences in support highlights the importance of recipients receiving culturally appropriate forms of support (e.g., familial support; Brannan, Biswas-Diener, Mohr, Mortazavi, & Stein, 2013; Dressler & Bindon, 2000).

The contextual processes in Figure 13.2 are also consistent with the life-span literature on the well-being of older adults. Age is typically associated with higher levels of received support (Lang & Carstensen, 1994; Martire et al., 1999). However, this may not always be a good thing as it may threaten the older adult's sense of independence and control (Baltes, 1995, 1997; Martire & Schulz, 2007). A distinction can be drawn between receiv-ing autonomy-enhancing and autonomy-decreasing support (Baltes, 1995; Martire & Schulz, 2007; Rowe & Kahn, 1987). Baltes (1995) argues that older adults appear to be subject to the dependency-support script in which their dependent behavior is rein-forced. In contrast, the independent behavior of the older adult is more likely to be ignored (i.e., independence-ignore script). Importantly, it is the autonomy-enhancing nature of received social support that may be beneficial (Martire & Schulz, 2007) and hence its absence is particularly detrimental to older adults.

The health implications of viewing received support as more of a situational factor are that the antecedent conditions and mediators may differ substantially from per-ceived support. As shown in Figure 13.2, the stressor context should play a more focal role in the effectiveness of coping options, only one of which includes receiving support as there may be other problem and emotion-focused coping strategies available (Carver et al., 1989). These contextual factors may then influence psychological processes such as one's sense of esteem/control in a positive or negative manner. For instance, receiving unsolicited support may be detrimental because it can threaten one's sense of esteem and competence (Bolger & Amarel, 2007). Hence, the skillful provision of "invisible sup-port" that is not noticed by the recipient but helpful nonetheless (e.g., doing extra chores temporarily so recipient can relax after a stressful day) is related to more positive out-comes (Bolger & Amarel, 2007; Howland & Simpson, 2010).

The influence of received support on chronic disease development should thus be attenuated because (a) of the variability associated with the effectiveness of received support and (b) it is just one of many coping options that could influence biological function. It is more likely that received support would primarily influence acute dis-ease susceptibility and the course of already diagnosed chronic disease. However, these associations can be either healthy or unhealthy depending on age-related contextual processes (Wallsten, Tweed, Blazer, & George, 1999). Although less data are available concerning these predictions, Selcuk and Ong (2013) recently found that receiving social support was related to higher mortality only if it was viewed as low in responsiveness. These data are consistent with other health studies that emphasize the crucial impor-tance of responsive social interactions (Slatcher, Selcuk, & Ong, 2015).

Finally, coping with a chronic disease is a significant stressor that influences not only the patient but also his or her close relationships and hence can have reciprocal influ-ences on the stress and coping context (Berg & Upchurch, 2007; Coyne & Smith, 1991). In one study, researchers directly tested this possibility by examining how support was influenced when couples attempted to cope with the diagnosis and treatment of breast cancer (Bolger, Foster, Vinokur, & Ng, 1996). These researchers found that, although support was initially mobilized in response to the diagnosis, the patient's distress was related to an erosion of received support from the spouse over time (also see Northouse, Templin, Mood, & Oberst, 1998). Thus, modeling reciprocal links between mechanisms and/or disease outcomes on the stress and coping contexts, especially dyadic-level processes, are important.

■ FUTURE DIRECTIONS AND APPLICATIONS OF THE THEORY

The life-span theory of support and health argues for the separability of perceived and received support based on different developmental antecedents and mediators (Uchino, 2009). It also makes more specific predictions about the role of these different facets of social support on disease development in comparison to its clinical course. Based on this view, there are a number of important future directions that warrant strong consideration, including linking the theory to health, expanding the domain of the theory, and novel intervention implications.

Linking the Theory to Health

Much of the data for this life-span theory of support and disease come from research on older adults given their greater vulnerability to physical health problems. This work is consistent with the SAVI model that highlights the potential negative influences of a loss of social resources in the elderly (Charles, 2010). For instance, low social support and feelings of loneliness are related to higher levels of blood pressure and cardiovascular reactivity, especially in older adults (Hawkley, Thisted, Masi, & Cacioppo, 2010; Ong & Allaire, 2005; Ong, Rothstein, & Uchino, 2012; Uchino, Holt-Lunstad, Uno, Betancourt, & Garvey, 1999). However, the life-span theory of social support and health also highlights the crucial role of the early family environment in the development of perceived support, which over time influences more downstream psychological, behavioral, and physiological pathways relevant to disease. The aforementioned studies are cross-sectional and hence cannot rule out whether these represent older adults' greater sensitivity to social losses or age-related changes that have their roots in the early family environment. A major challenge for future research would be to model these processes simultaneously over time to disentangle these theoretical predictions.

This life-span theory also suggests that a profile approach, which includes perceived support, would be useful for examining links to health. This represents an important alternative framework because most prior work is based on single psychosocial risk-factor modeling. Although such an approach is more tractable, it ignores the fact that many psychosocial processes appear to share common developmental antecedents (Shaw et al., 2004; Uchino, 2009). The theory suggests that there may be multiple components to this profile that range from social (e.g., social skills) to personal (e.g., personality, control) attributes that codevelop in the early family environment. At present, research has not delineated the main aspects of this profile that are health relevant. Future work examining multiple psychosocial risk factors using appropriate statistical modeling (e.g., latent profile analyses) will be needed to address these issues.

The theory also suggests that received support is more contextual and thus one needs to consider provider, recipient, and stressor factors. Because of these contextual factors, received support can have beneficial or detrimental influences on health depending on how these processes unfold. It also highlights the possibility that receiving low levels of support in some contexts may not be detrimental as individuals might be engaged in a broader set of effective coping behaviors (Carver et al., 1989). In such situations, it is possible that individuals would forego seeking support due to concerns about autonomy and/or relational threats. Indeed, as highlighted by other life-span models, such coping options may help to maintain beneficial levels of autonomy or control striving in the older adult (Baltes, 1997; Schulz & Heckhausen, 1996). Ideally, broader coping options would be enacted along with the receipt of autonomy-enhancing support, which is responsive to the context. Future work will be needed to determine the best balance of these coping options as well as which works best for what situations and for whom (e.g., individual differences).

One area that is in need of much more research is the predicted links in the model to different phases of the disease process. Given its early family roots and stability, it is hypothesized that perceived support should predict the development of chronic conditions such as cardiovascular disease that develop slowly over the life span. There is evidence consistent with the role of perceived support on lower cardiovascular disease incidence (André-Petersson, Hedblad, Janzon, & Ostergren, 2006; Orth-Gomér et al., 1993; Räikkönen et al., 2001). The theory would also predict that received support would not be associated with the development of chronic diseases. To date, there appears to be no research examining links between received support and the development of cardiovascular disease. However, less responsive received support is related to higher mortality rates, which is consistent with the contextual nature of the model (Selcuk & Ong, 2013). More generally, research is needed on the specificity of the links between perceived and received support to the development and course of cardiovascular disease, as well as other chronic and acute conditions (e.g., cancer, infectious diseases).

This framework also has implications for the concept of successful aging, which encompasses physical health, cognitive function, and social engagement (Rowe & Kahn, 1998). It predicts that individuals high in perceived support are more likely to have successfully aged in terms of their physical health (Horsten et al., 1999; Wang, Mittleman, & Orth-Gomer, 2005). In a series of studies, it was found that perceived support moderated age-related differences in resting blood pressure (Uchino et al., 1995, 1999). That is, older adults who were high in perceived support had resting blood pressure levels that were comparable to individuals almost 50 years younger than them (Uchino et al., 1995). Such data imply that individuals high in perceived support have more disease-free years with corresponding influences on the quality of their lives and relationships. There is also some evidence suggesting that perceived support predicts better cognitive (Gow, Corley, Starr, & Deary, 2013; Seeman, Lusignolo, Albert, & Berkman, 2001) and interpersonal (Bowen et al., 2013; Sarason et al., 1986) functioning. Thus, perceived support might be a central factor in successful aging and future work that better integrates these perspectives should be fruitful.

Demonstrating the Domain of the Theory

Although the life-span model of support postulates that crucial processes are occurring early in life and in older adults, data are needed on the proposed theoretical processes across the entire life span, including adolescence, emerging adulthood, and midlife. In adolescence, the establishment of strong peer groups in the context of one's own autonomy appears to be linked to better outcomes many years later (Allen & Loeb, 2015). These two factors (i.e., supportive peer groups and autonomy) may be influenced by the family context and hence part of a positive psychosocial profile that place individuals on healthier trajectories. In comparison, emerging adulthood is a time of greater residential change and associated disruptions in social networks (Arnett, 2000). Studies in this group would allow an examination of the continuity of perceived social support and how it facilitates the formation of new relationships and the receipt of support for such life-stage specific challenges. Finally, midlife is a time of heightened role responsibilities (e.g., family, work) and hence appears to be a time of relatively greater interpersonal stress (Blanchflower & Oswald, 2008; Darbonne, Uchino, & Ong, 2013). Midlife is also a time of vulnerability for comorbid chronic diseases (e.g., diabetes and cardiovascular disease; Booth, Kapral, Fung, & Tu, 2006) so variations in perceived and received social support may partly explain potential differences in midlife disease risk. In general, more theoretical work is needed to better specify the potential antecedents and mechanisms that are impacted by the unique challenges at specific stages of the life course.

Another future challenge is to more clearly detail the association between perceived support and social negativity (e.g., conflict, insensitivity; Brooks & Dunkel-Schetter, 2011; Rook, 2015). Although links between positive and negative social exchanges in the theory are explicit for received support, much less is known about how one might model the association between perceived support, social negativity, and health. For instance, are links between perceived support and health independent, mediated, or moderated by social negativity? Such modeling is important because social negativity is emerging as a robust predictor of health problems in its own right (DeVogli et al., 2007; Sneed & Cohen, 2014). In fact, some studies suggest that social negativity is a stronger predictor of future health problems compared to positive social interactions that is consistent with a negativity bias in social information processing (Rook, 2015; Taylor, 1991). However, there is good reason to suspect that the influence of perceived support is at least not confounded with social negativity. A large number of studies have shown that positivity and negativity in relationships are separable dimensions of social functioning with relatively unique antecedent and mediating processes (Finch, Okun, Barrera, Zautra, & Reich, 1989; Ruehlman & Karoly, 1991). This suggests more complex models linking relationship positivity and negativity that can be tested based on Figure 13.1. For instance, perceived support may be linked to lower amounts of negative social interactions over time (e.g., less stress exposure) caused by proactive coping or codeveloped social skills. Thus, social negativity may be a mediator of links between perceived support and health. However, few studies have contrasted broad measures of perceived support with similarly broad measures of social negativity so that future work would be needed to address these issues.

Although two distinct models were presented linking perceived and received support to health, more work is needed on how perceived and received support might interact in potentially important ways. For instance, what are the consequences of receiving support for individuals who are low versus high in perceived support? There is very little research that examines this issue, perhaps because of the conceptual overlap that is often assumed among these two support measures. One interesting possibility is, given their more positive interpersonal schemas, individuals high in perceived support may be more receptive and hence benefit more from received support. In comparison, the theoretical model suggests an alternative prediction. That is, because of the codevelopment of other positive psychosocial factors (e.g., self-esteem), when support is simply provided, individuals high in support may not benefit because it is deemed unnecessary (discounted) or could threaten their codeveloped sense of esteem or control. Several existing studies are consistent with this latter prediction (Lindner, Sarason, & Sarason, 1988; Sarason & Sarason, 1986), which is salient because of the proposed separability of these measures of support.

In a related point, there are other measurement approaches to social support that might reflect an integration of processes operating in both Figures 13.1 and 13.2. One important measurement strategy is relationship-specific measures of perceived support. Research by Lakey and colleagues (e.g., Lakey & Scoboria, 2005; Lakey, McCabe, Fisicaro, & Drew, 1996) suggests that relationship-specific measures are related, but distinct from general perceptions of support (also see Pierce, Sarason, & Sarason, 1991). Moreover, relationship-specific assessments appear to more strongly reflect trait X situational influences (Lakey et al., 1996). This suggests that such measures may be reflective of processes operating in both Figures 13.1 and 13.2. Consistent with this possibility, studies that focus on the quality of parental and marital relationships suggest more general links to biology, disease development, and its course (Miller et al., 2011; Robles, Slatcher, Trombello, & McGinn, 2014; Russek & Schwartz, 1997). Of course, for such measures to have an impact on health, it is probably necessary for it to be an important developmental relationship (e.g., parents, spouse, children). Future research will be needed to test these possibilities, along with the possible impact of relationship-specific negativity (e.g., support erosion, conflict; Bolger et al., 1996; Manne & Glassman, 2000).

Examining relationship-specific measures are also important because it raises issues regarding the relative importance of different relationships at distinct points in the life span. For instance, as attachment relationships are beginning to be transferred from parents to peers during adolescence, does parental support become less influential to health compared to peer support during this time? In regards to perceptions of parent versus friend support over time, researchers have found that parental support decreases and friend support increases, though greater perceived parental support was related to fewer emotional problems (e.g., less stress, better general well-being) throughout adolescence (Helsen, Vollebergh, & Meeus, 2000). In a study comparing the influence of sources of support on adolescent health, researchers found that perceived support from parents, other adults, and friends were all positively correlated with self-reported health (Vilhjalmsson, 1994). In subsequent models comparing the influence of these sources of support on various aspects of health, only friend and parental support were related to health behaviors. Whereby parental support predicted engagement in a range of good health behaviors (e.g., exercise, healthy diet), friend support was positively associated with the likelihood of smoking. Of all the tested sources of support, parents had the largest total effect on adolescents' self-reported health, with more support predicting better health.

Directly testing the predictions of the theory in different cultures will also be important to examine its boundary conditions and/or generalizability. Most of the work on culture and social support has focused on differences between individualistic and collective (especially Asian) cultures and psychological outcomes. In one of the few studies focusing on health-relevant outcomes, Chiang et al. (2013) found that perceived support predicted lower interleukin-6 (IL-6) levels (an inflammatory cytokine linked to poor health) in European Americans but not Asians (although there was a similar trend in Asian Americans). An examination of culture also highlights the more specific aspects of support that are important. For instance, there is a significant distinction between explicit (i.e., seeking and using support) and implicit (i.e., the comfort of simply having close relationships) support (Taylor, Welch, Kim, & Sherman, 2009). Because of relational concerns (e.g., concern about placing a burden on family who are obligated to be helpful), individuals from more collective cultures may benefit more from implicit forms of support during stress in which they simply feel more connected with others (Mojaverian & Kim, 2013; Taylor et al., 2009). Consistent with this possibility, Taylor et al. (2007) found that an implicit support manipulation was associated with lower cortisol reactions in Asians compared to European Americans. One limitation of prior work on culture and social support, however, is that it has focused mostly on Asian cultures and whether the same pattern would be found in other collective cultures (e.g., African American, Latino/Hispanic) is less clear. It is also important to note that prior epidemiological work does not provide strong evidence for cultural differences in the link between perceived support and health (Uchino, 2004). In the meta-analysis by Holt-Lunstad et al. (2010), perceived support predicted lower mortality and was not moderated by the geographic location of the study (also see meta-analysis by Shor et al., 2013). Nevertheless, given the general theoretical work on culture and social support (Taylor et al., 2009), future research will be needed to refine aspects of Figures 13.1 and 13.2 to make them more sensitive to cultural variations in support processes that are health relevant.

Finally, stronger integration with existing life-span models will be necessary to maximize theoretical development. For instance, given the different ways that older adults can cope with losses in primary control (Baltes, 1997; Heckhausen et al., 2010) what is the relative role of perceived and received support compared to other strategies? To what extent does a shift toward affect optimization, in contrast to complexity (Labouvie-Vief, 2008), influence perceptions of support that are thought to be rooted in the early family environment? To this point, it is interesting that many studies find that perceptions of support are lower as a function of age (Goodwin, 2006; Grav, Hellzèn, Romild, & Stordal, 2011; Wrosch, Rueggeberg, & Hoppmann, 2013; but see Ingersoll-Dayton & Antonucci, 1988). Because of the greater need for received support in older adults, do such differences reflect age-associated negative support interactions that gradually erode perceptions of support over time (Charles, 2010)? Or do these findings reflect the age-related loss of developmentally important relationships that are the basis for supportive schemas (i.e., parents)? More generally, these findings are at odds with other life-span perspectives that find older adults report (a) more satisfaction with their relationships, (b) a positivity bias after social interactions, and (c) better overall well-being (Charles & Carstensen, 2009; Fingerman, Hay, & Birditt, 2004; Story et al., 2007). Integration of theoretical perspectives in this case suggests "anomalies" that can aid in further theoretical development.

Intervention Implications of the Theory

The present framework also has intriguing intervention implications that could be pursued in future work. Although support interventions have had success in some areas (Hogan, Linden, & Najarian, 2002), it has had much less of an impact in other areas (The ENRICHD Investigators, 2003). The model suggests part of this variability might be improved by getting a more comprehensive assessment prior to performing support interventions. Are individuals high or low in perceived support? Are they experiencing deficits in received support? These questions are important because they might result in more specific interventions. For instance, if individuals are low in perceived support, they might be better candidates for a general cognitive behavioral intervention that focuses on a wider set of psychosocial processes that they may lack (e.g., support seeking skills, perceptions of control). However, those high in perceived support might be provided with choices regarding more specific interpersonal exchanges and information that fosters their general understanding of the stressor of interest (e.g., support groups for cancer patients). It may also be important to match particular people with specific network members to create support dyads that best meet the demands of the situation (Lakey & Orehek, 2011).

Most social support interventions also target individuals who are most at risk or who already have psychological, behavioral, or medical problems. An alternative way of thinking about support interventions is as a form of primary prevention that focuses on healthy individuals (Kaplan, 2000). Given that many chronic diseases have a long-term etiology and develop over decades (e.g., coronary artery disease), primary prevention efforts in social support interventions may be particularly important to consider. For instance, given the developmental antecedents of perceived support, it is clear that early familial interventions are an important starting point. Such interventions have been conducted mostly in at-risk populations and show promise in fostering more positive child outcomes (Alexander, Sexton, & Robbins, 2002). This life-span perspective on perceived support also raises the interesting possibility that interventions may be usefully applied early in children and adolescents to help them codevelop positive profiles that then place them on healthier trajectories (e.g., Eggert, Thompson, Herting, Nicholas, & Dicker, 1994). This literature has also focused on a different set of outcomes (e.g., social interactions, grade point average [GPA]); however, existing studies suggest that social-skills training in adolescents results in positive social and academic outcomes (Dirks, Treat, & Weersing, 2007). One meta-analysis estimated that such interventions were associated with a 12% increase in adolescent achievement (Durlak, Weissberg, & Pachan, 2010), although the long-term nature of such interventions needs further evaluation (Beelmann, Pfingsten, & Losel, 1994). One strength of the current framework for support interventions is that it makes salient differing potential entry points, as well as approaches, depending on whether one is focusing on perceived or received support.

The theory also suggests interesting intervention possibilities with older adults. Perceived support appears to be lower as a function of age (Goodwin, 2006; Wrosch, Rueggeberg, & Hoppmann, 2013). In fact, several studies suggest that support seeking more generally is lower with increasing age (Aldwin, Sutton, Chiara, & Spiro, 1996; Folkman, Lazarus, Pimley, & Novacek, 1987). Combined with the finding that older adults receive more support, this suggests that older individuals are receiving more unsolicited support that has been linked to negative outcomes (Bolger & Amarel, 2007). Perceived and received support are moderately correlated (Haber et al., 2007); so experiences with receiving support over time can influence perceptions of support, especially if some of these experiences are more negative in nature (Baltes, 1997). These data suggest that interventions aimed at mitigating age-related differences in perceived support over time may be helpful for the health of older adults. Interventions range from training close others to provide autonomy support (Baltes, 1997) to priming techniques that reinforce and strengthen perceptions of support (Carlisle et al., 2012). In recent work, implicit priming of positive aging stereotypes was associated with better self-perceptions of aging and physical functioning up to 3 weeks after the intervention (Levy et al., 2014). In fact, according to SAVI, such interventions in older adults should be especially powerful given age-related differences in sensitivity to social processes (Charles, 2010).

Finally, a more general issue is: Can interventions or later life experiences compensate for the predicted detrimental influence of a harsh, conflictual early family environment on health? The answer to this question is largely unknown but salient because of this life-span theory of social support. One recent study provides hope that perhaps interventions in adolescence can offset a harsh early environment. Miller, Brody, Yu, and Chen (2014) tested this idea in the Strong African Americans Families Project. Participants in this intervention were low socioeconomic status African American families who received training on nurturant parenting, monitoring, and communication skills when their child was 11 years old. At age 19 years, blood samples were taken from the now adult children to examine levels of inflammation. Impressively, the intervention was associated with lower levels of inflammation compared to the control group and corresponded to a large effect size (Cohen's $d = -.90$). Statistical mediational analyses also showed that part of this link was caused by the intervention-related improvements in parenting skills (Miller et al., 2014). These data are consistent with cross-sectional studies suggesting that despite adverse environments, nurturing parents are associated with better outcomes (Malecki & Demaray, 2006; Tracy, Zimmerman, Galea, McCauley, & Stoep, 2008). These data provide some of the first evidence that family interventions can potentially offset the negative health trajectories associated with harsh early life environments.

■ CONCLUSION

Social support is one of the most robust psychosocial factors influencing physical health outcomes. However, recent work is highlighting the complexity of such links when viewed from the lens of life-span development. This life-span theory of social support and health takes into account potentially important developmental processes influencing social support and its association to downstream mechanisms and health-relevant outcomes. This perspective is in need of stronger, direct tests of its premise and should be seen as complementary to existing broad models of life-span development. This complementarity implies that it can be informed by these broader models. It also implies that this life-span perspective on social support and health can inform broader perspectives on how these processes fit into the larger scheme of development, which includes health issues. After all, what is life without good health?

REFERENCES

Aldwin, C. M., Sutton, K. J., Chiara, G., & Spiro, A. (1996). Age differences in stress, coping and appraisal: Findings from the Normative Aging Study. *The Journals of Gerontology, Series B, 51*(4), 179–188.

Alexander, J. F., Sexton, T. L., & Robbins, M. (2002). The developmental status of family therapy in family psychology intervention science. In H. Liddle, D. Santisteban, R. Levant, & J. Bray (Eds.), *Family psychology science-based interventions*. Washington, DC: American Psychological Association.

Allen, J. P., & Loeb, E. L. (2015). The autonomy-connection challenge in adolescent peer relationships. *Child Development Perspectives, 9*(2), 101–105.

Anders, S. L., & Tucker, J. S. (2000). Adult attachment style, interpersonal communication competence, and social support. *Personal Relationships, 7*, 379–389.

André-Petersson, L., Hedblad, B., Janzon, L., & Ostergren, P. O. (2006). Social support and behavior in a stressful situation in relation to myocardial infarction and mortality: Who is at risk? Results from prospective cohort study "Men born in 1914," Malmö, Sweden. *International Journal of Behavioral Medicine, 13*(4), 340–347.

Antonucci, T. C., Ajrouch, K. J., & Birditt, K. S. (2014). The convoy model: Explaining social relations from a multidisciplinary perspective. *The Gerontologist, 54*, 82–92.

Antonucci, T. C., & Akiyama, H. (1987). Social networks in adult life and a preliminary examination of the convoy model. *Journal of Gerontology, 42*(5), 519–527.

Arnett, J. J. (2000). Emerging adulthood. A theory of development from the late teens through the twenties. *The American Psychologist, 55*(5), 469–480.

Aspinwall, L. G., & Taylor, S. E. (1997). A stitch in time: Self-regulation and proactive coping. *Psychological Bulletin, 121*(3), 417–436.

Baltes, M. M. (1995). Dependency in old age: Gains and losses. *Current Directions in Psychological Science, 4*, 14–19.

Baltes, P. B. (1997). On the incomplete architecture of human ontogeny. Selection, optimization, and compensation as foundation of developmental theory. *The American Psychologist, 52*(4), 366–380.

Barrera, M. (1986). Distinctions between social support concepts, measures, and models. *American Journal of Community Psychology, 14*, 413–445.

Barrera, M. (2000). Social support research in community psychology. In J. Rappaport & E. Seidman (Eds.), *Handbook of community psychology* (pp. 215–245). New York, NY: Kluwer Academic/Plenum Publishers.

Barth, J., Schneider, S., & von Känel, R. (2010). Lack of social support in the etiology and the prognosis of coronary heart disease: A systematic review and meta-analysis. *Psychosomatic Medicine, 72*(3), 229–238.

Beelmann, A., Pfingsten, U., & Losel, F. (1994). Effects of training social competence in children: A meta-analysis of recent evaluation studies. *Journal of Clinical Child Psychology, 23*(3), 260–271.

Berg, C. A., & Upchurch, R. (2007). A developmental-contextual model of couples coping with chronic illness across the adult life span. *Psychological Bulletin, 133*(6), 920–954.

Berkman, L. F., Glass, T., Brissette, I., & Seeman, T. E. (2000). From social integration to health: Durkheim in the new millennium. *Social Science and Medicine, 51*(6), 843–857.

Blanchard-Fields, F. (2007). Everyday problem solving and emotion. *Current Directions in Psychological Science, 16*, 26–31.

Blanchflower, D. G., & Oswald, A. J. (2008). Is well-being U-shaped over the life cycle? *Social Science and Medicine, 66*(8), 1733–1749.

Blazer, D. G. (1982). Social support and mortality in an elderly community population. *American Journal of Epidemiology, 115*(5), 684–694.

Bolger, N., & Amarel, D. (2007). Effects of social support visibility on adjustment to stress: Experimental evidence. *Journal of Personality and Social Psychology, 92*(3), 458–475.

Bolger, N., Foster, M., Vinokur, A. D., & Ng, R. (1996). Close relationships and adjustment to a life crisis: The case of breast cancer. *Journal of Personality and Social Psychology, 70*(2), 283–294.

Bolger, N., Zuckerman, A., & Kessler, R. C. (2000). Invisible support and adjustment to stress. *Journal of Personality and Social Psychology, 79*(6), 953–961.

Booth, G. L., Kapral, M. K., Fung, K., & Tu, J. V. (2006). Relation between age and cardiovascular disease in men and women with diabetes compared with non-diabetic people: A population-based retrospective cohort study. *The Lancet, 368*(9529), 29–36.

Bowen, K. S., Birmingham, W., Uchino, B. N., Carlisle, M., Smith, T. W., & Light, K. C. (2013). Specific dimensions of perceived support and ambulatory blood pressure: Which support functions appear most beneficial and for whom? *International Journal of Psychophysiology, 88*(3), 317–324.

Brannan, D., Biswas-Diener, R., Mohr, C. D., Mortazavi, S., & Stein, N. (2013). Friends and family: A cross-cultural investigation of social support and subjective well-being among college students. *The Journal of Positive Psychology, 8*, 65–75.

Brooks, K., & Dunkel-Schetter, C. (2011). Social negativity and health. *Social and Personality Psychology Compass, 5*, 904–918.

Carlisle, M., Uchino, B. N., Sanbonmatsu, D. M., Smith, T. W., Cribbet, M. R., Birmingham, W., . . . Vaughn, A. A. (2012). Subliminal activation of social ties moderates cardiovascular reactivity during acute stress. *Health Psychology: Official Journal of the Division of Health Psychology, American Psychological Association, 31*(2), 217–225.

Carstensen, L. L., Isaacowitz, D. M., & Charles, S. T. (1999). Taking time seriously: A theory of socioemotional selectivity. *The American Psychologist, 54*(3), 165–181.

Carver, C. S., Scheier, M. F., & Weintraub, J. K. (1989). Assessing coping strategies: A theoretically based approach. *Journal of Personality and Social Psychology, 56*(2), 267–283.

Cené, C. W., Loehr, L., Lin, F. C., Hammond, W. P., Foraker, R. E., Rose, K., . . . Corbie-Smith, G. (2012). Social isolation, vital exhaustion, and incident heart failure: Findings from the Atherosclerosis Risk in Communities Study. *European Journal of Heart Failure, 14*(7), 748–753.

Charles, S. T. (2010). Strength and vulnerability integration: A model of emotional well-being across adulthood. *Psychological Bulletin, 136*(6), 1068–1091.

Charles, S. T., & Carstensen, L. L. (2010). Social and emotional aging. *Annual Review Psychology, 61*, 383–409.

Chiang, J. J., Saphire-Bernstein, S., Kim, H. S., Sherman, D. K., & Taylor, S. E. (2013). Cultural differences in the link between supportive relationships and proinflammatory cytokines. *Social Psychological and Personality Science, 4*, 511–520.

Cohen, S. (2004). Social relationships and health. *The American Psychologist, 59*(8), 676–684.

Cohen, S., Mermelstein, R. J., Kamarck, T., & Hoberman, H. M. (1985). Measuring the functional components of social support. In I. G. Sarason & B. Sarason (Eds.), *Social support: Theory, research and applications* (pp. 73–94). The Hague, Holland: Martines Niijhoff.

Coyne, J. C., & Smith, D. A. (1991). Couples coping with a myocardial infarction: A contextual perspective on wives' distress. *Journal of Personality and Social Psychology, 61*(3), 404–412.

Craig, F. W., & Deichert, N. T. (2002). Can male-provided social support buffer the cardiovascular responsivity to stress in men? It depends on the nature of the support provided. *International Journal of Men's Health, 1*, 105–118.

Cutrona, C. E., & Russell, D. W. (1990). Type of social support and specific stress: Towards a theory of optimal matching. In B. R. Sarason, I. G. Sarason, & G. R. Pierce (Eds.), *Social support: An interactional view* (pp. 319–366). New York, NY: John Wiley and Sons.

Darbonne, A., Uchino, B. N., & Ong, A. D. (2013). What mediates links between age and well-being? A test of social support and interpersonal conflict as potential interpersonal pathways. *Journal of Happiness Studies, 14,* 951–963.

De Vogli, R., Chandola, T., & Marmot, M. G. (2007). Negative aspects of close relationships and heart disease. *Archives of Internal Medicine, 167*(18), 1951–1957.

DiMatteo, M. R. (2004). Social support and patient adherence to medical treatment: A meta-analysis. *Health Psychology: Official Journal of the Division of Health Psychology, American Psychological Association, 23*(2), 207–218.

Dirks, M. A., Treat, T. A., & Weersing, V. R. (2007). Integrating theoretical, measurement, and intervention models of youth social competence. *Clinical Psychology Review, 27*(3), 327–347.

Dong, M., Giles, W. H., Felitti, V. J., Dube, S. R., Williams, J. E., Chapman, D. P., & Anda, R. F. (2004). Insights into causal pathways for ischemic heart disease: Adverse childhood experiences study. *Circulation, 110*(13), 1761–1766.

Doucet, J., & Aseltine, R. H., Jr. (2003). Childhood family adversity and the quality of marital relationships in young adulthood. *Journal of Social and Personal Relationships, 20*(6), 818–842.

Dressler, W. W., & Bindon, J. R. (2000). The health consequences of cultural consonance: Cultural dimensions of lifestyle, social support, and arterial blood pressure in an African American community. *American Anthropologist, 102,* 244–260.

Dunkel-Schetter, C., & Bennett, T. L. (1990). Differentiating the cognitive and behavioral aspects of social support. In B. R. Sarason, I. G. Sarason, & G. R. Pierce (Eds.), *Social support: An interactional view* (pp. 267–296). New York, NY: John Wiley and Sons.

Durlak, J. A., Weissberg, R. P., & Pachan, M. (2010). A meta-analysis of after-school programs that seek to promote personal and social skills in children and adolescents. *American Journal of Community Psychology, 45*(3–4), 294–309.

Eggert, L. L., Thompson, E. A., Herting, J. R., Nicholas, L. J., & Dicker, B. G. (1994). Preventing adolescent drug abuse and high school dropout through an intensive school-based social network development program. *American Journal of Health Promotion, 8*(3), 202–215.

Engels, R. C. M. E., Dekovic, M., & Meeus, W. (2002). Parenting practices, social skills and peer relationships in adolescence. *Social Behavior and Personality, 30*(1), 3–18.

The ENRICHD Investigators. (2003). Effects of treating depression and low perceived social support on clinical events after myocardial infarction: The enhancing recovery in coronary heart disease patients (ENRICHD) randomized trial. *The Journal of the American Medical Association, 289,* 3106–3116.

Finch, J. F., Okun, M. A., Barrera, M., Zautra, A. J., & Reich, J. W. (1989). Positive and negative social ties among older adults: Measurement models and the prediction of psychological distress and well-being. *American Journal of Community Psychology, 17*(5), 585–605.

Fingerman, K. L., & Charles, S. T. (2010). It takes two to tango: Why older people have the best relationships. *Current Directions in Psychological Science, 19,* 172–176.

Fingerman, K. L., Hay, E. L., & Birditt, K. S. (2004). The best of ties, the worst of ties: Close, problematic, and ambivalent social relationships. *Journal of Marriage and Family, 66,* 792–808.

Flaherty, J. A., & Richman, J. A. (1986). Effects of childhood relationships on the adult's capacity to form social supports. *American Journal of Psychiatry, 143*(7), 851–855.

Flaherty, J. A, & Richman, J. A. (1989). Gender differences in the perception and utilization of social support: Theoretical perspectives and an empirical test. *Social Science and Medicine, 28*(12), 1221–1228.

Folkman, S., Lazarus, R. S., Pimley, S., & Novacek, J. (1987). Age differences in stress and coping processes. *Psychology and Aging, 2*(2), 171–184.

Forster, L. E., & Stoller, E. P. (1992). The impact of social support on mortality: A seven-year follow-up of older men and women. *Journal of Applied Gerontology, 11,* 173–186.

Gallo, L. C., & Smith, T. W. (1999). Patterns of hostility and social support: Conceptualizing psychosocial risk factors as characteristics of the person and the environment. *Journal of Research in Personality, 33,* 281–310.

Goodwin, R. (2006). Age and social support perception in Eastern Europe: Social change and support in four rapidly changing countries. *British Journal of Social Psychology, 45*(Pt. 4), 799–815.

Gow, A. J., Corley, J., Starr, J. M., & Deary, I. J. (2013). Which social network or support factors are associated with cognitive abilities in old age? *Gerontology, 59*(5), 454–463.

Grav, S., Hellzèn, O., Romild, U., & Stordal, E. (2011). Association between social support and depression in the general population: The HUNT study, a cross-sectional survey. *Journal of Clinical Nursing, 21*(1–2), 111–120.

Graves, P. L., Wang, N. Y., Mead, L. A., Johnson, J. V., & Klag, M. J. (1998). Youthful precursors of midlife social support. *Journal of Personality and Social Psychology, 74*(5), 1329–1336.

Haber, M. G., Cohen, J. L., Lucas, T., & Baltes, B. B. (2007). The relationship between self-reported received and perceived social support: A meta-analytic review. *American Journal of Community Psychology, 39*(1–2), 133–144.

Hardy, D. F., Power, T. G., & Jaedicke, S. (1993). Examining the relation of parenting to children's coping with everyday stress. *Child Development, 64*(6), 1829–1841.

Hawkley, L. C., Thisted, R. A., Masi, C. M., & Cacioppo, J. T. (2010). Loneliness predicts increased blood pressure: 5-year cross-lagged analyses in middle-aged and older adults. *Psychology and Aging, 25*(1), 132–141.

Heckhausen, J., Wrosch, C., & Schulz, R. (2010). A motivational theory of life-span development. *Psychological Review, 117*(1), 32–60.

Helsen, M., Vollebergh, W., & Meeus, W. (2000). Social support from parents and friends and emotional problems in adolescence. *Journal of Youth and Adolescence, 29,* 319–335.

Hogan, B. E., Linden, W., & Najarian, B. (2002). Social support interventions: Do they work? *Clinical Psychology Review, 22*(3), 383–442.

Holt-Lunstad, J., Smith, T. B., & Layton, J. B. (2010). Social relationships and mortality risk: A meta-analytic review. *PLoS Medicine, 7*(7), e1000316.

Holt-Lunstad, J., Uchino, B. N., Smith, T. W., & Hicks, A. (2007). On the importance of relationship quality: The impact of ambivalence in friendships on cardiovascular functioning. *Annals of Behavioral Medicine: A Publication of the Society of Behavioral Medicine, 33*(3), 278–290.

Horsten, M., Mittleman, M. A., Wamala, S. P., Schenck-Gustafsson, K., & Orth-Gomér, K. (1999). Social relations and the metabolic syndrome in middle-aged Swedish women. *Journal of Cardiovascular Risk, 6*(6), 391–397.

Howland, M., & Simpson, J. A. (2010). Getting in under the radar. A dyadic view of invisible support. *Psychological Science, 21*(12), 1878–1885.

Ikeda, A., Iso, H., Kawachi, I., Yamagishi, K., Inoue, M., & Tsugane, S.; JPHC Study Group. (2008). Social support and stroke and coronary heart disease: The JPHC study cohorts II. *Stroke: A Journal of Cerebral Circulation, 39*(3), 768–775.

Ingersoll-Dayton, B., & Antonucci, T. C. (1988). Reciprocal and nonreciprocal social support: Contrasting sides of intimate relationships. *Journal of Gerontology, 43*(3), S65–S73.

Kahn, R. L., & Antonucci, T. C. (1980). Convoys over the life course: Attachment, roles, and social support. In P. B. Baltes & O. Brim (Eds.), *Life-span development and behavior* (Vol. 3, pp. 253–268). New York, NY: Academic Press

Kaplan, R. M. (2000). Two pathways to prevention. *The American Psychologist, 55*(4), 382–396.

Krause, N. (1997). Received support, anticipated support, social class, and mortality. *Research on Aging, 19*, 387–422.

Labouvie-Vief, G. (2008). Dynamic integration theory: Emotion, cognition, and equilibrium in later life. In V. Bengtson, M. Silverstein, N. Putney, & D. Gans (Eds.), *Handbook of theories of aging* (pp. 277–293). New York, NY: Springer Publishing Company.

Lakey, B., McCabe, K. M., Fisicaro, S. A., & Drew, J. B. (1996). Environmental and personal determinants of support perceptions: Three generalizability studies. *Journal of Personality and Social Psychology, 70*(6), 1270–1280.

Lakey, B., & Orehek, E. (2011). Relational regulation theory: A new approach to explain the link between perceived social support and mental health. *Psychological Review, 118*(3), 482–495.

Lakey, B., & Scoboria, A. (2005). The relative contribution of trait and social influences to the links among perceived social support, affect, and self-esteem. *Journal of Personality, 73*(2), 361–388.

Lang, F. R., & Carstensen, L. L. (1994). Close emotional relationships in late life: Further support for proactive aging in the social domain. *Psychology and Aging, 9*(2), 315–324.

Levy, B. R., Pilver, C., Chung, P. H., & Slade, M. D. (2014). Subliminal strengthening: Improving older individuals' physical function over time with an implicit-age-stereotype intervention. *Psychological Science, 25*(12), 2127–2135.

Lindner, K. C., Sarason, I. G., & Sarason, B. R. (1988). Assessed life stress and experimentally provided social support. In C. D. Spielberger & I. G. Sarason (Eds.), *Stress & anxiety* (pp. 231–240). Washington, DC: Hemisphere.

Malecki, C. K., & Demaray, M. K. (2006). Social support as a buffer in the relationship between socioeconomic status and academic performance. *School Psychology Quarterly, 21,* 375–395.

Manne, S., & Glassman, M. (2000). Perceived control, coping efficacy, and avoidance coping as mediators between spouses' unsupportive behaviors and cancer patients' psychological distress. *Health Psychology: Official Journal of the Division of Health Psychology, American Psychological Association, 19*(2), 155–164.

Martire, L. M., & Schulz, R. (2007). Involving family in psychosocial interventions for chronic illness. *Current Directions in Psychological Science, 16,* 90–94.

Martire, L. M., Schulz, R., Mittelmark, M. B., & Newsom, J. T. (1999). Stability and change in older adults' social contact and social support: The cardiovascular health study. *The Journals of Gerontology, Series B, 54*(5), S302–S311.

Mechanic, D. (1980). The experience and reporting of common physical complaints. *Journal of Health and Social Behavior, 21*(2), 146–155.

Miller, G. E., Brody, G. H., Yu, T., & Chen, E. (2014). A family-oriented psychosocial intervention reduces inflammation in low-SES African American youth. *Proceedings of the National Academy of Sciences of the United States of America, 111*(31), 11287–11292.

Miller, G. E., & Chen, E. (2010). Harsh family climate in early life presages the emergence of a proinflammatory phenotype in adolescence. *Psychological Science, 21*(6), 848–856.

Miller, G. E., Lachman, M. E., Chen, E., Gruenewald, T. L., Karlamangla, A. S., & Seeman, T. E. (2011). Pathways to resilience: Maternal nurturance as a buffer against the effects of childhood poverty on metabolic syndrome at midlife. *Psychological Science, 22*(12), 1591–1599.

Mojaverian, T., & Kim, H. S. (2013). Interpreting a helping hand: Cultural variation in the effectiveness of solicited and unsolicited social support. *Personality & Social Psychology Bulletin, 39*(1), 88–99.

Northouse, L. L., Templin, T., Mood, D., & Oberst, M. (1998). Couples' adjustment to breast cancer and benign breast disease: A longitudinal analysis. *Psycho-Oncology, 7*(1), 37–48.

Ong, A. D., & Allaire, J. C. (2005). Cardiovascular intraindividual variability in later life: The influence of social connectedness and positive emotions. *Psychology and Aging, 20*(3), 476–485.

Ong, A. D., Rothstein, J. D., & Uchino, B. N. (2012). Loneliness accentuates age differences in cardiovascular responses to social evaluative threat. *Psychology and Aging, 27*(1), 190–198.

Orth-Gomér, K., Rosengren, A., & Wilhelmsen, L. (1993). Lack of social support and incidence of coronary heart disease in middle-aged Swedish men. *Psychosomatic Medicine, 55*(1), 37–43.

Pierce, G. R., Sarason, I. G., & Sarason, B. R. (1991). General and relationship-based perceptions of social support: Are two constructs better than one? *Journal of Personality and Social Psychology, 61*(6), 1028–1039.

Poon, C. Y., & Knight, B. G. (2013). Parental emotional support during emerging adulthood and Baby Boomers' well-being in midlife. *International Journal of Behavioral Development, 37*, 498–504.

Räikkönen, K., Matthews, K. A., & Kuller, L. H. (2001). Trajectory of psychological risk and incident hypertension in middle-aged women. *Hypertension, 38*(4), 798–802.

Reblin, M., Uchino, B. N., & Smith, T. W. (2010). Provider and recipient factors that may moderate the effectiveness of received support: Examining the effects of relationship quality and expectations for support on behavioral and cardiovascular reactions. *Journal of Behavioral Medicine, 33*(6), 423–431.

Reis, H. T. (2007). Steps toward the ripening of relationship science. *Personal Relationships, 14*, 1–23.

Repetti, R. L., Robles, T. F., & Reynolds, B. (2011). Allostatic processes in the family. *Development and Psychopathology, 23*(3), 921–938.

Robles, T. F., Slatcher, R. B., Trombello, J. M., & McGinn, M. M. (2014). Marital quality and health: A meta-analytic review. *Psychological Bulletin, 140*(1), 140–187.

Rook, K. S. (2015). Social networks in later life: Weighing positive and negative effects on health and well-being. *Current Directions in Psychological Science, 24*(1), 45–51.

Rowe, J. W., & Kahn, R. L. (1987). Human aging: Usual and successful. *Science, 237*(4811), 143–149.

Rowe, J. W., & Kahn, R. L. (1998). *Successful aging: The MacArthur Foundation study.* New York, NY: Pantheon Books.

Ruehlman, L. S., & Karoly, P. (1991). With a little flak from my friends: Development and preliminary validation of the test of negative social exchange (TENSE). *Psychological Assessment, 3*, 97–104.

Russell, D. W., & Cutrona, C. E. (1991). Social support, stress, and depressive symptoms among the elderly: Test of a process model. *Psychology and Aging, 6*(2), 190–201.

Russek, L. G., & Schwartz, G. E. (1997). Feelings of parental caring predict health status in midlife: A 35-year follow-up of the Harvard Mastery of Stress Study. *Journal of Behavioral Medicine, 20*(1), 1–13.

Sarason, B. R., Sarason, I. G., Hacker, A., & Basham, R. B. (1985). Concomitants of social support: Social skills, physical attractiveness, and gender. *Journal of Personality and Social Psychology, 49*(2), 469–480.

Sarason, I. G & Sarason, B. R. (1986). Experimentally provided social support. *Journal of Personality and Social Psychology, 50*, 1222–1225.

Sarason, I. G., Sarason, B. R., & Shearin, E. N. (1986). Social support as an individual difference variable: Its stability, origins, and relational aspects. *Journal of Personality and Social Psychology, 50*, 845–855.

Schulz, R., & Heckhausen, J. (1996). A life span model of successful aging. *The American Psychologist, 51*(7), 702–714.

Seeman, T. E., Lusignolo, T. M., Albert, M., & Berkman, L. (2001). Social relationships, social support, and patterns of cognitive aging in healthy, high-functioning older adults: MacArthur studies of successful aging. *Health Psychology: Official Journal of the Division of Health Psychology, American Psychological Association, 20*(4), 243–255.

Selcuk, E., & Ong, A. D. (2013). Perceived partner responsiveness moderates the association between received emotional support and all-cause mortality. *Health Psychology: Official Journal of the Division of Health Psychology, American Psychological Association, 32*(2), 231–235.

Shaw, B. A., Krause, N., Chatters, L. M., Connell, C. M., & Ingersoll-Dayton, B. (2004). Emotional support from parents early in life, aging, and health. *Psychology and Aging, 19*(1), 4–12.

Shor, E., Roelfs, D. J., & Yogev, T. (2013). The strength of family ties: A meta-analysis and meta-regression of self-reported social support and mortality. *Social Networks, 35*, 626–638.

Slatcher, R. B., Selcuk, E., & Ong, A. D. (2015). Perceived partner responsiveness predicts diurnal cortisol profiles 10 years later. *Psychological Science, 26*(7), 972–982.

Sneed, R. S., & Cohen, S. (2014). Negative social interactions and incident hypertension among older adults. *Health Psychology: Official Journal of the Division of Health Psychology, American Psychological Association, 33*(6), 554–565.

Story, T. N., Berg, C. A., Smith, T. W., Beveridge, R., Henry, N. J., & Pearce, G. (2007). Age, marital satisfaction, and optimism as predictors of positive sentiment override in middle-aged and older married couples. *Psychology and Aging, 22*(4), 719–727.

Symister, P., & Friend, R. (2003). The influence of social support and problematic support on optimism and depression in chronic illness: A prospective study evaluating self-esteem as a mediator. *Health Psychology: Official Journal of the Division of Health Psychology, American Psychological Association, 22*(2), 123–129.

Taylor, S. E. (1991). Asymmetrical effects of positive and negative events: The mobilization-minimization hypothesis. *Psychological Bulletin, 110*(1), 67–85.

Taylor, S. E., Welch, W. T., Kim, H. S., & Sherman, D. K. (2007). Cultural differences in the impact of social support on psychological and biological stress responses. *Psychological Science, 18*(9), 831–837.

Testa, M., & Collins, R. L. (1997). Alcohol and risky sexual behavior: Event-based analyses among a sample of high-risk women. *Psychology of Addictive Behavior, 11*, 190–201.

Thoits, P. A. (1986). Social support as coping assistance. *Journal of Consulting and Clinical Psychology, 54*(4), 416–423.

Tracy, M., Zimmerman, F. J., Galea, S., McCauley, E., & Stoep, A. V. (2008). What explains the relation between family poverty and childhood depressive symptoms? *Journal of Psychiatric Research, 42*(14), 1163–1175.

Uchino, B. N. (2004). *Social support and physical health: Understanding the health consequences of our relationships*. New Haven, CT: Yale University Press.

Uchino, B. N. (2009). Understanding the links between social support and physical health: A life-span perspective with emphasis on the separability of perceived and received support. *Perspectives on Psychological Science: A Journal of the Association for Psychological Science, 4*(3), 236–255.

Uchino, B. N., Cacioppo, J. T., Malarkey, W., Glaser, R., & Kiecolt-Glaser, J. K. (1995). Appraisal support predicts age-related differences in cardiovascular function in women. *Health Psychology: Official Journal of the Division of Health Psychology, American Psychological Association, 14*(6), 556–562.

Uchino, B. N., Holt-Lunstad, J., Uno, D., Betancourt, R., & Garvey, T. S. (1999). Social support and age-related differences in cardiovascular function: An examination of potential mediators. *Annals of Behavioral Medicine: A Publication of the Society of Behavioral Medicine, 21*(2), 135–142.

Uchino, B. N., Vaughn, A. A., Carlisle, M., & Birmingham, W. (2012). Social support and immunity. In S. Segerstrom (Ed.), *The Oxford handbook of psychoneuroimmunology* (pp. 214–233). New York, NY: Oxford University Press.

van Tilburg, T. (1998). Losing and gaining in old age: Changes in personal network size and social support in a four-year longitudinal study. *The Journals of Gerontology, Series B, 53*(6), S313–S323.

Vilhjalmsson, R. (1994). Effects of social support on self-assessed health in adolescence. *Journal of Youth and Adolescence, 23,* 437–452.

Wallsten, S. M., Tweed, D. L., Blazer, D. G., & George, L. K. (1999). Disability and depressive symptoms in the elderly: The effects of instrumental support and its subjective appraisal. *International Journal of Aging and Human Development, 48*(2), 145–159.

Wang, H. X., Mittleman, M. A., & Orth-Gomer, K. (2005). Influence of social support on progression of coronary artery disease in women. *Social Science and Medicine, 60*(3), 599–607.

Wills, T. A., & Shinar, O. (2000). Measuring perceived and received social support. In S. Cohen, L. Gordon, & B. Gottlieb (Eds.), *Social support measurement and intervention: A guide for health and social scientists* (pp. 86–135). New York, NY: Oxford University Press.

Wrosch, C., Rueggeberg, R., & Hoppmann, C. A. (2013). Satisfaction with social support in older adulthood: The influence of social support changes and goal adjustment capacities. *Psychology and Aging, 28*(3), 875–885.

CHAPTER 14

Age Stereotypes' Influence on Health: Stereotype Embodiment Theory

Brad A. Meisner and Becca R. Levy

Over the past few hundred years, sociocultural norms have increasingly disparaged older adults and pathologized the aging process (Ng, Allore, Trentalange, Monin, & Levy, 2015). During this period, in an era that prioritized industrial labor, there developed a focus on the limitations that come with increasing age. Simultaneously, positive qualities of aging were rendered less important as oral histories and traditions, which fostered ideals of wisdom and resilience, were thought to be less relevant to the creation of a productive society (Nelson, 2005). There is empirical research to support these changing beliefs about aging throughout history. Using a large historical literary database of 400 million words from 1810 to 2009, a recent study found aging representations were, for the most part, positive in 1810; however, they became increasingly more negative over the subsequent 200 years (Ng et al., 2015). This historico-cultural shift has resulted in a largely biomedicalized idea of what it means to be "old" that is still present today. It is important to note that these changing standards of aging are often based on biased belief structures, rather than on accurate evidence-based knowledge of aging processes. More than 50 years ago, Kent recognized that "there exists today a chasm between our perceptions of aging and the facts" (Kent, 1965, p. 51).

There is growing evidence that these views on aging have a significant impact on multiple domains, pathways, and outcomes related to health in later life (Levy, 2003, 2009; Levy, Slade, Murphy, & Gill, 2012; Meisner, 2012). Given that common representations and understandings of aging are overly and overtly negative, and that the proportion of older adults in the population is increasing at an unprecedented rate, therein lies a critical health-related problem that warrants not only an explanation, but also a solution.

In this chapter, the increasing number of studies that pertain to the stereotype embodiment theory (SET) are integrated and reflected upon to represent the current state of this theoretical perspective and how it can help explain age stereotypes' contributions to health and aging (Levy, 2003, 2009; Meisner, 2012; Westerhof et al., 2014). The first part of this chapter describes the history, cultural context, and nature of age stereotypes and age self-stereotypes in a largely ageist society. The second part presents SET (Levy, 2009), which provides a framework for explaining how age stereotypes are acquired to subsequently influence health outcomes. Replication studies conducted in different countries, as well as meta-analyses, are described and discussed to demonstrate the validity of this theory as well as to illustrate the meaning and impact of its components.

The final part of this chapter entails an illustration of how SET may be applied to shape future healthy aging research, policy, and practice.

■ AGE STEREOTYPES AND AGE SELF-STEREOTYPES: CONTENT, VALENCE, AND DIVERSITY

Age stereotypes are defined as beliefs about older people as a generalized group (Levy, 2003, 2009). Early research on age stereotypes focused on generating and classifying the cognitive structural categories of age stereotype content to apply the findings to the social perception of, and behavior toward, older adults. First, Brewer, Dull, and Lui (1981) differentiated three elderly subgroup prototypes perceived by college-aged younger adults (i.e., grandmother, elder statesman, and senior citizen). Then, two subsequent studies found that there are many more subgroup types, including much more diverse age stereotype traits, within the general category of "elderly" (Hummert, 1990; Schmidt & Boland, 1986). This early evidence demonstrated that age stereotypes are not simple and insular. Instead, they are complex and multifaceted. People can demonstrate numerous and varied age stereotypes that are usually positive or negative in valence. There is an extensive body of research showing that age stereotypes are indeed mixed as older adults are often described as being friendly, good-natured, sincere, and warm while simultaneously being incapable, incompetent, unintelligent, and unskilled (Cuddy & Fiske, 2002).

Within these mixed age stereotypes, negative age stereotypes tend to outnumber positive ones. For instance, the studies of Schmidt and Boland (1986) and Hummert (1990) found more negative subgroups than positive subgroups, which were represented by more negative traits than positive traits. To illustrate, Hummert (1990) found 3 positively defined subgroups including 31 traits, but 7 negatively defined subgroups including 53 traits. Further evidence comes from two meta-analyses performed by Kite and her colleagues (Kite & Johnson, 1988; Kite, Stockdale, Whitley, & Johnson, 2005) that show old-age stereotypes are mixed and, for the most part, negative—especially in comparison to young-age stereotypes. In addition, the fact that these two meta-analyses were published 17 years apart connotes the pervasive and persistent nature of negative age stereotypes (Cuddy, Norton, & Fiske, 2005; Levy, Slade, Chung, & Gill, 2015; Nelson, 2005; Ng et al., 2015).

Most of the early research on age stereotypes focused on beliefs held among younger adults—who belong to a "young" in-group, reflecting upon an older out-group. Since then, an increasing number of researchers have focused on the stereotypes that older adults have about aging—who belong to, and are reflecting upon, an "old" in-group (i.e., age self-stereotypes; Levy & Langer, 1994). It could be hypothesized that members of the out-group may have more negatively biased beliefs than members of an in-group. If so, the negative stereotypes about aging held by younger adults would not be generalizable to older people. Indeed, it seems logical that older adults would exhibit a more positive image of their own group; however, that does not appear to be the case (Levy & Banaji, 2002). For instance, following a research protocol that was similar to their previous study on younger adults' age stereotypes, Hummert, Garstka, Shaner, and Strahm (1994) conducted another study to generate and categorize age stereotype content among younger (18–22 years of age), middle-aged (35–51 years of age), and older adult groups (60–85 years of age). At that point in time, it was not clear whether older adults would endorse the same sort of negatively-biased age stereotypes that were found within their younger counterparts. Results demonstrated that, similar to younger adults, middle-aged and older adult age groups reported both negative and positive age stereotypes and that negative age stereotypes predominated over positive ones.

Additionally, there is a growing body of research that explores the variability and diversity in age stereotypes cross-culturally. It has become apparent that some age stereotypes differ by culture whereas others are more universal. The most comprehensive empirical evidence to demonstrate a global-age stereotype perspective comes from a study by Löckenhoff and 47 of her international colleagues (2009). Together, they collected data from 3,435 people within 26 different cultures across the world to compare and contrast age stereotype content between and among countries. In this study, transcultural positive age stereotypes included increased levels of *knowledge, wisdom,* and *respect with aging*, whereas transcultural negative age stereotypes included decreased *attractiveness, functional ability to complete everyday tasks,* and *ability to learn new things*. Thus, there are certain stereotypes that are common across cultures, in both the East and West. In addition, despite the mixture of positive and negative age stereotypes reported around the world, it was found that most cultures viewed aging in a negative light. Countries with the strongest negative age stereotypes were Argentina, Czech Republic, Serbia, and the United Kingdom. Other countries demonstrated more neutral or somewhat positive age stereotypes, including India, Mainland China, Malaysia, New Zealand, and Russia. The subtle cultural variances in age stereotypes are important because these differences can have an impact on older individuals' health and well-being, as described in the following section.

■ STEREOTYPE EMBODIMENT THEORY (SET): KEY PRINCIPLES

Most of the early research on the impact of age stereotypes focused on how they influenced younger individuals' behaviors toward older individuals rather than how they impacted older individuals themselves. Since then, there has been considerable work done to authenticate this latter relationship. However, in this developing research, there lacked a theory to explain how age stereotypes could influence the health of older adults. To fill this gap, SET was developed (Levy, 2009).

The overall premise of SET is that age stereotypes can, and do, impact older individuals' health, recognizing that both negative and positive age stereotypes have a self-fulfilling influence on health and disease processes that occur with aging. SET posits that the influence of age stereotypes on health-related outcomes manifests via two key directional mechanisms: first, through a top-down direction, such that age stereotypes are assimilated from the culture to influence the individual (i.e., from society to self); second, through a developmental approach that occurs over time, such that age stereotypes are assimilated over an individual's life span (i.e., from young childhood to old age). SET draws on a considerable amount of evidence, including numerous experimental laboratory and longitudinal epidemiological studies that demonstrate age stereotypes' influence on a range of health and disease outcomes as well as other aspects of the aging process.

A meta-analysis by Meisner (2012) examining experimental age stereotyping research found clear evidence that negative and positive age stereotypes operate through self-fulfilling prophecies in the direction of the age stereotype. Generally, negative age stereotypes cause reliable impairments in biopsychosocial outcomes among older adults, whereas positive age stereotypes promote these same factors. Thus, older adults who have more negative age self-stereotypes are shown to have numerous impairments in health and increased risks of disease, whereas older adults with more positive age self-stereotypes experience better health and decreased risks of disease.

In the following subsections, the overall supposition of SET, which is that age stereotypes are assimilated to influence older individuals' health, is reviewed. Research evidence on this topic is synthesized and presented in three sections. The first section presents research that shows age stereotypes can influence physical and functional outcomes, the second section that they influence cognitive and mental health outcomes, and the third section that these age self-stereotype effects are stronger when there is a correspondence between the domain of the stereotype and the health-related outcome (i.e., the stereotype matching effect; Levy & Leifheit-Limson, 2009). Succeeding these three sections, research findings relating to the four components of SET are presented to demonstrate ways that age stereotypes may become embodied to influence health-related outcomes in later life.

Age Stereotypes' Influence on Physical and Functional Health Outcomes

A number of studies have found that older individuals' age stereotypes can impact physical and functional health outcomes. For example, Hausdorff, Levy, and Wei (1999) investigated whether walking performance was influenced by implicit priming of age stereotypes. Pre- to posttest analyses revealed that older adults who were positively primed demonstrated a significant increase in walking speed and balance. The effect size of this result is robust as it is similar to the effectiveness of a multiple month-long exercise intervention program. In addition to this evidence involving gross motor skills as an indicator of functioning, there appears to be a similar influence on fine motor skills. For instance, Levy (2000) found that a number of handwriting characteristics were modified by implicit positive and negative age stereotypes. Following the experimental manipulation, the older adults' handwriting in the positive prime group was assessed to be more *accomplished* and *confident* by blinded adjudicators, whereas the handwriting among those in the negative prime group was assessed to be more *deteriorated* and *shaky*. Thus, after exposure to the primes, the older adults in these two experiments demonstrated behaviors that are representative of the age stereotype itself.

Further to these experimental findings, studies conducted in the community and over time have also found an association between self-perceptions of aging and functional health. Levy, Slade, and Kasl (2002) compared older individuals with positive versus negative self-perceptions of aging and discovered that those with negative self-perceptions of aging experienced significantly worse functional health for more than an 18-year period. In this particular study, self-perceptions of aging had a greater impact on functional health than did self-rated health, gender, race, and social status, which are all known predictors of functional health. These findings were replicated and extended by Sargent-Cox, Anstey, and Luszcz (2012) who studied data from older participants in the Australian Longitudinal Study of Aging to show a predictive relationship of self-perceptions of aging on physical functioning up to 16 years later. They also found support for the directionality of aging self-perceptions' influence on physical function rather than vice versa. More specifically, consistent with SET, self-perceptions of aging significantly predicted physical function, but physical function did not predict self-perceptions of aging over time (Sargent-Cox et al., 2012).

It is also found that age beliefs held early in development can influence physical health outcomes in later life. Levy, Zonderman, Slade, and Ferrucci (2009) explored whether negative age stereotypes reported earlier in adulthood would increase the risk of experiencing an adverse cardiovascular event during the aging process. In this study, participants were between the ages of 18 and 49 years at baseline and were followed for almost four decades. It was found that, 30 years after baseline, 25% of the participants with negative age stereotypes had experienced a cardiovascular event compared to 13% of those participants with positive age stereotypes. In addition, it has been found that older adults with more positive age self-stereotypes, compared to those with more negative age self-stereotypes, have better recovery expectations and actual physical recovery following a life-threatening experience (e.g., an acute myocardial infarction; Levy, Slade, May, & Caracciolo, 2006) and that they are 44% more likely to fully recover from severe disability (Levy, Slade, Murphy, & Gill, 2012).

The overall SET premise that age stereotypes can impact physical health is supported by a recent meta-analysis of 19 longitudinal studies involving age stereotypes' impact on health outcomes among older adults that found a significant and reliable relationship between aging beliefs and outcomes such as survival and functional health (Westerhof et al., 2014). The findings were similar across participant samples from a number of countries including Australia, Finland, Germany, Hong Kong, Switzerland, and the United States. These experimental, longitudinal, and meta-analytical studies confirm the detrimental and beneficial physical health outcomes among older adults caused by negative and positive age stereotypes, respectively. They also highlight the utility of positive age stereotypes in health promoting physical and functional health following adverse health events.

Age Stereotypes' Influence on Cognitive and Mental Health Outcomes

The connection between cognitive health and age stereotypes was first examined experimentally by Levy (1996). In her study, 90 people, aged 60 years or greater, came into a laboratory to take part in a study that involved a subliminal priming paradigm that flashed either positive or negative age stereotype words at a speed that was sufficient for participants to be aware of the word's general location on the computer screen, but not enough time for participants to perceive the word and be aware of its meaning. Pre- to posttest results showed that participants who were implicitly primed with negative age stereotypes had significantly impaired memory, whereas those primed with the positive age stereotypes had significantly improved memory. This study demonstrated that age stereotypes can impact older individuals' cognitive performance and that this process can occur implicitly. The finding that age stereotypes can impact older individuals' cognition has been replicated by Hess and his colleagues (Hess, Auman, Colcombe, & Rahhal, 2003; Hess, Hinson, & Statham, 2004) as well as by a meta-analysis on age stereotypes relevant to memory that found a strong effect size in support of the relationship between negative age stereotypes and impaired memory performance among older adults (Horton, Baker, Pearce, & Deakin, 2008). However, these effects extend beyond the walls of the laboratory and are shown to have long-term outcomes. Levy, Zonderman, Slade, and Ferrucci (2012) found that, compared to older adults with more positive age stereotypes, those with more negative age stereotypes had worse visual recall memory over a 38-year time period. This effect was greater among participants who indicated that the negative age stereotype was directly relevant to themselves.

Regarding mental health outcomes, recently Levy, Pilver, and Pietrzak (2014) explored the relationship between age stereotyped expectations and a number of mental health outcomes, specifically suicidal ideation, anxiety, and posttraumatic stress disorder

(PTSD). It was found that older adults who fully accepted negative age stereotypes were significantly more likely to report experiencing all three adverse mental health conditions. However, those who were more resistant to negative age stereotypes had significantly lower prevalence rates. Another recent study using data from the English Longitudinal Study of Ageing found that age stereotypes and aging expectations are associated with another mental health outcome in later life, which is loneliness. Among adults older than 50 years, Pikhartova, Bowling, and Victor (2015) found that those who believed old age was a time of loneliness were 1.5 times more likely to report feelings of loneliness over time (i.e., lacking companionship as well as social exclusion and isolation), compared to those who did not endorse this statement. In addition, those who reported that they expected to get lonelier with age were 2.4 times more likely to report these same loneliness outcomes over time, again compared to those who did not have this aging expectation. Also pertinent to mental health, age stereotypes influence older adults' will to live. In two implicit age stereotype priming experimental studies, older participants who were exposed to negative age stereotype primes were more likely to refuse hypothetical life-prolonging interventions compared to those who were exposed to positive age stereotype primes (Levy, Ashman, & Dror, 1999–2000; Marques, Lima, Abrams, & Swift, 2014). This finding may help explain decreased longevity among those who embody negative age stereotypes (Kotter-Grühn, Kleinspehn-Ammerlahn, Gerstorf, & Smith, 2009; Levy, Slade, Kunkel, & Kasl, 2002; Sargent-Cox, Anstey, & Luszcz, 2014).

Matching Effect of Age Stereotype to Domain of Health Outcome

In the previous two subsections, research evidence supporting the basis of SET demonstrates that the presence and activation of generalized positive or negative age stereotypes can lead to better or worse health-related outcomes among older individuals, respectively. However, considering that individuals hold multiple age stereotypes, a new line of research has examined whether age stereotype effects among older individuals' health outcomes are stronger when there is a correspondence between the domain of age stereotype activated and the domain of the outcome that is influenced. Indeed, there is proof of such a "stereotype matching effect" (Levy & Leifheit-Limson, 2009).

To examine the stereotype matching effect, Levy and Leifheit-Limson (2009) generated a list of positive and negative cognitive and physical age stereotype traits and then used them in an implicit priming task among adults older than 60 years. The dependent variables of interest in this study were a photo-recall task (i.e., memory performance as a cognitive measure) and a timed chair-stand task (i.e., balance performance as a physical measure). Results supported the age stereotype matching effect such that the impact of both positive and negative age stereotypes on cognitive and physical performance was greatest when the age stereotype content was directly relevant to the outcome of that stereotype domain.

There is observational survey–based research that also demonstrates a matching effect between age-stereotypical beliefs and specific health-related outcomes among older adults. In two studies using the Expectations Regarding Aging (ERA) survey (Sarkisian, Steers, Hays, & Mangione, 2005), Meisner and his colleagues found that middle-aged and older adults who believed that the aging process brings inevitable and unavoidable decline were less likely to receive a preventive routine checkup from their doctor and were also less likely to be engaging in health-promoting physical activity (Meisner & Baker, 2013; Meisner, Weir, & Baker, 2013). However, a closer inspection of the ERA subscales within these studies revealed that mental health ERA was the main predictor of receiving a routine checkup and that physical health ERA was the main predictor of the association found for physical activity. The experimental and observational research shows that the general self-relevance of age stereotypes to the general category of "old" results in significant effects upon individuals after they enter later life; however, the direct relevance and specificity of age stereotype domains to the individual who hosts these beliefs are even more prominent.

■ SET: FOUR CORE COMPONENTS

The evidence and findings have demonstrated that age stereotypes influence multiple health outcomes in later life and throughout adult development. To clarify the process by which age stereotypes influence health outcomes, SET includes four key components: (a) age stereotypes become internalized across the life span; (b) age stereotypes can operate unconsciously; (c) age stereotypes gain salience from self-relevance; and (d) age stereotypes utilize multiple pathways. In the following four sections, each of the core components of SET is discussed, and evidence is integrated to support, build upon, and explain how the health outcome findings reviewed in the previous sections may occur. It is important to note that these four components reflect the two-dimensional directionality of how age stereotypes operate in a top-down manner and manifest themselves over time to influence health outcomes.

SET Component One: Age Stereotypes Become Internalized Across the Life Span

To understand the process in which age stereotypes influence older adults, SET takes a life-course developmental approach, starting in early childhood. A literature review of children's age stereotypes concluded that children as young as 3 years of age demonstrate negative attitudes and prejudicial behaviors against "old" categories and that the validity and reliability of these effects increase among children between the ages of 5 to 8 years, indicating that age stereotypes become more specific and precise as childhood progresses (Gilbert & Ricketts, 2008). Children and adolescents are naturally vulnerable to the biased stereotypes that exist not only in the larger society and in day-to-day exchanges, but also in educational and entertainment programming specifically intended for this young age group. For example, older characters are often missing from children's picture story books and Disney animated films; however, when they are present, they often reinforce negative aspects of age (Danowski & Robinson, 2012; Robinson, Callister, Magoffin, & Moore, 2007)—either directly (e.g., Scrooge) or indirectly (e.g., a nurturing, but frail, grandmother).

Additionally, negative age stereotype development is self-sustaining. To illustrate, an effect of age stereotypes is for children and young adults to actively avoid older adults (North & Fiske, 2012; Pasupathi & Löckenhoff, 2002). Thus, once negative age stereotypes and attitudes are formed among children, they may be more likely to engage in distancing behaviors, keeping them away from meaningful, prolonged interactions with older adults. Yet, these interactions are the most effective for promoting children's positive age stereotypes and reducing intergenerational prejudice (e.g., Kwong See & Nicoladis, 2010). This young–old divide is further emphasized within larger social structures that segregate younger and older adults within various systems such as school, employment, and personal social networks (Hagestad & Uhlenberg, 2005). These subtle and overt forms of personal and institutional ageist behavior reduce or eliminate new and future opportunities for children and adolescents to engage with potential positive exemplars of aging that would counter any overgeneralized negative age stereotypes.

Although age stereotypes are first internalized during childhood, the development of age stereotypes extends beyond these early years of life. In fact, SET stipulates that age stereotypes are reinforced throughout a person's life span. Younger people spend over six decades of their lives existing in a society that popularizes negative images of aging. Before becoming older adults, younger individuals are particularly vulnerable to negative age stereotype formation because it contributes to their in-group worth and member self-esteem (Levy, 2003; Tajfel & Turner, 1979). These representations are assimilated from the environment to reflect a personal understanding of the collective cultural view on aging (Löckenhoff et al., 2009). This age stereotype assimilation approach explains why older adults often have relatively more negative age self-stereotypes than positive ones—despite now belonging to the older in-group.

A recent observational study provides support for this developmental internalization process of age stereotypes. Kornadt and Rothermund (2012) were interested in examining the path by which age stereotypes become internalized into the aging self. They generated a randomized sample of 769 community-dwelling adults between the ages of 30 and 80 years. With these participants, they administered a previously tested questionnaire that assessed multiple dimensions of age stereotypes relating to eight domain groups (Kornadt & Rothermund, 2011). When analyzing these age stereotype domains across decade-stratified age groups, it was found that all age stereotypes were strongest among the older adults of the sample and weakest among the younger adults. The authors noted that this finding provides support for the notion that internalization of age stereotypes increases with advancing age.

SET Component Two: Age Stereotypes Can Operate Unconsciously

Most of the earlier studies examining age stereotypes focused on explicit, conscious beliefs. However, as found with other types of stereotypes (e.g., race; Devine, 1989), age stereotypes also operate below the level of conscious awareness as a function of automatic information processing (Levy, 1996; Levy & Banaji, 2002). Studies that investigate the automaticity of age stereotypes use implicit techniques. One prominent technique is the Implicit Associations Test (IAT; Greenwald, McGhee, & Schwartz 1998). The age-IAT assesses the strength of associations between *young* and *old* concepts and evaluates how relatively *good* or *bad* they are. The association strength is determined by the lapsed time latency indicator between being exposed to a concept object (e.g., photo of an older or younger face) and the evaluation of it, such that a greater strength is indicated by less time. Multiple studies using the age-IAT show strong young–good and old–bad pairings that indicate an implicit preference for younger adults and an implicit negative bias against older adults. Once again, these findings are true for both younger and older adults (Axt, Ebersole, & Nosek, 2014; Levy & Banaji, 2002).

The second implicit technique that is commonly used is a subliminal age stereotype priming task. The first study to show that age stereotypes can be activated in older individuals without their awareness, and that age stereotypes can influence their health-related outcomes, was performed by Levy (1996). As described earlier in the section on age stereotypes' influence on cognitive and mental health outcomes, Levy (1996) discovered that older individuals who are exposed to implicit negative age stereotypes, which were presented at fast, subliminal speeds to allow for unconscious perception, demonstrated a decline in memory performance. However, those exposed to implicit positive age stereotypes tended to demonstrate an improvement in memory performance.

The utility of these implicit approaches versus explicit ones is important when thinking about how age stereotypes may exert their impact. Methodologically, implicit techniques have the advantage of reducing the discomfort people may have in reporting age stereotypes and prejudice. People may believe in one thing, but say another due to the corrective tendencies of controlled conscious thought (Devine, 1989). Thus, implicit methods are believed to be more representative of an individual's true beliefs. Indeed, implicit age stereotypes are more negative than explicit ones from childhood until late in life (Nosek, Banaji, & Greenwald, 2002). Because older individuals are not aware of these implicit negative age self-stereotypes, it is difficult for them to defend themselves against their damaging effects. Rather, they may misattribute any experienced detrimental health outcomes to old age itself, thereby representing the self-fulfilling prophetic nature of age stereotype effects (Levy, Ashman, & Slade, 2009; Meisner, 2012).

SET Component Three: Age Stereotypes Gain Salience From Self-Relevance

From a stereotyping perspective, the aging process is unique. Characteristics such as race, gender, and sexual orientation that are ascribed around birth have group memberships that are usually constant over the life span (Nelson, 2002). Conversely, old-age group membership is the one that is achieved if people are fortunate enough to have longevity. Thus, over one's life span, age stereotypes become age self-stereotypes by virtue of the natural aging process (Levy, Slade, Kunkel, & Kasl, 2002). Internalized age stereotypes, either positive or negative, have few reliable influences on behavioral outcomes among younger people (Hess, Hinson, & Statham, 2004); however, after the younger-to-older group membership transition takes place, age stereotypes are then more self-relevant and elicit their effects. The general finding that age stereotypes do not influence outcomes among younger adults, but do among older adults, supports self-relevance as a key aspect of how age stereotypes influence health-related outcomes in later life.

According to SET (Levy, 2009) and some early contributions to the development of this theory (Levy, 2003), there are a number of personal and social factors that likely contribute to age stereotypes' self-relevance. First, over time, age identity shifts as individuals develop an awareness of their advanced age. This change in identity may come sooner for some compared to others depending on the extent to which their negative age stereotypes outnumber or outweigh the positive stereotypes. Second, self-relevance may be strengthened in varying degrees by the extent to which individuals are targeted by ageism. Ageism may be encountered in such areas as ageist jokes, infantilizing communication, forced retirement, and discrimination in health care. Thus, even if a person does not feel old per se, his or her larger environment often indicates otherwise, which may ultimately shape his or her identity into old age (Eibach, Mock, & Courtney, 2010; Kotter-Grühn & Hess, 2012). Empirical evidence supports the importance of age stereotype self-relevance among older adults. A longitudinal study by Levy, Zonderman, Slade, and Ferrucci (2012) found that age self-stereotypes' influence on memory over time was even more pronounced when the age stereotypes were identified as self-relevant.

SET Component Four: Age Stereotypes Utilize Multiple Pathways

SET proposes that the influence age self-stereotypes have on health outcomes occurs through three intermediary pathways that operate in tandem. These pathways operate via psychological, behavioral, and physiological processes into, and throughout, later life (Levy, 2009). Research is presented in the following paragraphs to highlight the relevance and importance of each pathway.

PSYCHOLOGICAL PATHWAY

Several psychological mechanisms that demonstrate age stereotypes' impact on health outcomes have been identified in experimental and longitudinal studies. For example, using experimental methods, Levy (1996) found not only that implicit age stereotypes influence older individuals' memory performance, but that memory self-efficacy mediates that relationship. That is, mirroring the findings on memory, older adults in the negative age stereotype priming group had decreased levels of self-efficacy, whereas the opposite was found for those in the positive age stereotype priming group. Longitudinal observational studies corroborate these findings. For example, Wurm, Tesch-Römer, and Tomasik (2007) showed that older adults who believed physical decline was an inevitable part of aging demonstrated lower control beliefs, whereas those who believed aging can bring continued growth and development had a stronger sense of control, self-efficacy, and hope for the future. Wurm et al. (2007) demonstrated that varying levels of these psychological factors were operating along the causal relationship between age self-stereotypes and health-related outcomes. Furthermore, Sargent-Cox, Anstey, and Luszcz (2012) found that both high-control expectancies and self-esteem protected older adults from the damaging effects of age self-stereotypes. Lastly, Levy (2008) found that more negative age stereotypes at baseline resulted in more negative age self-perceptions in the following 18 years. Taken together, the beliefs that we have about older adults become embedded into what we think our old-age experience will be like, which, in turn, modifies our actual current and future selves in age stereotype congruent ways.

BEHAVIORAL PATHWAY

To date, five studies, conducted with four different samples, have found that age beliefs impact health-related behaviors. In the first study, Levy and Myers (2004) found that positive self-perceptions of aging predicted health-related behavioral practices, including exercise and eating a balanced diet, 20 years later. Additionally, as discussed earlier, Meisner and his colleagues found significant associations between aging expectations and two important health-promoting behaviors: seeking a routine checkup from a health care professional (Meisner & Baker, 2013) and engaging in physical activity (Meisner, Weir, & Baker, 2013). In the fourth study, the authors found that positive self-perceptions of aging predicted increased reports of having received cholesterol screening among older adults as well as mammograms among the female participants or prostate exams among the male participants (Kim, Moored, Giasson, & Smith, 2014). In the fifth study, Beyer, Wolff, Warner, Schüz, and Wurm (2015) conducted a longitudinal study with older adults aged 65 years and found that positive self-perceptions of aging at baseline significantly predicted improved self-rated health 2.5 years later. Relevant to the behavioral pathway, the authors also found that increased participation in physical activity at 6 months was a significant mediator of this longitudinal relationship.

PHYSIOLOGICAL PATHWAY

Research on how age stereotypes influence the functioning of a person has found evidence that the stress response and cardiovascular reactivity during stress-inducing tasks may act as physiological mediators. In two experimental studies involving implicit age self-stereotyping, Levy, Hausdorff, Hencke, and Wei (2000) examined the impact of both negative and positive age stereotypes on a number of outcomes, such as blood pressure. In the first study, older participants' physiological assessments were taken both before and after negative or positive implicit age stereotype priming and stress-inducing tasks. Compared to baseline, participants in the negative age stereotype-priming group demonstrated significant increases in three of the four outcomes. Conversely, positive age stereotypes appeared to protect individuals from experiencing stress. That is, those in the positive age stereotype-priming group did not demonstrate a significant increase in these physiological stress responses. Given that this first study involved mostly White participants, Levy, Ryall, Pilver, Sheridan, Wei, and Hausdorff (2008) then investigated whether these same associations were found among Black older adults. Replicating the aforementioned results, it was found that exposure to negative age stereotypes causes significantly higher cardiovascular responses to stress than do positive age stereotypes. These findings show that negative age stereotypes reinforce or perhaps exaggerate the stress response to environmental cues, whereas positive age stereotypes provide protection from these responses.

■ FUTURE RESEARCH, APPLICATION, POLICY, AND PRACTICE

Although research exists to support the key principles and core components of SET among diverse sets of participants from numerous countries, there are still numerous beneficial questions that could be explored in future studies. An important area to examine is the breadth of SET's relevance to additional health outcomes. There is clear evidence that age stereotypes are diverse and mixed; however, to date, the health domains examined have concentrated mostly on physical and/or functional and cognitive and/or mental health. Given that there are many other common and strong age stereotypes (e.g., appearance, personality, religion, work) (Kite et al., 1988, 2005; Kornadt & Rothermund, 2011), a broader examination of additional aging self-stereotypes will generate a more complete picture of their overall impact. To aid in this exploratory pursuit, the inclusion of qualitative studies would be beneficial. Currently, the preponderance of research on aging self-stereotypes is quantitative, using mostly experimental and longitudinal designs. Undoubtedly, there is great benefit in using these particular methods to study impact and determine cause-and-effect relationships; however, they are restricted by the inability of including a wide range of the lived experiences relating to aging self-stereotypes among older individuals. With future multimethod studies, a deeper and more comprehensive knowledge base will develop that is essential to understand the total impact of age stereotypes on the health and lives of older adults.

Considering the evidence that shows the formation, presence, activation, application, and frequency of negative age stereotypes pose a health-related concern (because they tend to consistently exacerbate decline), there is a clear need for interventions to interrupt negative age self-stereotype operation. One potentially efficient approach is to reinforce positive age stereotypes (because they support health) to help mitigate the impact of negative age stereotypes. Drawing on laboratory- and community-based evidence, such interventions could employ explicit or implicit positive age stereotypes. For example, Levy, Pilver, Chung, and Slade (2014) developed an 8-week age stereotype intervention with 100 community-dwelling older adults to examine whether sustained activation of positive age stereotypes would protect older adults from the damaging effects of negative age self-stereotypes. Results indicated that the implicit positive age stereotyping not only improved physical function over time, but also weakened negative age stereotypes. Additionally, future interventions would be particularly beneficial if older adults who have, or who are at high risk of developing, strong and persistent negative age stereotypes were targeted. Thus, future research ought to explore the characteristics and circumstances that increase the likelihood of being more susceptible to negative age stereotypes.

There is also great potential value in applying SET to policy and practice. In fact, addressing negative age stereotypes through social policies is particularly appropriate considering that age stereotypes operate in a top–down fashion—from society to self (Levy, 2009). In many societies, the aging process is still too often represented as a process that brings inevitable and undesirable decline (Löckenhoff et al., 2009). Additionally, older people are too often represented as existing in states of disease, decrepitude, and dependency (Cuddy, Norton, & Fiske, 2005). Meanwhile, positive representations of aging and older people are underrepresented or are often missing completely. Biased portrayals of aging can be found in advertisements and marketing (Hurd Clarke, Bennett, & Liu, 2014; Low & Dupuis-Blanchard, 2013), television programs (Donlon, Ashman, & Levy, 2005), movies (Malone & Meisner, 2015), and social media networks (Levy, Chung, Bedford, & Navrazhina, 2014). The resulting skewed cultural standards of aging create a larger social environment that condones, promotes ageism that infiltrates our daily lives, and reinforces negative age stereotypes, whether we are aware of it or not. Therefore, the health and well-being of our current and future older adults would dramatically benefit from a cultural shift. To facilitate this social change, changes should be made at higher levels—within communities, aging-related organizations, public health agencies, and governments. This collective strategy would help address age stereotype and health issues more broadly. Age stereotype research should play an important role in this process to provide appropriate evidence-based knowledge on the detrimental health consequences of not curtailing negative age stereotypes.

Additionally, it would be beneficial if future applied research and policy work could be tailored to address contemporary social issues pertaining to age- and health-related inequalities and disparities such as the mental health of veterans and those older adults who belong to additional marginalized groups (Meisner & Hynie, 2009). These social issues are currently insufficiently studied in relation to age stereotypes. Another potentially important application of SET would be within health care settings to discern how age stereotypes are supported or deconstructed within these systems. By knowing more about how age stereotypes contribute to social-level problems, the utility and application of SET to the development of public policy would be strengthened.

Even small and subtle changes made within social structures, policies, systems, communities, and institutions could have meaningful effects on the lives and experiences of older adults within those settings. A multilevel approach would not only help raise awareness of the impact that age stereotypes have on health with aging, but may also reduce ageism within each one of these levels. Such initiatives would involve active multisectorial collaborations among researchers, policy makers, health practitioners, community partners, and older adults as key stakeholders in the promotion of positive and healthy aging at individual-to-social levels. Examining these various areas would provide useful direction for future research and policies to mitigate the condition and effects of age-related marginalization.

■ CONCLUSION

This chapter provides the current context of how age stereotypes and self-stereotypes are formed, organized, explicitly understood, implicitly activated, and applied intra-individually. In addition, there is a necessary consideration of the larger environmental context of aging individuals, across their life-span development, to add interpersonal, sociocultural, and temporal dimensions. SET provides an illustration of how socialized age norms become age stereotypes (i.e., via internalization) and then become aging self-stereotypes (i.e., via continued internalization and self-relevance) (Levy, 2009). Connections are made, supported by evidence, to highlight the importance of these processes to show that age stereotypes can significantly contribute to health-related outcomes. Consistently, the effects that positive- and negative-aging self-stereotypes have on health and disease occur through similar, parallel psychological, behavioral, and physiological pathways. Considering these processes, SET demonstrates the means by which aging self-stereotypes affect the health and aging of older adults.

SET sheds light on how sociocultural norms that exist about aging shape our minds and bodies throughout our lives to ultimately contribute to the older adult we become. Examinations of the overall impact that age stereotypes have on health and well-being among older adults should continue and these issues should be raised publicly to generate social awareness. Innovative ways to effectively negate or reduce the damaging effects on health brought about by negative age stereotypes must be discovered, while simultaneously finding ways to support the health-promoting properties of positive age stereotypes. This will require a narrowing of the gap between what we *believe* about aging and what is *actually known* (Kent, 1965). To facilitate these long- and short-term goals, SET provides an operational framework for exploring how age stereotypes influence health. Ideally, the result will be a widespread recognition that aging and health cannot be solely understood through biomedical approaches. Instead, there must be an acknowledgment of aging as a psychosocial construct, which interacts with the biomedical, to manifest itself in self-fulfilling ways over time.

REFERENCES

Axt, J. R., Ebersole, C. R., & Nosek, B. A. (2014). The rules of implicit evaluation by race, religion, and age. *Psychological Science, 25*(9), 1804–1815.

Beyer, A. K., Wolff, J. K., Warner, L. M., Schüz, B., & Wurm, S. (2015). The role of physical activity in the relationship between self-perceptions of ageing and self-rated health in older adults. *Psychology & Health, 30*(6), 671–685.

Brewer, M., Dull, V., & Lui, L. (1981). Perceptions of the elderly: Stereotypes as prototypes. *Journal of Personality and Social Psychology, 41,* 656–670.

Cuddy, A. J. C., & Fiske, S. T. (2002). Doddering, but dear: Process, content, and function in stereotyping of elderly people. In T. D. Nelson (Ed.), *Ageism: Stereotyping and prejudice against older persons.* Cambridge, MA: MIT Press.

Cuddy, A. J. C., Norton, M. I., & Fiske, S. T. (2005). This old stereotype: The pervasiveness and persistence of the elderly stereotype. *Journal of Social Issues, 61,* 265–283.

Danowski, J., & Robinson, T. (2012). The portrayal of older characters in popular children's picture books in the US: A content analysis from 2000 to 2010. *Journal of Children and Media, 6,* 333–350.

Devine, P. (1989). Stereotypes and prejudice: Their automatic and controlled components. *Journal of Personality and Social Psychology, 56*, 5–18.

Donlon, M. M., Ashman, O., & Levy, B. R. (2005). Re-vision of older television characters: A stereotype-awareness intervention. *Journal of Social Issues, 61*, 307–319.

Eibach, R. P., Mock, S. E., & Courtney, E. (2010). Having a "senior moment": Induced aging phenomenology, subjective age, and susceptibility to ageist stereotypes. *Journal of Experimental Social Psychology, 46*, 643–649.

Gilbert, C. N., & Ricketts, K. G. (2008). Children's attitudes towards older adults and aging: A synthesis of research. *Educational Gerontology, 34*, 570–586.

Greenwald, A. G., McGhee, D. E., & Schwartz, J. L. (1998). Measuring individual differences in implicit cognition: The implicit association test. *Journal of Personality and Social Psychology, 74*(6), 1464–1480.

Hagestad, G. O., & Uhlenberg, P. (2005). The social separation of old and young: A root of ageism. *Journal of Social Issues, 61*, 343–360.

Hausdorff, J. M., Levy, B. R., & Wei, J. Y. (1999). The power of ageism on physical function of older persons: Reversibility of age-related gait changes. *Journal of the American Geriatrics Society, 47*(11), 1346–1349.

Hess, T. M., Auman, C., Colcombe, S. J., & Rahhal, T. A. (2003). The impact of stereotype threat on age differences in memory performance. *The Journals of Gerontology, Series B, 58*(1), P3–11.

Hess, T. M., Hinson, J. T., & Statham, J. A. (2004). Explicit and implicit stereotype activation effects on memory: Do age and awareness moderate the impact of priming? *Psychology and Aging, 19*(3), 495–505.

Horton, S., Baker, J., Pearce, G. W., & Deakin, J. M. (2008). On the malleability of performance: Implications for seniors. *Journal of Applied Gerontology, 27*, 446–465.

Hummert, M. L. (1990). Multiple stereotypes of elderly and young adults: A comparison of structure and evaluations. *Psychology and Aging, 5*(2), 182–193.

Hummert, M. L., Garstka, T. A., Shaner, J. L., & Strahm, S. (1994). Stereotypes of the elderly held by young, middle-aged, and elderly adults. *Journal of Gerontology, 49*(5), P240–P249.

Hurd Clarke, L., Bennett, E. V., & Liu, C. (2014). Aging and masculinity: Portrayals in men's magazines. *Journal of Aging Studies, 31*, 26–33.

Kent, D. P. (1965). Aging—fact and fancy. *The Gerontologist, 5*, 51–56.

Kim, E. S., Moored, K. D., Giasson, H. L., & Smith, J. (2014). Satisfaction with aging and use of preventive health services. *Preventive Medicine, 69*, 176–180.

Kite, M. E., & Johnson, B. T. (1988). Attitudes toward older and younger adults: A meta-analysis. *Psychology and Aging, 3*(3), 233–244.

Kite, M. E., Stockdale, G. D., Whitley, B. E., Jr., & Johnson, B. T. (2005). Attitudes toward younger and older adults: An updated meta-analytic review. *Journal of Social Issues, 61*, 241–266.

Kornadt, A. E., & Rothermund, K. (2011). Contexts of aging: Assessing evaluative age stereotypes in different life domains. *The Journals of Gerontology, Series B, 66*(5), 547–556.

Kornadt, A. E., & Rothermund, K. (2012). Internalization of age stereotypes into the self-concept via future self-views: A general model and domain-specific differences. *Psychology and Aging, 27*(1), 164–172.

Kotter-Grühn, D., & Hess, T. M. (2012). The impact of age stereotypes on self-perceptions of aging across the adult lifespan. *The Journals of Gerontology, Series B, 67*(5), 563–571.

Kotter-Grühn, D., Kleinspehn-Ammerlahn, A., Gerstorf, D., & Smith, J. (2009). Self-perceptions of aging predict mortality and change with approaching death: 16-year longitudinal results from the Berlin Aging Study. *Psychology and Aging, 24*(3), 654–667.

Kwong See, S. T., & Nicoladis, E. (2010). Impact of contact on the development of children's positive stereotyping about aging language competence. *Educational Gerontology, 36*, 52–66.

Levy, B. (1996). Improving memory in old age through implicit self-stereotyping. *Journal of Personality and Social Psychology, 71*(6), 1092–1107.

Levy, B., Ashman, O., & Dror, I. (1999–2000). To be or not to be: The effects of aging stereotypes on the will to live. *Omega, 40*(3), 409–420.

Levy, B., & Langer, E. (1994). Aging free from negative stereotypes: Successful memory among the American deaf and in China. *Journal of Personality and Social Psychology, 66*, 935–943.

Levy, B. R. (2000). Handwriting as a reflection of aging self-stereotypes. *Journal of Geriatric Psychiatry, 33*, 81–94.

Levy, B. R. (2003). Mind matters: Cognitive and physical effects of aging self-stereotypes. *The Journals of Gerontology, Series B, 58*(4), P203–P211.

Levy, B. R. (2008). Rigidity as a predictor of older persons' aging stereotypes and self-perceptions of aging. *Social Behavior and Personality: An International Journal, 36*, 559–570.

Levy, B. R. (2009). Stereotype embodiment: A psychosocial approach to aging. *Current Directions in Psychological Science, 18*, 332–336.

Levy, B. R., Ashman, O., & Slade, M. D. (2009). Age attributions and aging health: Contrast between the United States and Japan. *The Journals of Gerontology, Series B, 64*(3), 335–338.

Levy, B. R., & Banaji, M. R. (2002). Implicit ageism. In T. D. Nelson (Ed.), *Ageism: Stereotyping and prejudice against older persons*. Cambridge, MA: MIT Press.

Levy, B. R., Chung, P. H., Bedford, T., & Navrazhina, K. (2014). Facebook as a site for negative age stereotypes. *The Gerontologist, 54*(2), 172–176.

Levy, B. R., Hausdorff, J. M., Hencke, R., & Wei, J. Y. (2000). Reducing cardiovascular stress with positive self-stereotypes of aging. *The Journals of Gerontology, Series B, 55*(4), P205–P213.

Levy, B. R., & Leifheit-Limson, E. (2009). The stereotype-matching effect: Greater influence on functioning when age stereotypes correspond to outcomes. *Psychology and Aging, 24*(1), 230–233.

Levy, B. R., & Myers, L. M. (2004). Preventive health behaviors influenced by self-perceptions of aging. *Preventive Medicine, 39*(3), 625–629.

Levy, B. R., Pilver, C. E., Chung, P. H., & Slade, M. D. (2014). Subliminal strengthening: Improving older individuals' physical function over time with an implicit-age-stereotype intervention. *Psychological Science, 25*(12), 2127–2135.

Levy, B. R., Pilver, C. E., & Pietrzak, R. H. (2014). Lower prevalence of psychiatric conditions when negative age stereotypes are resisted. *Social Science and Medicine, 119*, 170–174.

Levy, B. R., Ryall, A. L., Pilver, C. E., Sheridan, P. L., Wei, J. Y., & Hausdorff, J. M. (2008). Influence of African American elders' age stereotypes on their cardiovascular response to stress. *Anxiety, Stress, and Coping, 21*(1), 85–93.

Levy, B. R., Slade, M. D., Chung, P. H., & Gill, T. M. (2015). Resiliency over time of elders' age stereotypes after encountering stressful events. *The Journals of Gerontology, Series B, 70*(6), 886–890.

Levy, B. R., Slade, M. D., & Kasl, S. V. (2002). Longitudinal benefit of positive self-perceptions of aging on functional health. *The Journals of Gerontology, Series B, 57*(5), P409–P417.

Levy, B. R., Slade, M. D., Kunkel, S. R., & Kasl, S. V. (2002). Longevity increased by positive self-perceptions of aging. *Journal of Personality and Social Psychology, 83*(2), 261–270.

Levy, B. R., Slade, M. D., May, J., & Caracciolo, E. A. (2006). Physical recovery after acute myocardial infarction: Positive age self-stereotypes as a resource. *International Journal of Aging and Human Development, 62*(4), 285–301.

Levy, B. R., Slade, M. D., Murphy, T. E., & Gill, T. M. (2012). Association between positive age stereotypes and recovery from disability in older persons. *The Journal of the American Medical Association, 308*(19), 1972–1973.

Levy, B. R., Zonderman, A. B., Slade, M. D., & Ferrucci, L. (2009). Age stereotypes held earlier in life predict cardiovascular events in later life. *Psychological Science, 20*(3), 296–298.

Levy, B. R., Zonderman, A. B., Slade, M. D., & Ferrucci, L. (2012). Memory shaped by age stereotypes over time. *The Journals of Gerontology, Series B, 67*(4), 432–436.

Löckenhoff, C. E., De Fruyt, F., Terracciano, A., McCrae, R. R., De Bolle, M., Costa, P. T. Jr., ... Yik, M. (2009). Perceptions of aging across 26 cultures and their culture level associates. *Psychology and Aging, 24*, 941–954.

Low, J., & Dupuis-Blanchard, S. (2013). From Zoomers to Geezerade: Representations of the aging body in ageist and consumerist society. *Societies, 3*, 52–65.

Malone, M. R., & Meisner, B. A. (2015). Nebraska: Oscar® winning representations of aging and older adults. *Journal of Ethics in Mental Health, 10*(1), 1–5.

Marques, S., Lima, M. L., Abrams, D., & Swift, H. (2014). Will to live in older people's medical decisions: Immediate and delayed effects of aging stereotypes. *Journal of Applied Social Psychology, 44*, 399–408.

Meisner, B. A. (2012). A meta-analysis of positive and negative age stereotype priming effects on behavior among older adults. *The Journals of Gerontology, Series B, 67*(1), 13–17.

Meisner, B. A., & Baker, J. (2013). An exploratory analysis of aging expectations and health care behavior among aging adults. *Psychology and Aging, 28*(1), 99–104.

Meisner, B. A., & Hynie, M. (2009). Ageism with heterosexism: Self-perceptions, identity, and psychological health in older gay and lesbian adults. *Gay & Lesbian Issues & Psychology Review, 5,* 51–58.

Meisner, B. A., Weir, P. L., & Baker, J. (2013). The relationship between aging expectations and various modes of physical activity among aging adults. *Psychology of Sport and Exercise, 14,* 569–576.

Nelson, T. D. (Ed.). (2002). *Ageism: Stereotyping and prejudice against older people.* Cambridge, MA: MIT Press.

Nelson, T. D. (2005). Ageism: Prejudice against our feared future self. *Journal of Social Issues, 61,* 207–221.

Ng, R., Allore, H. G., Trentalange, M., Monin, J. K., & Levy, B. R. (2015). Increasing negativity of age stereotypes across 200 years: Evidence from a database of 400 million words. *PloS One, 10*(2), e0117086.

North, M. S., & Fiske, S. T. (2012). An inconvenienced youth? Ageism and its potential intergenerational roots. *Psychological Bulletin, 138*(5), 982–997.

Nosek, B. A., Banaji, M. R., & Greenwald, A. G. (2002). Harvesting intergroup attitudes and beliefs from a demonstration website. *Group Dynamics, 6,* 101–115.

Pasupathi, M., & Löckenhoff, C. E. (2002). Ageist behavior. In T. D. Nelson (Ed.), *Ageism: Stereotyping and prejudice against older persons.* Boston, MA: MIT Press.

Pikhartova, J., Bowling, A., & Victor, C. (2015). Is loneliness in later life a self-fulfilling prophecy? *Aging and Mental Health, 25,* 1–7.

Robinson, T., Callister, M., Magoffin, D., & Moore, J. (2007). The portrayal of older characters in Disney animated films. *Journal of Aging Studies, 21,* 203–213.

Sargent-Cox, K. A., Anstey, K. J., & Luszcz, M. A. (2012). The relationship between change in self-perceptions of aging and physical functioning in older adults. *Psychology and Aging, 27*(3), 750–760.

Sargent-Cox, K. A., Anstey, K. J., & Luszcz, M. A. (2014). Longitudinal change of self-perceptions of aging and mortality. *The Journals of Gerontology, Series B, 69*(2), 168–173.

Sarkisian, C. A., Steers, W. N., Hays, R. D., & Mangione, C. M. (2005). Development of the 12-item expectations regarding aging survey. *The Gerontologist, 45*(2), 240–248.

Schmidt, D. F., & Boland, S. M. (1986). Structure of perceptions of older adults: Evidence for multiple stereotypes. *Psychology and Aging, 1*(3), 255–260.

Tajfel, H., & Turner, J. C. (1979). An integrative theory of intergroup conflict. In W. G. Austin & S. Worchel (Eds.), *The social psychology of intergroup relations* (pp. 33–47). Monterey, CA: Brooks/Cole.

Westerhof, G. J., Miche, M., Brothers, A. F., Barrett, A. E., Diehl, M., Montepare, J. M., Wahl, H. W., & Wurm, S. (2014). The influence of subjective aging on health and longevity: A meta-analysis of longitudinal data. *Psychology and Aging, 29*(4), 793–802.

Wurm, S., Tesch-Römer, C., & Tomasik, M. J. (2007). Longitudinal findings on aging-related cognitions, control beliefs, and health in later life. *The Journals of Gerontology, Series B, 62*(3), P156–P164.

CHAPTER 15

Terminal Decline of Function
Gizem Hülür, Nilam Ram, and Denis Gerstorf

The last years of life are typically characterized by decrements in function in multiple domains, a phenomenon typically referred to as "terminal decline." In studies of terminal decline, developmental trajectories are modeled as a function of closeness to death (i.e., time left to live) as opposed to other time metrics such as chronological age (i.e., time lived; see Ram, Gerstorf, Fauth, Zarit, & Malmberg, 2010). Individual development in late life is heterogeneous and reflects the influence of a multitude of factors, including age-, pathology-, and mortality-related processes (see Birren & Cunningham, 1985; Gerstorf, Ram, Röcke, Lindenberger, & Smith, 2008; Ram et al., 2010).

Although there is substantial conceptual and empirical overlap among these processes, notions of terminal decline (Berg, 1996; Birren & Cunningham, 1985; Kleemeier, 1962; Riegel & Riegel, 1972) highlight the prominence of mortality-related processes as primary drivers of changes in function in the very last years of life. However, the exact timing of the transition into terminal decline is not always clear. In preterminal phases of adulthood, mortality-related processes have not yet set in and individual development in multiple domains of functioning is often characterized by relative stability or rather mild forms of functional decline. In the terminal phase, mortality-related processes have set in and exert their influence, producing pronounced and rapid forms of functional decline. Thus, individual development may be reasonably well characterized at a descriptive level by chronological age across most phases of the life span, whereas closeness to death might be a better proxy for developmental processes that occur at the end of life.

Our objective in this chapter is to highlight key issues in the study of terminal decline. First, we review research on terminal decline in multiple domains of function and consider the extent to which terminal decline pervades and cuts across many different domains of function. Second, although late life is typically characterized by extensive functional declines, there are considerable individual differences in terminal decline trajectories (see Gerstorf & Ram, 2013). Working through the existing literature, we evaluate what is known regarding the key predictors of individual differences in terminal decline. Third, terminal decline may not only affect levels of function in multiple domains, but also affect their covariation (see Gerstorf & Ram, 2015). We illustrate this aspect of terminal decline and highlight areas of research where such covariations have been observed. Fourth, as with other phases of development, terminal decline is influenced by the context in which it proceeds. Focusing on the role of the historical context, we consider how terminal decline differs and/or is changing across cohorts. Finally, we outline some open questions and avenues for future inquiry.

■ TERMINAL DECLINE IN DIFFERENT DOMAINS OF FUNCTION

Historically, research on terminal decline has focused primarily on end-of-life changes in cognitive function (for an overview, see Bäckman & MacDonald, 2006). More recently, researchers have started examining terminal decline in other domains as well, including motor function (e.g., Wilson, Segawa, Buchman, et al., 2012), sensory function (e.g., Gerstorf, Ram, Lindenberger, & Smith, 2013), physical health (e.g., Diehr, Williamson, Burke, & Psaty, 2002), and psychosocial function (e.g., Gerstorf, Ram, Röcke, et al., 2008; Gerstorf et al., 2013). Panel A of Figure 15.1 illustrates trajectories of terminal decline in different domains of function (cognitive function: performance on the Digit Symbol test; psychosocial function: perceived control; physical function: grip strength) for a hypothetical individual based on average trajectories reported by Gerstorf et al. (2013).

Although function in these three domains shows mortality-related decrements in proximity of death, theoretical notions and empirical evidence suggest that terminal decline is not uniform across all life domains. For example, terminal decline in cognitive function amounted to more than a full standard deviation (SD) unit per decade, whereas terminal increase in loneliness was much weaker and amounted to about half a SD unit over a decade (Gerstorf et al., 2013). Terminal decline is also not uniform within a domain (see Diehr et al., 2002): For example, in the physical domain, people's ability to engage in activities of daily living was found to show more pronounced mortality-related decline (0.66 SD units in men and 0.79 SD units in women over a time span of 5 years; Diehr et al., 2002) than walking speed (women: 0.13 SD units over a time span of 5 years; men: 0.19 SD units more than 5 years). In examining these differences more fully, we review literature on terminal decline in multiple domains.

Cognition

An accumulating body of evidence over the recent decades has documented that cognitive abilities decline in proximity of death (for an overview, see Bäckman & MacDonald, 2006). Research suggests that terminal decline in the cognitive domain is pervasive and can be observed in multiple cognitive abilities, including general cognition, episodic memory, and perceptual speed (e.g., Batterham, Mackinnon, & Christensen, 2011; Thorvaldsson, Hofer, & Johansson, 2006; Wilson, Beckett, Bianias, Evans, & Bennett, 2003). Terminal decline is typically seen across measures of both fluid and crystallized intelligence (see Bäckman & MacDonald, 2006).

A number of studies have examined the timing of cognitive decline, that is, when the transition toward a terminal period characterized by rapid declines takes place. Although some studies reported that terminal decline of cognitive function begins in the last 2.5 to 4 years before death (Wilson et al., 2003; Wilson, Beck, Bienias, & Bennett, 2007; Wilson, Segawa, Hizel, Boyle, & Bennett, 2012), others have found that individuals enter the terminal phase much earlier, ranging from about 6 years to more than 8 years before death (Batterham, Mackinnon, & Christensen, 2011; Muniz-Terrera, Minett, Brayne, & Matthews, 2014; Muniz-Terrera, van den Hout, Piccinin, Matthews, & Hofer, 2013; Sliwinski et al., 2006; Thorvaldsson et al., 2008). It is yet unclear how differences in study design (e.g., number of data points, length of follow-up intervals) and statistical modeling (e.g., inclusion of individuals who have died vs. individuals who were still alive) contributed to these discrepant findings.

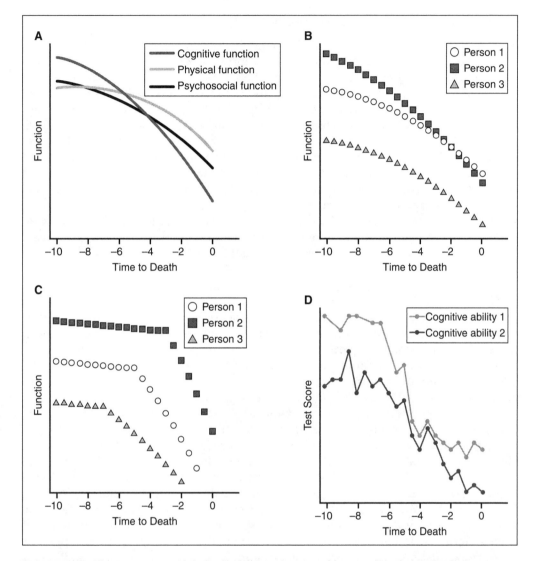

FIGURE 15.1 Illustrating terminal decline in different domains of function (Panel A); individual differences in levels and rates (Panel B); onset (Panel C); and covariation in terminal decline (Panel D). Panel A: Terminal decline trajectories of cognitive (performance in the Digit Symbol test), physical (grip strength), and psychosocial (perceived control) function for a hypothetical individual based on average trajectories in Gerstorf, Ram, Lindenberger, and Smith (2013). Panel B: Individual differences in levels and rates of decline for three hypothetical individuals. Person 1 and Person 2 do not differ in levels of function 2 years before death; however, Person 2 shows steeper terminal decline. On the other hand, Person 1 and Person 3 do not differ in rates of decline; however, Person 3 shows lower levels of function. Panel C: Individual differences in onset of decline for three hypothetical individuals. Person 1 experiences terminal decline 5 years before death, Person 2 experiences terminal decline 3 years before death, and Person 3 experiences terminal decline 7 years before death. Panel D: Coupling of two different cognitive abilities across time to death for a hypothetical individual. In line with the dedifferentiation hypothesis, cognitive abilities were more closely associated in closeness to death at the within-person level.

Sensory, Motor, and Physical Function

Several studies converge in reporting that a number of bodily functions decline in proximity of death, including sensory function (Gerstorf et al., 2013), motor function (Wilson, Segawa, Buchman, et al., 2012), physical function (Gerstorf et al., 2013), and functional health (Diehr et al., 2002). For example, Gerstorf et al. (2013) reported that sensory function, as indicated by close vision, declined by 1.6 SD units per decade in proximity of death. Another indicator of sensory function, hearing acuity, declined about 0.9 SD units per decade over distance to death (Gerstorf et al., 2013). Terminal decline was also observed for various indicators of physical function, including grip strength and maximum walking distance (Gerstorf et al., 2013). To date, few studies have examined the onset of terminal decline in sensory, motor, and physical functions. In one of the few exceptions, Wilson, Segawa, Buchman, et al. (2012) examined terminal decline in motor function as indicated by 11 performance measures including tests of grip strength, gait, and balance. They found that the onset of terminal decline was on average 2.5 years before death (Wilson, Segawa, Buchman, et al., 2012).

Psychosocial Function

Terminal decline is not only found in domains assessed through objective or performance-based measures (e.g., cognition, sensory function, and health), but also observed in psychosocial domains typically assessed using self-report measures. Research on psychosocial function in old age has mainly focused on subjective well-being and the so-called stability-despite-loss-paradox (see Berg, 2014) wherein both cognitive-evaluative (e.g., Diener & Suh, 1998) and affective (e.g., Mroczek & Kolarz, 1998) components of subjective well-being remain stable across adulthood and into old age while health and cognition decline. However, when looking at the very end of life, both cognitive-evaluative (e.g., life satisfaction: Berg, Hassing, Thorvaldsson, & Johansson, 2011; Gerstorf, Ram, Estabrook, et al., 2008; Gerstorf, Ram, Mayraz, et al., 2010; Gerstorf, Ram, Röcke, et al., 2008; Palgi et al., 2010) and affective (e.g., positive affect: Vogel, Schilling, Wahl, Beekman, & Penninx, 2013; negative affect: Palgi et al., 2010; Schilling, Wahl, & Wiegering, 2013; Vogel et al., 2013; vitality and mental health: Burns, Byles, Magliano, Mitchell, & Anstey, 2015) components of well-being do appear to exhibit terminal decline. Terminal decline in well-being was substantial, amounting to, for example, 0.75 SD units per decade for life satisfaction (Gerstorf, Ram, Röcke, et al., 2008) and to 0.44 and 0.25 SD units over a decade for positive affect and negative affect, respectively (Vogel et al., 2013). Studies that have examined the onset of terminal decline have found that terminal decline in various aspects of subjective well-being typically falls into a time window ranging from about 4 years (life satisfaction: Gerstorf, Ram, Estabrook, et al., 2008; Gerstorf, Ram, Röcke, et al., 2008; negative affect: Vogel et al., 2013) to about 6 years before death (positive affect; Vogel et al., 2013).

Recent evidence suggests that terminal decline also manifests in other aspects of psychosocial function, including social function and sense of control (Gerstorf et al., 2013). Theoretical notions and empirical evidence on social relationships in old age suggest that, although quantitative aspects of one's social life (e.g., the number of people in one's social network) may change across the life span, qualitative (e.g., support quality of relationships) aspects of social life remain rather stable though adulthood and old age (see Antonucci, Ajrouch, & Birditt, 2006; Antonucci, Birditt, & Akiyama, 2009). However, when looking specifically at the last years of life, social life does appear to change. For example, analyses of the Berlin Aging Study indicate that emotional loneliness increased about half a SD unit in the last decade of life (Gerstorf et al., 2013). Evidence for terminal decline was also found in perceived control (i.e., the extent to which individuals think they can influence what is happening in their lives; see Bandura, 1977; Lachman, 2006). Theories of perceived control propose that individuals' sense of control may deteriorate with increasing burdens and constraints (Brandtstädter & Greve, 1994; Heckhausen & Schulz, 1995). Thus, perceived control can be expected to deteriorate in similar manner to the terminal declines seen in other domains. Initial evidence suggests that the extent of terminal decline in perceived control is similar to the extent of terminal decline in physical function or subjective health (Gerstorf et al., 2013). In contrast, self-esteem, which is usually defined as global evaluations and feelings of a person's self-worth (Brown & Marshall, 2006), appears to be relatively stable through old age, all the way to death, suggesting that some aspects of the self-system remain relatively robust (Wagner, Gerstorf, Hoppmann, & Luszcz, 2013; Wagner, Hoppmann, Ram, & Gerstorf, 2015). As best as we can tell, no studies have yet specifically examined timing of the onset of terminal decline in psychosocial functions (other than subjective well-being as mentioned earlier).

■ INDIVIDUAL DIFFERENCES IN TERMINAL DECLINE

Like other developmental processes, mortality-related processes do not play out in the same way for all individuals; rather, there are substantial individual differences in terminal decline trajectories (see Gerstorf & Ram, 2013). First, individuals may differ in levels of function. That is, some individuals may be more cognitively fit than others in the last years of life. Second, individuals may differ in the rate of terminal decline. For example, some individuals' cognitive abilities may decline more rapidly than others'. Panel B of Figure 15.1 illustrates individual differences in levels and rates of terminal decline. Third, individuals may differ in the onset of cognitive decline: Although some individuals may begin exhibiting terminal declines of cognitive function many years before death, others may not enter the terminal decline phase until a year or some months before death. Panel C of Figure 15.1 illustrates individual differences in the onset of terminal decline. Investigation of the differences shown in Panels B and C typically seeks to identify associations with other individual difference factors. In reviewing this work, we note that the factors being identified in this literature are not specific to terminal decline, per se, but are also often related to levels of function and age-related changes in function throughout the aging literature.

Individual Differences in Terminal Decline of Cognitive Function

Individuals differ in trajectories of late-life cognitive function (see Bäckman & MacDonald, 2006). One of the central predictors of cognitive function is education: Education is crucial for the development of many cognitive abilities in childhood (Cahan & Cohen, 1989; Ceci, 1991) and continues to be associated with cognitive function throughout the adult life span, including old age (e.g., Tucker-Drob, Briley, Starr, & Deary, 2014). Theories of cognitive reserve propose that education serves as a buffer against pathology-related damages to the brain (Stern, 2002). In line with this reasoning, many studies have found that higher education is associated with higher levels of function in the last years of life (e.g., Gerstorf, Ram, Hoppmann, Willis, & Schaie, 2011; Hülür, Infurna, Ram, & Gerstorf, 2013). If education can compensate for negative effects of pathology, individuals with more education should enter the terminal phase later in time (i.e., closer to death), and spend fewer years in the terminal phase. Thus far, however, the evidence is mixed. A previous study by Batterham, Mackinnon, and Christensen (2011) did not find evidence for a protective effect of education to shorten the terminal phase, whereas a recent study showed that completing education at a later age was associated with a delayed onset of terminal decline (Muniz-Terrera et al., 2014). Muniz-Terrera et al. (2014) have found that being 1 year older when leaving school was associated with 0.4 years delayed onset of terminal decline. However, rates of cognitive decline in the terminal phase were steeper for those with more education (Muniz-Terrera et al., 2014). This finding is consistent with previous work on cognitive reserve in Alzheimer's disease (AD) that suggests that clinical disease onset is delayed for more educated individuals but that they experience more rapid declines after being diagnosed (e.g., Stern, Albert, Tang, & Tsai, 1999).

Evidence is also accumulating that genetic risk factors are related to individual differences in onset and rate of terminal decline in the cognitive domain. The apolipoprotein E (APOE) ε4 allele is a well-established risk factor for late-onset AD (Corder et al., 1993) and is associated with AD pathology (Bennett et al., 2003). Longitudinal studies have demonstrated that the APOE ε4 allele is associated with the onset and rates of terminal decline (Praetorius, Thorvaldsson, Hassing, & Johansson, 2013; Wilson et al., 2007; Yu et al., 2013), suggesting that AD pathology may contribute to terminal decline observed in the cognitive domain. Wilson et al. (2007) observed that APOE ε4 carriers showed steeper rates of terminal decline than noncarriers, even though they did not differ in baseline cognitive ability or rate of change before the terminal period. Moreover, terminal decline of cognitive function was not observed among noncarriers (Wilson et al., 2007). Another recent study by Praetorius et al. (2013) corroborated these findings by showing that APOE ε4 carriers showed steeper rates of terminal decline. The effects of APOE ε4 became largely insignificant after controlling for dementia incidence, suggesting that the APOE ε4 effect is related to dementia (Praetorius et al., 2013). Yu et al. (2013) extended these findings by showing that carriers of the APOE ε4 allele showed an earlier onset of terminal decline. Although the onset of terminal decline started 3.2 years before death for noncarriers, APOE ε4 carriers started experiencing terminal decline of cognitive function about 9 months earlier (Yu et al., 2013). This effect of the APOE ε4 allele was no longer significant after controlling for AD pathology, underlining the role of AD pathology for terminal cognitive decline (Yu et al., 2013).

Very old age is often characterized by dysfunctionalities and vulnerabilities (see Baltes & Smith, 2003; Suzman, Manton, & Willis, 1992), perhaps because humans are evolutionarily not prepared to survive into very old ages (incompleteness of the genetic architecture; see Baltes, 1997). In line with the increased dysfunction and vulnerability, higher age at death is typically associated with lower levels of function and steeper rates of terminal decline of cognitive function (see Bäckman & MacDonald, 2006; Gerstorf et al., 2013). This set of relations might be viewed from a different angle by explicitly examining the proportion of lifetime that individuals spend outside of terminal decline. For example, an individual who lived 90 years and showed terminal decline of cognitive function during the last 5 years would have been cognitively fit for 96% of his or her life. In contrast, a person who lived 70 years and spent 4 years in terminal decline would have been cognitively fit for 94% of his or her life. Thus, although the 90-year-old spent more absolute time in terminal decline (5 vs. 4 years), he or she spent less relative time in terminal decline (4% vs. 6%). The alternative perspective provides for additional consideration of the implications of the research findings for social policy. Do we, as a society seek a terminal decline phase that is shorter in absolute time or shorter relative the length of lifetime (absolute vs. relative compression of morbidity; see Fries, 2005)?

Individual Differences in Terminal Decline of Sensory, Motor, and Physical Function

Several factors have been associated with interindividual differences in terminal decline of sensory, motor, and physical function. Mirroring findings in the cognitive domain (see Bäckman & MacDonald, 2006), higher age at death is associated with lower levels of sensory (Gerstorf et al., 2013), physical (Gerstorf et al., 2013), and motor function (Wilson, Segawa, Buchman, et al., 2012) before death. Higher socioeconomic status is associated with higher levels of sensory and physical function late in life, suggesting that socioeconomic resources support individuals' function over the entire life span (Gerstorf et al., 2013). Health is also associated with terminal decline of physical and motor function, but we note that there are some conceptual (and/or practical) over-laps between indicators of health and indicators of physical and sensory function. First, comorbidity (i.e., having multiple diseases) is associated with lower levels and steeper declines of physical function (Gerstorf et al., 2013). Second, neuropathological burden (as indicated by plaques and tangles, Lewy bodies, and cerebral infarction) is associated with lower levels of motor function before death (Wilson, Segawa, Buchman, et al., 2012). Furthermore, plaques and tangles predicted an earlier onset of terminal decline of motor function (Wilson, Segawa, Buchman, et al., 2012). In line with these findings, suspected dementia was associated with lower levels of physical function before death (Gerstorf et al., 2013). However, vascular risk factors (e.g., diabetes, hypertension, and smoking) and vascular conditions (e.g., claudication, stroke, and heart attack) were not associated with trajectories of terminal decline of motor function (Wilson, Segawa, Buchman, et al., 2012).

Research on gender differences in morbidity and mortality has demonstrated that older women typically show lower levels of functional health (e.g., Crimmins, Kim, & Solé-Auró, 2011), although they live longer than men (Vaupel, 2010). In line with these findings, gender is typically a predictor of physical and motor function and health in the last years of life. Diehr et al. (2002) reported that women showed steeper age-related declines of functional health and walking speed than men, although men and women did not differ in rates of terminal decline. Men showed steeper terminal decline in body mass index and in the self-reported frequency of number of blocks walked in the pre-vious week (Diehr et al., 2002). Taken together, these findings suggest the presence of some gender specificity in the mortality-related processes influencing motor and phys-ical function.

Individual Differences in Terminal Decline of Psychosocial Function

Many of the same factors that are associated with individual differences in terminal decline in the cognitive, sensory, physical, motor, and health domains are also related to individual differences in terminal decline in the psychosocial domain. First, in line with theoretical notions and empirical evidence suggesting less favorable late-life develop-ment for those surviving into advanced old ages (see Baltes & Smith, 2003), a higher age at death was associated with lower levels of psychosocial function before death, as indi-cated by higher emotional loneliness and less perceived control (Gerstorf et al., 2013). These findings suggest that dysfunctionalities in very old age also influence subjective function (i.e., self-reports). Bluntly, people generally seem to know they are dying. Second, in line with research documenting gender inequalities in old age (see Moen, 1996), women showed lower levels of psychosocial function before death, as indicated by higher loneliness and less perceived control (Gerstorf et al., 2013). Some studies did not find gender differences in late-life trajectories of subjective well-being (e.g., Berg et al., 2011; Diehr et al., 2002). In studies that found gender differences, men typically report higher levels of subjective well-being (e.g., Hülür, Ram, & Gerstorf, 2015; Vogel et al., 2013). Third, worse health is associated with lower levels of psychosocial function in late life. For example, comorbidity was associated with lower levels of life satisfaction (Berg et al., 2011; Gerstorf, Ram, Estabrook, et al., 2008) and higher levels of loneliness (Gerstorf et al., 2013), whereas disability predicted lower levels of perceived control (Gerstorf et al., 2013). Berg et al. (2011) found that the association between comorbidity and life satisfaction was weaker among individuals with higher levels of perceived control, suggesting that perceived control may possibly buffer deleterious effects of comorbidity on life satisfaction. Fourth, socioeconomics is associated with the level of psychosocial function in late life. For example, higher socioeconomic status as indicated by education, occupation, and income is associated with lower levels of loneliness (Gerstorf et al., 2013). Fifth, personality is related to late-life psychosocial function. Berg et al. (2011) reported that higher levels of extraversion and lower levels of neuroticism were related to higher levels of life satisfaction in the last years of life. In sum, interindividual differences in trajectories of terminal decline are related to many of the same factors (e.g., SES, health, gender) that are associated with both differential development earlier in the life span and differential survival (e.g., age at death).

■ COVARIATION IN TERMINAL DECLINE

As outlined in the previous sections, terminal decline is a pervasive phenomenon that manifests in multiple domains of function. So far, only a few studies have analyzed how terminal decline unfolds simultaneously or time-lagged fashion across multiple domains of function, or how terminal decline manifests in the covariation among subfacets of the same domain (e.g., cognitive dedifferentiation). In the following three sections, we review theory and previous findings on mortality-related changes in covariation within the (a) cognitive; (b) sensory, motor, and physical; and (c) psychosocial domains.

Covariation Among Terminal Declines of Cognitive Functions

Life-span researchers have long been interested in ontogenetic changes in covariation between different cognitive abilities (Baltes, Cornelius, Spiro, Nesselroade, & Willis, 1980; Reinert, 1970). According to notions of cognitive dedifferentiation, covariation between cognitive abilities increases in old age (Baltes et al., 1980). Several mechanisms have been proposed to underlie such a development as we have discussed earlier (for an overview, see Hülür, Ram, Willis, Schaie, & Gerstorf, 2015). All of these proposals share the view that deteriorations in biological resources (e.g., sensory, central nervous system [CNS], and motor functions; Baltes, Reuter-Lorenz, & Rösler, 2006; Schaie, Maitland, & Willis, 2000) or more basal cognitive processes that can be considered cognitive primitives (e.g., processing speed: Hertzog & Bleckley, 2001; constituent cognitive processes: Li et al., 2004) propel dedifferentiation of cognitive abilities. Studies have typically examined cognitive dedifferentiation across age (e.g., Baltes & Lindenberger, 1997; Tucker-Drob, 2009) and were almost exclusively based on analyses of covariation from a between-person difference perspective. For example, evidence of dedifferentiation might be derived from findings that intertest correlations are higher for an older adult sample, as compared to a younger adult sample. From a within-person perspective, dedifferentiation would be indicated by an individual scoring lower in one cognitive test on occasions where he or she scored lower on other tests, and that this covariation would increase as that individual gets older or closer to death (see Hülür, Ram, Willis, et al., 2015). Panel D of Figure 15.1 illustrates mortality-related cognitive dedifferentiation at the within-person level.

As summarized elsewhere, some studies have examined the role of pathology and mortality in cognitive dedifferentiation (for an overview, see Hülür, Ram, Willis, et al., 2015). For example, Sliwinski, Hofer, and Hall (2003) examined cognitive dedifferentiation in two groups of individuals, those who eventually developed dementia and those who did not. Rates of changes in different cognitive domains were more closely associated in the dementia group (rs ranging from .45 to .51) as compared to the group that remained cognitively healthy (rs ranging from .07 to .18). These findings suggest that disease progression plays an important role in cognitive dedifferentiation. Using cross-sectional data, Batterham, Christensen, and Mackinnon (2011) showed that cognitive dedifferentiation was stronger across time-to-death as compared to age. Furthermore, dedifferentiation effects were no longer significant after controlling for dementia, suggesting that processes related to pathology may be one key underlying source of cognitive dedifferentiation. Wilson, Segawa, Hizel, et al. (2012) examined terminal dedifferentiation of four cognitive abilities and reported that correlations between rates of cognitive change were higher in the terminal period (rs ranging from .83 to .89) than in the preterminal period (rs ranging from .25 to .46). A recent study (Hülür, Ram, Willis, et al., 2015) extended these findings by examining cognitive dedifferentiation from a within-person perspective. Our findings showed that cognitive abilities moved toward a dedifferentiated structure with increasing proximity of death (Hülür, Ram, Willis, et al., 2015). Taken together, research supports the view that closeness to death is associated with cognitive dedifferentiation. However, the mechanisms underlying cognitive dedifferentiation are not yet well understood. For example, the role of pathology-related processes could be examined more closely by comparing individuals who died from different terminal illnesses on the extent of cognitive dedifferentiation. Notably, much greater numbers of repeated assessments of the biological resources and cognitive primitives (e.g., perceptual speed) are needed to test the hypothesis that changes in those primitives are a major driving force for cognitive dedifferentiation at the within-person level (Hertzog & Bleckley, 2001).

Covariation Among Terminal Declines in Sensory, Motor, and Physical Functions

Wilson, Segawa, Buchman, et al. (2007) have examined covariation of terminal decline in motor function with terminal decline in cognitive function from a between-person difference perspective. They found that the onset of motor decline was highly correlated with the onset of cognitive decline ($r = .94$), suggesting that those who experience an early onset of terminal decline in motor function also enter the terminal phase of decline in the cognitive domain earlier than others (Wilson, Segawa, Buchman, et al., 2007). Moreover, rates of terminal decline in cognitive and motor function were modestly associated ($r = .34$; Wilson, Segawa, Buchman, et al., 2007). A recent study by Burns, Mitchell, Shaw, and Anstey (2014) examined covariation between terminal decline of self-rated physical health (operationally defined with the physical health subscale of the SF-36) and terminal decline of well-being (operationally defined with the vitality and mental health subscales of the SF-36). Within-person changes in physical health accounted for terminal decline in both indicators of well-being (Burns et al., 2014). Taken together, these findings underscore the interrelatedness of terminal decline in motor function and physical health with terminal decline in cognition and psychosocial function. However, these associations have been examined only from a between-person perspective. Inference to within-person covariation must be done very cautiously.

Covariation Among Terminal Declines in Psychosocial Function

Theoretical notions propose that covariation among affective responses might change in proximity of death. According to the Dynamic Model of Affect, individuals strive to gain a nuanced understanding of situations, including their affective reactions to events (Davis, Zautra, & Smith, 2004; Zautra, Affleck, Tennen, Reich, & Davis, 2005). Toward this end, relatively independent positive affect and negative affect allow people to achieve maximum information about their affective state and understand both positive and negative aspects of a situation (Davis et al., 2004; Zautra et al., 2005). In typical daily life, positive affect and negative affect are moderately correlated (e.g., $r = -.35$: Carstensen et al., 2000; $r = -.29$: Hülür, Hoppmann, Ram, & Gerstorf, 2015). However, when individuals are in stressful and uncertain situations, they will process information (about their affective states) more rapidly than deeply (Davis et al., 2004; Zautra et al., 2005). In these situations, a highly inverse association of positive affect and negative affect would emerge, given that clear distinction of positive and negative information reduces uncertainty.

Empirical evidence largely supports this Dynamic Model of Affect by showing that the covariation between positive affect and negative affect was more negative in times of stress (Scott, Sliwinski, Mogle, & Almeida, 2014; Zautra, Berkhof, & Nicolson, 2002) and pain (Zautra, Smith, Affleck, & Tennen, 2001). Given pervasive declines in multiple domains of function as summarized in previous sections, late life is typically characterized by the presence of chronic stressors. In line with these expectations, Palgi et al. (2014) have found that the within-person covariation between positive affect and negative affect becomes increasingly negative as individuals get closer to death. Interestingly, not only actual but also perceived closeness to death was associated with a more negative covariation between positive affect and negative affect (Palgi et al., 2014). Taken together, the findings of Palgi et al. (2014) showed that both level of affect and the covariance structure of affect change with proximity to death. What is less well understood, however, is how the within-person covariation of positive affect and negative affect is related to developmental outcomes late in life (for an overview, see Hülür, Hoppmann, et al., 2015). For example, although some studies have found that a less-negative within-person covariation was associated with more positive developmental outcomes in old age (e.g., better physical health: Hershfield et al., 2013; less neuroticism, less daily stress, better resilience: Ong & Bergeman, 2004), the same and other studies did not find significant associations with depressive symptoms (Grühn, Lumley, Diehl, & Labouvie-Vief, 2013), life satisfaction (Grühn et al., 2013; Ong & Bergeman, 2004), and physical health (Ong & Bergeman, 2004). More research is needed to understand how positive and negative affect move toward a more inversely associated structure late in life and what this change implies with regard to developmental outcomes.

■ THE ROLE OF HISTORICAL CONTEXT

Life-span researchers have long been interested in how individual development is shaped by the historical and societal contexts in which people live (Baltes, Cornelius, & Nesselroade, 1979; Riley, 1973; Ryder, 1965; Schaie, 1965). Extending these notions into the last phase of life, evidence is accumulating that terminal decline is shaped by the historical contexts. In the following sections, we focus on reviewing research on the effects of historical contexts on terminal decline of function and highlight three possible scenarios that could lead to the emergence of cohort differences late in life.

Cohort Differences in Terminal Decline of Cognitive Function

The increase in fluid cognitive performance over the past century has been well documented (e.g., Flynn, 1987, 2007). These historical increases in levels of cognitive performance have been argued to have resulted from improvements in a wide range of cultural factors (broadly defined), including material and economic environments, health care, educational, and media systems, as well as individual resources such as reading, writing, and computer literacy (Alwin & McCammon, 2001; Blair, Gamson, Thorne, & Baker, 2005; Hauser & Huang, 1997; Rönnlund, Nyberg, Bäckman, & Nilsson, 2005).

As discussed earlier, it is an open question whether the historical improvements observed over most of the life span (including old age: Christensen et al., 2013; Dodge, Zhu, Lee, Chang, & Ganguli, 2014; Matthews et al., 2013; Sacuiu et al., 2010; Zelinski & Kennison, 2007) also manifest during the very last years of life (for an overview, see Gerstorf et al., 2015; Hülür et al., 2013). On the one hand, these same factors could lead to the maintenance of cognition in old age and in the last years of life. As a consequence, later cohorts should exhibit less terminal decline than earlier cohorts. On the other hand, although improvements in medical care may help individuals to survive into higher ages, the increase in length of life may be achieved at the cost of late-life function (see Olshansky, Hayflick, & Carnes, 2002). Thus, the secular advantage of the later cohorts should be reduced or no longer apparent during terminal decline. The available evidence supports the second scenario: Gerstorf et al. (2011) examined cohort differences in age-related and mortality-related trajectories of cognitive change between an earlier-born (1886–1913) and a later-born (1914–1948) cohort in the Seattle Longitudinal Study. Although cohort differences favoring the later-born cohort emerged in age-related trajectories of cognitive abilities, the later-born cohort showed steeper cognitive declines in proximity of death. Using data from the Gerontological and Geriatric Population Studies in Gothenburg, Sweden (birth-year cohorts: 1901, 1906, and 1930), Karlsson, Thorvaldsson, Skoog, Gudmundsson, and Johansson (2015) reported similar findings: Later-born cohorts showed higher levels of cognitive performance, but they also exhibited steeper declines of cognitive performance with age relative to earlier-born cohorts. A study by Hülür et al. (2013) corroborated and extended these findings. To focus on factors that shape terminal decline, Hülür et al. defined cohorts not based on year of birth, but based on year of death and compared two cohorts of Asset and Health Dynamics among the Oldest Old (AHEAD) study participants who have died in the 1990s versus in the 2000s. No differences favoring the later-deceased cohort could be found in age-related or mortality-related trajectories of memory performance. Taken together, these rather disconcerting findings suggest that historical improvements in cognition that are apparent throughout much of the life span do not extend into the end of life. We are, however, only at the very beginning of understanding why historical trends in cognitive performance are not also appearing in terminal decline.

Cohort Differences in Terminal Decline of Sensory, Motor, and Physical Function

Research suggests that physical function has improved among older adults across recent decades (for an overview, see Crimmins & Beltrán-Sánchez, 2011). For example, Spiers, Jagger, and Clarke (1996) reported that the odds of being dependent on others to complete basic activities of daily living were lower among older adults in 1988 as compared to same-aged individuals in 1981. A more recent study by Christensen et al. (2013) reported that, at approximately the same age, Danish 90+-year-olds born in 1915 showed fewer disabilities with activities of daily living and faster gait speed than those born in 1905. No cohort differences were found in grip strength and chair stand tests (Christensen et al., 2013). To date, it is less clear whether these historical improvements in physical function are also happening in terminal decline.

Cohort Differences in Terminal Decline of Psychosocial Function

The same factors that may have led to historical improvements of cognitive function are also expected to have led to historical improvements in well-being, as we have argued earlier (for an overview, see Gerstorf et al., 2015; Hülür, Ram, & Gerstorf, 2015). First, higher socioeconomic status, as typically indicated by education and income, is associated with higher subjective well-being (for a meta-analysis, see Pinquart & Sörensen, 2000). Research indicates that socioeconomic conditions of older adults have improved across cohorts (Cribier, 2005). Second, individuals in better health report higher levels of well-being (for reviews, see Chida & Steptoe, 2008; Ong, 2010). Research has reported mixed evidence for historical improvements in health (for an overview, see Crimmins & Beltrán-Sánchez, 2011). For example, although common diseases such as heart disease or arthritis have become less disabling, the prevalence of heart disease remained stable or even increased across recent decades (see Crimmins & Beltrán-Sánchez, 2011). Third, educational attainment is related to higher well-being (e.g., Blanchflower & Oswald, 2004) and has increased considerably across cohorts over the past century (e.g., Schaie, Willis, & Pennak, 2005).

Research on cohort differences in well-being has yielded rather inconclusive findings, with some studies reporting evidence favoring earlier-born cohorts (e.g., Schilling, 2005) and other studies reporting evidence favoring later-born cohorts (e.g., Gerstorf et al., 2015; Sutin et al., 2013). The reason for this discrepancy is not yet clear, but might be based on methodological factors (see Hülür, Ram, & Gerstorf, 2015), including the nature of the samples (e.g., volunteer vs. representative), country of residence of participants, age ranges (e.g., life span vs. old adult samples), the period of assessment, the testing situation, and the measures of well-being (e.g., cognitive-evaluative vs. affective). One recent study examined whether cohorts differed in trajectories of well-being in old age and late in life using data from two national samples, Health and Retirement Study in the United States and the German Socio-Economic Panel (Hülür, Ram, & Gerstorf, 2015). As expected, based on historical improvements in education, economic prosperity, and medical care, later-born individuals (1940s) showed higher levels of well-being in old age. However, a comparison of death-year cohorts (1990s vs. 2000s) who mainly differed in circumstances in the last years of life revealed no differences favoring the later-deceased cohort, and even a partial reversal. In line with notions of manufactured survival (Olshansky et al., 2002), secular improvements in well-being are not appearing in the last years of life. Together with reports of similar trends in late-life trajectories of cognition, these findings suggest that the pervasiveness of terminal decline might minimize or even reverse cohort differences based on historical improvements that are visible in adulthood and old age.

Possible Scenarios for Cohort Differences in Late-Life Development

We conclude from the earlier description that cohort differences favoring later cohorts are apparent throughout most of the life span in multiple domains, including cognition and well-being, but these advantages are not manifesting in the last years of life. To reconcile this set of findings, we outline three scenarios that could explain how cohort differences manifest late in life (see Gerstorf et al., 2015). A graphical representation of these scenarios can be found in Figure 15.2. All scenarios share three underlying assumptions: First, in line with conclusive evidence over recent decades (see Vaupel, 2010), it is hypothesized that later-born cohorts live longer and die at higher ages than earlier-born cohorts. Second, based on notions and empirical evidence on terminal decline as outlined in this chapter, it is hypothesized that the last years of life are characterized by rapid decline in multiple domains of function. Third, it is assumed that cohorts do not

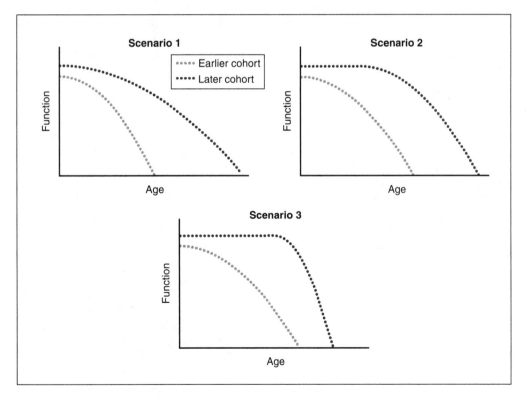

FIGURE 15.2   Illustrating three scenarios for cohort differences late in life. Scenario 1: Cohorts do not differ in onset, but in rate of decline. The later cohort shows slower declines over time. Scenario 2: Cohorts do not differ in rate, but in the onset of decline: The later cohort shows a later onset of decline. Scenario 3: Cohorts differ both in onset and rate of decline. The later cohort experiences a later onset of decline and shows steeper declines, thus spending less time in the decline period.

differ in levels of function at the time of death, that is, that the cohorts were not sick or healthier when facing death. Working from these assumptions, three possible scenarios are plausible.

According to the first scenario, the age at the onset of terminal decline has not changed across cohorts, but the rate of terminal decline is less steep for later-born cohorts. Thus, later-born cohorts experience a slower and longer decline process. According to the second scenario, the onset of terminal decline occurs later for later-born cohorts, but rates of terminal decline do not differ across cohorts. In this scenario, the mortality-related processes driving terminal decline are not different, they are simply being postponed to a later age. According to the third scenario, both the onset of terminal decline and the rate of terminal decline differ across cohorts: Later-born cohorts enter terminal decline at a later age and decline more steeply than earlier-born cohorts. Thus, later-born cohorts spend less and less absolute time in the terminal phase. This scenario is in line with notions of compression of morbidity (Fries, 1980) according to which functional declines are historically compressed into an increasingly shorter period of time at the very end of life.

Empirical data has not yet provided conclusive evidence supporting any one of these three scenarios. We have argued earlier (Gerstorf et al., 2015) that the first scenario is least likely because it is difficult to explain the tremendous differences found at cross-section among cohorts by a slowing of mortality-related process alone. However, although research has conclusively demonstrated that mortality has been prolonged to later ages, it is less clear whether debility and senescence have also been delayed (see Vaupel, 2010). This is partly due to the fact that health or other indicators of function are relatively difficult to measure as compared to post hoc time of death (Vaupel, 2010).

■ OPEN QUESTIONS

Terminal decline describes development at the very end of the life span. Typically, changes in function are modeled retrospectively as a function of proximity to death. It is an open question whether insights gained from this descriptive approach can ever be used in a prospective manner to support healthy and successful aging. Joint analyses of longitudinal trajectories and survival (e.g., Ghisletta, 2008; Ghisletta, McArdle, & Lindenberger, 2006; Muniz-Terrera, Piccinin, Johansson, Matthews, & Hofer, 2011; Sabia et al., 2014) offer a promising route for future research. Although studies of the terminal decline phenomenon typically describe (individual differences in) trajectories of function across distance to death, studies using shared parameter growth and survival models use individual differences in trajectories of function to predict survival over a specific time interval. Studies taking this approach have convincingly demonstrated that rates of change in cognition (Ghisletta, 2008; Ghisletta et al., 2006; Muniz-Terrera et al., 2011), physical function (Sabia et al., 2014), and well-being (Chui, Gerstorf, Hoppmann, & Luszcz, 2015) are predictive of mortality among older adults. As these findings are replicated and extended, we shall learn more about the specific pathways and mechanisms that link developmental change to mortality.

Along these lines, late-life development has been conceptualized as reflecting the influence of aging, pathology, and mortality-related processes (see Birren & Cunningham, 1985; Gerstorf, Ram, Roecke, et al., 2008; Ram et al., 2010). Age-related processes are assumed to be normative, whereas pathology-related processes are associated with specific diseases, and mortality-related processes operate in the last years of life. Currently, little is known about how these processes are distinguished from one another. For example, are "mortality-related processes" a distinct category, or is terminal decline merely a combination of normative age-related and pathology-related processes that happens to end in death? For example, a study by Laukka, MacDonald, and Bäckman (2006) showed that, after excluding participants with (preclinical) dementia, accelerated declines were no longer observed for individuals in close proximity of death as compared to survivors. Similarly, a study by Piccinin, Muniz, Matthews, and Johansson (2011) has found that cognitive decline before death was much weaker among individuals without preclinical dementia. Taken together, these findings suggest that pathology-related processes related to (preclinical) dementia might be the driver of terminal declines of cognitive function. Future research needs to disentangle these processes so as to move toward understanding the specific mechanisms that lead to phenomena of terminal decline.

Recent evidence indicates that late-life development is also shaped by the geographic context (Gerstorf, Ram, Goebel, et al. 2010; Gerstorf & Wagner, 2010). For example, Gerstorf, Ram, Goebel, et al. (2010) have demonstrated that 8% of the between-person variation in late-life trajectories of well-being could be explained by county-level variables, including gross domestic product, rate of unemployment, and number of medical doctors. Although 8% explained variance may not seem overwhelming at first, two points are to be noted (see Gerstorf & Ram, 2013): First, the amount of variance explained by geographical factors (8%) exceeds effect sizes for individual difference factors such as education and personality (around 4%) and is comparable to the effect size of health that is estimated at around 10% (for a meta-analysis, see DeNeve & Cooper, 1998). Furthermore, the study by Gerstorf, Ram, Goebel, et al. (2010) included a national sample of Germany with relatively small regional differences and obligatory health insurance. Thus, future research should examine regional differences in late-life trajectories of function in countries with greater geographical variability, such as the United States, where the effect of the geographical context can be expected to be more pronounced (see Gerstorf & Ram, 2013).

To better understand the mechanisms underlying terminal decline, more studies are needed that examine how late-life changes take place simultaneously or in a time-lagged fashion across multiple domains of function. Taking this approach will lead to more insight on whether terminal decline in one domain of function (e.g., health) predicts subsequent terminal decline in other domains (e.g., cognition, psychosocial function). Furthermore, studies examining the role of (terminal) diseases for late-life function in multiple domains may help to better understand how age-, pathology-, and mortality-related processes simultaneously influence individual development late in life. In addition, more tightly spaced assessments in different domains of function in the last years of life are necessary to understand the timing of terminal decline and to identify individual difference or context factors that are associated with compressed morbidity.

■ CONCLUSION

In this chapter, we have outlined what is known about terminal decline in multiple domains of function. Terminal decline is a pervasive process that can be observed in multiple domains of function, including cognitive, sensory, motor, physical, and psychosocial function. There are substantial individual differences in trajectories of terminal decline in these domains that are related to many of the same factors that are associated with differential development in other phases of the life span (Ram et al.,

2015). For example, research indicates that, although the APOE ε4 allele might serve as a risk factor for cognitive decline in late life (Praetorius et al., 2013; Wilson et al., 2007; Yu et al., 2013), education might be a protective factor (Muniz-Terrera et al., 2014). Furthermore, terminal decline in average levels of function may be accompanied by changes in structure, as indicated by differences in the patterns of covariation among cognitive, physical, sensory, and psychosocial functions (see Gerstorf & Ram, 2015; Ram & Gerstorf, 2009). Looking at historical context, evidence suggests that the cohort-to-cohort increase in cognitive function and subjective well-being found throughout most of the life span does not appear at the very end of the life. In outlining scenarios that might describe this pattern of finding (see Gerstorf et al., 2015), we note the utility of studying cohort differences in terminal decline. Critically needed are more mechanisms-oriented lines of inquiry and moving from post hoc description of change toward prospective prediction of change.

■ ACKNOWLEDGMENTS

We are indebted to Ulman Lindenberger who has helped us (and many others) tremendously to structure our thinking about the nature and implications of cohort differences by suggesting these scenarios to us. This work was supported by the Penn State Social Science Research Institute, the National Institutes of Health (grant numbers R01 HD076994 and R24 HD041025), and the National Center for Advancing Translational Sciences (grant number UL TR000127). The authors gratefully acknowledge the support provided by the German Research Foundation (Grant, GE 1896/3-1). The content is solely the responsibility of the authors and does not necessarily represent the official views of the funding agencies.

REFERENCES

Alwin, D. F., & McCammon, R. J. (2001). Aging, cohorts, and verbal ability. *The Journals of Gerontology, Series B, 56*(3), S151–S161.

Antonucci, T. C. Ajrouch, K. J., & Birditt, K. (2006). Social relations in the third age. In J. B. James & P. Wink (Eds.), *The crown of life: Dynamics of the early post-retirement period. Annual review of Gerontology and Geriatric* (Vol. 26, pp. 193–210).

Antonucci, T. C., Birditt, K. S., & Akiyama, H. (2009). Convoys of social relations: An interdisciplinary approach. In V. Bengtson, M. Silverstein, N. Putney, & D. Gans (Eds.), *Handbook of theories of aging*. New York, NY: Springer Publishing Company.

Bäckman, L., & MacDonald, S. W. S. (2006). Death and cognition: Synthesis and outlook. *European Psychologist, 11*, 224–235.

Baltes, P. B., & Lindenberger, U. (1997). Emergence of a powerful connection between sensory and cognitive functions across the adult life span: A new window to the study of cognitive aging? *Psychology and Aging, 12*(1), 12–21.

Baltes, P. B., Cornelius, S. W., & Nesselroade, J. R. (1979). Cohort effects in developmental psychology. In J. R. Nesselroade & P. B. Baltes (Eds.), *Longitudinal research in the study of behavior and development* (pp. 61–87). New York, NY: Academic Press.

Baltes, P. B., Cornelius, S. W., Spiro, A., Nesselroade, J. R., & Willis, S. L. (1980). Integration vs. differentiation of fluid-crystallized intelligence in old age. *Developmental Psychology, 16*, 625–635.

Baltes, P. B., Reuter-Lorenz, P. A., & Rösler, F. (Eds.). (2006). *Lifespan development and the brain: The perspective of biocultural co-constructivism.* New York, NY: Cambridge University Press.

Baltes, P. B., & Smith, J. (2003). New frontiers in the future of aging: From successful aging of the young old to the dilemmas of the fourth age. *Gerontology, 49*(2), 123–135.

Bandura, A. (1977). Self-efficacy: Toward a unifying theory of behavioral change. *Psychological Review, 84*(2), 191–215.

Batterham, P. J., Christensen, H., & Mackinnon, A. J. (2011). Comparison of age and time-to-death in the dedifferentiation of late-life cognitive abilities. *Psychology and Aging, 26*(4), 844–851.

Batterham, P. J., Mackinnon, A. J., & Christensen, H. (2011). The effect of education on the onset and rate of terminal decline. *Psychology and Aging, 26*(2), 339–350.

Bennett, D. A., Wilson, R. S., Schneider, J. A., Evans, D. A., Aggarwal, N. T., Arnold, S. E., . . . Bienias, J. L. (2003). Apolipoprotein E epsilon4 allele, AD pathology, and the clinical expression of Alzheimer's disease. *Neurology, 60*(2), 246–252.

Berg, A. I. (2014). Life satisfaction in the oldest old. In A. C. Michalos (Ed.), *Encyclopedia of quality of life and well-being research* (pp. 3589–3591). New York, NY: Springer Publishing Company.

Berg, A. I., Hassing, L. B., Thorvaldsson, V., & Johansson, B. (2011). Personality and personal control make a difference for life satisfaction in the oldest-old: Findings in a longitudinal population-based study of individuals 80 and older. *European Journal of Ageing, 8*, 13–20.

Berg, S. (1996). Aging, behavior, and terminal decline. In J. E. Birren & K. W. Schaie (Eds.), *Handbook of the psychology of aging* (4th ed., pp. 323–337). San Diego, CA: Academic Press.

Birren, J. E., & Cunningham, W. (1985). Research on the psychology of aging: Principles, concepts, and theory. In J. E. Birren & K. W. Schaie (Eds.), *Handbook of the psychology of aging* (2nd ed., pp. 3–34). New York, NY: Van Nostrand Reinhold.

Blair, C., Gamson, D. A., Thorne, S., & Baker, D. P. (2005). Rising mean IQ: Cognitive demand of mathematics education for young children, population exposure to formal schooling, and the neurobiology of the prefrontal cortex. *Intelligence, 33*, 93–106.

Blanchflower, D. G., & Oswald, A. J. (2004). Well-being over time in Britain and the USA. *Journal of Public Economics, 88*, 1359–1386.

Brandtstädter, J., & Greve, W. (1994). The aging self: Stabilizing and protective processes. *Developmental Review, 14*, 52–80.

Brown, J. D., & Marshall, M. A. (2006). The three faces of self-esteem. In M. Kernis (Ed.), *Self-esteem: Issues and answers* (pp. 4–9). New York, NY: Psychology Press.

Burns, R. A., Byles, J., Magliano, D. J., Mitchell, P., & Anstey, K. J. (2015). The utility of estimating population-level trajectories of terminal well-being decline within a growth mixture modelling framework. *Social Psychiatry and Psychiatric Epidemiology, 50*(3), 479–487.

Burns, R. A., Mitchell, P., Shaw, J., & Anstey, K. J. (2014). Trajectories of terminal decline in the well-being of older women: The DYNOPTA project. *Psychology and Aging, 29*(1), 44–56.

Cahan, S., & Cohen, N. (1989). Age versus schooling effects on intelligence development. *Child Development, 60*(5), 1239–1249.

Carstensen, L. L., Pasupathi, M., Mayr, U., & Nesselroade, J. R. (2000). Emotional experience in everyday life across the adult life span. *Journal of Personality and Social Psychology, 79*(4), 644–655.

Ceci, S. J. (1991). How much does schooling influence general intelligence and its cognitive components? A reassessment of the evidence. *Developmental Psychology, 27*, 703–722.

Chida, Y., & Steptoe, A. (2008). Positive psychological well-being and mortality: A quantitative review of prospective observational studies. *Psychosomatic Medicine, 70*(7), 741–756.

Christensen, K., Thinggaard, M., Oksuzyan, A., Steenstrup, T., Andersen-Ranberg, K., Jeune, B.,...Vaupel, J. W. (2013). Physical and cognitive functioning of people older than 90 years: A comparison of two Danish cohorts born 10 years apart. *The Lancet, 382*(9903), 1507–1513.

Chui, H., Gerstorf, D., Hoppmann, C. A., & Luszcz, M. A. (2015). Trajectories of depressive symptoms in old age: Integrating age-, pathology-, and mortality-related changes. *Psychology and Aging, 30*(4), 940–951.

Corder, E. H., Saunders, A. M., Strittmatter, W. J., Schmechel, D. E., Gaskell, P. C., Small, G. W.,...Pericak-Vance, M. A. (1993). Gene dose of apolipoprotein E type 4 allele and the risk of Alzheimer's disease in late onset families. *Science, 261*(5123), 921–923.

Cribier, F. (2005). Changes in the experiences of life between two cohorts of Parisian pensioners, born in circa 1907 and 1921. *Ageing and Society, Series B, 25*, 637–654.

Crimmins, E. M., & Beltrán-Sánchez, H. (2011). Mortality and morbidity trends: Is there compression of morbidity? *The Journals of Gerontology, Series B, 66*(1), 75–86.

Crimmins, E. M., Kim, J. K., & Solé-Auró, A. (2011). Gender differences in health: Results from SHARE, ELSA and HRS. *European Journal of Public Health, 21*(1), 81–91.

Davis, M. C., Zautra, A. J., & Smith, B. W. (2004). Chronic pain, stress, and the dynamics of affective differentiation. *Journal of Personality, 72*(6), 1133–1159.

DeNeve, K. M., & Cooper, H. (1998). The happy personality: A meta-analysis of 137 personality traits and subjective well-being. *Psychological Bulletin, 124*(2), 197–229.

Diehr, P., Williamson, J., Burke, G. L., & Psaty, B. M. (2002). The aging and dying processes and the health of older adults. *Journal of Clinical Epidemiology, 55*(3), 269–278.

Diener, E., & Suh, M. E. (1998). Subjective well-being and age: An international analysis. In K. W. Schaie & M. P. Lawton (Eds.), *Annual review of gerontology and geriatrics: Vol. 17. Focus on emotion and adult development* (pp. 304–324). New York, NY: Springer Publishing Company.

Dodge, H. H., Zhu, J., Lee, C. W., Chang, C. C., & Ganguli, M. (2014). Cohort effects in age-associated cognitive trajectories. *The Journals of Gerontology, Series A, 69*(6), 687–694.

Flynn, J. R. (1987). Massive IQ gains in 14 nations: What IQ tests really measure. *Psychological Bulletin, 101,* 171–191.

Flynn, J. R. (2007). Solving the IQ puzzle. *Scientific American Mind, 18,* 24–31.

Fries, J. F. (1980). Aging, natural death, and the compression of morbidity. *The New England Journal of Medicine, 303*(3), 130–135.

Fries, J. F. (2005). The compression of morbidity. 1983. *The Milbank Quarterly, 83*(4), 801–823.

Gerstorf, D., Hülür, G., Drewelies, J., Eibich, P., Duezel, S., Demuth, I.,…Lindenberger, U. (2015). Secular changes in late-life cognition and well-being: Towards a long bright future with a short brisk ending? *Psychology and Aging, 30*(2), 301–310.

Gerstorf, D., & Ram, N. (2013). Inquiry into terminal decline: Five objectives for future study. *The Gerontologist, 53*(5), 727–737.

Gerstorf, D., & Ram, N. (2015). A framework for studying mechanisms underlying terminal decline in well-being. *International Journal of Behavioral Development, 39,* 210–220.

Gerstorf, D., Ram, N., Estabrook, R., Schupp, J., Wagner, G. G., & Lindenberger, U. (2008). Life satisfaction shows terminal decline in old age: Longitudinal evidence from the German Socio-Economic Panel Study (SOEP). *Developmental Psychology, 44*(4), 1148–1159.

Gerstorf, D., Ram, N., Goebel, J., Schupp, J., Lindenberger, U., & Wagner, G. G. (2010). Where people live and die makes a difference: Individual and geographic disparities in well-being progression at the end of life. *Psychology and Aging, 25*(3), 661–676.

Gerstorf, D., Ram, N., Hoppmann, C., Willis, S. L., & Schaie, K. W. (2011). Cohort differences in cognitive aging and terminal decline in the Seattle Longitudinal Study. *Developmental Psychology, 47*(4), 1026–1041.

Gerstorf, D., Ram, N., Lindenberger, U., & Smith, J. (2013). Age and time-to-death trajectories of change in indicators of cognitive, sensory, physical, health, social, and self-related functions. *Developmental Psychology, 49*(10), 1805–1821.

Gerstorf, D., Ram, N., Mayraz, G., Hidajat, M., Lindenberger, U., Wagner, G. G., & Schupp, J. (2010). Late-life decline in well-being across adulthood in Germany, the United Kingdom, and the United States: Something is seriously wrong at the end of life. *Psychology and Aging, 25*(2), 477–485.

Gerstorf, D., Ram, N., Röcke, C., Lindenberger, U., & Smith, J. (2008). Decline in life satisfaction in old age: Longitudinal evidence for links to distance-to-death. *Psychology and Aging, 23*(1), 154–168.

Gerstorf, D., & Wagner, G. G. (2010). Lebenszufriedenheit am Ende des Lebens in Ost- und Westdeutschland: Die DDR wirft noch einen langen Schatten [Life satisfaction at the end of life in East- and West-Germany: East-Germany is casting a long shadow]. In I. Ostner & P. Krause (Eds.), *Leben in Ost- und Westdeutschland: Eine sozialwissenschaftliche Bilanz der deutschen Einheit 1990–2010* [Living in East- and West-Germany: A Review of German Reunification 1990–2010 from a Social Science Perspective] (pp. 429–445). Berlin, Germany: Campus.

Ghisletta, P. (2008). Application of a joint multivariate longitudinal-survival analysis to examine the terminal decline hypothesis in the Swiss Interdisciplinary Longitudinal Study on the Oldest Old. *The Journals of Gerontology, Series B, 63*(3), P185–P192.

Ghisletta, P., McArdle, J. J., & Lindenberger, U. (2006). Longitudinal cognition-survival relations in old and very old age: 13-year data from the Berlin Aging Study. *European Psychologist, 11,* 204–223.

Grühn, D., Lumley, M. A., Diehl, M., & Labouvie-Vief, G. (2013). Time-based indicators of emotional complexity: Interrelations and correlates. *Emotion, 13*(2), 226–237.

Hauser, R. M., & Huang, M.-H. (1997). Verbal ability and socioeconomic success: A trend analysis. *Social Science Research, 26,* 331–376.

Heckhausen, J., & Schulz, R. (1995). A life-span theory of control. *Psychological Review, 102*(2), 284–304.

Hershfield, H. E., Scheibe, S., Sims, T. L., & Carstensen, L. L. (2013). When feeling bad can be good: Mixed emotions benefit physical health across adulthood. *Social Psychological and Personality Science, 4,* 54–61. doi: 10.1177/1948550612444616

Hertzog, C., & Bleckley, M. K. (2001). Age differences in the structure of intelligence: Influences of information processing speed. *Intelligence, 29,* 191–217.

Hülür, G., Hoppmann, C. A., Ram, N., & Gerstorf, D. (2015). Developmental associations between short-term variability and long-term changes: Intraindividual correlation of positive and negative affect in daily life and cognitive aging. *Developmental Psychology, 51*(7), 987–997.

Hülür, G., Infurna, F. J., Ram, N., & Gerstorf, D. (2013). Cohorts based on decade of death: No evidence for secular trends favoring later cohorts in cognitive aging and terminal decline in the AHEAD study. *Psychology and Aging, 28*(1), 115–127.

Hülür, G., Ram, N., & Gerstorf, D. (2015). Historical improvements in well-being do not hold in late life: Birth- and death-year cohorts in the United States and Germany. *Developmental Psychology, 51*(7), 998–1012.

Hülür, G., Ram, N., Willis, S. L., Schaie, K. W., & Gerstorf, D. (2015). Cognitive dedifferentiation with increasing age and proximity of death: Within-person evidence from the Seattle Longitudinal Study. *Psychology and Aging, 30*(2), 311–323.

Karlsson, P., Thorvaldsson, V., Skoog, I., Gudmundsson, P., & Johansson, B. (2015). Birth cohort differences in fluid cognition in old age: Comparisons of trends in levels and change trajectories over 30 years in three population-based samples. *Psychology and Aging, 30*(1), 83–94.

Kleemeier, R. W. (1962). Intellectual changes in the senium. *Proceedings of the Social Statistics Section of the American Statistical Association, 1,* 290–295.

Lachman, M. E. (2006). Perceived control over aging-related declines: Adaptive beliefs and behaviors. *Current Directions in Psychological Science, 15,* 282–286.

Laukka, E. J., MacDonald, S. W., & Bäckman, L. (2006). Contrasting cognitive trajectories of impending death and preclinical dementia in the very old. *Neurology, 66*(6), 833–838.

Li, S. C., Lindenberger, U., Hommel, B., Aschersleben, G., Prinz, W., & Baltes, P. B. (2004). Transformations in the couplings among intellectual abilities and constituent cognitive processes across the life span. *Psychological Science, 15*(3), 155–163.

Matthews, F. E., Arthur, A., Barnes, L. E., Bond, J., Jagger, C., Robinson, L., & Brayne, C.; Medical Research Council Cognitive Function and Ageing Collaboration. (2013). A two-decade comparison of prevalence of dementia in individuals aged 65 years and older from three geographical areas of England: Results of the Cognitive Function and Ageing Study I and II. *The Lancet, 382*(9902), 1405–1412.

Moen, P. (1996). Gender, age, and the life course. In R. H. Binstock & L. K. George (Eds.), *Handbook of aging and the social sciences* (4th ed., pp. 230–238). New York, NY: Academic Press.

Mroczek, D. K., & Kolarz, C. M. (1998). The effect of age on positive and negative affect: A developmental perspective on happiness. *Journal of Personality and Social Psychology, 75*(5), 1333–1349.

Muniz-Terrera, G., Minett, T., Brayne, C., & Matthews, F. E. (2014). Education associated with a delayed onset of terminal decline. *Age and Ageing, 43*, 26–31.

Muniz-Terrera, G., van den Hout, A., Piccinin, A. M., Matthews, F. E., & Hofer, S. M. (2013). Investigating terminal decline: Results from a UK population-based study of aging. *Psychology and Aging, 28*(2), 377–385.

Olshansky, S. J., Hayflick, L., & Carnes, B. A. (2002). Position statement on human aging. *The Journals of Gerontology, Series A, 57*(8), B292–B297.

Ong, A. D. (2010). Pathways linking positive emotion and health in later life. *Current Directions in Psychological Science, 19*, 358–362.

Ong, A. D., & Bergeman, C. S. (2004). The complexity of emotions in later life. *The Journals of Gerontology, Series B, 59*, 55–60.

Palgi, Y., Shrira, A., Ben-Ezra, M., Spalter, T., Kavé, G., & Shmotkin, D. (2014). Age-related and death-related differences in emotional complexity. *Psychology and Aging, 29*(2), 284–296.

Palgi, Y., Shrira, A., Ben-Ezra, M., Spalter, T., Shmotkin, D., & Kavé, G. (2010). Delineating terminal change in subjective well-being and subjective health. *The Journals of Gerontology, Series B, 65*(1), 61–64.

Piccinin, A. M., Muniz, G., Matthews, F. E., & Johansson, B. (2011). Terminal decline from within- and between-person perspectives, accounting for incident dementia. *The Journals of Gerontology, Series B, 66*(4), 391–401.

Pinquart, M., & Sörensen, S. (2000). Influences of socioeconomic status, social network, and competence on subjective well-being in later life: A meta-analysis. *Psychology and Aging, 15*(2), 187–224.

Praetorius, M., Thorvaldsson, V., Hassing, L. B., & Johansson, B. (2013). Substantial effects of apolipoprotein E e4 on memory decline in very old age: Longitudinal findings from a population-based sample. *Neurobiology of Aging, 34*(12), 2734–2739.

Ram, N., Gatzke-Kopp, L., Gerstorf, D., Coccia, M., Morack, J., & Molenaar, P. C. M. (2015). Intraindividual variability across the life span: Moving towards a computational developmental science. In M. Diehl, K. Hooker, & M. Sliwinski (Eds.), *Handbook of intraindividual variability across the lifespan* (pp. 16–34). New York, NY: Routledge.

Ram, N., & Gerstorf, D. (2009). Time-structured and net intraindividual variability: Tools for examining the development of dynamic characteristics and processes. *Psychology and Aging, 24*(4), 778–791.

Ram, N., Gerstorf, D., Fauth, E., Zarit, S., & Malmberg, B. (2010). Aging, disablement, and dying: Using time-as-process and time-as-resources metrics to chart late-life change. *Research in Human Development, 7*(1), 27–44.

Reinert, G. (1970). Comparative factor analytic studies of intelligence throughout the human life-span. In L. R. Goulet & P. B. Baltes (Eds.), *Life-span developmental psychology* (pp. 467–484). New York, NY: Academic Press.

Riegel, K. F., & Riegel, R. M. (1972). Development, drop, and death. *Developmental Psychology, 6*, 306–419.

Riley, M. W. (1973). Aging and cohort succession: Interpretations and misinterpretations. *Public Opinion Quarterly, 37*, 35–49.

Rönnlund, M., Nyberg, L., Bäckman, L., & Nilsson, L. G. (2005). Stability, growth, and decline in adult life span development of declarative memory: Cross-sectional and longitudinal data from a population-based study. *Psychology and Aging, 20*(1), 3–18.

Ryder, N. B. (1965). The cohort as a concept in the study of social change. *American Sociological Review, 30*(6), 843–861.

Sabia, S., Dumurgier, J., Tavernier, B., Head, J., Tzourio, C., & Elbaz, A. (2014). Change in fast walking speed preceding death: Results from a prospective longitudinal cohort study. *The Journals of Gerontology, Series A, 69*(3), 354–362.

Sacuiu, S., Gustafson, D., Sjögren, M., Guo, X., Ostling, S., Johansson, B., & Skoog, I. (2010). Secular changes in cognitive predictors of dementia and mortality in 70-year-olds. *Neurology, 75*(9), 779–785.

Schaie, K. W. (1965). A general model for the study of developmental problems. *Psychological Bulletin, 64*, 92–107.

Schaie, K. W., Maitland, S. B., & Willis, S. L. (2000). *Longitudinal studies of cognitive dedifferentiation in older adults.* Paper presented at the Cognitive Aging Conference, Atlanta, GA.

Schaie, K. W., Willis, S. L., & Pennak, S. (2005). An historical framework for cohort differences in intelligence. *Research in Human Development, 2*(1–2), 43–67.

Schilling, O. K. (2005). Cohort- and age-related decline in elder's life satisfaction: Is there really a paradox? *European Journal of Ageing, 2*, 254–263.

Schilling, O. K., Wahl, H. W., & Wiegering, S. (2013). Affective development in advanced old age: Analyses of terminal change in positive and negative affect. *Developmental Psychology, 49*(5), 1011–1020.

Scott, S. B., Sliwinski, M. J., Mogle, J. A., & Almeida, D. M. (2014). Age, stress, and emotional complexity: Results from two studies of daily experiences. *Psychology and Aging, 29*(3), 577–587.

Sliwinski, M. J., Hofer, S. M., & Hall, C. (2003). Correlated and coupled cognitive change in older adults with and without preclinical dementia. *Psychology and Aging, 18*(4), 672–683.

Sliwinski, M. J., Stawski, R. S., Hall, R. B., Katz, M., Verghese, J., & Lipton, R. B. (2006). On the importance of distinguishing pre-terminal and terminal cognitive decline. *European Psychologist, 11*, 172–181.

Spiers, N., Jagger, C., & Clarke, M. (1996). Physical function and perceived health: Cohort differences and interrelationships in older people. *The Journals of Gerontology, Series B, 51*(5), S226–S233.

Stern, Y. (2002). What is cognitive reserve? Theory and research application of the reserve concept. *Journal of the International Neuropsychological Society, 8*(3), 448–460.

Stern, Y., Albert, S., Tang, M. X., & Tsai, W. Y. (1999). Rate of memory decline in AD is related to education and occupation: Cognitive reserve? *Neurology, 53*(9), 1942–1947.

Sutin, A. R., Terracciano, A., Milaneschi, Y., An, Y., Ferrucci, L., & Zonderman, A. B. (2013). The effect of birth cohort on well-being: The legacy of economic hard times. *Psychological Science, 24*(3), 379–385.

Suzman, R. M., Manton, K. G., & Willis, D. P. (1992). Introducing the oldest old. In M. Suzman, D. P. Willis, & K. G. Manton (Eds.), *The oldest old* (pp. 3–14). New York, NY: Oxford University Press.

Terrera, G. M., Piccinin, A. M., Johansson, B., Matthews, F., & Hofer, S. M. (2011). Joint modeling of longitudinal change and survival: An investigation of the association between change in memory scores and death. *GeroPsych, 24*(4), 177–185.

Thorvaldsson, V., Hofer, S. M., Berg, S., Skoog, I., Sacuiu, S., & Johansson, B. (2008). Onset of terminal decline in cognitive abilities in individuals without dementia. *Neurology, 71*(12), 882–887.

Thorvaldsson, V., Hofer, S. M., & Johansson, B. (2006). Ageing and late life terminal decline: A comparison of alternative modeling approaches. *European Psychologist, 11*, 196–203.

Tucker-Drob, E. M. (2009). Differentiation of cognitive abilities across the life span. *Developmental Psychology, 45*(4), 1097–1118.

Tucker-Drob, E. M., Briley, D. A., Starr, J. M., & Deary, I. J. (2014). Structure and correlates of cognitive aging in a narrow age cohort. *Psychology and Aging, 29*(2), 236–249.

Vaupel, J. W. (2010). Biodemography of human ageing. *Nature, 464*(7288), 536–542.

Vogel, N., Schilling, O. K., Wahl, H. W., Beekman, A. T., & Penninx, B. W. (2013). Time-to-death-related change in positive and negative affect among older adults approaching the end of life. *Psychology and Aging, 28*(1), 128–141.

Wagner, J., Gerstorf, D., Hoppmann, C., & Luszcz, M. A. (2013). The nature and correlates of self-esteem trajectories in late life. *Journal of Personality and Social Psychology, 105*(1), 139–153.

Wagner, J., Hoppmann, C., Ram, N., & Gerstorf, D. (2015). Self-esteem is relatively stable late in life: The role of resources in the health, self-regulation, and social domains. *Developmental Psychology, 51*(1), 136–149.

Wilson, R. S., Beck, T. L., Bienias, J. L., & Bennett, D. A. (2007). Terminal cognitive decline: Accelerated loss of cognition in the last years of life. *Psychosomatic Medicine, 69*(2), 131–137.

Wilson, R. S., Beckett, L. A., Bienias, J. L., Evans, D. A., & Bennett, D. A. (2003). Terminal decline in cognitive function. *Neurology, 60*(11), 1782–1787.

Wilson, R. S., Segawa, E., Buchman, A. S., Boyle, P. A., Hizel, L. P., & Bennett, D. A. (2012). Terminal decline in motor function. *Psychology and Aging, 27*(4), 998–1007.

Wilson, R. S., Segawa, E., Hizel, L. P., Boyle, P. A., & Bennett, D. A. (2012). Terminal dedifferentiation of cognitive abilities. *Neurology, 78*(15), 1116–1122.

Yu, L., Boyle, P., Schneider, J. A., Segawa, E., Wilson, R. S., Leurgans, S., & Bennett, D. A. (2013). APOE e4, Alzheimer's disease pathology, cerebrovascular disease, and cognitive change over the years prior to death. *Psychology and Aging, 28*(4), 1015–1023.

Zautra, A. J., Affleck, G. G., Tennen, H., Reich, J. W., & Davis, M. C. (2005). Dynamic approaches to emotions and stress in everyday life: Bolger and Zuckerman reloaded with positive as well as negative affects. *Journal of Personality, 73*(6), 1511–1538.

Zautra, A. J., Berkhof, H., & Nicolson, N. (2002). Changes in affect interrelations as a function of stressful life events. *Cognition and Emotion, 16*, 309–318.

Zautra, A., Smith, B., Affleck, G., & Tennen, H. (2001). Examinations of chronic pain and affect relationships: Applications of a dynamic model of affect. *Journal of Consulting and Clinical Psychology, 69*(5), 786–795.

Zelinski, E. M., & Kennison, R. F. (2007). Not your parents' test scores: Cohort reduces psychometric aging effects. *Psychology and Aging, 22*(3), 546–557.

PART IV

Social Science Theories and Concepts

ADVANCES IN SOCIAL SCIENCE THEORIES OF AGING
Richard A. Settersten, Jr.

As social scientists arrived at the study of aging in the middle of the past century, they naturally relied on their toolbox of classical and contemporary theories: theories of functionalism, social conflict, social interaction and exchange, symbolic interactionism, and phenomenology and social constructivism. Central starting points for developing theories were also found in social gerontology, especially disengagement and modernization theories in the 1960s and 1970s. At about the same time, the age stratification framework, which drew inspiration from earlier works of sociologists and anthropologists of age status, would emerge as a key heuristic device for advancing inquiry into the social, and especially structural, aspects of aging.

Each of these theorists, in his or her own way, emphasized that aging is a social process and that age is a structural feature of societies, with both people and roles allocated based on it. They also pointed to the dynamic aspects of aging, emphasizing that new cohorts of people are born, grow up and older together, and move through the age structure of the population as a group. These themes would also become central hallmarks of the life course perspective. Other major traditions would as well emerge in the social sciences and aging, especially informed by political economy, feminist, and critical gerontology perspectives.

Today, social science research continues to be one of the most active areas of research on aging. This is because the concerns in this area range so broadly, from global aging and the changing age distributions of societies and populations down to the personal meanings that individuals create themselves and with others to make sense of aging experiences. A central focus of recent theorizing has been to explain social and economic inequalities or "disparities" between groups for issues such as physical and mental health statuses, economic status, and reactions to stress. This has also notably involved a shift toward social genomics. Another focus has been to theorize the connection between aging and social relationships and networks, and to relate aging to social integration and to the social capital that individuals have accumulated by their later years.

WORKING AND RETIREMENT: TRUST AND THE SOCIAL CONTRACT

In Chapter 16, Melissa Hardy and Adriana Reyes address theories of work and retirement with an eye to matters of culture, trust, and the social contract. The authors note that theories of work and retirement can be constructed at (a) institutional, (b) organizational, and (c) personal levels. Institutionally, work and retirement are periods of life that have cultural meanings and expectations and are associated with formal rules and regulations related to eligibility. Organizationally, they sort people according to labor force statuses and are "market signals" for many products and services. Personally, they matter for identity and the rhythm and goals of daily life and future planning. Therefore, a complete understanding of retirement must incorporate theories at and across these levels.

As the nature and meaning of work and retirement have been so radically altered, trust has become a critical new issue to be nurtured in theories of aging. Contracts between employers and employees require some level of trust on entering into an agreement, and require some level of public trust in government. The erosion of trust increases individual risk and transforms "simple exchanges into highly problematic negotiations."

The later-life experiences of workers with discontinuous employment histories, self-employed workers, and contingent workers are part of the "untold story" of retirement. In revealing these stories, researchers will have to revise existing theories or build new ones to account for these realities. Theories of culture, trust, and the social contract are important gateways to doing so.

THE IMPORTANCE OF FAMILY-LEVEL APPROACHES TO AGING

Another major social institution that shapes the structure and experience of aging and the life course is the family, to which Rosemary Blieszner and Marieke Voorpostel (Chapter 17) turn. Most adults live with and grow old among family members. Relationships exist across multiple generations, and these family members come from different cohorts. There is great need to generate dynamic and holistic theories that treat families as complex and diverse kinship units that change in form and function over time.

Blieszner and Voorpostel emphasize the need to theorize family life with a long view in mind—for example, to examine the effects of early family experiences on later health and well-being. They also stress the need to theorize bidirectional influences across generations—for example, not only to explain how parents shape children but also how children shape parents. Advancing theories of resilience, which lie at the intersection between psychology and sociology, would seem an especially promising focus for theory development in family gerontology, as would a focus on "relational flourishing" in whole families.

The authors also elaborate on two key points of theoretical development in family gerontology: (a) on "intergenerational solidarity and conflict" and (b) on "intergenerational ambivalence." With respect to intergenerational solidarity and conflict, they suggest that theories go beyond parent–adult child dyads to other types of intergenerational relationships, including dynamics across more than two generations (e.g., how the parent generation plays roles in the grandparent–grandchild relationship) and how intergenerational solidarity and conflict vary over contexts and populations. So, too, do they emphasize how family relationships in turn affect societies, particularly in reproducing social inequality through the investments that family members are able to make in one another (or not).

Blieszner and Voorpostel point out that theories of intergenerational relationships in adulthood have largely focused on *either* solidarity or conflict. However, family relationships are often characterized by *both* solidarity and conflict—thereby creating conditions of *sociological* ambivalence (e.g., in which the diversity of family relationships and roles may lead to contradictory expectations) or *psychological* ambivalence (e.g., in which there is a simultaneous subjective experience of positive and negative emotions toward the same individual). Given the complexity of family life today, these forms of ambivalence are surely common and fertile ground for theoretical development.

◾ SOCIAL INEQUALITIES, AGING, AND HEALTH

Two chapters focus on inequalities in health and aging, which are pressing concerns for policymakers and practitioners and preoccupations of social science researchers. In Chapter 18, Jaclyn Wong and Linda Waite note that differences in social relationships and support account for some of these inequalities. Theories of social capital have therefore been central to inquiry in this area because relationships are viewed as resources on which individuals can draw to achieve their goals.

When it comes to how social relationships may influence health and well-being, there have been two dominant approaches: (a) the "main effects" model, which suggests that relationships may lead to better health through a variety of cognitive, emotional, behavioral, and biological pathways; and (b) the "stress-buffering" model, which suggests that relationships provide a variety of resources that can prevent damaging responses or promote adaptation to life's stressors.

Where specific relationships are concerned, greatest attention has been paid to the marital relationship, and then to parent–child relationships (which were addressed in Chapter 17). Yet, larger social networks beyond the family are also important points of theory development (e.g., changes in network size and composition, volume or frequency of contact, substitutions in the face of network "turnover," and specific types of activity that may be health promoting or health harming).

Advances in theory development also rest on inquiry into (a) the social integration and engagement of elders in their local communities, (b) the *subjective* perceptions of social connectedness, which may also carry an independent and sizable effect on health and well-being in old age alongside the objective aspects of social relationships and networks, and (c) *why* and *how* exposure to stress is unequally distributed (i.e., experienced significantly more by) for women, racial and/or ethnic minorities, unmarried persons, and working-class and poor individuals. Social capital and other coping resources are disproportionately low among these groups, which only accentuates the disadvantages they already face.

Anticipating new frontiers in social theories of aging, Wong and Waite point to social genomics. Here, research must explore how social forces affect gene expression, especially in making elders more or less prone to inflammatory diseases, which are tied directly to cardiovascular and respiratory diseases of aging. Consistent with the life course perspective, the authors also note the surge of research that attempts to link childhood adversity and later life outcomes. Although these empirical connections are just being established, there is a need to develop theories to explain the processes or mechanisms that bring about these effects.

In Chapter 19, Angela O'Rand reviews major theoretical programs that have emerged over two decades to address the "seemingly inextricable" relationships among health, aging, and social inequality across the life course. These are: (a) the "education-health research program," which is focused on explaining the robust relationship between years of schooling and later health; (b) the "fundamental cause program," which argues that socioeconomic status (SES) is an underlying, pervasive phenomenon that propels the aging process via multiple mechanisms over time that cannot be captured by commonly used "surface indicators" of SES; (c) the "cumulative advantage–cumulative disadvantage theory" (CAD), which draws attention to time-related processes that generate inequality; and, relatedly, (d) the "cumulative inequality program," which attempts to expand theories of CAD into a broader theory of aging inequality that incorporates health and human agency.

Like Wong and Waite, O'Rand points to social genomics as a new frontier for advancing theories of inequality and aging. One example of this, she says, is the potential contribution of biosocial research to the understanding of the origins of health inequalities in early life and the subsequent trajectories of health and aging as individuals successively encounter unequal social risks and resources over their lives. New possibilities of integrating genomic, physiological, and clinical data with social survey data have made this line of investigation central to aging theory.

■ SOCIAL CONSTRUCTIONS OF AGE AND AGING

In Chapter 20, Victor Marshall, Anne Martin-Matthews, and Julie McMullin turn attention to the "interpretive" perspective, which is largely anchored in the symbolic interactionism tradition in sociology. This tradition views individuals not as simply acting out prescribed and internalized social roles, but as actively *taking* and *making* social roles that carry significant meaning for them and for society.

In probing the interpretive perspective, Marshall and colleagues classify theories across three levels of analysis: (a) interpretive-micro, (b) interpretive-macro, and (c) interpretive-linking. In gerontology, *interpretive-micro* perspectives focus on aging individuals and the meaning they attribute to various aspects of social life and identity. *Interpretive-macro* perspectives emphasize the fact that the structures in which individuals exist are socially constructed. Two examples in gerontology are the political economy and life course perspectives that emphasize the role of social institutions and policies in structuring individual meaning and action. *Interpretive-linking* perspectives seek to theorize phenomena in ways that connect micro and macro levels of analysis. This is nicely illustrated with the life course perspectives as well as feminist and cultural theories. Given the rapid social changes that have affected aging and the life course, the interpretive perspective is a powerful tool for advancing social science theories.

■ CONCLUSION

The chapters in this section provide a rich sample of social theories of age and aging. These theories are especially important to our field because they repeatedly remind us of the need to keep in view explanations of aging that go beyond the individual level, sometimes far beyond it. From issues of social capital in retirement negotiations to how individuals interpret the changes of aging, there is an underlying theme of social integration, and of how individuals and age groups develop or maintain integration in the face of the challenges that accompany aging. These issues provide a fertile context for theorizing *social* causes and outcomes, and *social* variability and inequalities, in aging and later life.

CHAPTER 16

Theories of Work and Retirement:
Culture, Trust, and the Social Contract

Melissa Hardy and Adriana M. Reyes

Work and retirement are simultaneously constructed at the institutional, organizational, and individual levels. At the institutional level, they reflect life stages imbued with cultural meanings and expectations and are incorporated into formal rules and regulations as a basis for both entitlement and disqualification. Our lives are organized around them. They are linked to the goals we pursue and the aspirations we hope to realize. At the organizational level, they sort people according to labor force statuses, industries, and occupations; define categories of activities and income; structure group memberships; and operate as market signals for all sorts of products and services. At the personal level, they are important facets of identity and the roles we play day to day; they set constraints on the time we devote to those roles; and we associate them with different stages of our lives. Whereas retirement had been viewed as the culmination of a working lifetime, work now has become the means to achieving a good retirement. Before careers are fully launched, young workers consider how any given move might affect their retirement (Ekerdt, 2004). Therefore, a complete understanding of retirement interweaves theories of corporations and pensions, employment policy and social insurance, expectations and shared meanings, and agency and structure. From a leisure status that was available only to a select group, retirement was expanded and institutionalized as a period of late-life, post-employment independence for the middle class and as a late-life elevation out of poverty for the working poor. In the past several decades, retirement has been transformed once again as political and economic discourse reframes the social vocabulary of contribution and reward into one of assets and liabilities.

The historical narrative separates retirement into three eras. In the pre–World War II environment, employers had considerable discretion in determining when and how retirement could occur, whether it would be associated with pension benefits, and how long those benefits would last. On the whole, however, retirement and pensions were primarily for high-income or white-collar workers rather than the rank and file (Graebner, 1980; Quadagno, 1988; Achenbaum, 1983). For most workers, old age unemployment or disability followed decades of demanding labor, unless they died on the job. The second era of retirement was marked by the passage of Social Security and the expansion of employer-sponsored pensions. This expansion was particularly strong in the public sector and that part of the private sector that was unionized (Dobbin, 1992; Myles, 1984; Jacoby, 1985). Social Security benefits alone made for a grim retirement. The finishing touch to this expansion occurred in the 1970s, when fundamental changes in the benefit structure of Social Security enhanced the affordability of early retirement, significantly increased the real level of benefits and secured their long-term purchasing power. By the time those accomplishments were in place, the groundwork for the transition to the third era was already underway. This most-recent era begins about 1980 and extends to the present. In that sense, the "new" retirement is decades old.

Because these relationships are dynamic, with the nexus of work and retirement being amended in both small and profound ways, theories of work and retirement must also explain social change in the construction of retirement and how change becomes embedded across the multiple levels of social organization. They must help us understand how it is that retirement—as status, transition, late-career process, demographic category, and identity—means one thing for one series of birth cohorts, and then means something quite different for the next. Or, why nations construct and support retirement and retirement security in different ways. Perhaps most important, we need to develop theories that allow us to anticipate how the future of retirement will be challenged and how these challenges can be resolved.

Scholars have conceptualized these processes at different levels of analysis. In current research, much of the focus is on individual behavior and how workers are adapting to the new rules of retirement. In one branch practiced primarily within economics and oriented toward prediction, higher levels of social organization are treated as context. Workers' behaviors, which are assumed to reflect their preferences, effectively signal endorsement of any new circumstances by accepting job or pension offers. Perhaps more important, the behavioral space is monetized, with work–and–retirement decisions being driven by individual (or household) budgets (Lumsdaine & Mitchell, 1999). The theoretical models predict behavioral responses to economic conditions that shape budget constraints. In addressing broader social conditions, the emphasis is placed on gauging the effects of economic shocks, such as changes in the housing market, declines in stock values, or higher unemployment rates on delaying or speeding up retirement (Coile & Levine, 2006, 2007; Coronado & Perozek, 2003; Poterba, Venti, & Wise, 2012).

In constructing explanations for the variation in retirement pathways, sociologists contextualize transition sequences relative to characteristics associated with advantage or disadvantage as an indirect approach to opportunity structures. In addition, comparative studies use variation at the organizational or institutional levels to demonstrate how features of the macro environment can shape behavior. Some arguments have extended stratification theories to draw out the implications for inequality and cumulative disadvantage, particularly those patterns of inequality that adhere to gender, race and/or ethnicity, or low socioeconomic status (Ekerdt, 2009).

A second theoretical perspective more often applied to questions of work than retirement examines the changes in employer–employee relationships, jobs, labor markets, and corporate structures that have accompanied occupational and industrial reorganization (Baron & Bielby, 1980, 1984; DiMaggio & Powell, 1983; Dobbin, 1994; Fligstein & Dauber, 1989; Fligstein & Markowitz, 1993; Jacoby, 1985; Kalleberg et al., 1997). The distinction in types of jobs, whether through segmented labor markets, closed versus open positions, long-term versus spot market contracts, "good" jobs versus "bad" jobs, sets the stage for a stratified view of retirement. Retirement transitions that were forced or voluntary, included private pension benefits or only Social Security, allowed total retirement or required (or allowed) part-time work sorted retirees into different types of retirement as they had sorted workers into different types of jobs (Riley, 1987; Sorensen, 1994, 1998).

At the institutional level, studies have highlighted the connections between political ideologies, the modern welfare state, public policy, and age-specific rates of retirement. Comparative studies of the welfare state called attention to "American exceptionalism," which was generally attributed to its common law traditions, weak central government, and enthusiasm for a distinctly American version of individualism (Estes, 1991; Quadagno, 1988; Myles, 1991; Meyer, 2008). Because the modern nation state had become the central social institution, prominent institutional actors were identified as elected leaders in their role as policy makers or appointed officials responsible for implementation. Through this lens, public policy became the primary expression of institutional structure.

A third approach uses the organizing concept of the life course to study retirement (Han & Moen, 1999; Henretta, 2003; O'Rand & Henretta, 1999; Dannefer, 2003; Settersten & Mayer, 1997). The societal implications of retrenchment are seen in the replacement of age-graded entitlements with programs that have erased many of the age-based behavioral markers. The turn away from age grading has been viewed in both positive and negative terms. On the one hand, the erosion of the age-graded life course and its potential replacement with an age-integrated one held the promise of reducing age stereotypes and providing people with more flexibility in how they distributed periods of education, work, and leisure across their lives. Participating in societal institutions that previously had been sharply age segmented could create new opportunities for interaction and personal development. The more rigid sequencing of work following the completion of education, and retirement following the termination of work, could be amended to allow parallel tracks. Adults could more easily return to school and change careers. Retirees could "un"retire. With more flexible employer expectations, adults could reallocate time from work to family while their children were young (Riley & Riley, 1994).

On the other hand, removing these age boundaries also undermines people's expectations of what to do and when to do it. The age-standardized life course had provided clear societal direction for individual behavior and a template for personal plans (Mayer & Schoepflin, 1989; Riley, 1987). Further, although the abstract characterization of fewer age constraints created an impression of institutional and organizational openness, access might be restricted in other ways. Without that age-based sequencing, life course transitions become blurred and their timing less uniform. Although the age-integrated life course spoke in terms of possibilities, the reality was likely to be riddled with uncertainties and constraints. Employers, for example, preferred a more one-sided flexibility that could be granted at their discretion (Hardy, 2008).

Considerable empirical evidence has documented the increasing variation in the timing of retirement transitions, the reversibility of those transitions, and difficulty encountered by older workers who want to keep their jobs (O'Rand, 2010; Warner, Hayward, & Hardy, 2010). These observations have led some to conclude that retirement (and the life course more generally) is being deinstitutionalized (Han & Moen, 1999) and that the likely result will be an exacerbation of existing inequality (O'Rand & Henretta, 1999). The deinstitutionalization argument points to a weakening of social norms that define retirement behavior. Less compact distributions of age at retirement and increasing difficulty in designating the start of retirement support this claim.

Disparate behaviors also can signal a transitional stage, a temporary blurring of boundaries before a new pattern emerges. To the extent that retirement continues to be the anticipated end game, the timing of retirement may reflect something other than age at entry, and the status of retirement may involve a broad range of formal and informal activity. In these ways, entry into the "new" retirement may be governed more by account balances than age. Social Security may become more important as wage subsidy than as wage replacement. Access to a financially secure old age may become more restricted. Among the poor, options to supplement retirement income may require growth in the grey economy when jobs in the formal economy are unavailable.

In accounting for these changes, our attention has been directed primarily to state policies, shifts in political power, the service-based economy, and globalization. Receiving less attention are the cultural meanings and moral understandings of how retirement fits into the U.S. landscape. In questioning this cultural dimension, we search for the mechanisms that carry social change across the individual, organizational, and institutional levels and provide either forward momentum to new constructions or a more negative reaction to the new institutional logics being promoted.

Our goal in this chapter is to explore that cultural dimension by analyzing the role of "trust" as a key underlying cultural concept in the social construction of retirement. Trust is an element central to all social exchange. Cultural understandings of work and retirement require both intertemporal and intergenerational features of exchange relationships. The strength of the social contract and by extension the efficacy of state policy depends on public trust in the legitimacy of the federal government. Contracts between employers and employees require some level of trust between the parties entering into the agreement. One feature of trust in the contractual arrangements supporting retirement involves the longer time horizon over which that trust must be sustained.

A second feature of these contractual arrangements is the power imbalance involved in ending any long-term commitment. Because corporate welfare policies are entirely voluntary, changes in corporate structure and key personnel allow space for reinterpreting previously made agreements. To the extent that the enforcement of any retirement agreement is contingent on prevailing economic conditions, workers whose long-term planning is based on trust in the firm's future behavior may find their plans upended. The balance between trust and risk is therefore central to the understanding of how retirement has changed.

At the extreme, the absence of trust turns simple exchanges into highly problematic negotiations. People cannot have confidence in their expectations, nor can they rely on help from any quarter. Because trust has a temporal dimension, with longer time horizons requiring greater trust in the original understandings and in those entering into those understandings, a decline in trust implies the need to shift to shorter time horizons in the interest of self-protection. These quicker exchanges collapse the time interval between the initiation and completion of the terms of the agreement. Even if the actors remain the same, any long-term agreement is broken into pieces that are abbreviated in duration and scope, and therefore also of limited commitment and exposure.

In the conversion of the U.S. economy from manufacturing to service, the nature of work was transformed and, since retirement has operated as the post-work stage of the career, the nature of retirement also changed. The rapid termination of defined benefit (DB) pension plans and their replacement with defined contribution (DC) plans has become emblematic of that conversion (Hardy, 2011; O'Rand, 2010), although the motivations for and consequences of that conversion are still disputed. To the extent that workers' trust in their employers has been eroded and institutionally deconstructed, then the risk inherent in that relationship has created the need for a different approach to risk management. In that workers now own their pension accounts—at least in the cases where workers have such accounts—the argument has been one of risk transfer from the employer to the worker. Because risk management is a collective enterprise, however, the new strategy must transfer trust from one organizational and/or institutional context to another. To the extent that modernity requires an increasing vesting of trust in anonymous others, the counterpoint to individual risk management is anonymous trust relationships. The trust-building mechanisms required to accomplish this transference relied, at least in part, on discursive practices that promoted the trustworthiness of the new arrangement (including the science behind it and the expertise required to enact it) while undermining confidence in the old (Ekerdt, 1998; Giddens, 1990; Ocasio & Joseph, 2005; Quadagno, 1996).

In the sections of the chapter that follow, we take up three questions. First, we question the changes in trust relationships the DB–DC transition signaled. Second, we question how risk management of retirement income was reframed. Third, we address the changes in the structure of the labor market and the nature of work that have coincided with the third era of retirement. Our goal is to provide both a conceptual argument for the importance of cultural understandings as a central consideration in theories of work and retirement and empirical observations that invite further exploration relative to this claim. The empirical fingerposts are suggestive rather than formal tests of these propositions. We hope to convince the reader that addressing these types of questions can provide a different and important perspective on possible futures of retirement.

■ BREAKING THE TRUST

Most scholars view the change in employer-sponsored pension plans as the key event in redefining retirement for the 21st century. Explanations for this fundamental restructuring of pensions are more varied. Within neoclassical theory, individuals as agents motivate change at both the organizational and the individual level. Organizationally, increased federal regulation and oversight restricted firms' flexibility in managing corporate accounts and added to the administrative costs of DB plans. Increased global competition required that firms be more agile in adapting their internal labor forces to changing markets. Finally, the longtime horizon over which benefits would be paid introduced a financial strain that compromised the competitive position firms needed to occupy to stay in business.

Workers' preferences changed accordingly. A desire for greater portability and more control over pension assets translated into greater acceptance of employment contracts that provided DC coverage. The equation of behavior with realized preference is a central theoretical assumption. If workers accepted jobs with DC plans, they must have chosen DC jobs (or the DC option) over other alternatives; to choose a DC plan, workers must have decided that DC plans served their interests; to make that decision, workers must have a preference for DC plans. On the whole, the change in pension structure was the efficient response to a changing market environment, where the rational actors were both corporations and individual workers, and environmental contexts were largely made up of market forces.

Sociological explanations drew more on conflict theory, emphasizing the weakening of labor unions, the growing power of corporations, the widening gap in wealth and income, and federal regulations and court decisions that made it more difficult to challenge corporate practices. From one perspective, these newer developments represented a postindustrial version of the class conflicts of earlier eras. Control over resources, exploitation, the influence of wealth in political contests, and the resurgence of individual over collective approaches to social problems were evident, albeit in a 21st-century guise. Attitudinal evidence of shifting cultural understandings was more common than explanations of the underlying social processes behind these cultural changes.

In developing explanations for these social changes, therefore, one approach has been to emphasize individual-level causal pathways that imply that actors are "socially organized" primarily through markets. The causal effects are rooted in interior characteristics of the individual, particularly in the pursuit of self-interest. A second approach is to view causal effects as rooted in collective, complex networks of interaction, or other features we equate with social structure (Jepperson & Meyer, 2011). The explanation for individual (or organizational) behaviors thereby invokes culturally legitimized "action scripts." If the institutional logic behind the action script acts as a blueprint for rational behavior, then the behavior may "look" rational, not because of some elemental feature of human nature, but because of a socially constructed valuation of a particular form of rationality. By that interpretive framework, the rapid replacement of DB with DC plans within U.S. industry was shaped by a shift in institutional logics in the wider environment (Meyer & Rowan, 1977).

Institutional logics prescribe formal and informal rules of action, interaction, and interpretation (Ocasio, 1997). At the same time, they privilege certain values and beliefs that influence the formulation of the problem, the menu of potential solutions that are considered, and the reasoning that recommends a solution. They comprise both strategies of action and strategies of decision making—what to attend to and what to ignore, what to prioritize, and how to interpret what happens next. These logics may exist within organizational fields (DiMaggio & Powell, 1983) and influence employer–employee relationships (Thornton & Ocasio, 1999), executive power and executive replacement (Fligstein, 1990; Jackall, 1988), organizational control (Westphal, Gulati, & Shortell, 1996), and organizational dynamics (Meyer, 2008).

The role of institutional logics is largely implicit in sociological theories of retirement, perhaps because we have fairly recently begun to consider retirement as an embedded feature of the work career rather than as the beginning of the post-career life stage. By conceptually aligning the retirement transition with other relational features of employment and working life, we expand the relevance of organizational and institutional actors beyond the terms of pensions and retirement policies. In other words, we embed workers in more complex systems of social organization rather than defining their organizational context by demographic categories or individualized incentive structures derived from pension policies.

■ THE CHANGING LOGICS OF DEFINED BENEFITS

Whereas military pensions have a long history, in the modern era public sector employees (civil servants) were among the first group of workers to receive pension coverage. Teachers, firefighters, and police officers had pensions in the early 1900s. In 1920, Congress passed universal coverage for federal civil servants, and state and local governments followed as early adopters (Clark & Craig, 2003). Although coverage of private sector workers stalled at about 50%, coverage of public sector workers is higher. In 2006, for example, 76% of state and local workers aged 25-64 had pension coverage compared to 43% of private sector workers (Munnell & Soto, 2007). Union workers in the private sector also fare better than nonunion workers. By 2011, defined benefit plans covered 67% of union workers compared to 13% of nonunion workers (Wiatrowski, 2012).

In 1975, 44.5 million workers participated in pension plans, with almost three- quarters in DB plans. By 2013, of the 131.6 million participants, 70% were in DC plans. During that same time period, real DB pension assets grew by 240% (to $2.9 trillion), whereas assets in DC plans increased more than 12-fold, to $5 trillion (Table A1. Employee Benefits Security Administration, U.S. Department of Labor, 2015). Nevertheless, residual pockets of DB plans remain among firms with collective bargaining agreements and most prominently among public sector workers (Clark & Craig, 2003; Craig, 1995).

By entering into a DB contract, workers agreed that their potential benefits would accumulate in a "pension trust" over which they had no control and that they could begin collecting these benefits 30 or more years in the future. DB pensions therefore involved three major risks. The first was introduced by workers' willingness to accept some of their pay as deferred compensation, which required them to trust that they would receive future benefits and a secure retirement. This strategy of deferred compensation took advantage of the tax law at the time. When DB plans gained acceptance in the private sector, individuals received no tax benefit for pension contributions. Corporations, however, could take a tax write-off for making those contributions on workers' behalf.

The second risk involved the survival of the firm. Because their hard work would not save a poorly run business, they had to trust the managers and corporate executives to make sound business decisions. The third involved the security of the pension trust. Workers had to trust that employers would manage the pension fund in good faith and that the federal government or the unions would protect their interests. The favored tax status afforded corporate pension trusts was of concern to early lawmakers. If tax exempt contributions could be invested and then the proceeds pulled back into corporate earnings accounts at any future time, the tax exemption would subsidize corporate accumulation of tax-sheltered investments rather than workers' pensions. In other words, Congress did not fully trust corporations to use the funds as intended and feared they would exploit the tax exemption. Considering all contributions to the pension trust as irrevocable would have been the strongest step to take to protect workers' benefits, thereby making it impossible for corporations to ever take funds from the pension account. Through the 1938 Revenue Act, Congress decided instead to restrict the diversion of plan assets until "all liabilities" had been paid (Revenue Act of 1938, §165[a][2]), a constraint which was elaborated in 1939 to allow "recover[y] at termination of the trust and only at termination of the trust, any balance which is due to erroneous actuarial computation" (Reg. § 1.401–2[b][1]). [The regulatory history on which we draw has been carefully documented and presented by Stein (1989). His argument relies on both the original regulatory text as well as supporting documents that provide persuasive evidence as to legislative intent. The key point he makes with regard to the 1939 interpretation is that the House argued that the extension of privileged tax status made sense only if the pension trust was outside the employer's control and contributions to that trust were irrevocable. The Senate changed the language (after being heavily lobbied)].

This implicit contract benefitted workers only if they stayed with the same employer. In that sense, the long-term commitment from workers and the promised future reward were in the relational aspects of the contract rather than in the letter of the signed document. The terms of pension entitlement and the formula for calculating pension benefits reinforced that relational understanding with two disincentives. Workers needed to complete vesting periods to be entitled to any benefits, which meant moving required that they restart the vesting clock. Second, once workers were vested, the value of their benefits at any point in time was far less than the value expected at retirement. The pension cost of leaving was particularly high during the middle years, when workers could receive a fraction of the expected benefits without any hope of recovering the difference. The contract provided employers with enforcement incentives throughout the workers' careers; however, workers' expectations were not tested until retirement. Cohort succession was a necessary component to the trust relationship. To the extent that older cohorts of workers were treated according to expectations, workers' future expectations were validated.

In addition, typical DB formulas reproduced key features of the Social Security benefit structure. Both plans required some minimum years of work before becoming eligible for future benefits; both assigned far greater weight to later career salary levels than earlier ones; and both rewarded continuous work histories. Although the trust in the federal system could be attributed to the government's taxing authority, during these postwar decades, trust in the federal government was relatively high in general. The trust in the private system lay in employers' promises to maintain an adequate pension account and in governmental oversight. In unionized industries where DB plans were the strongest, workers had additional insurance in the power of the union itself. Workers knew that a failure to follow through would mean a strike and a lawsuit. The union could ensure a swift and coordinated response so long as the firm avoided bankruptcy. In addition, annual wage increases and job security relative to seniority were also required topics of collective bargaining and important long-term considerations.

In the public sector, unions also play a role. However, because changes to pensions have to be enacted by elected officials, politicians could be held accountable in election years. From this standpoint, the dynamics of DB pensions appear to differ across organizational contexts (Munnell, Haverstick, & Soto, 2007). Much of our attention is on the private sector, and as rates of unionization decline, that means studying retirement in an increasingly nonunionized work force. Options for protest among nonunion private sector workers are limited to complaints registered through human resources departments or, if that option fails, to legal action. Among public sector workers, rates of unionization are much higher, and changing pensions requires legislative action. The political context can highlight differences in competing institutional logics, since these logics form one basis for the campaign to change or retain the current pension structure. In addition, because voters decide which institutional logic prevails, the importance of cultural patterns of reasoning, valuing, prioritizing, and trusting either the statement or the speaker are in the forefront.

■ RISK MANAGEMENT

Risk management is an inherently collective enterprise. Risk is based on probabilities and losses, and insurance companies use these probabilities of negative events and estimated losses to determine whom to insure and how much to charge for the policies. These charges vary across people, depending on expected payout and conditional probabilities based on their characteristics. The insurance paradigm works to the extent that risks are exogenous (or if endogenous, the self-sorting process is known and the information needed to calculate individual values can be collected) and independent. Dependent risks occur when an exogenous shock creates a cascade of losses.

Although risk management is now considered to be a measurable component of an investment strategy, risk also has a strong cultural component and is conceptually bound by trust. Risk management strategies are therefore culturally embedded practices that allow peace of mind under certain social conditions and fear of loss under others. The overall risk management strategy under DB plans was one of mutual investment. Employers reduced the risk of quits, minimized the costs of labor replacement, hired workers who shared an interest in profitability, and secured the workers' consent to be paid in future dollars. Workers reduced their risk of job loss or lay off, of reaching retirement age with insufficient retirement savings, and of running out of funds if they lived longer than expected.

The mechanism for risk management of the pension fund was collective investment. Since all contributions were held in a single account and managed by an independent financial institution, usually banks or insurance companies with an independent auditor, the portfolio of investments could be diversified in terms of types of investments and time horizons, two basic strategies of risk management. Contributions would continue to be made and payouts would increase gradually as the pension fund grew and more workers retired. In other words, responsibility for handling the investment, inflation, and longevity risk of total DB assets was assigned to pension-fund managers, but long-term losses had to be covered by the employer.

Two important dimensions of this arrangement were that pension funds often invested in the parent company, and that as the fiduciary agents of that fund, fund managers held the voting rights to any stock held in the trust. When corporate governance issues were contested, the shares generally were voted in support of current management (Stein, 1989). However, these arrangements distanced both workers and management from control. Although contributions to the fund were made on behalf of workers, the fund itself was owned by the corporation. To ensure that management did not take money from the fund, the financial management of the trust was external to the corporation. In this way, neither workers nor management could exercise the voting rights of the shares.

One further understanding made the implicit contract sustainable in the private sector. The workers trusted that "if the firm is successful, the plan will not be terminated, and workers [will] receive the full value of their ongoing benefits" (Ippolito, 1997, p. 7). To say that workers did not share the investment risk is to argue that payment of pension benefits would continue even if the contributions required by the pension fund led to bankruptcy. Certainly the expectation was that employers would have to assign some amount of corporate earnings to the pension fund on a routine basis. But the likelihood that the pension trust could weather a spell of low investment returns was increased by its size and diversity of assets. Fund managers had the flexibility to combine higher risk with lower risk investments, longer term with shorter term payouts. In addition, fund managers were conservative investors. Given the fiduciary responsibility they had for protecting pension assets, their investments were relatively risk averse (Ippolito, 1990, 2003). In this sense, workers and management had entered into a mutually beneficial exchange relationship (Blau, 1964). Both invested in the success of the business, and business success allowed the work-and-retirement relationship to hold. Workers' risks were arguably greater than those of management, since their financial circumstances were far less forgiving. Further, although unions could protect workers' interests in contract negotiations, they could not eliminate the risk of bankruptcy.

In retrospect, the trust that workers placed in these relationships held for about one generation—long enough for another generation of workers to be somewhere in the work-and-retirement pipeline. During the 1960s and early 1970s, a series of pension terminations among underfunded plans placed pension regulation on the Congressional agenda. The most visible example was the bankruptcy of Studebaker in 1963 and the discovery that, while the pension trust could purchase annuities for those aged 60 and older, the firm could not pay the accrued benefits to workers younger than 60 years of age (Wooten, 2001). These failures made visible the weaknesses in the oversight of pension funds. That Studebaker workers were part of the United Auto Workers also put unions on notice. They could do little to ensure workers' pensions if firms shorted the accounts and made poor decisions.

The passage of the Employee Retirement Income Security Act (ERISA) in 1974 was the legislative response to workers' and retirees' loss of benefits through plan defaults. Although the legal remedies did not apply retroactively, ERISA was supposed to reinforce workers' rights to their pensions. Most assessments either promote ERISA as a victory for workers or claim that mandated insurance, funding formulas, and reporting requirements made DB plans too expensive for employers. The rapid decline in DB plans that began after ERISA is often used as evidence of the negative effects of federal regulation, since DC plans were not subject to ERISA.

Consider these events from a different angle. Corporate pensions have always been voluntary in the United States, which was a primary reason for the tax incentives for employers to create them. From that standpoint, employers had always been able to terminate the plans at will (except when part of a collective bargaining agreement). ERISA reiterated the voluntary nature of the private pension system, noting that employers could adopt, modify, or terminate their plans at any time and for any reason, except where collective bargaining agreements were in place (Anenson & Lahey, 2007). When ERISA was passed, many pensions had enough assets to pay all future benefits, which meant they had calculated their liabilities on the basis of the implicit contract. They assumed workers would stay, wages would rise, and the retirement-level benefits would be paid.

Before 1980, plan terminations for reasons other than bankruptcy were rare, but the number of hostile corporate takeovers was increasing. Not only were the 1980s the era of pension reversions, but they also were the "heyday of corporate raiders" (Futrelle, 2012). In the 1960s, a loophole in federal regulation revived the strategy of the hostile takeover, and firms with large DB pension funds were prime targets. The securities that were owned by pension trusts were voted by pension-fund trustees, who had been reliable allies of management. Then they switched sides, voting to accept the offer and realize a short-term gain as fulfillment of their fiduciary responsibility to beneficiaries (Hablutzel & Selmer, 1988). The organizational diffusion of pension replacement occurred rapidly. Whether an expression of opportunism or mimicry, from 1980 to 1988, almost 1,700 financially healthy DB plans were terminated for large (more than $1 million) reversions, affecting 1.9 million participants and pulling $18.5 billion (45% of total pension assets) back into corporate accounts (Stein, 1989). These plan reversions were accomplished by terminating the plan and paying workers the value of the benefits they had accrued to that point. Whatever remained in the pension trust was then reclaimed by the corporation (Ippolito, 2003).

Recall that we listed three major risks associated with DB plans when we considered the multiple vectors of trust that were required for the implicit contract to work (Blau, 1964). Here we add two more. First is the risk that the legislative intent of laws passed in a different era would no longer be recognized. Second is the risk that the independent fund managers—the banks or the insurance companies Congress had charged with protecting pension funds—would apply a fundamentally different institutional logic in meeting their fiduciary responsibility (Hablutzel & Selmer, 1988). The interpretations of legislative intent can be skewed by ideology. Understandings of an implicit contract, or the enforceable terms of any contract, are subject to the emphasis placed on the letter versus the spirit of an agreement.

The dissimilarity in institutional logics that adhere to different historical eras can be reinforced at different levels by actors in different domains (Thornton & Ocasio, 1999). Over time, organizational leadership will change. The new executives often bring new approaches to evaluation and compensation, a new vocabulary of problems and solutions, and a different lens for interpreting the decisions of the officers they replace. Underlying the disjuncture, however, is a fundamental cultural change that allows people to view the more recent logic as acceptable, justified, and legitimate.

The law as a part of institutional structure exists in its shared meaning. Because interpretations are produced by people who view the law from a particular vantage point, understand the spirit of the law in different ways, and determine compliance versus violation within a cognitive framework, the law itself changes. It changes not only because it can be amended or repealed or superseded by subsequent acts, but because it is reconstructed as meaning something different as well. The earlier Revenue Act included a definition for pension funds that would qualify for corporate reclamation. Once the Internal Revenue Service approved the methodology for calculating benefits that were owed to workers upon plan termination (Ippolito, 1997), what remained in the account, by definition, was *not* owed to the workers. Instead, the IRS and the corporations agreed on a different classification: erroneous actuarial calculation. The broader business climate in which all this occurred, however, deemed these actions legitimate.

After appeals on the basis of the 1938–1939 Revenue Acts failed, pension plan reversions were challenged as a form of age discrimination. Workers who were early in their careers but not yet vested lost years to eligibility, but they had longer to recover. Workers on the verge of retirement were approaching their high point in service and wages, so their losses were relatively small. The workers who lost the most were past midcareer, often in their 40s or 50s. Their year-to-year increase in accrued benefits was just beginning to accelerate, and they were old enough that even smart investment would fall far short of matching what they had been promised. Because the age group covered by the Age Discrimination in Employment Act included those 45 and older, the argument that the negative impact fell disproportionately on older workers was made.

Different courts rendered different decisions in these disputes, which itself is an indicator of normative ambiguity. Some agreed that older workers could lose as much as half of their expected retirement benefit and that basing termination benefits on the amount currently accrued did discriminate against older workers. Other judges ruled that employers were obligated to pay only benefits earned to that date. Lawyers for the workers argued the importance of the relational contract, equating pensions with deferred wages. Ultimately, workers lost.

In thinking about institutional structure, even the more formal rules contained in laws and regulations rely on culturally shared meanings, which make any policy an ongoing project of interpretation and implementation. At the time of the enactment, there appear to be winners and losers. The contest, however, continues. Staff must execute the policy as circumstances change. Incumbents occupying an office at different times under different managers work with redefined criteria and guidelines. Incoming and outgoing administrations have more or less enthusiasm for enforcement mechanisms. Congress allocates varying levels of funding dedicated to policy administration. And the cultural understandings of what the policy does, why it was passed, and whether it still makes sense can change as well. The promulgation of rules, definitions, or classifications to address specific issues on which the legislation was silent creates openings for either strengthening or weakening the policy's reach. The inevitable series of lawsuits and legal actions filed by businesses, unions, or people (either as individual or class actions) give the courts an opening to influence the meaning of any policy. Courts can narrow or broaden the policy's reach, change rules of evidence in determining compliance, or declare certain practices outside the scope of the law. All of these factors create a dynamic interpretive field around any policy. Although the words on the page may be the same, many other things will not be.

■ RISK MANAGEMENT IN THE DC ERA

As owners of individual pension accounts, workers needed a different strategy of risk management. In other words, they needed a new organizational form to collectivize the process—to pool individual accounts, diversify investments, and keep workers apprised of the fit between the amount they needed to retire and projections of their account balances when they would reach retirement age. In offering DC plans, firms designate a financial management firm to provide this guidance. The general structure of the arrangement is the same as it was with the DB plan, except that, rather than manage one account, the financial firm now manages as many accounts as there are individual participants, collecting management fees from each one.

Each worker and/or investor learns that investing in a single stock or even a few stocks is riskier than diversifying investments across a wider range of companies. Individual accounts are too small to follow this strategy unless they invest in mutual funds, which are themselves like companies that pool people's savings to purchase stocks, bonds, and other securities. Firms offering financial management of pension accounts have developed their own menu of mutual funds. The unsurprising result is that pension accounts managed by a given firm tend to be heavily invested in that firm's mutual funds. By buying mutual funds, people own shares in mutual fund companies, but they do not own the stocks held by the mutual funds. Once again, workers' pensions rely on the management decisions of companies in whose stock they are invested. However, they are distanced from actual ownership of these shares, with the mutual fund operating as intermediary. Therefore, workers cannot exercise the voting rights of their shares.

The change in pension structure provided an alternative to stimulating demand in a postindustrial economy. In a manufacturing economy, the role of workers was to produce goods that would be sent to stores for consumers to buy (Fontenelle, 2015). One concern with the ups and downs of the business cycle was how to maintain consumption that could then spur economic recovery. The Keynesian solution was to transfer funds to households through social programs, such as unemployment insurance, to allow people to continue to make purchases. An important economic feature of Social Security and DB benefits was providing a reliable basis for continued consumption among the growing population or retirees. The enhancements to retirement income through the 1970s raised the standard of living of retirees and increased the amount of goods that people could purchase.

In contrast, the diffusion of DC plans has spurred growth in the financial sector by turning workers-with-pension accounts into consumers of financial services (Jung & Dobbin, 2012). Immediately after the war, the financial sector accounted for 2.3% of GDP. By 1980, the proportion had grown to 4.9%, reaching 8.3% in 2006 (Greenwood & Scharfstein, 2013; Philippon, 2008). Since 1980, growth in the financial sector accounted for almost one fourth of total service sector growth, with a rate of growth significantly above the trend line (Greenwood & Scharfstein, 2013). Disproportionate increases in average wages of finance sector employees mirrored this trend. In 1980, their earnings were roughly equivalent to those of employees in other industries; however, wages for employees in financial services are now 70% higher (Philippon & Reshef, 2009). Employers designate management firms to handle workers' pension accounts, and financial managers channel individual investors into mutual funds, thereby reconstructing the collective approach to investment diversification used in pension trust funds. One key difference, however, is that saving for retirement has become an act of consumption, generating jobs and expanding the financial services sector.

Rather than trusting the employer, workers now must trust the financial management firms and the market. Workers must trust that their advisers act in accordance with the workers' best interests and that the recommendations are sound; that the fees are fair; and that the business practices are ethical. Putting trust in the market may be more difficult, which could explain the conservatism of many investors. When covered by DB plans, regulatory protections for workers focused on employment policy, contract enforcement, and pension law. Protection for those with DC plans must focus on consumer safeguards and regulating the finance industry.

■ DISCUSSION

During the past century, the social constructions of retirement have occurred within the multidimensional space that connects individual, organizational, and institutional actors. In the transformation from an agricultural to an industrial economy, labor was moved from family farms to urban factories, and cities became the financial centers of economic activity. The need to develop reliable institutional and organizational mechanisms for wage replacement created one friction in this transitional period. The efforts that followed were grounded in cultural constructions of the elderly as poor, ill, and needy within a broader sense of political and economic vulnerability. The sense of old age security that was built in the postwar decades relied on the federal government and the employer–employee relationship, supported by workers' collective representation through unions. These relationships required workers' trust in long-term benefits in exchange for loyalty.

In the transformation from the nation-based manufacturing to the globalized service economy, these relationships were fundamentally reconfigured. Cultural understandings of aging more often invoked an "alarming" increase in the 65 and older population. Through political rhetoric, these demographic developments were then causally linked to negative economic consequences. As new marketing strategies targeted older consumers, the social construction of older people was as independent, healthier, and wealthier than any other age group—people who faced lower risks of poverty than children. The tone of national discussions began to change from one of support to a minor chord of resentment around any form of "redistribution." During this same period, a change in the cultural meanings attached to social insurance and DB pensions was signaled by a new terminology, with "deferred wages" and "earned benefits" replaced by "wage replacement" and "government transfer." When the equation of retirement benefits to welfare showed little traction, monthly benefits were reformulated in actuarial terms such as "pension wealth" and "Social Security wealth." This reassignment of expected monthly income to current net worth substantially altered the wealth profile of older households, which, to that time, had been described in very modest terms, particularly when home equity was not included.

Through mandatory retirement policies and DB pensions, corporations had appropriated age as an indicator of employability. Instead of entitlement age, DC-based retirement is informed by account balances, which fluctuate with the market. Since retirement planning coordinates the timing of retirement with the balance needed to fund retirement, changes in market valuation are reflected in frequently amended possible retirement ages. To the extent that investments are conservative (less susceptible to market fluctuation), retirement expectations will be less variable, but reaching the target balance may take longer. By combining the monthly income desired with life expectancy and projected levels of inflation, retirement advisers determine the target account balance. Therefore, current age relative to life expectancy factors into these actuarial calculations by defining the available period of accumulation relative to the number of years of spending. The erosion of age norms in the timing of retirement have been replaced by a normative process of retirement saving and investment. This process spans the adult lifetime. One is either investing the savings for retirement or spending one's retirement savings. Both require financial advisers and investment managers. Rather than trusting in the benefits promised by employers, workers must now trust the market process and rely on financial advisers to help them navigate it.

Variability in the timing of retirement for those with DC pensions reflects household differences in saving rates, investment portfolios, and retirement income targets, all relative to their market behavior. Even so, DC plans provide workers with more limited choices than the rhetoric suggests. At the same time, the management contracts allow financial firms considerable influence over investment strategies. The new version of risk management, therefore, has turned saving into consumption—the longer we live, the more financial services we must consume.

The consequences of globalization for workers and retirees within the broader contexts of national and multinational corporations have been seismic. The time–space compression in the connection of production to consumption has transformed the nature of exchange, and, insofar as exchange is trust based, has necessarily recast trust relationships. Instead of the reliability of localized trust relationships based on face-to-face interaction or personal recommendations, trust is diffused through interconnected networks. Exchanges then rely on the actions of any number of anonymous actors under the assumption that these actors will behave honestly and ethically. One irony in this transformation is that the diffusion of trust to anonymous others is combined with claims of increased control, enhanced agency, greater choice, and therefore greater opportunity for the individual, now constructed as a highly reflexive rational actor (Meyer & Jepperson, 2000).

Within this globalized environment, a key goal was to guarantee the flow of money, goods, and people (Wallerstein, 1989). Tax policy, minimal federal regulations, trade agreements, and treaties to open new markets have led to corporations accounting for more than half of the world's top 100 financial entities (Reich, 2007). One step in this process was to "free" financial capital from the constraints of conservatively managed pension funds. Attempts continued to relocate savings-through-taxes currently invested by the Social Security trust fund in U.S. treasury bills. A second step was to increase labor flexibility, which is more easily accomplished with a peripheral contingent labor force and without unions. The U.S. response to the challenges and opportunities of globalization, therefore, had a distinct pro-business tilt. Federal policy facilitated the transfer and accumulation of trillions in pension savings to financial management firms. Risk-management strategies channeled the savings into the mutual funds and other investment vehicles these firms created. Restrictive legislation and conservative court decisions have undermined unions in the private sector, quieting workers' combined voices, and dismantling the organizational structure conducive to collective action. DB plans are now limited primarily to public sector workers, who also happen to be highly unionized. Replacement of their DB plans with DC plans has also been proposed, particularly in states that have prioritized lower tax rates and the elimination of public sector unions over making timely pension contributions. In that sense, concerns that the Supreme Court decision in Friedrichs *vs.* California Teachers Association could overturn 30 years of labor law precedent are well founded.

In recent decades, the risk associated with employment and retirement has been shifted from indirect (via the employer) to direct exposure to the marketplace. To the extent that employers figure into these plans, it is by providing workers with access to pretax savings accounts and in some cases, making contributions to these accounts. The financial responsibility for addressing retirement income risk, therefore, was placed with individuals and their families. As a result, risk management strategies have become an individual goal and risk factors are individual traits that can ostensibly be "managed" through proper behavior (O'Rand, 2010). This perspective allows the labeling of those with insufficient financial resources in retirement as being "poor planners" or retiring "too early." By concentrating on individual agents, the rhetoric surrounding retirement planning, pensions, and retirement transitions reinforces a perception that "ownership" of pension accounts signals control over retirement futures.

The emphasis on individual choice has been accompanied not only by a discourse that undermines relationships of trust, but also by corporate and institutional actors that challenge the trustworthiness of elected officials or chief executive officers (CEOs). Not surprisingly, public opinion regarding the trustworthiness of institutions has become more negative over this same period. Trust in financial companies and government officials dropped to an all-time low after 2010. In the mid-1970s, 31.4% of the public had a great deal of confidence in banks and financial institutions, 13.2% in Congress. By 2012, those numbers had dropped to 11.8% and 6.6% respectively, with the concomitant change showing up in trusting them "hardly at all" (Smith & Sun, 2013)—yet these are the very actors on which the future of retirement depends.

Insofar as our theories of retirement link both status and transition to the coupling of social insurance and corporate pensions, we address only part of the population. As the proportion of contingent workers increases, that segment can only grow. Those left out of our theoretical frames include a disproportionate number of racial and/or ethnic minorities, immigrants, and women. By omitting these segments of the paid and unpaid labor force, we miss an important dimension of this process, and we limit our understanding of how changing expectations for financing retirement affect those whose work histories differ from a normative career. Theories of political economy and cumulative disadvantage speak directly to these issues of marginalization and economic exclusions (Estes & Phillipson, 2002; O'Rand & Henretta, 1999), pointing to patterns of resource distribution through social structural processes of allocation.

The later-life experiences of workers with discontinuous work histories, self-employed workers, and contingent workers are part of the untold story of retirement. To the extent that research includes these workers, they are studied within the same theoretical context as career workers or not studied at all. Workers' job histories may display discontinuities introduced by spells of unemployment, injury, or illness. Employment also may be interrupted by spells of informal, unpaid work. One of the fundamental structural inequalities in the definition of work relates to this gendered definition of activities that qualify for payment. The empirical literature on childcare and elder care has documented the central role women play in providing this care in both formal and informal contexts. Among the poor or near-poor, these informal arrangements significantly reduce the demand for Medicaid-funded assistance. Even so, those who make commitments to unpaid family work are treated in equivalent fashion to those out of the labor force for reasons other than retirement or disability. Therefore, these interludes compromise both current- and future-income security (Estes, 2004). In addition, workers who remain in part-time positions or full-time work in low-wage jobs that do not offer pensions will have continuous work histories, but will accumulate little to fund their retirement. In all these ways, those with weaker connections to the labor market are marginalized at the same time that the proportion of workers in "alternative" work arrangements is growing (GAO, 2015). The standard definitions of retirement may not fit their experiences, and the challenges they face at older ages may reflect different life course patterns (Calasanti, 1996b; Gibson, 1987; Zsembik & Singer, 1990).

Retirement for those at the top of the income distribution also receives limited attention. Although the poor and middle class can be monitored through administrative records, the wealthy are more difficult to observe. Our theories of cumulative advantage are thereby theories of relative advantage among those who comprise the vast majority of the population but control a minority of income or wealth. Congress argues over the minimum wage, whereas compensation for corporate executives grows exponentially (Murphy, 2012; Schultz, 2011).

Because pensions build over the decades of working life, the retirement consequences of the DC regime are just beginning to unfold. As they do, one must wonder whether another transition is already underway. Millennials, after all, are being asked to save for retirement at the same time they are paying off student loans and trying to buy homes. In an economy where wages have remained flat but debt has grown, the future of a retirement that relies on personal savings yet spans decades of later life seems difficult to imagine—even more difficult if social insurance programs are abandoned. As we consider the alternative futures of retirement, we must keep in mind that the widening gap in later-life inequality that we observe for current cohorts of retirees reflects the careers launched in the 1980s or earlier. Since the 1970s, top-income shares in the United States have increased enormously (Atkinson & Piketty, 2006; Kopczuk & Saez, 2004). At the same time, inequality in educational opportunities and importance of family origins have increased, the likelihood of moving out of poverty has declined, and wages for the middle class have stagnated (Corak, 2013). Given current conditions, retirement security for many workers will be difficult to achieve.

REFERENCES

Achenbaum, A. W. (1983). *Shades of gray: Old age, American values, and federal policies since 1920.* Boston, MA: Little, Brown.

Anenson, T. L., & Lahey, K. E. (2007). The Crisis in Corporate America: Private Pension liability and proposals for reform. *U. PA. Journal of Labor and Employment Law, 9*(3), 495–529.

Atkinson, A., & Piketty, T. (2006). *Top incomes over the twentieth century.* Oxford, UK: Oxford University Press.

Baron, J. N., & Bielby, W. T. (1980). Bringing the firms back in: Stratification, segmentation, and the organization of work. *American Sociological Review, 45,* 737–765.

Baron, J. N., & Bielby, W. T. (1984). The organization of work in a segmented economy. *American Sociological Review, 49*, 454–473.

Blau, P. (1964). *Exchange and power in social life*. New York, NY: John Wiley and Sons.

Calasanti, T. M. (1996a). Gender and life satisfaction in retirement: An assessment of the male model. *The Journals of Gerontology, Series B, 51*(1), S18–S29.

Calasanti, T. M. (1996b). Incorporating diversity: Meaning, levels of research, and implications for theory. *The Gerontologist, 36*(2), 147–156.

Clark, R. L., & Craig, L. A. (2003). *A history of public sector pensions*. Philadelphia, PA: University of Pennsylvania Press.

Coile, C. C., & Levine, P. B. (2006). Bulls, bears, and retirement behavior. *Industrial and Labor Relations Review, 59* (3), 408–429.

Coile, C. C., & Levine, P. B. (2007). Labor market shocks and retirement: Do government programs matter? *Journal of Public Economics, 91*(10), 1902–1919.

Corak, M. (2013). Income inequality, equality of opportunity, and intergenerational mobility. *Journal of Economic Perspectives, 27*(3), 79–102.

Coronado, J., & Perozek, M. (2003). Wealth effects and the consumption of leisure: Retirement decisions during the stock market boom of the 1990s. *Board of Governors of the Federal Reserve System, Finance and Economics Discussion Series, #2003–20.*

Craig, L. A. (1995). The political economy of public-private compensation differentials: The case of federal pensions. *Journal of Economic History, 55*, 304–320.

Dannefer, D. (2003). Cumulative advantage/disadvantage and the life course: Cross-fertilizing age and social science theory. *The Journals of Gerontology, Series B, 58*(6), S327–S337.

DiMaggio, P. J., & Powell, W. W. (1983). The iron cage revisited: Institutional isomorphism and collective rationality in organizational fields. *American Sociological Review, 48*, 147–160.

Dobbin, F. R. (1992). The origins of private social insurance: Public policy and fringe benefits in America, 1920–1950. *American Journal of Sociology, 97*(5), 1416–1450.

Dobbin, F. R. (1994). Cultural models of organization: The social construction of rational organizing principles. In D. Crane (Ed.), *The sociology of culture: Emerging theoretical perspectives* (pp. 117–141). Cambridge, MA: Blackwell.

Ekerdt, D. J. (1998). Entitlements, generational equity, and public-opinion manipulation in Kansas City. *The Gerontologist, 38*(5), 525–536.

Ekerdt, D. J. (2004). Born to retire: The foreshortened life course. *The Gerontologist, 44*(1), 3–9.

Ekerdt, D. J. (2009). Population retirement patterns. In P. Uhlenberg (Ed.), *International handbook of population aging* (pp. 471–491). New York, NY: Springer.

Estes, C. L. (1991). The new political economy of aging: Introduction and critique. In M. Minkler, & C. Estes (Eds.), *Critical perspective on aging: The political and moral economy of growing old* (pp. 19–36). Amityville, NY: Baywood.

Estes, C. L. (2004). Social Security privatization and older women: A feminist political economy perspective. *Journal of Aging Studies, 18*, 9–26.

Estes, C. L., & Phillipson, C. (2002). The globalization of capital, the welfare state, and old age policy. *International Journal of Health Services: Planning, Administration, Evaluation, 32*(2), 279–297.

Fligstein, N. J. (1990). *The transformation of corporate control.* Cambridge, MA: Harvard University Press.

Fligstein, N. J., & Dauber, K. (1989). Structural change in corporate organization. *Annual Review of Sociology, 15,* 73–96.

Fligstein, N. J., & Markowitz, L. (1993). Financial reorganization of American corporations in the 1980s. In W. J. Wilson (Ed.), *Sociology and the public agenda* (pp. 185–206). Newbury Park, CA: Sage.

Fontenelle, I. A. (2015). Organizations as producers of consumers. *Organization, 22*(5), 644–660.

Futrelle, D. (2012, November 7). Corporate raiders beware: A short history of the "poison pill" takeover defense. *Time.*

GAO. (2015). Contingent Workforce: Size, Characteristics, Earnings, and Benefits, GAO-15-168R. Washington, DC.

Gibson, R. C. (1987). Reconceptualizing retirement for Black Americans. *The Gerontologist, 27*(6), 691–698.

Giddens, A. (1990). *The consequences of modernity.* Stanford, CA: Stanford University Press.

Graebner, W. (1980). *A history of retirement: The meaning and function of an American institution.* New Haven, CT: Yale University Press.

Greenwood, R., & Scharfstein, D. (2013). The growth of finance. *Journal of Economic Perspectives, 27*(2), 3–28.

Hablutzel, P. N., & Selmer, D. R. (1988). Hostile corporate takeovers: History and overview. *Northern Illinois University Law Review,* 203–235.

Han, S.-K., & Moen, P. (1999). Clocking out: Temporal patterning of retirement. *American Journal of Sociology, 105,* 191–236.

Hardy, M. (2008). Making work more flexible: Opportunities and evidence. *American Association of Retired Persons.* Insights on the Issues, No. 11, November, 2008. AARP Public Policy Institute.

Hardy, M. (2011). Rethinking Retirement. In R. A. Settersten, & J. L. Angel (Eds.), *Handbook of sociology of aging* (pp. 213–227). New York, NY: Springer.

Henretta, J. C. (2003). The life-course perspective on work and retirement. In R. A. Settersten (Ed.), *Invitation to the life course* (pp. 85–105). Amityville, NY: Baywood.

Ippolito, R. A. (1990). Toward explaining earlier retirement after 1970. *Industrial and Labor Relations Review, 43,* 556–569.

Ippolito, R. A. (1997). *Pension plans and employee performance: Evidence, analysis & policy.* Chicago, IL: University of Chicago Press.

Ippolito, R. A. (2003). *Tenuous property rights: The unraveling of defined benefit pension contracts in the United States.* George Mason Law & Economics Research Paper. Number 03–06.

Jackall, R. (1988). *Moral mazes: The world of corporate managers.* New York, NY: Oxford University Press.

Jacoby, S. M. (1985). *Employing bureaucracy: Managers, unions, and the transformation of work in American industry, 1900–1945.* New York, NY: Columbia University Press.

Jepperson, R., & Meyer, J. W. (2011). Multiple levels of analysis and the limitations of methodological individualisms. *Sociological Theory, 29*, 54–73.

Jung, J., & Dobbin, F. (2012). Finance and institutional investors. In K. K. Cetina, & A. Preda (Eds.), *The sociology of finance* (pp. 52–74). New York, NY: Oxford University Press.

Kalleberg, A. L., Rassell, E., Cassirez, N., Reskin, B. F., Hudson, K., Webster, D.,… Appelbaum, E. (1997). *Nonstandard work, substandard jobs: Flexible work arrangements in the U.S.* Washington, DC: Economic Policy Institute.

Kopczuk, W., & Saez, E. (2004). Top wealth shares in the United States, 1916–2000. *National Tax Journal, 57*(2), 445–87.

Lumsdaine, R., & Mitchell, O. (1999). New developments in the economic analysis of retirement. In O. Ashenfelter & R. Layard (Eds.), *Handbook of labor economics* (Vol. 3, pp. 3261–3308). New York, NY: North-Holland.

Mayer, K. U., & Schoepflin, U. (1989). The state and the life course. *Annual Review of Sociology, 15*, 187–209.

Meyer, J. W. (2008). Reflections on institutional theories of organizations. In R. Greenwood, C. Oliver, K. Sahlin, & R. Suddaby (Eds.), *The Sage handbook of organizational institutionalism* (pp. 790–811). London, UK: Sage.

Meyer, J. W., & Jepperson, R. (2000). The "actors" of modern society: The cultural construction of social agency. *Sociological Theory, 18*(1), 100–120.

Meyer, J. W., & Rowan, B. (1977). Institutionalized organizations: Formal structure as myth and ceremony. *American Journal of Sociology, 83*, 440–463.

Munnell, A. H., & Soto, M. (2007). *State and Local Pensions are Different from Private Plans.* Boston, MA: Center for Retirement Research.

Munnell, A. H., Haverstick, K., & Soto, M. (2007). *Why have defined benefit plans survived in the public sector?* Boston, MA: Center for Retirement Research.

Murphy, K. (2012). Executive compensation: Where we are, and how we got there. In G. Constantinides, M. Harris, & R. Stulz (Eds.), *Handbook of the economics of finance.* The Netherlands: Elsevier Science (North Holland).

Myles, J. F. (1984). *Old age in the welfare state.* Boston, MA: Little, Brown.

Myles, J. F. (1991). Postwar capitalism and the extension of social security into a retirement wage. In M. Minkler, & C. L. Estes (Eds.), *Critical perspectives on aging: The political and moral economy of growing old* (pp. 293–309). Amityville, NY: Baywood.

Ocasio, W. (1997). Towards an attention-based view of the firm. *Strategic Management Journal, 18*, 189–206.

Ocasio, W., & Joseph, J. (2005). Cultural adaptation and institutional change: The evolution of vocabularies of corporate governance, 1972–2003. *Poetics, 33*, 163–178.

O'Rand, A. M. (2010). SSS presidential address: The devolution of risk and the changing life course in the United States. *Social Forces, 90*, 1–16.

O'Rand, A. M., & Henretta, J. C. (1999). *Age and inequality: Diverse pathways through alter life.* Boulder, CO: Westview.

Philippon, T. (2008). Why has the U.S. financial sector grown so much? The role of corporate finance. *NBER Working Paper No. 13405.* http://www.nber.org/papers/w13405

Philippon, T., & Reshef, A. (2009). Wages and human capital in the U.S. financial industry, 1909–2006. *NBER Working Paper 14644. http://www.nber.org/papers/w14644*

Poterba, J., Venti, S. F., & Wise, D. A. (2012). Were they prepared for retirement? Financial status at advanced ages in the HRS and AHEAD cohorts. In D. A. Wise (Ed.), *Investigations in the economics of aging*. Chicago, IL: University of Chicago Press.

Quadagno, J. S. (1988). *The transformation of old age security: Class and politics in the American welfare state*. Chicago, IL: University of Chicago Press.

Quadagno, J. S. (1996). Social Security and the myth of the entitlement "crisis." *The Gerontologist, 36*(3), 391–399.

Reich, R. B. (2007). *Supercapitalism: The transformation of business, democracy, and everyday life*. New York, NY: Alfred Knopf.

Riley, M. W. (1987). On the significance of age in sociology. *American Sociological Review, 52*, 1–14.

Riley, M. W., & Riley, J. W. (1994). Structural lag: Past and future. In M. W. Riley, R. L. Kahn, & A. Foner (Eds.), *Age and structural lag* (pp. 15–36). New York, NY: Wiley.

Schultz, E. E. (2011). *Retirement heist: How companies plunder and profit from the nest eggs of American workers*. New York, NY: Penguin Group.

Settersten, R. A., & Mayer, K. U. (1997). The measurement of age, age structuring, and the life course. *Annual Review of Sociology, 23*, 233–261.

Smith, T. W., & Sun, J. (2013). *General social survey 2012 final report: Trends in public attitudes about confidence in institutions*. Chicago, IL: NORC.

Sorensen, A. B. (1994). Firms, wages and incentives. In N. J. Smelser & R. Swedberg (Eds.), *Handbook of economic sociology* (pp. 504–528). Princeton, NJ: Princeton University Press.

Sorensen, A. B. (1998). Career trajectories and the older worker. In K. W. Schaie & C. Schooler (Eds.), *Impact of work on older adults* (pp. 207–234). New York, NY: Springer Publishing Company.

Stein, N. P. (1989). Reversions from pension plans: History, policies, and prospects. *N.Y.U. Tax Law Review, 44*, 259–334.

Thornton, P. H., & Ocasio, W. (1999). Institutional logics and the historical contingency of power in organizations: Executive succession in the higher education publishing industry 1958–1990. *American Journal of Sociology, 105*, 801–843.

U.S. Department of Labor. (2015). Private pension Plan Bulletin: Abstract of 2013 Form 5500 Annual Reports (Data extracted on 6/2/2015). U.S. Department of Labor, Employee Benefits Security Administration, September 2015.

Wallerstein, I. (1989). The capitalist world-economy: Middle-run prospects. *Alternatives: Global, Local, Political, 14*, 279–288.

Warner, D. F., Hayward, M. D., & Hardy, M. A. (2010). The retirement life course in America at the dawn of the twenty-first century. *Population Research and Policy Review, 29*(6), 893–919.

Westphal, J. D., Gulati, R., & Shortell, S. M. (August 1996). The institutionalization of total quality management: The emergence of normative adoption and the consequences for organizational legitimacy and performance. *Academy of Management Proceedings*, 249–253.

Wiatrowski, W. W. (2012). The last private industry pension plans: A visual essay. *Monthly Labor Review*, December, 3–18.

Wooten, J. A. (2001). The most glorious story of failure in the business: The Studebaker-Packard corporation and the origins of ERISA. *Buffalo Law Review, 49,* 683.

Zsembik, B. A., & Singer, A. (1990). The problem of defining retirement among minorities: The Mexican Americans. *The Gerontologist, 30*(6), 749–757.

CHAPTER 17

Families and Aging: Toward an Interdisciplinary Family-Level Approach

Rosemary Blieszner and Marieke Voorpostel

Most adults live with and grow old among family members, often including multiple generations (representing family lineage) and cohorts (representing different age groups). It seems crucial, then, to study the family context of aging by using theories and research methods that pertain to a family level of analysis. That statement might appear to be a truism, but a historical look at work in the field of family gerontology reveals many studies that actually encompassed a narrower perspective. An interesting compendium of family gerontology research exists in the series of "decade review" articles commissioned by the National Council on Family Relations for publication in its *Journal of Marriage and Family* beginning in 1971 and continuing through the most recent version in 2010 (Allen, Blieszner, & Roberto, 2000; Brubaker, 1990; Silverstein & Giarusso, 2010; Streib & Beck, 1980; Troll, 1971). Looking back to the first review's discussion of theory, Troll (1971) noted that the preponderance of research in family studies in general and hence in family gerontology to that point in time had adopted static institutional or structural–functional frameworks to guide exploratory investigations of family and aging topics. Likewise, Troll cited various studies that had presented conclusions about marital quality and other domains of family life based on cross-sectional interviews with just one person in each family, and examined individual-level concepts to the exclusion of relational concepts. This is not to say that Troll's review included no mention of interactional theories and concepts, dyadic analyses, or experimental designs; she did cite some. However, awareness of the need to study relational and family-level variables in combination with individual-level variables has grown steadily over the ensuing years, and stronger statements of family-level theories to guide predictions related to those variables have emerged over time as well. These trends are particularly emphasized in the more recent decade reviews (Allen et al., 2000; Silverstein & Giarusso, 2010). The movement toward a true *family* gerontology perspective has been accompanied by employment of longitudinal designs and dyadic analysis methods, further contributing to discovery of deeper insights about family interaction patterns in later life than were available in the past.

Advocating for true family-level studies makes it important to define "family." Silverstein and Giarusso (2010) pointed out that, although many specific family relationships have been investigated (e.g., romantic relations, sibling relations, parent–child relations, grandparent–grandchild relations), a holistic approach to studying families as complex kinship units is still rare. As discussed by Blieszner and Bedford (2012), traditional demographic and sociological definitions of family do not reflect very well the lived experiences of older adults and their families in contemporary society. Thus, they recommended an inclusive definition of family that incorporates dual perspectives on older adults within families, namely, older adults as persons with various kinds of family ties, and older adults as relatives of those belonging to other generations:

> *Family* is a set of relationships determined by biology, adoption, marriage, and...social designation and existing even in the absence of contact or affective involvement, and, in some cases, even after the death of certain members. (p. 4)

By focusing the definition of family on its structure, we do not intend to imply that the functions of and interpersonal processes within families are homogeneous or are unimportant research considerations. Rather, our intention is to challenge investigators to adopt an inclusive stance as to who is examined in their research projects on family functions and interactions and to assess a wider range of family members, as defined by study participants, than has been examined in the past. This definition permits study not only of family structures, functions, and relational processes found in traditional nuclear families, but also study of those aspects within increasingly common pluralistic family structures that incorporate new types of members and relationships within broader definitions of family than were typical in the past (Roberto & Blieszner, 2015). Further, an inclusive definition prompts study of families over time, in recognition of the influence of personal developmental change on family ties and reciprocally, the influence of family composition and relationship changes on individual and collective outcomes experienced by family members. It also conveys the need to study family dyads, triads, and larger constellations, because as Simons, Whitbeck, Conger, and Chyi-In (1991) explained, "no single family member has the best or most valid perspective on family processes...Rather, each family member presents a partially correct picture as filtered through his or her personal biases and emotions" (p. 162). Finally, who belongs to a person's family is not always apparent to external observers, so a methodological implication of this definition is the need to ask research participants to identity the members of their family themselves, rather than researchers assuming the composition of the kinship unit.

We believe using this conceptualization of family when focusing on older adults and their kin ties will encourage more family-level studies of multiple dimensions of these important bonds in the later years of life. Our goal for this chapter is to examine theories that are useful for guiding such research, thus yielding broader and deeper understanding of the ways older adults and their relatives negotiate family roles, responsibilities, and interactions in the context of both traditional and pluralistic family configurations. Taking a cue from the acknowledgment of change in the definition of "family," we begin with analysis of life-span development and life-course perspectives as applied to research on older adults and their families. These perspectives are especially useful because they accommodate study of micro- and macro-level change pertinent to family relationships and can be linked with other theories as sensitizing constructs for investigating change over time. Next is examination of the promise and problems associated with two key theoretical approaches that have been particularly effective in guiding family gerontology research in recent years, intergenerational solidarity and conflict, and intergenerational ambivalence. These approaches are strong in their own right and have the further advantage of linking well with life-span development and life-course perspectives. We focus on their theoretical tenets and principles, empirical applications, and strengths and limitations, with a critical assessment throughout. The last section of the chapter considers theoretical and empirical directions for future research in family gerontology.

■ LIFE-SPAN DEVELOPMENT AND LIFE-COURSE PERSPECTIVES

Tenets and Principles

Life-span development theories, typically grounded in a psychological perspective, extend early theories of development focused on children and adolescents to the study of adult development. The tenets of the life-span development framework posit that growth and change occur throughout the life cycle, different categories of behavior follow different developmental trajectories, functional growth or gains as well as declines or losses occur across all the years, behavior is modifiable throughout life, and historical and situational contexts interact with ontogeny to influence developmental outcomes (Baltes, 1987; Baltes, Lindenberger, & Staudinger, 2006). The life-course framework, evincing a sociological perspective, focuses on the social and historical contexts of development, including the social meanings of age and cohort, the organization of social roles, the timing and order of life transitions, the intersection of personal and social changes both within and across cohorts, the effects of agency on choices and actions, and the influence of interdependent lives on life-course outcomes (Elder & Shanahan, 2006). Considered together, these complementary perspectives offer a comprehensive set of constructs and hypotheses for assessing personal development over the years as well as family-related topics throughout both individual and family life cycles.

Both perspectives can be extended from the individual to the family level of analysis. Family development theory (Gavazzi, 2011; Rodgers & White, 1993) complements the life-span development framework. It focuses on transitions into and out of family roles across the family life cycle. The timing of transitions may be normative or nonnormative with respect to stages of personal development and the sequencing of family stages and events. As with a life-span development focus, these notions of timing and sequencing imply differential effects on personal and family outcomes according to extent of conformity with social expectations. Attention is given to tasks and challenges associated with transitions family members face and how they manage and adapt to transitions. Dyadic relations, the family as a group, and the intersection of families and societies all can be examined within a longitudinal context that acknowledges change over time.

Bengtson and Allen (1993) provided a comprehensive extension of the life-course perspective to families, focusing on consideration of the influences of generational and historical time, as well as social locations and diversity, on family interactions. Attending to generational time acknowledges that, not only does age (as a proxy for both ontogeny and the range of experiences one has acquired) influence behavior, so does placement in the family's generational lineage, which shifts over time with birth and death of one's relatives. Many dimensions of family interaction patterns are transmitted across generations, with potential for fostering both continuity of the family itself and adaptation to internal and external changes that have an impact on family interactions and well-being.

Although life-span development and life-course frameworks originated in different disciplines and traditionally emphasized different research questions, these perspectives are complementary. Both focus on the importance of studying the societal and historical contexts of family life and both promote the study of family members as developing people and families as dynamic, evolving groups.

Typical Applications

Early research emanating from a family development theoretical stance was concerned with describing common features of different stages of the family life cycle and the timing and sequencing of transitions into and out of roles associated with those stages (Rodgers & White, 1993). Many topics were explored, ranging as widely as marital satisfaction (Rollins & Cannon, 1974), time spent in housework (Rexroat & Shehan, 1987), and family life cycle effects on church membership (Stolzenberg, Blair-Loy, & Waite, 1995). Scholars came to realize, however, that the family life cycle approach assumed a conventional nuclear family, what Smith (1993) called the "Standard North American Family (SNAF)" (p. 25), that was demographically rare and did not reflect the lived experiences of modern families (Roberto & Blieszner, 2015). Hence, a variety of studies attempting to assess consequences of the intersecting and evolving realities of personal and family experiences aside from family life cycle stages emerged.

For example, one approach has been to examine the effects of early family experiences on personal health and well-being later on, which in turn can influence family life throughout adulthood. Research on the intergenerational transmission of parenting styles reveals long-term effects of how offspring are treated by parents. Using a prospective design, Chen and Caplan (2001) focused on transmission of constructive parenting. They demonstrated that adolescents who reported experiencing positive parenting were able, when they were middle-aged parents, to extend the same benefits to their own children. In contrast, Simons et al. (1991) used a dyadic design incorporating both parent retrospective data of how they were treated during their own adolescence and self-reports of how they treat their children, along with their adolescents' reports of the parents' behavior. This study showed that harsh parenting tends to be passed down the generational line from grandparents to parents to (grand)children, with gender and socioeconomic status affecting the likelihood of the middle-generation parents employing strategies they had themselves experienced when young. Luecken, Roubinov, and Tanaka (2013) cited extensive evidence showing that stressful family environments and negative parent–child relationships during childhood can impede development of crucial skills and abilities, such as social competence and emotion regulation, which are essential for managing stress and achieving supportive relationships in adolescence and beyond. Impaired ability to establish healthy relationships and cope with difficulties interferes with both psychological and physiological functioning and foretells a cycle of negative outcomes in adulthood.

Not all childhood family adversity impairs adult family relationships, however. A longitudinal follow-up investigation of middle-aged women who had experienced a poor relationship with one or both of their parents in childhood or adolescence showed differential effects on adult partnerships. Women who displayed insecure attachment styles had significantly greater negative functioning in romantic relationships, whereas those with secure attachment, despite their childhood difficulties, were more successful in adult relationships (McCarthy, 1999). Furthermore, research points to continuity of positive early family experiences throughout the life course. A prospective longitudinal study revealed that persons who had reported warm and trusting relationships with their parents during their adolescent years were likely to express satisfaction with their partner relationships in midlife (Möller & Stattin, 2001).

In keeping with the linked lives tenet of the life-course perspective, not only do parents affect children's outcomes, offspring have an impact on the well-being of older family members as well. With respect to effects on grandparents, Arpino and Bordone (2014) found some evidence that caring for grandchildren is positively associated with grandparents' cognitive functioning, pointing to the cognitive benefit of social interaction with younger relatives. Westphal, Poortman, and Van der Lippe (2015) revealed that parents' divorce affected grandparents' opportunities to interact with their grandchildren, depending on with which parent the grandchildren resided. Looking at parenthood, Umberson, Pudrovska, and Reczek (2010) reviewed the effects of being a parent on adults from a life-course perspective, showing the impact of contextual factors such as offspring age, evolving types of family structures, and a complex array of sociodemographic characteristics intersecting with cumulative advantages and disadvantages over time. They called for more longitudinal research, a greater variety of dependent variables, and more studies of intertwining trajectories across generations. An example of this kind of research, from the vantage point of linked lives, is a study by Kiecolt, Blieszner, and Savla (2011) of changes in parental ambivalence over time as adolescent and emerging adult offspring faced normative transitions related to leaving home, getting married, becoming parents, and achieving educational and work success. These researchers found a decline in parents' ambivalent feelings over 14 years of the study. However, not all of the decline could be explained by offspring's transitions because the pattern of attaining adult statuses was not straightforward. Some of the expected associations between adult children completing transitions successfully and reduced ambivalence were not supported by the data. Nevertheless, parental ambivalence about their children did affect parental well-being.

A life-course perspective informs understanding of other relationships as well. Sassler's (2010) review of research on romantic partnering from adolescence to old age highlights the changing forms of intimate relationships in contemporary society and the increasing fluidity of these ties over the adult years. The ways partners develop and enact relationships at one stage in life have implications for the nature of partnering at future stages. In the context of intimate bonds, personal life events affect not only the partner experiencing the event but also the other partner. For example, Wickrama, O'Neal, and Lorenz (2013) developed a conceptual framework that integrates life-course and stress-process perspectives to analyze the effects of midlife transitions such as retirement on later life outcomes such as marital quality. The framework takes into account the cumulative effects of genetics, family of origin experiences, personal dispositions, spousal interaction patterns, chronic adversities, health, family structure, and other factors on marital interactions and marital quality. Assessing these features in midlife provides the backdrop for examining their long-term impact on the aftermath of a transition such as retirement. A focus on the retirement transition, for example, would lead to examining aspects of work and the family's financial status over time, such as positive or negative work experiences, economic conditions, and the respective timing of spouses' retirements. This integrative framework could be applied to other relationships and outcomes; investigations would need to specify links between personal background and dispositional characteristics, dyadic influences, and anticipated outcomes as they all evolve over time.

Critical Assessment and New Directions

The life-span development and life-course perspectives offer investigators a broad and deep array of concepts and intersecting influences on lives over time, and by extension, on generations and families over time. Developmental tasks can be articulated for individuals at all stages of life, along with factors contributing to and hindering achievement of such tasks (McCormick, Kuo, & Masten, 2011). It is important to recognize, though, that life stages are fluid, not rigidly constructed, allowing for a variety of patterns and sequences (Smith-Osborne, 2007). At the same time, societies have norms and expectations of functions to be accomplished by families for their different generations, and family members exert a profound and pervasive influence on one another through-out life (Repetti, Flook, & Sperling, 2011). The life-course perspective is especially useful for examining the intersecting influences of individuals and families on development and well-being over time (Bengtson & Allen, 1993).

Settersten (2009) analyzed the potential benefits and challenges associated with inte-gration of the life-course and life-span perspectives. A key critique of the life-span per-spective is insufficient attention to the social structures in which individuals develop and the ways institutions affect developmental opportunities and constraints. In turn, a key critique of the life-course perspective is failure to examine the effects of personal characteristics on opportunities and constraints that individuals experience. If family gerontologists were more attuned to both the influences of personal dispositions and the influences of social structure on individual and family development, uniting these two perspectives could give rise to a creative synergy in research that addresses import-ant questions about family interactions and their outcomes over time more thoroughly than ever.

An emerging focus on resilience in the later years of life provides promising theo-retical guidance for such creative synergy in family gerontology research. Resilience signifies the ability of individuals to respond to adversity with positive adaptation that promotes not mere surviving, but thriving (Ryff & Singer, 2000; Smith-Osborne, 2007). It reflects the life-span principles of intraindividual plasticity in development (Smith & Hayslip, 2012) and ongoing potential for development, implying that resilience can be manifest throughout life. Moreover, resilience implies resistance to external risks and challenges, invoking life-course principles related to the impact of environmen-tal and contextual factors on development, including both risk factors and protective factors, and the cumulative effects of adversity as well as advantage (Nelson-Becker, 2013). Resilience is also a characteristic of families (Hawley & DeHaan, 1996; Walsh, 2012), evident when immediate and extended kin can identify resources and processes that enable the family not only to cope with challenges, but also to grow and flourish as a result of adversity. Here, the notion of linked lives is very apparent, both in the sense that one family member's difficulties are likely felt by others in the family and in the sense that family members can rally to support the member or members in distress.

Key theoretical considerations in the study of family resilience in the later years of life include assessment of risk factors pertaining both to older family members' function-ing and to the characteristics of other relatives, whose needs and problems may affect the older members. Risk factors are also associated with family contextual conditions such as generational structure and economic status. Likewise, protective factors may be found within individuals and the family group (e.g., personal attributes, knowledge of resources and past experiences, quality of interpersonal relationships, supportive environments). Protective factors serve to buffer the effects of adverse events and cir-cumstances, thereby promoting positive adaptation. The timing of adverse events and situations in relation to the ages of family members and normative expectations for role transitions and events is another key consideration in examining resilience in families (Nelson-Becker, 2013; Smith & Hayslip, 2012; Smith-Osborne, 2007; Walsh, 2012).

The application of a resilience perspective to family gerontology research can enhance investigation of developmental outcomes for family members and the family as a whole. Ryff and Singer (2000) focused on the contribution of resilience to relational flourishing, which in turn affects the health and psychological well-being of family members. They advocated studying social support as a multidimensional construct and examining receiving as well as giving support. They also called for deeper investigation of the role of positive and negative emotions in buffering stressors and contributing to both family resilience and high-quality close relationships. Within this vein, several researchers have studied family ties and family responses to typical challenges in old age. For example, prospective research by Be, Whisman, and Uebelacker (2013) illustrated the reciprocal relationship between marital satisfaction and life satisfaction in midlife and old age, including demonstration of cross-partner effects on longitudinal changes in marital adjustment and life satisfaction. These findings help explain the strong influence of positive family relationships on health and psychological well-being (Ryff & Singer, 2000). In another example, Coon (2012) assessed research on resilience in the context of challenges associated with family caregiving for relatives with dementia and for custodial grandchildren. Although many variables affect resilience under these often stressful circumstances, availability of social support from family and friends was a common factor in sustaining caregivers' resilience and hence, their health and well-being. These and other authors endorse the value of studying resilience in late-life families and call for incorporation of resilience-related constructs in many domains of family gerontology research where mechanisms influencing outcomes are not well characterized.

In summary, life-span development and life-course conceptual frameworks can be extended from the individual to the family level of analysis, with fruitful outcomes for adding to understanding of families as dynamic groups that influence the quality of life for all members, including the oldest ones, over time. Incorporating a focus on resilience and relational flourishing into such research permits examination of new variables that have not been thoroughly explored in attempts to explain the connections among individual characteristics or actions and the collective characteristics or actions of the family as a whole. In the following sections, we address two theoretical frameworks that are closely tied to this developmental and resilience-focused approach, intergenerational solidarity and conflict and intergenerational ambivalence. Taken together, these theories provide strong underpinning for a robust family gerontology research agenda.

■ INTERGENERATIONAL SOLIDARITY AND CONFLICT

Tenets and Principles

The theoretical framework of intergenerational solidarity and conflict originated in the idea that the family constitutes a social group, with solidarity as the basis for its social order and a prerequisite for its continued existence. Solidarity is seen as "the engine driving the pursuit of the common good within families" (Roberts, Richards, & Bengtson, 1991, p. 12). This theoretical perspective puts intergenerational relationships in adulthood at the core of the family, designating them as central ties beyond the nuclear family (Katz, Lowenstein, Phillips, & Daatland, 2005; Silverstein & Bengtson, 1997). Based on early sociological and social psychological theories on solidarity (notably Dürkheim, Tönnies, Homans, and Heider), the initial model defined six dimensions of solidarity: normative integration (standards for and expectations about the relationship), functional interdependence (the exchange of support), similarity or consensus in values, mutual affection, interaction, and family structure (the opportunity structure for interaction, such as geographical proximity), and also defined how the solidarity dimensions are linked (Bengtson & Schrader, 1982; Roberts et al., 1991). By jointly assessing these dimensions of solidarity and conflict, intergenerational relationships can be captured in all their complexity, and not simply be characterized by the presence or absence of specific solidarity domains (Bengtson, Giarusso, Marby, & Silverstein, 2002).

The initial model was criticized for its limitation to measuring positive aspects of intergenerational relationships, which painted a normative picture of how intergenerational relations "should be" (Lüscher, 2000). With scant attention to negative aspects of intergenerational solidarity, the model was thought to provide little insight into conflictual relationships (Bengtson et al., 2002; Katz et al., 2005). In response, Bengtson et al. revised the solidarity model to incorporate conflict explicitly (Bengtson et al., 2002; Bengtson, Rosenthal, & Burton, 1995). Moreover, they pointed out that the solidarity dimensions are meant to capture both positive and negative aspects of family relationships by treating them as dialectics reflecting: (a) intimacy and distance (affectual solidarity), (b) agreement and dissent (consensual solidarity), (c) dependency and autonomy (functional solidarity), (d) integration and isolation (associational solidarity), (e) opportunities and barriers for interaction (family structure), and (f) familism and individualism (normative solidarity). Finally, they stated that the framework also allows for potential negative consequences of positive scores on the solidarity dimensions, which can be "too much of a good thing" (Silverstein, Chen, & Heller, 1996).

Typical Applications

Over the last decades, research has shown that the framework of intergenerational solidarity and conflict is a reliable and valid tool for studying intergenerational relationships, including those between grandparents and grandchildren, most notably because of its attention to the multidimensionality of intergenerational relationships (Lin, Bryant, Boldero, & Dow, 2015; Moorman & Stokes, 2014). Moreover, the model is applicable to various ethnic groups and cross-national contexts (Katz et al., 2005). The main application of the model has been to describe parent–adult child relationships using several (although rarely all) dimensions of solidarity. This has been done in different countries, such as the Netherlands (Hogerbrugge & Komter, 2012) and Germany (Szydlik, 2008), or by comparing various European countries (Daatland & Lowenstein, 2005; Szydlik, 2012), and also for specific ethnic groups such as Chinese immigrants in the United States (Lin et al., 2015).

Although the origins of the model of intergenerational solidarity and conflict lie in theoretical work on small groups, its general use has usually been limited to the study of a single relationship, most typically between parents and adult children. However, other intergenerational relationships, such as the grandparent–grandchild bond, have received attention as well. For example, Moorman and Stokes (2014) linked solidarity between grandparents and grandchildren to depression in either party and showed the complex nature of these ties: For both grandparents and grandchildren, greater affinity was associated with fewer depressive symptoms, whereas more contact was associated with more symptoms. The authors concluded that the average grandparent–adult grandchild relationship is a source of both support and strain to both generations.

Hoff (2007) focused on functional solidarity and examined it among three generations in Germany: grandparents, parents, and children. He found a greater imbalance in support exchange in the relationship grandparents had with their grandchildren compared to the relationship with their children. Hoff did not directly address the mediating role the middle generation plays in the grandparent–grandchild relationship. The relationship the grandparent has with the parent as well as events occurring in the lives of the parents have their bearing on the grandparent–grandchild relationship

(Silverstein, Giarrusso, & Bengtson, 1998). Incorporating the ways in which the parent generation plays a role in the grandparent–grandchild relationship will move the framework beyond the level of dyadic ties to address the family as a more complex set of interdependent relationships.

A few studies using the solidarity and conflict perspective explicitly connected several family dyads. Voorpostel and Blieszner (2008) linked support between two adult siblings to solidarity displayed in the parent–child relationship. Examining the effects of the relationship with the parents on support between adult siblings, they studied how affinity, association, and value similarity in the relationship with the parent were associated with giving and receiving practical and emotional support in the sibling dyad. They discovered both compensatory processes, where a poor relationship and low contact frequency with the parent were compensated by increased emotional support exchange in the sibling dyad, and processes of reinforcement, where increased parental support coincided with higher levels of sibling support. Focusing on another family bond, Milardo (2009) addressed solidarity within and across generations by showing that the relationships aunts and uncles have with their nieces and nephews are situated in the relational context of the family.

Applying the intergenerational solidarity and conflict framework at the family level can also occur by including the network characteristics of a family in the investigation. Van Gaalen, Dykstra, and Flap (2008) examined how the sibling network affected intergenerational contact in a Dutch sample. They found that having sisters, having stepsiblings, a larger geographical distance between the siblings, and lower levels of network cohesion were associated with less contact in the parent–adult child dyad. Although this study focused only on contact and not on intergenerational solidarity in all its complexity, it does show that, not only do other family relationships affect the parent–child bond, but also the constellation of those family relationships as a whole matter.

Moving beyond the context of the family, some European studies have linked the intergenerational solidarity and conflict model to the macro context of a country. Intergenerational solidarity and conflict vary over contexts and populations, implying that they are affected by social circumstances and social structures. In turn, families also have an impact on society, notably in the way they reproduce social inequality. As family members help each other, especially as parents invest in their children, more advantaged families provide better chances for their children compared to those in lower social classes, which contributes to inequality in society (Szydlik, 2012). Research by Daatland and Lowenstein (2005) and by Szydlik (2008, 2012) tested two hypotheses regarding the relationship of welfare state provisions with family caregiving, the "crowding out" hypothesis, according to which the welfare state displaces the family, and the "crowding in" hypothesis, which states that welfare services facilitate family care and help adults provide for their children, or at the very least do not decrease family involvement in caregiving. Szydlik's model of intergenerational solidarity includes affectual solidarity, associational solidarity, and functional solidarity as outcomes, with opportunity structures (e.g., geographical proximity), need structures (e.g., financial needs or frailty), family structures (e.g., family size, composition and norms), and cultural–contextual structures (e.g., welfare state regulations) as determinants of solidarity, thereby explicitly placing the intergenerational relationship in a societal context (Szydlik, 2008, 2012). Daatland and Lowenstein (2005) distinguished associational solidarity, affectual solidarity, functional solidarity, and normative solidarity, but did not explicitly state the determinants of these solidarity dimensions. Both studies included various European countries in the analysis and both showed that stronger welfare states are positively associated with intergenerational practical support such as household chores or home repairs, and negatively with intergenerational personal care, such as help with bathing or eating. They concluded that social services alleviate the burden on family members of providing intensive personal care and free up family resources to provide intergenerational help with practical matters.

Linking the framework of intergenerational solidarity and conflict to the life-course and life-span perspectives brings the process of aging more to the foreground. Solidarity and conflict in relationships at a given moment in time can provide only a snapshot of the situation (Silverstein & Bengtson, 1997; Van Gaalen & Dykstra, 2006), which is the state of most of the research in this area. But an important question is: How do solidarity and conflict change over the life course? Family relationships develop over time and life events may trigger changes in the relationships among family members, potentially influencing solidarity and conflict. So far, little research has addressed family diversity or variation in trajectories when using the solidarity and conflict model. In one of the few longitudinal studies employing this framework, Hogerbrugge and Komter (2012) analyzed two waves from a large Dutch longitudinal study and showed that affection, association, and support were mutually reinforcing dimensions of solidarity over time, whereas conflict affected subsequent levels of associational and functional solidarity. Hogerbrugge and Komter concluded that associational, affectional, and functional solidarity can be regarded as the core dimensions, whereas structural solidarity and conflict should be regarded as exogenous to the other dimensions. Such an assessment of change over time allows the further specification and testing of the intergenerational solidarity and conflict model.

Critical Assessment and New Directions

Over the last two decades, the framework of intergenerational solidarity and conflict developed by Bengtson and colleagues has proven useful as an approach for studying the complexity of intergenerational relationships. More recently, researchers have realized that this model is not only relevant for intergenerational relationships but also can be extended to other family relationships and can include multiple relationships examined simultaneously. How do family members beyond the parent–adult child dyad create and maintain solidarity and experience conflict in relationships with each other? How can researchers address the family, in all its diverse forms, with all its changes over time, as a group or as a set of interdependent relationships? We have highlighted several ways in which the scope of the solidarity and conflict framework can be broadened to address the family as a complex kinship unit. Incorporating multiple family relationships and their mutual influences, and integrating network characteristics when studying intergenerational solidarity and conflict, are promising directions for future work. Every family relationship is interrelated with other ties in the family network, implying that solidarity and conflict in any given family dyad do not exist in isolation.

More work linking the framework of intergenerational solidarity and conflict to the life-course perspective will advance knowledge on how intergenerational solidarity and conflict change over time and how life events shape solidarity and conflict in various family relationships. In addition, research in this direction would enhance understanding of the process of aging in relation to family life. An example of a life event that affects multiple family members in a kinship network is the transition to retirement. In the process of adapting to this transition psychologically and financially, as well as in terms of the changed demands in their daily lives, individuals may have to renegotiate their relationships with family members (Damman, Henkens, & Kalmijn, 2015; Henkens, 1999). This adaptive process has potential consequences for the content of their family relationships in terms of conflict and solidarity. Study of other, less normative transitions would also be fruitful. For example, as older adults experience divorce themselves or divorce of their offspring, personal and relational adaptation is necessary and family ties become more complex. Research could address the implications of the adaptive processes and relationship changes for solidarity and conflict and in turn, for older adults' well-being. Furthermore, how life events and transitions affect intergenerational solidarity and conflict can be linked to features of social structure in different societal and cultural contexts. Resources for coping and managing transitions vary across individuals, families, and populations. How individuals are situated in the social structure in terms of gender, age, ethnicity, and socioeconomic status has bearing on their options for managing evolving family relationships in ways that are supportive and emotionally satisfying. Adding a resilience perspective to research on these questions would provide more information on available resources at the individual, family, and societal levels and the extent to which such resources are employed productively to aid in managing these changes.

■ INTERGENERATIONAL AMBIVALENCE

Tenets and Principles

Lüscher and Pillemer (1998) introduced the concept of intergenerational ambivalence in family studies. They pointed out that theoretical work on intergenerational relationships in adulthood had been focused on either solidarity or conflict separately, whereas family relationships are often characterized by both aspects simultaneously, which creates ambivalence. They defined intergenerational ambivalence as "contradictions in relationships between parents and adult offspring that cannot be reconciled" (Lüscher & Pillemer, 1998, p. 416). Their formulation of intergenerational ambivalence distinguished two dimensions. The first, "sociological ambivalence," refers to discrepant views of a relationship that follow from incompatible normative expectations. Contemporary family relationships have become more diverse, and traditional normative expectations associated with specific family roles have lost clarity. Different roles both within the family and in society may be associated with contradictory norms, creating ambivalence. The second form, "psychological ambivalence," is a subjective feeling. This form of ambivalence refers to the simultaneous experience of positive and negative emotions toward the same individual. Given the complexity of intimate relationships, it is likely that these forms of ambivalence are fairly common across family ties.

Connidis and McMullin (2002b) further developed the sociological ambivalence dimension (renaming it "structured ambivalence") by using it as a bridging concept between social structure and individual action, made evident in social interaction. Their definition of structured ambivalence goes beyond competing normative expectations at the individual level, explicitly positioning family relationships in a broader social structure. They argued that ambivalence "is created by the contradictions and paradoxes that are embedded in sets of structured social relations (e.g., class, age, race, ethnicity, gender) through which opportunities, rights, and privileges are differentially distributed" (Connidis & McMullin, 2002b, p. 565). The social structure in which relationships are embedded creates differences in the ability to exercise agency. Individuals with fewer resources at their disposal have fewer options available to manage ambivalence (Connidis & McMullin, 2002a, 2002b). This influence between agency and social structure goes in both directions: not only does the social structure limit or facilitate individual agency, the ways that individuals negotiate their family ties, in turn, influence the social world around them (Connidis, 2015).

The development of intergenerational ambivalence prompted renewed discussion on the solidarity and conflict model discussed previously. Although Lüscher and Pillemer (1998) introduced ambivalence as an alternative to the intergenerational solidarity and conflict model, proponents of the latter model proposed to integrate ambivalence into the intergenerational solidarity and conflict model. This would expand the original model to include social–structural factors, hence linking family solidarity to the larger societal level of analysis. Such an extension would address the intersection of institutional domains with family life, which in turn has implications for intergenerational solidarity and conflict (Bengtson et al., 2002). The ambivalence concept can broaden the explanatory power of the solidarity and conflict framework by providing a link to the positioning in the social structure of society, producing inequality in the structured distribution of resources. In their response to this proposal, Connidis and McMullin (2002a) stressed that ambivalence and intergenerational solidarity do not occur at the same level of analysis; whereas ambivalence is thought to motivate personal action and as such helps to explain how relationships are negotiated, intergenerational solidarity captures the conditions of intergenerational relationships as they exist in the larger social domain.

Following this debate, Hogerbrugge and Komter (2012) compared the intergenerational solidarity and conflict model and the concept of ambivalence using longitudinal data, and did not find strong support for the idea that ambivalence is a driving force behind processes of change in relationships. Although high levels of psychological ambivalence were associated with decreasing levels of contact, none of the other solidarity domains were affected. They found that structural relations among the dimensions of solidarity better explained changes in family relationships. In line with this result, Lendon, Silverstein, and Giarusso (2014) found only few individual and health-related variables significantly associated with ambivalence. Although the concept of ambivalence is a useful interpretive device, these findings have raised questions about whether the notion of ambivalence is more useful as a heuristic device than as an empirical predictor.

Typical Applications

The concept of ambivalence has been addressed in studies on various family relationships (for an overview, see Connidis, 2015). Yet, the vast majority of studies so far have examined psychological ambivalence rather than the multilevel conception of structured ambivalence. The focus on psychological ambivalence is limited to the study of individual perceptions of family relationships. Although studies on psychological ambivalence provide insight into the kind of ambivalent feelings people experience, they generally do not address the structural conditions under which older adults are more or less likely to experience such feelings, or the structural conditions under which such feelings have negative consequences. Thus, this approach misses the opportunity to link contradictions in family relationships to the larger social structure (Connidis, 2015). A notable exception is the study by Neuberger and Haberkern (2014) who demonstrated, using data from various European countries, that grandparents experienced lower quality of life if they did not care for grandchildren in countries where normative expectations of grandparent support are high. In countries where such norms were weak, not providing support did not affect grandparents' quality of life. This study explicitly addressed how the macro-level of the country can create socially structured ambivalence.

Lüscher and Pillemer proposed three aspects of parent–adult child relationships that are likely to generate ambivalence: ambivalence between dependence and autonomy, ambivalence resulting from conflicting norms on intergenerational relationships, and ambivalence resulting from solidarity. Several studies have demonstrated ambivalence related to dependence versus autonomy. For example, a desire for personal independence together with the emotional satisfaction derived from receiving care from adult children was a source of ambivalent feelings for older adults (Spitze & Gallant, 2004). Other studies addressed contradictory feelings of older parents regarding their offspring's independence. Aging parents were more likely to experience ambivalence toward children who encounter problems or fail to make several normative transitions in the life course such as getting married and finding a job (Birditt, Fingerman, & Zarit, 2010; Pillemer et al., 2007). Also, the tension between children leading busy lives, signifying their success and independence, and the desire to spend more time with them produced ambivalent feelings among older adults (Peters, Hooker, & Zvonkovic, 2006).

The majority of recent studies on ambivalence focused on the parent–child relationship (e.g., Birditt et al., 2010; Gilligan, Suitor, Feld, & Pillemer, 2015), but ambivalence in other family bonds has also received some research attention. Fingerman, Hay, and Birditt (2004) examined a broad range of relationships, both within the family and non-family ties. Ambivalence was more common in close family ties than in more distant ones and, in general, closeness was associated with ambivalence regardless of relationship type. Ambivalence was less common among older adults compared to younger adults, however. Connidis (2007) investigated ambivalence in two qualitative studies on adult sibling relationships. She found evidence of ambivalence when sibling dyads, which are generally seen as based on equality, were characterized by socioeconomic inequality. The concepts of role ambiguity and boundary ambiguity are insightful for understanding in which relationships ambivalence is likely to arise (Sarkisian, 2006). In the absence of clear societal expectations for a role (i.e., role ambiguity), or when there is disagreement or uncertainty (either among family members or within an individual) about who is part of the family and who is not (i.e., boundary ambiguity), people have to choose from several potentially contradictory norms or courses of action, which may lead to ambivalence.

Grandparents may experience role ambiguity, as their potential level of involvement may vary from complete absence of contact or occasional contact with grandchildren to being their main care provider. Mason, May, and Clarke (2007) showed in their qualitative study that grandparents experienced ambivalence around two predominant norms of grandparenting. First, the boundary between the norm of "not interfering" and that of being involved in child rearing created difficulties, which was related to the fact that grandparents to one generation simultaneously occupy the role of parent to another generation. This finding fits well with Lüscher and Pillemer's (1998) expectation that ambivalence arises when norms on intergenerational relationships are in conflict with each other. Second, the norm of "being there" for their grandchildren conflicted with a need for self-determination and control (Mason et al., 2007). Role ambiguity may also play a role in in-law relationships. Willson, Shuey, and Elder (2003) found ambivalence to be more common in relationships with in-laws than in relationships with parents. Boundary ambiguity may arise in stepfamily relationships, where members report more ambivalence on who is part of the family compared to people in nondivorced families (Widmer, 2010).

Several recent studies of ambivalence focused on potential negative outcomes, in keeping with research showing that ambivalence has negative consequences for well-being. The study by Kiecolt and colleagues (2011), described previously, showed that, even though ambivalence declined over the course of 14 years, it had a persistent negative effect on well-being. Suitor, Gilligan, and Pillemer (2011) found that ambivalence predicted depressive symptoms and positive affect among a sample of older mothers, but they did not find such a relationship among adult children. Trying to explain this negative effect, Gilligan et al. (2015) tested three mechanisms that may be at work in the relation between ambivalence and well-being: positive feelings exacerbate the impact of negative feelings on well-being, positive feelings work as a buffer against the impact of negative feelings, or positive feelings have no effect at all on well-being. They found support for only the latter mechanism, suggesting it may not so much be ambivalent feelings that lower well-being, but rather it is the experience of negative feelings regardless of any positive feelings that affects well-being. This brings into question the contribution of ambivalence to well-being, if the negative impact on well-being arises from negative affect rather than from ambivalence itself. Given that ambivalence is seen as a source of relationship change, tracking the longitudinal development of positive and negative feelings may enhance understanding of the connections among relationship changes, ambivalence, and well-being over time.

Critical Assessment and New Directions

Although most often applied to the parent–adult child bond, there is no compelling reason to assume that ambivalence cannot arise in other family relationships. Not only do parents and adult children experience ambivalence, it is likely that siblings, grandparents, and grandchildren, and romantic partners also experience contradictory normative expectations in their relationships over time and have conflicting feelings. Thus, theory about intergenerational ambivalence can be extended to investigation of ambivalence in other family relationships beyond the parent–child dyad.

Moreover, the concept of ambivalence has great potential to address interactions at the family level. One new direction is to study ambivalence as it pertains to performing different family roles and clusters of roles. Ambivalence may arise as individuals manage multiple family relationships simultaneously, as was demonstrated by Mason and colleagues (2007) in their study on grandparents. The middle generation of parents of younger children may be faced with contradictory courses of action as well, when managing their roles as both parents to young children and offspring of aging parents. Another example is the notion of collective ambivalence, which refers to mixed feelings across multiple children, and can be seen as a collective feature of a family (Ward, 2008; Ward, Deane, & Spitze, 2008). The concepts of role ambiguity and boundary ambiguity (Sarkisian, 2006) are also promising in linking ambivalence to the family level. Within one family, different members can hold different perspectives on who belongs to the family and what role is expected of them; these views may be even more discrepant when looking across nonadjacent generations and cohorts with greatly different life experiences. Assessing role and boundary ambiguity this way reveals the complexity of the family as experienced by different members.

Stepfamilies may also experience this kind of within-family ambivalence, as boundary ambiguity is likely to arise in stepfamily relationships where normative expectations and roles are not clear-cut (Schmeeckle, Giarrusso, Feng, & Bengtson, 2006; Widmer, 2010). Acknowledging that ambivalence can occur as multiple family members manage interdependent family relationships can further the study of how individuals together navigate their roles in the larger family.

Ambivalence fits very well with the life-course perspective. Like the life-course approach, it also explicitly addresses how social structure matters for family experiences and affects the resources available to resolve it. Moreover, transitions over the life course may trigger ambivalence and reciprocally, conflicted feelings may lead to personal and relational decisions that have an impact on family ties. Finally, the concept of linked lives can help to move ambivalence beyond the individual or single dyadic relationship level of analysis to the family level. The study of how ambivalence is experienced and managed over the life course and in relation to (and from the perspective of) multiple family members will further understanding of how the family contributes or is detrimental to older adults' well-being. Linking attempts to manage ambivalence to individual and family resilience could yield new insights into strengths that reside in family ties despite the occurrence of conflicting feelings among the members.

■ CONCLUSION

In crafting this overview of theoretical perspectives for family gerontology research, our goal was to highlight the importance of analyzing the family as a whole when seeking answers about changes over time in this vital unit of society and when developing recommendations for aiding families to achieve optimal functioning. Toward that end, we challenge researchers to embrace greater complexity in conceptualizing family matters, which in turn has implications for the research designs required to work at a family level of analysis.

Theoretical Issues and Implications for Research

Family gerontology addresses family interactions and outcomes from the dual perspectives of older adults and their relationships with relatives in younger generations as well as younger family members and their relationships with those in older generations. More research is needed on topics that influence individual and family well-being by simultaneously studying family members from multiple generations. The purpose would be to assess shared values and attitudes despite cohort differences that may point to protective factors in the family, as well as generational differences that may affect family processes, family support, family resilience, and family well-being.

Recognizing that the traditional notion of family life cycle stages does not fit well with the pluralistic forms of family structures and functions in contemporary society leads to novel questions about definitions of family and identification of significant family events and transitions. Emphasizing the need to determine who it is individuals consider as family members or like family to them highlights our contention that "family" means more than its structure or household, as traditionally defined. It signifies a set of relationships that may be broader than demographers have assumed and not completely apparent to outsiders, yet may offer many important forms of assistance and support. Moreover, in theorizing about "family," it is important to recognize the fluidity of family (Finch, 2007) on several levels. First, different family members are likely to hold varying perceptions of who belongs to that family. Second, the constellation of family relationships changes over time, just as perceptions of who belongs to the family may change. Third, the very meaning of family may change over the life course both within individual members and differentially across various members.

This focus on multiple aspects of difference and change means that the occurrence, timing, and sequencing of family events and transitions may vary along many dimensions of family structure and social location that remain to be mapped via longitudinal designs. New criteria are needed for determining how and when to assess significant events and transitions, given that family milestones are likely to affect the health and well-being of family members and perhaps even the stability of the family unit itself. With increasing fluidity of families over time, examining how people "do family" is more important than ever. People display many kinds of behaviors and engage in many actions to show others whom they consider part of their family and what makes these relationships meaningful (Finch, 2007). Their decisions and behaviors affect the availability of resources that can aid in coping with events and transitions, such as emotional and instrumental support.

Advocating for a broader range of family-level studies, focused on family members beyond romantic and parent–child dyads, leads to questions about the interactions within larger family groups and among extended kin ties and how they vary across cultural subgroups. Calling for an expanded set of focal variables to include concepts related to resilience and positive outcomes leads to questions about family strengths instead of deficits. As these observations suggest, it would be productive to ask: Who belongs to the family, when, and for how long? How do families incorporate new members and release current members from the family? What expectations do family members hold for one another; how are those expectations conveyed; and how do they change over time? What is the role of personal agency in the context of various family structures that are more fluid now than in the past? How do people manage multiple family relationships that are both interdependent and fluid over time?

This notion of interdependence is at the heart of the linked lives concept in the life-course perspective. A family-level approach recognizes that the linkages are not necessarily continuous nor always with the same persons, and this type of fluidity will vary across family members. As a result, the characteristics of intergenerational solidarity and conflict as well as intergenerational ambivalence are also likely to be fluid over time within and between family members. As solidarity or conflict increases or decreases, as ambivalence intensifies or subsides, outcomes for various family members will fluctuate. Under what circumstances might conflict enhance rather than diminish solidarity? When and for whom is ambivalence consequential or negligible?

Another aspect of linked lives is that intergenerational solidarity and conflict, and intergenerational ambivalence, are not solely properties of individuals. Rather, they are influenced by and influence the content of other family relationships as well. For example, the relationship older parents have with their adult children will affect the relationship these children have among themselves as siblings and how they socialize their own offspring, setting the stage for interactions among the siblings when they themselves become old and for how their offspring will treat them. A family-level approach both captures contemporary interaction patterns and foretells the outcomes of intergenerational transmission of attitudes, values, and behaviors.

In acknowledging that families are diverse and subjective to change, it is important not to neglect the influence of societal structure on how family solidarity, conflict, and ambivalence affect individual outcomes. Moreover, dimensions of social location, such as gender and racial ethnic status, have not yet been investigated thoroughly in research on intergenerational solidarity and conflict and intergenerational ambivalence. How do solidarity, conflict, and ambivalence take shape and change over the life course for women and for men and in various racial ethnic groups? In what ways does intersectionality, or the cumulative effects of age, class, race, ethnicity, and sexual orientation, affect solidarity, conflict, and ambivalence processes over time among older and younger family members? Are some structural features of persons and families more strongly associated than others with the experience of ambivalence, its negative outcomes, and the resources required to manage or resolve it? Simultaneously, it is important to recognize the interplay of family members' personality traits and other personal characteristics with their social location characteristics in examining processes associated with solidarity, conflict, ambivalence, and resilience in families with older members. How do level of maturity, interpretation of experiences, and traits such as anxiety or openness to new experiences affect family members' efforts to sustain affective, supportive, and instrumental ties with one another? How do they contribute to skills needed for managing and resolving conflict and ambivalence? To what extent does personal hardiness in the face of challenges affect family-level management of elder care tasks so all generations can flourish in the face of aging-related needs among those in the latter part of the life span?

These are only a few of the many possible directions that arise from the convergence of life-span and life-course perspectives with a resilience framework and theories about intergenerational solidarity and conflict and intergenerational ambivalence. Better understanding of the role of families in the process of aging requires theorizing on the family level, rather than at the level of a single family relationship at one moment in time. This integrative approach to conceptualizing family holds great promise for advancing the field of family gerontology.

REFERENCES

Allen, K. R., Blieszner, R., & Roberto, K. A. (2000). Families in the middle and later years: A review and critique of research in the 1990s. *Journal of Marriage and Family, 62,* 911–926.

Arpino, B., & Bordone, V. (2014). Does grandparenting pay off? The effects of child care on grandparents' cognitive functioning. *Journal of Marriage and Family, 76,* 337–351.

Baltes, P. B. (1987). Theoretical propositions of life-span developmental psychology: On the dynamics between growth and decline. *Developmental Psychology, 23,* 611–626.

Baltes, P. B., Lindenberger, U., & Staudinger, U. M. (2006). Life span theory in developmental psychology. In W. Damon & R. M. Lerner (Eds.), *Handbook of child psychology: Vol. 1. Theoretical models of human development* (6th ed., pp. 569–664). New York, NY: John Wiley.

Be, D., Whisman, M. A., & Uebelacker, L. A. (2013). Prospective associations between marital adjustment and life satisfaction. *Personal Relationships, 20,* 728–739.

Bengtson, V. L., & Allen, K. R. (1993). The life course perspective applied to families over time. In P. G. Boss, W. J. Doherty, R. LaRossa, W. R. Schumm, & S. K. Steinmetz (Eds.), *Sourcebook of family theories and methods* (pp. 469–499). New York, NY: Plenum.

Bengtson, V. L., Giarusso, R., Marby, J. B., & Silverstein, M. (2002). Solidarity, conflict, and ambivalence: Complementary or competing perspectives on intergenerational relationships? *Journal of Marriage and Family, 64*, 568–576.

Bengtson, V. L., Rosenthal, C. J., & Burton, L. M. (1995). Paradoxes of families and aging. In R. H. Binstock & L. K. George (Eds.), *Handbook of aging and the social sciences* (4th ed., pp. 253–282). San Diego, CA: Academic Press.

Bengtson, V. L., & Schrader, S. S. (1982). Parent-child relations. In D. J. Mangen & W. A. Peterson (Eds.), *Social roles and social participation* (Vol. 2, pp. 115–186). Minneapolis: University of Minnesota Press.

Birditt, K. S., Fingerman, K. L., & Zarit, S. H. (2010). Adult children's problems and successes: Implications for intergenerational ambivalence. *The Journals of Gerontology, Series B, 65*, 145–153.

Blieszner, R., & Bedford, V. H. (2012). The family context of aging: Trends and challenges. In R. Blieszner & V. H. Bedford (Eds.), *Handbook of families and aging* (2nd ed., pp. 3–8). Westport, CT: Praeger.

Brubaker, T. H. (1990). Families in later life: A burgeoning research area. *Journal of Marriage and Family, 52*, 959–981.

Chen, Z., & Kaplan, H. B. (2001). Intergenerational transmission of constructive parenting. *Journal of Marriage and Family, 63*, 17–31.

Connidis, I. A. (2007). Negotiating inequality among adult siblings: Two case studies. *Journal of Marriage and Family, 69*, 482–499.

Connidis, I. A. (2015). Exploring ambivalence in family ties: Progress and prospects. *Journal of Marriage and Family, 77*, 77–95.

Connidis, I. A., & McMullin, J. A. (2002a). Ambivalence, family ties, and doing sociology. *Journal of Marriage and Family, 64*, 594–601.

Connidis, I. A., & McMullin, J. A. (2002b). Sociological ambivalence and family ties: A critical perspective. *Journal of Marriage and Family, 64*, 558–567.

Coon, D. W. (2012). Resilience and family caregiving. *Annual Review of Gerontology and Geriatrics, 32*, 231–249.

Daatland, S., & Lowenstein, A. (2005). Intergenerational solidarity and the family–welfare state balance. *European Journal of Ageing, 2*, 174–182.

Damman, M., Henkens, K., & Kalmijn, M. (2015). Missing work after retirement: The role of life histories in the retirement adjustment process. *The Gerontologist, 55*, 802–813.

Elder, G. H., Jr., & Shanahan, M. J. (2006). The life course and human development. In W. Damon & R. M. Lerner (Eds.), *Handbook of child psychology: Vol. 1. Theoretical models of human development* (6th ed., pp. 665–715). New York, NY: John Wiley.

Finch, J. (2007). Displaying families. *Sociology, 41*, 65–81.

Fingerman, K. L., Hay, E. L., & Birditt, K. S. (2004). The best of ties, the worst of ties: Close, problematic, and ambivalent social relationships. *Journal of Marriage and Family, 66*, 792–808.

Gavazzi, S. M. (2011). Family development theory. In R. J. R. Levesque (Ed.), *Encyclopedia of adolescence* (pp. 925–930). New York, NY: Springer Science + Business Media, LLC.

Gilligan, M., Suitor, J. J., Feld, S., & Pillemer, K. (2015). Do positive feelings hurt? Disaggregating positive and negative components of intergenerational ambivalence. *Journal of Marriage and Family, 77*, 261–276.

Hawley, D. R., & DeHaan, L. (1996). Toward a definition of family resilience: Integrating life-span and family perspectives. *Family Process, 35*, 283–298.

Henkens, K. (1999). Retirement intentions and spousal support: A multi-actor approach. *The Journals of Gerontology, Series B, 54*, S63–S73.

Hoff, A. (2007). *Functional solidarity between grandparents and grandchildren in Germany. Working Paper 307.* Oxford, UK: University of Oxford, Oxford Institute of Aging.

Hogerbrugge, M. J. A., & Komter, A. E. (2012). Solidarity and ambivalence: Comparing two perspectives on intergenerational relations using longitudinal panel data. *The Journals of Gerontology, Series B, 67*, 372–383.

Katz, R., Lowenstein, A., Phillips, J., & Daatland, S. O. (2005).Theorizing intergenerational family relations: Solidarity, conflict, and ambivalence in cross-national contexts. In V. L. Bengtson, A. C. Acock, K. R. Allen, P. Dilworth-Anderson, & D. M. Klein (Eds.), *Sourcebook of family theory & research* (pp. 393–420). Thousand Oaks, CA: Sage.

Kiecolt, K. J., Blieszner, R., & Savla, J. (2011). Long-term influences of intergenerational ambivalence on midlife parents' psychological well-being. *Journal of Marriage and Family, 73*, 369–382.

Lendon, J. P., Silverstein, M., & Giarrusso, R. (2014). Ambivalence in older parent–adult child relationships: Mixed feelings, mixed measures. *Journal of Marriage and Family, 76*, 272–284.

Lin, X., Bryant, C., Boldero, J., & Dow, B. (2015). Older Chinese immigrants' relationships with their children: A literature review from a solidarity–conflict perspective. *The Gerontologist, 55*, 990–1005.

Luecken, L. J., Roubinov, D. S., & Tanaka, R. (2013). Childhood family environment, social competence, and health across the lifespan. *Journal of Social and Personal Relationships, 30*, 171–178.

Lüscher, K. (2000). Ambivalence: A key concept for the study of intergenerational relations. In S. Trnka (Ed.), *Family issues between gender and generations: Seminar report of the European Observatory on Family Matters* (pp. 11–25). Vienna, Austria: Austrian Institute for Family Studies.

Lüscher, K., & Pillemer, K. (1998). Intergenerational ambivalence: A new approach to the study of parent-child relations in later life. *Journal of Marriage and Family, 60*, 413–425.

Mason, J., May, V., & Clarke, L. (2007). Ambivalence and the paradoxes of grandparenting. *The Sociological Review, 55*, 687–706.

McCarthy, G. (1999). Attachment style and adult love relationships and friendships: A study of a group of women at risk of experiencing relationship difficulties. *British Journal of Medical Psychology, 72*, 305–321.

McCormick, C. M., Kuo, S. I.-C., & Masten, A. S. (2011). Developmental tasks across the life span. In K. L. Fingerman, C. A. Berg, J. Smith, & T. C. Antonucci (Eds.),

Handbook of life-span development (pp. 117–140). New York, NY: Springer Publishing Company.

Milardo, R. M. (2009). *The forgotten kin: Aunts and uncles.* Cambridge, UK: Cambridge University Press.

Möller, K., & Stattin, H. (2001). Are close relationships in adolescence linked with partner relationships in midlife? A longitudinal, prospective study. *International Journal of Behavioral Development, 25,* 69–77.

Moorman, S. M., & Stokes, J. E. (2014). Solidarity in the grandparent–adult grandchild relationship and trajectories of depressive symptoms. *The Gerontologist.* Advance online publication.

Nelson-Becker, H. (2013). Resilience in aging: Moving through challenge to wisdom. In D. S. Becvar (Ed.), *Handbook of family resilience* (pp. 339–357). New York, NY: Springer Science + Business Media.

Neuberger, F., & Haberkern, K. (2014). Structured ambivalence in grandchild care and the quality of life among European grandparents. *European Journal of Ageing, 11,* 171–181.

Peters, C. L., Hooker, K., & Zvonkovic, A. M. (2006). Older parents' perceptions of ambivalence in relationships with their children. *Family Relations, 55,* 539–551.

Pillemer, K., Suitor, J. J., Mock, S. E., Sabir, M., Pardo, T. B., & Sechrist, J. (2007). Capturing the complexity of intergenerational relations: Exploring ambivalence within later-life families. *Journal of Social Issues, 63,* 775–791.

Repetti, R., Flook, L., & Sperling, J. (2011). Family influences on development across the life span. In K. L. Fingerman, C. A. Berg, J. Smith, & T. C. Antonucci (Eds.), *Handbook of life-span development* (pp. 745–775). New York, NY: Springer Publishing Company.

Rexroat, C., & Shehan, C. (1987). The family life cycle and spouses' time in housework. *Journal of Marriage and Family, 49,* 737–750.

Roberto, K. A., & Blieszner, R. (2015). Diverse family structures and the care of older persons. *Canadian Journal on Aging, 34,* 305–320.

Roberts, R. E. L., Richards, L. N., & Bengtson, V. L. (1991). Intergenerational solidarity in families: Untangling the ties that bind. *Marriage and Family Review, 16,* 11–46.

Rodgers, R. H., & White, J. M. (1993). Family development theory. In P. G. Boss, W. J. Doherty, R. LaRossa, W. R. Schumm, & S. K. Steinmetz (Eds.), *Sourcebook of family theories and methods* (pp. 225–254). New York, NY: Plenum Press.

Rollins, B. C., & Cannon, K. L. (1974). Marital satisfaction over the family life cycle: A reevaluation. *Journal of Marriage and Family, 36,* 271–282.

Ryff, C. D., & Singer, B. (2000). Interpersonal flourishing: A positive health agenda for the new millennium. *Personality and Social Psychology Review, 4,* 30–44.

Sarkisian, N. (2006). "Doing family ambivalence": Nuclear and extended families in single mothers' lives. *Journal of Marriage and Family, 68,* 804–811.

Sassler, S. (2010). Partnering across the life course: Sex, relationships, and mate selection. *Journal of Marriage and Family, 72,* 557–575.

Schmeeckle, M., Giarrusso, R., Feng, D., & Bengtson, V. L. (2006). What makes someone family? Adult children's perceptions of current and former stepparents. *Journal of Marriage and Family, 68*, 595–610.

Settersten, R. A., Jr. (2009). It takes two to tango: The (un)easy dance between life-course sociology and life-span psychology. *Advances in Life Course Research, 14*, 74–81.

Silverstein, M., & Bengtson, V. L. (1997). Intergenerational solidarity and the structure of adult child–parent relationships in American families. *American Journal of Sociology, 103*, 429–460.

Silverstein, M., Chen, X., & Heller, K. (1996). Too much of a good thing? Intergenerational social support and the psychological well-being of older parents. *Journal of Marriage and Family, 58*, 970–982.

Silverstein, M., & Giarrusso, R. (2010). Aging and family life: A decade review. *Journal of Marriage and Family, 72*, 1039–1058.

Silverstein, M., Giarrusso, R., & Bengtson, V. L. (1998). Intergenerational solidarity and the grandparent role. In M. E. Szinovacz (Ed.), *Handbook on grandparenthood* (pp. 144–158). Westport, CT: Greenwood.

Simons, R. L., Whitbeck, L. B., Conger, R. D., & Chyi-In, W. (1991). Intergenerational transmission of harsh parenting. *Developmental Psychology, 27*, 159–171.

Smith, D. E. (1993). The Standard North American Family: SNAF as an ideological code. *Journal of Family Issues, 14*, 50–65.

Smith, G. C., & Hayslip, B., Jr. (2012). Resilience in adulthood and later life: What does it mean and where are we heading? *Annual Review of Gerontology and Geriatrics, 32*, 3–28.

Smith-Osborne, A. (2007). Life span and resiliency theory: A critical review. *Advances in Social Work, 8*, 152–168. Retrieved from https://journals.iupui.edu/index.php/advancesinsocialwork/article/view/138

Spitze, G., & Gallant, M. P. (2004). "The bitter with the sweet": Older adults' strategies for handling ambivalence in relations with their adult children. *Research on Aging, 26*, 387–412.

Stolzenberg, R. M., Blair-Loy, M., & Waite, L. J. (1995). Religious participation in early adulthood: Age and family life cycle effects on church membership. *American Sociological Review, 60*, 84–103.

Streib, G. F., & Beck, W. R. (1980). Older families: A decade review. *Journal of Marriage and Family, 42*, 937–956.

Suitor, J. J., Gilligan, M., & Pillemer, K. (2011). Conceptualizing and measuring intergenerational ambivalence in later life. *The Journals of Gerontology, Series B, 66*, 769–781.

Szydlik, M. (2008). Intergenerational solidarity and conflict. *Journal of Comparative Family Studies, 39*, 97–114.

Szydlik, M. (2012). Generations: Connections across the life course. *Advances in Life Course Research, 17*, 100–111.

Troll, L. E. (1971). The family of later life: A decade review. *Journal of Marriage and Family, 33*, 263–290.

Umberson, D., Pudrovska, T., & Reczek, C. (2010). Parenthood, childlessness, and well-being: A life course perspective. *Journal of Marriage and Family, 72*, 612–629.

Van Gaalen, R. I., & Dykstra, P. A. (2006). Solidarity and conflict between adult children and parents: A latent class analysis. *Journal of Marriage and Family, 68*, 947–960.

Van Gaalen, R. I., Dykstra, P. A., & Flap, H. (2008). Intergenerational contact beyond the dyad: The role of the sibling network. *European Journal of Ageing, 5*, 19–29.

Voorpostel, M., & Blieszner, R. (2008). Intergenerational solidarity and support between adult siblings. *Journal of Marriage and Family, 70*, 157–167.

Walsh, F. (2012). Successful aging and family resilience. *Annual Review of Gerontology and Geriatrics, 32*, 153–172.

Ward, R. A. (2008). Multiple parent–adult child relations and well-being in middle and later life. *The Journals of Gerontology, Series B, 63*, S239–S247.

Ward, R. A., Deane, G., & Spitze, G. (2008). Ambivalence about ambivalence: Reply to Pillemer and Suitor. *The Journals of Gerontology, Series B, 63*, S397–S398.

Westphal, S. K., Poortman, A., & Van der Lippe, T. (2015). What about the grandparents? Children's postdivorce residence arrangements and contact with grandparents. *Journal of Marriage and Family, 77*, 424–440.

Wickrama, K. A. S., O'Neal, C. W., & Lorenz, F. O. (2013). Marital functioning from middle to later years: A life course–stress process framework. *Journal of Family Theory & Review, 5*, 15–34.

Widmer, E. (2010). *Family configurations: A structural approach to family diversity.* Burlington, VT: Ashgate Publishing.

Willson, A. E., Shuey, K. M., & Elder, G. H. (2003). Ambivalence in the relationship of adult children to aging parents and in-laws. *Journal of Marriage and Family, 65*, 1055–1072.

CHAPTER 18

Theories of Social Connectedness and Aging

Jaclyn S. Wong and Linda J. Waite

Inequality in health and aging is a key concern for scholars, policy makers, and practitioners. Traditional biomedical models of health that view aging as a process of physiological decline fail to account for variations in trajectories of health and aging. We argue here that a holistic understanding of the last third of life requires careful consideration of the many differences in the social worlds that people inhabit and the ways that these affect and are affected by health. Trajectories of well-being and aging differ across national contexts (Steptoe, Deaton, & Stone, 2015), and across social categories such as race (Krueger, Saint Onge, & Chang, 2011) and socioeconomic status (Miech, Pampel, Kim, & Rogers, 2011), for example. Furthermore, differences in social ties and social support seem to account for some of the variation in health outcomes and mortality (Holt-Lundstad, Smith, & Layton, 2010).

■ THEORIES OF SOCIAL CAPITAL

Scholars studying social connectedness draw on the sociological theory of social capital (Coleman, 1988). Coleman (1988) defines social capital as aspects inherent to the structure of social relations that facilitate individuals' actions. Social relationships create capital in various ways: (a) by fostering obligations, expectations, and trust; (b) by acting as information channels; (c) by enforcing norms and imposing sanctions; and (d) by enabling the flow of goods and services. Thus, social connections are resources that individuals can draw on to achieve their goals. According to the social capital framework, those with more and better social connections will have greater resources and can navigate the life course more successfully.

In recent years, social scientists have proposed theoretical and conceptual models to explore the role of social connectedness in the specific context of aging. There are two general theoretical models that explicate the processes through which social relationships may influence health: the main effects model and the stress-buffering model (Cohen, Gottlieb, & Underwood, 2000; Holt-Lundstad et al., 2010; Thoits, 2011). Both are grounded in the overarching proposition that social connections facilitate successful action, drawn from social capital theory.

The main effects model suggests that social relationships may lead to better health through various cognitive, emotional, behavioral, and biological pathways. For example, social relationships may directly encourage health behaviors through social influence or control, and indirectly through providing role-based purpose and meaning or a sense of belonging, increasing self-esteem, and bolstering a sense of control. Social connections may provide care when one is sick, or information about treatments. Thus, the main effects model suggests that social connections directly promote better health and well-being at older ages.

The stress-buffering model, on the other hand, proposes that social relationships—both perceived and objective—provide informational, emotional, or tangible resources that promote adaptive behavioral or neuroendocrine responses to acute or chronic stressors such as illness, life events, and life transitions. According to this model, social support prevents health-damaging responses to stressful events; by slowing or otherwise altering declines in health and well-being, social relationships contribute to more successful aging.

■ CURRENT RESEARCH

Guided by these key lines of thought, recent research in the social sciences has assessed the ways social connections affect aging. This research provides support for the social capital framework, but suggests that the effects of social connectedness on health can vary depending on the number, type, and quality of those relationships. This research points to both direct effects of social relationships and to stress-buffering effects. In proceeding, we discuss marriage, social networks, and social participation, and how they influence health in the last third of life.

Marriage and Romantic Partnership

The biopsychosocial model conceives of health as produced in a social context, most often the intimate dyad (Lindau, Laumann, Levinson, & Waite, 2003). The benefits of marriage and partnership for health are well documented (Waite & Gallagher, 2001), but the effects depend on one's marital biography—transitions into and out of marriage, age at first marriage, and marital exposure (Hughes & Waite, 2009; McFarland, Hayward, & Brown, 2013). Those who have experienced marital loss and those who have been married for fewer years tend to have worse physical health, worse emotional health, and more functional limitations. Recent research has linked marital dissolution for women to metabolic risk and years married to lower cardiovascular risk. Among men, those who married at younger ages were more likely to experience chronic inflammation than those who married at later ages (McFarland et al., 2013).

This research suggests that experiences of marriage and marital loss get under the skin through different mechanisms and into different bodily systems over different time scales. Total time spent married may be especially important for health conditions that develop slowly, such as cardiovascular risk or other chronic conditions. On the other hand, marital transitions may influence health characteristics that change quickly, such as emotional health or metabolic risk, because getting married or marital loss may induce rapid changes in diet, physical activity, and stress. In sum, these findings support the main effects model of social relationships, which suggests that social connections directly promote well-being. More broadly, these findings support the proposition from social capital theory that those with social ties are advantaged compared to their disconnected counterparts, and that loss of close ties damages health.

Although research points to several benefits associated with being married, marital *status* in itself may not be as important to health and aging as marital *quality*. Those in high-quality marriages seem to be protected from declines in cardiovascular health, functional limitations, and emotional well-being. Alternatively, a poor quality marriage may cause stress and lead directly to health problems. Higher relationship satisfaction and supportive spouse behaviors appear to moderate the effects of poor vision on functional limitations and on depressive symptoms (Bookwala, 2011), and also offer protection from the negative effects of disability on loneliness (Warner & Kelley-Moore, 2012). Marital strain, on the other hand, increases the chances of poor cardiovascular health, especially for women and at older ages (Liu & Waite, 2014). These findings provide evidence to support the stress-buffering model, and further, add nuance to the general argument that social relationships are beneficial: It seems that high-quality relationships are especially beneficial to successful aging and poor quality ones are harmful.

Marriage also seems to be a *unique* social context for the production of health at older ages. Supportive network ties do not appear to buffer the effects of an unhappy marriage or being unmarried on physical health, suggesting that the spousal relationship is more influential than other relationships (Holt-Lundstad, Birmingham, Brandon, & Jones, 2008). Marriage also seems irreplaceable in dealing with the functional impairments that frequently develop at older ages. These impairments increase risk of loneliness in older adults, and both nonmarital and marital relationships independently affect loneliness. However, only the marital relationship seems to moderate the effect of disablement on loneliness. Supportive nonspousal relationships do not compensate for the negative effects of a weak marital relationship for functionally impaired older adults. That is, although physically disabled older adults in higher quality marriages were buffered from loneliness, supportive nonmarital relationships do not appear to offset elevated loneliness among those in low-quality marriages (Warner & Adams, 2012).

Research on the links between marriage, marital quality, and health adds detail and nuance to the social capital framework. Although having relationships seems to be better than not having any (e.g., McFarland et al., 2013), and having high-quality relationships is better than having low-quality ones (Bookwala, 2011; Warner & Kelley-Moore, 2012), recent research suggests that certain kinds of relationships—in this case, marriage—are better than others in promoting well-being in late life (Holt-Lundstad et al., 2008; Warner & Adams, 2012).

Social Networks

Although marital relationships seem to play a central role in the health and well-being of elderly individuals, the network of people with whom we exchange information, affection, social support, and social contact is also key in theoretical frameworks on aging. Recent data on the social networks of older adults paint a rich picture of the individual, or egocentric, social networks of the elderly community-dwelling population. Measures of social networks from the National Social Life Health and Aging Project (NSHAP), a nationally representative longitudinal study of more than 3,000 older adults, provide one example. NSHAP's network measures ask each respondent to name and characterize each of the people with whom he or she has discussed important matters over the past year. Characteristics of each individual and their connections to the respondent and to each other are obtained. The detailed social network information from NSHAP sheds light on the various kinds of social capital available to elderly Americans.

One surprising set of findings shows that, contrary to some theories (emotional selectivity), the availability of social capital both increases and decreases over the life course, depending on the type of capital being measured. Network size declines with age, but the volume or frequency of contact with network members is U-shaped: the young–old and the oldest old have similar levels of contact with network members, while those in the middle have less (Cornwell, Laumann, & Schumm, 2008). This U-shaped pattern may reflect changes older adults face at different ages. Contact declines in the middle-aged group as social roles dissipate because of retirement, bereavement, and health declines. However, the greater volume seen among the oldest old may indicate adaptation to the loss of social roles, friends, or family members.

Longitudinal studies of social networks also paint a brighter picture of aging than some theoretical perspectives would suggest. Cornwell and Laumann (2013) use Waves 1 and 2 of NSHAP to assess how older adults' social networks changed between 2005/2006 and 2010/2011. Respondents "lost" a network member if they named a person in Wave 1 but not in Wave 2. The most common reason respondents gave for losing a network member had to do with geographic distance (either the respondent or the confidant moved, or the respondent felt that the confidant lived "too far away," 23.4%). Another common response was that the confidant died during the study period (17.1%). Otherwise, respondents reported that they were "still in touch" with the confidant, but presumably not on the same level they had been at Wave 1 (15.3%), or that they just "drifted apart" (14.8%). In line with Cornwell and colleagues' (2008) descriptive cross-sectional findings detailed previously, these responses suggest that networks are not static at older ages, and that elders are likely to lose family members, friends, and spouses over time.

However, these losses do not typically result in a shrinkage of network size. Instead, older adults seem to actively rebuild their networks in a process of "network turnover"; when respondents lost confidants, they tended to add the same or a greater number of new ones (Cornwell & Laumann, 2013). Thirty-eight percent of people saw a net expansion of their networks, compared to 26.6% who experienced a net decrease in network size. Of those who showed no net change in network size, 80.6% showed some change in the people in their networks. Regardless of whether network size changed between waves, 81.8% of respondents named a confidant at Wave 2 whom they had not named at Wave 1. Only 7% of respondents reported complete stability in their networks—no changes in network size or members.

Not only do elders' networks change over 5 years, Cornwell and Laumann find that older adults who cultivate new ties appear to enjoy health benefits. As the number of confidants added at Wave 2 increases, the risk of functional impairment declines; the odds of reporting better health increase; and the probabilities of reporting depression decrease. They hypothesize that cultivating new network members may increase physical and cognitive activity to an extent that benefits immune and cardiovascular health. Or, the addition of new confidants may boost self-esteem and reduce depression, which can have a variety of downstream health benefits. Taken together, Cornwell and Laumann's (2013) study offers support for the main effects and stress-buffering models of social connectedness and health, and more broadly offers support for the social capital framework. Cultivating social ties—creating more sources of social capital—may lead to physiological, cognitive, and emotional benefits.

In addition to the changing availability of social capital at older ages, specific characteristics of a social network appear to have implications for health and aging. For example, Shiovitz-Ezra and Litwin (2012) show that network type affects health behaviors. They identified five types of networks among the elderly:

1. "Diverse" networks—high contact with family, friends, and organized groups
2. "Friends" networks—a large number of friends
3. "Congregant" networks—frequent attendance at religious services

4. "Family" networks—a large number of children
5. "Restricted" networks—low sociability with few family or extrafamilial ties

Shiovitz-Ezra and Litwin then show that older people embedded in family and restricted networks, the network types with the fewest resources, were more likely than others to report alcohol abuse, physical inactivity, and less use of complementary and alternative medicine. The authors propose that people exposed to the control of a variety of social agents are more apt to experience positive pressure to adopt health-promoting behaviors, and more often receive informal sanctions that discourage health-damaging habits.

Specific activities within a social network may influence health outcomes at older ages, but the effects may depend on the characteristics of the network. For example, having a large network is beneficial for management of hypertension only if the individual is likely to discuss health with network members (York Cornwell & Waite, 2012). Those with larger networks face lower chances of having uncontrolled hypertension (diagnosed, but unmedicated hypertension) if the network discusses health. The less likely those in the network are to have health discussions, the greater the risk that those with a large network tend to have *worse* health. These findings contradict the general hypothesis that having more social relationships is beneficial; having a large social network that does not support positive health behaviors may be worse for an individual's health than having a smaller but more resourceful or supportive network.

These research examples provide support for the main effects model of social connectedness and aging, and offer further nuance to social capital theory. Shiovitz-Ezra and Litwin's (2012) study suggests that variety in one's social relationships is beneficial; those exposed to social control from different kinds of people may experience more positive pressure to adopt health-promoting behaviors, and may receive more informal sanctions that discourage health-damaging habits, than people without extensive networks or those with homogeneous networks. York Cornwell and Waite (2012) suggest that having a social network that discusses health promotes positive health management behaviors, which again, highlights the importance of considering the particular behaviors of one's social groups in studying social capital.

Social Participation

In addition to maintaining interpersonal social networks, older adults are connected to their communities through socializing with neighbors, and through religious, volunteer, and organized group participation (Cornwell et al., 2008). Interestingly, the oldest adults appear most connected to the community. Compared to their younger counterparts, the oldest old have the greatest odds of socializing with neighbors on a weekly basis, attending religious services at least once a week, and volunteering every week. This pattern of social participation among the elderly suggests that individuals actively cultivate social capital, and compensate for changes or losses in their interpersonal social networks by becoming more involved in other social activities.

This engagement in the community appears to be adaptive in the aging process. Several studies on religious participation using NSHAP data provide an instructive example of the positive effects of social participation on health at older ages. These studies show that religious attendance is negatively associated with a host of physiological issues such as inflammation, metabolic state, and cardiovascular status (Das & Nairn, 2014), and negative emotional states such as loneliness (Rote, Hill, & Ellison,

2013). Religious attendance may protect against poor physical and psychological health by integrating older adults into supportive social networks, by providing shared goals, and by giving life meaning beyond oneself.

Sustaining high levels of social integration over time may be particularly beneficial for mental and physical health. Older individuals who have stably high or increasing social engagement experience lower levels of physical and cognitive limitations over time (Thomas, 2011). For instance, continuous participation in activities such as going out to do shopping; community or volunteer work; paid employment; going to a movie, restaurant, or sporting event; playing cards, games, or bingo; attending religious services; and participating in social and community groups is associated with fewer depressive symptoms (Glass, Mendes De Leon, Bassuk, & Berkman, 2006). More importantly, the least engaged groups of older adults have steeper increases in depression over time compared to more socially engaged elderly individuals (Glass, Mendes De Leon, Bassuk, & Berkman, 2006). Those who are more socially integrated may be likely to experience more motivation or pressure, or receive better information, to take care of their health compared to those who are socially disengaged. This research provides particularly clear evidence in support of the buffering model of social connectedness: individuals who maintain high levels of social capital as they age appear to experience slower declines in well-being over time.

Objective and Subjective Social Relationships

As this section demonstrates, there is a great amount of literature showing that the objective characteristics (e.g., quantity, type) of social relationships influence health and aging. However, research shows that *subjective* perceptions of social connectedness exert an independent and sizable effect on health and well-being in old age. Objective social disconnectedness is not always accompanied by feelings of isolation, so the two types of social isolation are conceptually distinct and independently associated with health. Social disconnectedness, the *objective* lack of contact with others because of situational factors like small networks or lack of participation in social activities, and perceived isolation or loneliness, the *subjective* experience of shortcomings of one's social resources, both exert an independent effect on the likelihood of reporting poorer self-rated physical and mental health (York Cornwell & Waite, 2009). Furthermore, the effect of perceived isolation may be especially great on mental health.

Other research shows that perceptions of isolation are uniquely linked to outcomes such as impaired cognition (Shankar, Hamer, McMunn, & Steptoe, 2013) and mortality (Luo, Hawkley, Waite, & Cacioppo, 2012). Loneliness may impact these outcomes by affecting sleep (Cacioppo et al., 2002), reducing physical activity (Hawkley, Thisted, & Cacioppo, 2009), and impairing physiological function (Hawkley, Masi, Berry, & Cacioppo, 2006). These studies highlight the importance of accounting for both objective measures of social relationships (i.e., number of confidants, network density) and subjective evaluations of those relationships when studying social connectedness and aging. Perceived availability of social capital may well be as important as actual social resources in producing health and well-being in late life.

■ VARIABILITY AND DIVERSITY IN AGING

Thus far, the chapter has introduced the theory of social capital, and detailed the main effects and stress-buffering models of social connectedness and health. In describing empirical studies on aging, we have enumerated the ways research has pushed social capital theory forward. Starting with the basic principle that social relationships are a resource that help produce health and well-being, scholars have contributed work that broadens our lines of inquiry. Not only do social connections matter, we know that the quality, kind, and number of social relationships matter in different ways. Access to a variety of types of social connections matters. The activities in which one's social group engages matter. Sustaining sources of social capital over time matters. Finally, both actual and perceived access to social relationships matter.

Although a wealth of literature documents the ways in which social connectedness influences aging, researchers are increasingly asking how this relationship may vary across different social groups. Leading scholars such as Thoits (2010) point out that exposure to stress is unequally distributed in the general population: women, racial/ethnic minorities, unmarried persons, and working-class and poor individuals are exposed to a wider variety of stressors than had been previously measured, including the additional stress of discrimination. Furthermore, social capital and other coping resources are disproportionately low among these groups, exacerbating the disadvantages they already face. Research in sociology emphasizes the importance of understanding differences across social groups when developing theories of aging.

Numerous studies on the variability in social capital and health and aging have focused on gender differences. When confronted by stressful situations, women are more likely than men to seek and use social support (Taylor, 2011) and to benefit from social support (Taylor et al., 2000). This pattern suggests that models of social connections and health may apply more readily to women than men, and that the social capital framework may be especially useful for understanding women's experiences of aging. However, other research suggests that men might just respond differently to social support and isolation than women do: Yang, McClintock, Kozloski, and Li (2013) find that social isolation is correlated with more adverse inflammatory responses in men than women. The authors hypothesize that the physiological response typical of women (the tend-and-befriend pattern) acts to downregulate innate immune responses such as inflammation, but men do not respond similarly. Further research is needed to continue documenting the ways the connection between social capital and health may vary by gender.

In addition to gender differences, some scholars have explored racial and ethnic variation in social capital at older ages and have found that social networks vary in size, type, and quality across groups (e.g., Umberson & Montez, 2010). However, few researchers explicitly examine whether the main effects or stress-buffering models apply as well to these groups, and it is unclear whether social connectedness is related to health and aging in the same way across different populations. One study documents a *lack* of association between social connectedness and health among Black men: Black men had smaller networks than White men, but network size did not have any significant linkages with blood sugar or cardiovascular health among Black men (Das, 2013). Instead, chronic inflammation, a biological marker of long-term stress exposure, more consistently accounted for Black men's worse metabolic health. Nevertheless, social relationships, inflammation, and health are likely to be interrelated, and more research is required to explore these theories across different social groups.

Moving forward, theory and research should (a) pay attention to structural factors that affect different groups' social relationships and (b) account for possible differences in biological processes that link social connectedness to health outcomes in order to better describe the role of social connectedness in producing health at older ages across different social groups.

■ NEW THEORIES AND CONCEPTS

Although social capital theory has effectively guided empirical research, new ideas and concepts in aging research are generating interest among scholars, and are taking the field in innovative directions. We discuss several of these exciting new research areas subsequently.

Social Genomics

Scholars have successfully integrated social factors into theories of aging, and researchers are now turning to the question of how the social and biological are linked. The field of social genomics studies the ways in which social experiences regulate gene activity (Cole, 2009; Shanahan, 2013). Scholars in this area examine how social experiences affect the way information contained in DNA is transcribed into messenger RNA (mRNA), the molecular building block essential to all biological processes in the cell. Understanding how social forces affect gene expression will help determine the causal link between the social and the biophysical. Current research suggests that social stressors alter genetic expression by influencing the inflammatory responses of the immune system. The glucocorticoid insensitivity hypothesis posits that chronically stressed individuals become insensitive to the anti-inflammatory actions of glucocorticoids, the steroids that regulate the inflammatory response system. In other words, those exposed to ongoing stress are less able to reduce inflammation, which makes them prone to inflammatory diseases such as cardiovascular and respiratory disease.

Research on social isolation provides an illustrative example of the work in social genomics. Scholars have found that isolation, a stressful state of disconnectedness in social species, increases glucocorticoid resistance, which suppresses the immune system and increases inflammatory responses. Together, these two processes result in negative health outcomes in social mammals, and more specifically, contribute to higher rates of morbidity and mortality in older adults (Cacioppo, Hawkley, Norman, & Berntson, 2011). In sum, social genomics research suggests that social connections might produce well-being in late life via biophysical pathways.

Childhood Adversity and the Life-Course Perspective

Accumulating empirical evidence documenting a relationship between childhood experiences and biological exposures has led researchers to more closely examine the link between very early life stages and later ones. Research in aging that employs the life-course perspective (Mayer, 2009) considers unique trajectories of aging that result from biological processes, personal biography, linked lives, and institutional policies situated in historical time. The life-course framework calls for a longer view of aging, and longitudinal data collection efforts such as the National Longitudinal Surveys (NLS), the Health and Retirement Study (HRS), and the National Longitudinal Study of Adolescent Health (Add Health) have enabled researchers to develop this model by more rigorously exploring individual trajectories over time.

For example, poor health in childhood affects family income, household wealth, individual earnings, and labor supply many years later (Smith, 2009). Similarly, psychological problems and substance abuse in childhood have large effects on individuals' later educational outcomes, their ability to work, the likelihood of family formation, and the amount of family assets (Smith & Smith, 2010), all of which are in turn associated with successful aging. Thus, experiences in childhood can be consequential for outcomes later in life.

New research in this area documents the importance of conditions as early as in utero for outcomes in aging. For example, poor maternal nutrition may predispose a woman's children to later disease (for a review, see Gluckman, Hanson, Cooper, & Thornburg, 2008), including conditions that develop at older ages like cancer (Grotmol, Weiderpass, & Tretli, 2006). Scholars in this field suggest that adverse intrauterine environments increase the likelihood of aberrant phenotypes in the offspring: in utero conditions prime an individual's biological processes to react to and protect against unhealthy environments even though conditions may change after birth. The life-course perspective's call to take a longer view of aging will help scholars illuminate the processes and experiences over the life course that produce disparities in old age.

The Environment

Scholars have also begun focusing their attention on the environmental contexts of health and social connectedness. It is important to consider space in research on aging because environmental conditions (a) shape the ways individuals access resources and experience the social world and (b) influence individuals' exposure to pollutants that are detrimental to health.

Urban sociologists suggest that the neighborhoods in which elders live and conduct their everyday activities affect the experience of aging. Most research on the neighborhood context of health is guided by social disorganization theory, which suggests that neighborhood structural characteristics such as concentrated poverty, racial/ethnic composition, and residential instability influence the capacity of residents to achieve common goals, develop neighborhood ties and social networks, and participate in voluntary organizations that benefit the community. A number of studies suggests that neighborhood socioeconomic status is linked to health in late life: poverty and socioeconomic disadvantage at the neighborhood level are associated with individual-level self-rated health (Cagney, Browning, & Wen, 2005), mental health (Aneshensel et al., 2007), and mortality (Diez Roux, Borrell, Haan, Jackson, & Schultz, 2004). However, a growing body of research shows that the social environment of the neighborhood—levels of collective efficacy, participation in volunteer organizations and supportive neighborhood social networks—can be protective against adverse conditions (e.g., Browning, Feinberg, Wallace, & Cagney, 2006).

In addition to the social characteristics of the neighborhood, the built environment, the physical features of the neighborhood, and the available amenities affect aging by facilitating or inhibiting activity and social interaction. For example, features like walkable sidewalks, adequate lighting, and the availability of local businesses may become more influential on aging-related outcomes as older adults develop physical limitations and lose the ability to perform activities like driving a car (Clarke, Ailshire, & Lantz, 2009).

Recent research guided by principles in public health and epidemiology has begun to consider the effects of other environmental conditions on health in late life. Racial/ethnic minorities and the poor are more likely to live near environmentally hazardous facilities (for a review, see Brulle & Pellow, 2006), and the elderly in these communities may bear a disproportionate share of the health burden from exposures to toxins. A series of studies based on the Veterans Affairs Normative Aging Study (NAS), an ongoing study of aging established in 1963, documents a relationship between air pollution and various health conditions such as increased blood pressure (Wilker et al., 2010) and inflammation (Madrigano et al., 2010). Other research links air pollutants to increased hospital admissions for cardiovascular disease, congestive heart failure, and ischemic heart disease (Suh, Zanobetti, Schwartz, & Coull, 2011). This new body of work suggests that environmental and atmospheric conditions are consequential to health and aging, and scholars in this field are continuing to identify the specific pollutants that are associated with various health outcomes, and the mechanisms linking them.

In short, research on neighborhood and environmental factors suggests that space and place shape aging. Understanding the physical context in which the elderly conduct their lives points to an additional set of factors that produces inequality in health and well-being in late life.

■ FUTURE DEVELOPMENT AND APPLICATION OF THEORY

In addition to continuing research in these areas and documenting variability in social connectedness and aging, researchers can continue developing other concepts to ensure viable theories of social capital in aging in the decade ahead. We discuss some ideas subsequently.

Negative Social Relationships

We noted previously that relationship quality often matters more than simply the existence of a social relationship, and although it is shown that high-quality relationships exert a positive influence on health outcomes (e.g., Bookwala, 2011; Warner & Kelley-Moore, 2012), fewer studies specifically examine the impact of negative relationships on aging. Stressful and demanding social relationships may be just as harmful as supportive relationships are beneficial. For example, one study finds that marital strain accelerates the decline in self-rated health over time, especially at older ages (Umberson, Williams, Powers, Liu, & Needham, 2006). Furthermore, negative social interactions with family members and friends might be linked to depression, and the ill effects of negative interactions may not be buffered by positive interactions (Stafford, McMunn, Zaninooto, & Nazroo, 2011). Researchers should continue studying the relationship between negative social capital and outcomes in aging in order to account for relationship quality in the main effects and stress-buffering models of social connectedness and health.

Relationship Between Objective and Subjective Social Connections

Although studies show that perceived social support is just as important as actual, objective social support for health (e.g., Luo et al., 2012; York Cornwell & Waite, 2009), little research identifies how objective social connections and perceived social support are related. Why do some older adults feel lonely even when they are surrounded by family and friends, while others are not adversely affected by a lack of social resources? A theory of optimal matching (Cutrona & Russell, 1990), in which social support must match the specific needs of an individual facing a specific stressful event in order to be efficacious, has been advanced to explain the connection between objective and subjective evaluations of social connections, but the hypothesis has not been rigorously, empirically tested. In addition, a variety of factors such as personality characteristics or broader social context may affect how relationships are perceived or how social resources are assessed and used, but little is known about the topic at this time.

Social Connectedness Over the Life Course: Trajectories of Social Relationships and Health

Social relationships and health change over time, and research needs to account for the dynamic nature of these processes in aging. Several recent studies point to the importance of examining changes in and trajectories of social relationships in order to understand how social connections shape trajectories of health (Cornwell & Laumann, 2013; Thomas, 2011). Employing the life-course perspective to theorize changes in connectedness would add a crucial level of nuance to the main effects and stress-buffering models of social relationships and health.

These emerging research ideas may be explored with the development of better measures and better analytic methods. Precise measures of both positive and negative relationship quality, as well as objective social connections and subjective evaluations of social relationships, would allow for a deeper understanding of how different facets of social relationships uniquely influence health and aging. Longitudinal studies like NSHAP would provide researchers with detailed information about social relationships and health over time, enabling more accurate analyses of the dynamic relationship between social connectedness and health. Better measures, longitudinal data, and advances in computing and analytic techniques would facilitate our efforts to understand the causal pathway between social relationships and health.

Theories of social capital and research in social connectedness and aging point to several areas in which policy and practice can improve well-being in the last third of life. Because quality relationships promote good health, identifying those at risk for social isolation is the first step in increasing well-being at older ages. Doctors and social workers should ask about older individuals' partners, families, friends, and network members, and ask about any stressors or strains in these relationships. Social workers can then provide resources for enhancing social skills, increasing social support, increasing opportunities for social interaction, and addressing maladaptive social cognition (Hawkley & Cacioppo, 2010). Second, as neighborhoods and the built environment shape health outcomes, city and community leaders can invest in increasing and improving the amenities that facilitate elders' ability to access social and material resources, such as safe, walkable sidewalks, and local shops and community centers. Finally, any policy or intervention should take into account the diversity of the older population and tailor practices to meet the varying needs of the elderly in the community.

REFERENCES

Aneshensel, C. S., Wight, R. G., Miller-Martinez, D., Botticello, A. L., Karlamangla, A. S., & Seeman, T. E. (2007). Urban neighborhoods and depressive symptoms among older adults. *The Journals of Gerontology, Series B, 62*(1), S52–S59.

Bookwala, J. (2011). Marital quality as a moderator of the effects of poor vision on quality of life among older adults. *The Journals of Gerontology, Series B, 66*(5), 605–616.

Browning, C. R., Feinberg, S. L., Wallace, D., & Cagney, K. A. (2006). Neighborhood social processes, physical conditions, and disaster-related mortality: The case of the 1995 Chicago heat wave. *American Sociological Review, 71*(4), 661–678.

Brulle, R. J., & Pellow, D. N. (2006). Environmental justice: Human health and environmental inequalities. *Annual Review of Public Health, 27*, 103–124.

Cacioppo, J. T., Hawkley, L. C., Berntson, G. G., Ernst, J. M., Gibbs, A. C., Stickgold, R., & Hobson, J. A. (2002). Do lonely days invade the nights? Potential social modulation of sleep efficiency. *Psychological Science, 13*, 385–388.

Cacioppo, J. T., Hawkley, L. C., Norman, G. J., & Berntson, G. G. (2011). Social isolation. *Annals of the New York Academy of Sciences, 1231*, 17–22.

Cagney, K. A., Browning, C. R., & Wen, M. (2005). Racial disparities in self-rated health at older ages: What difference does the neighborhood make? *The Journals of Gerontology, Series B, 60*(4), S181–S190.

Clarke, P., Ailshire, J. A., & Lantz, P. (2009). Urban built environments and trajectories of mobility disability: Findings from a national sample of community-dwelling American adults (1986–2001). *Social Science and Medicine, 69*(6), 964–970.

Cohen, S., Gottlieb, B. H., & Underwood, L. G. (2000). Social relationships and health. In S. Cohen, L. G. Underwood, & B. H. Gottlieb (Eds.), *Measuring and intervening in social support* (pp. 3–25). New York, NY: Oxford University Press.

Cole, S. W. (2009). Social regulation of human gene expression. *Current Directions in Psychological Science, 18*, 132–137.

Coleman, J. S. (1988). Social capital in the creation of human capital. *American Journal of Sociology, 94*, S95–S120.

Cornwell, B., & Laumann, E. O. (2013). The health benefits of network growth: New evidence from a national survey of older adults. *Social Science and Medicine, 125*, 94–106.

Cornwell, B., Laumann, E. O., & Schumm, L. P. (2008). The social connectedness of older adults: A national profile. *American Sociological Review, 73*(2), 185–203.

Cutrona, C. E., & Russell, D. (1990). Type of social support and specific stress: Toward a theory of optimal matching. In B. R. Sarason, I. G. Sarason, & G. R. Pierce (Eds.), *Social support: An interactional view* (pp. 319–366). New York, NY: John Wiley.

Das, A. (2013). How does race get "under the skin"? Inflammation, weathering, and metabolic problems in late life. *Social Science and Medicine, 77*, 75–83. doi:10.1016/j.socscimed.2012.11.007

Das, A., & Nairn, S. (2014). Religious attendance and physiological problems in late life. *The Journals of Gerontology, Series B*, Advance online publication.

Diez Roux, A. V., Borrell, L. N., Haan, M., Jackson, S. A., & Schultz, R. (2004). Neighbor-hood environments and mortality in an elderly cohort: Results from the Cardiovascular Health Study. *Journal of Epidemiology and Community Health, 58*, 917–923.

Glass, T. A., Mendes De Leon, C. F., Bassuk, S. S., & Berkman, L. F. (2006). Social engagement and depressive symptoms in late life: Longitudinal findings. *Journal of Aging and Health, 18*, 604–628.

Gluckman, P. D., Hanson, M. A., Cooper, C., & Thornburg, K. L. (2008). Effect of in utero and early-life conditions on adult health and disease. *New England Journal of Medicine, 359*, 61–73.

Grotmol, T., Weiderpass, E., & Tretli, S. (2006). Conditions in utero and cancer risk. *European Journal of Epidemiology, 21*, 561–570.

Hawkley, L. C., & Cacioppo, J. T. (2010). Loneliness matters: A theoretical and empirical review of consequences and mechanisms. *Annals of Behavioral Medicine, 40*, 218–227.

Hawkley, L. C., Masi, C. M., Berry, J. D., & Cacioppo, J. T. (2006). Loneliness is a unique predictor of age-related differences in systolic blood pressure. *Psychology and Aging, 21*, 152–164.

Hawkley, L. C., Thisted, R. A., & Cacioppo, J. T. (2009). Loneliness predicts reduced physical activity: Cross-sectional and longitudinal analyses. *Health Psychology, 28*, 354–363.

Holt-Lundstad, J., Birmingham, B. S., Brandon, Q., & Jones, B. S. (2008). Is there something unique about marriage? The relative impact of marital status, relationship quality, and network social support on ambulatory blood pressure and mental health. *Annals of Behavioral Medicine, 35*(2), 239–244.

Holt-Lundstad, J., Smith, T. B., & Layton, J. B. (2010). Social relationships and mortality risk: A meta-analytic review. *PLoS Medicine, 7*, 1–20.

Hughes, M. E., & Waite, L. J. (2009). Marital biography and health at mid-life. *Journal of Health and Social Behavior, 50*, 344–358.

Krueger, P. M., Saint Onge, J. M., & Chang, V. W. (2011). Race/ethnic differences in adult mortality: The role of perceived stress and health behaviors. *Social Science and Medicine, 73*, 1312–1322.

Lindau, S. T., Laumann, E. O., Levinson, W., & Waite, L. J. (2003). Synthesis of scientific disciplines in pursuit of health: The Interactive Biopsychosocial Model. *Perspectives in Biology and Medicine, 46*, S74–S86.

Liu, H., & Waite, L. (2014). Bad marriage, broken heart? Age and gender differences in the link between marital quality and cardiovascular risks among older adults. *Journal of Health and Social Behavior, 55*, 403–423.

Luo, Y., Hawkley, L. C., Waite, L. J., & Cacioppo, J. T. (2012). Loneliness, health, and mortality in old age: A national longitudinal study. *Social Science and Medicine, 74*, 907–914.

Madrigano, J., Baccarelli, A., Wright, R. O., Suh, H., Sparrow, D., Vokonas, P. S., & Schwartz, J. (2010). Air pollution, obesity, genes, and cellular adhesion molecules. *Occupational and Environmental Medicine, 67*, 312–317.

Mayer, K. U. (2009). New directions in life course research. *Annual Review of Sociology, 35*, 413–433.

McFarland, M. J., Hayward, M. D., & Brown, D. (2013). I've got you under my skin: Marital biography and biological risk. *Journal of Marriage and Family, 75*, 363–380.

Miech, R., Pampel, F., Kim, J., & Rogers, R. G. (2011). The enduring association between education and mortality: The role of widening and narrowing disparities. *American Sociological Review, 76*, 913–934.

Rote, S., Hill, T. D., & Ellison, C. G. (2013). Religious attendance and loneliness in later life. *The Gerontologist, 53*, 39–50.

Shanahan, M. J. (2013). Social genomics and the life course: Opportunities and challenges for multilevel population research. In L. J. Waite & T. J. Plewes (Eds.), *New directions in the sociology of aging* (pp. 255–276). Washington, DC: National Academies Press.

Shankar, A., Hamer, M., McMunn, A., & Steptoe, A. (2013). Social isolation and loneliness: Relationships with cognitive function during 4 years of follow-up in the English Longitudinal Study of Ageing. *Psychosomatic Medicine, 75*, 161–170.

Shiovitz-Ezra, S., & Litwin, H. (2012). Social network type and health-related behaviors: Evidence from an American national survey. *Social Science and Medicine, 75*, 901–904.

Smith, J. P. (2009). The impact of childhood health on adult labor market outcomes. *Review of Economics and Statistics, 91*, 478–489.

Smith, J. P., & Smith, G. C. (2010). Long-term economic costs of psychological problems during childhood. *Social Science and Medicine, 71*, 110–115.

Stafford, M., McMunn, A., Zaninotto, P., & Nazroo, J. (2011). Positive and negative exchanges in social relationships as predictors of depression: Evidence from the English Longitudinal Study of Aging. *Journal of Aging and Health, 23*, 607–628.

Steptoe, A., Deaton, A., & Stone, A. A. (2015). Subjective wellbeing, health, and ageing. *The Lancet, 385*, 640–648.

Suh, H. H., Zanobetti, A., Schwartz, J., & Coull, B. A. (2011). Chemical properties of air pollutants and cause-specific hospital admissions among the elderly in Atlanta, Georgia. *Environmental Health Perspectives, 119*, 1421–1428.

Taylor, S. E. (2011). Social support: A review. In H. S. Friedman (Ed.), *The Oxford handbook of health psychology* (pp. 189–214). New York, NY: Oxford University Press.

Taylor, S. E., Klein, L. C., Lewis, B. P., Gruenewald, T. L., Gurung Regan, A. R., & Updegraff, J. A. (2000). Biobehavioral responses to stress in females: Tend-and-befriend, not fight-or-flight. *Psychological Review, 107*, 411–429.

Thoits, P. A. (2010). Stress and health: Major findings and policy implications. *Journal of Health and Social Behavior, 51*, S41–S53.

Thoits, P. A. (2011). Mechanisms linking social ties and support to physical and mental health. *Journal of Health and Social Behavior, 52*, 145–161.

Thomas, P. A. (2011). Trajectories of social engagement and limitations in late life. *Journal of Health and Social Behavior, 52*, 430–443.

Umberson, D., & Montez, J. K. (2010). Social relationships and health: A flashpoint for health policy. *Journal of Health and Social Behavior, 51*, S54–S66.

Umberson, D., Williams, K., Powers, D. A., Liu, H., & Needham, B. (2006). You make me sick: Marital quality and health over the life course. *Journal of Health and Social Behavior, 47*, 1–16.

Waite, L. J., & Gallagher, M. (2001). *The case for marriage: Why married people are happier, healthier, and better off financially.* New York, NY: Broadway Books.

Warner, D. F., & Adams, S. A. (2012). Widening the social context of disablement among married older adults: Considering the role of nonmarital relationships for loneliness. *Social Science Research, 41*, 1529–1545.

Warner, D. F., & Kelley-Moore, J. (2012). The social context of disablement among older adults: Does marital quality matter for loneliness? *Journal of Health and Social Behavior, 53*, 50–66.

Wilker, E. H., Baccarelli, A., Suh, H., Vokonas, P., Wright, R. O., & Schwartz, J. (2010). Black carbon exposures, blood pressure, and interactions with single nucleotide polymorphisms in microRNA processing genes. *Environmental Health Perspectives, 118*, 943–948.

Yang, Y. C., McClintock, M. K., Kozloski, M., & Li, T. (2013). Social isolation and adult mortality: The role of chronic inflammation and sex differences. *Journal of Health and Social Behavior, 54*, 183–203.

York Cornwell, E., & Waite, L. J. (2009). Social disconnectedness, perceived isolation, and health among older adults. *Journal of Health and Social Behavior, 50*, 31–48.

York Cornwell, E., & Waite, L. J. (2012). Social network resources and management of hypertension. *Journal of Health and Social Behavior, 53*(2), 215–231.

CHAPTER 19

Long, Broad, and Deep: Theoretical Approaches in Aging and Inequality

Angela M. O'Rand

The development of theories of inequality over the life courses of aging cohorts is arguably the core theoretical enterprise driving most of aging research over the last two decades. The origins and interdependent trajectories of inequality with age across life domains including race/ethnicity, gender, family, education, socioeconomic status (SES), and health are the predominant foci represented in research journals, books, and book chapters. Life chances from birth to death and life styles related to social perceptions and behaviors and their life-course consequences pervade this literature. The problematic long-term cumulative dynamics among race/ethnicity, class of origin (especially poverty in childhood), education, and health with age have assumed a central position in this research and unleashed a robust conversation about age and inequality, and particularly about how inequality "gets under the skin"—putatively to accelerate the aging process, to constrain the quality of life, and to yield wide variations in (healthy) life expectancy.

The focus on health has been generated, in part, by the integration of biological with social data that has introduced new, and potentially transformative, sources for theoretical elaboration. Genomic, physiological biomarker, and clinical and other administrative data collected as repeated observations over the life course are raising questions about gene–environment interactions and about *how* social exposures to stressors such as sustained poverty; to economic shocks such as unemployment; and to social losses such as late-life loneliness affect the aging process. Research on aging and inequality before the mid-1990s largely could not get under the skin per se, although it identified important surface manifestations of environmental conditions and subjective responses that influenced aging through processes of inequality. Also, longitudinal data were only beginning to capture mid- to late-life processes of aging that could link earlier to later life conditions and establish associations (and possible causal linkages) of inequality across the life course.

This chapter focuses specifically on this ascendant research area, although the field of aging and inequality is a broader one. In my judgment, this research area provides an opportunity to examine theory development and how it proceeds as a product of the interaction of preexisting theories, new data, and innovative methods for their analysis. Specifically, with the integration of maturing longitudinal panel data including social and biological measures over longer periods of the life course with time-sensitive methods of data analysis, aging is now observable as a continuous lifelong process, not as disjunctive and strictly age dependent. Institutional factors matter, even those that stratify populations by age, but the dynamics of inequality are continuous, cumulative, and pervasive leading to inequalities and disparities whose mechanisms are problematic and motivate new theories.

■ LONG, BROAD, AND DEEP: WHAT AGING IS AND *WHY* AND *HOW* IT OCCURS

The lifelong manifold process of aging implicates biological, psychological, social, and environmental factors that interact over time and across place in complex ways to direct and temporally organize the shapes and boundaries of lives (O'Rand, 2009). As such, aging is a long, broad, and deep process: *long*, because it occurs continuously across the life span (probably starting before birth); *broad*, because it continuously integrates diverse factors from across levels of observation (from the molecular to the social to the global); *deep*, because it is never fully and directly observable as an ongoing generative process. The patterns in which these interactions occur lead to variations in the pace of aging that are only partially evident in patterns of inequality that include widening socioeconomic stratification and the differential onsets and trajectories of health decline and mortality rates observable within aging cohorts. Some but not all major empirical generalizations that have emerged as components of the phenomena of aging include lifelong cumulative patterns of sequential contingency (or selection) in which earlier outcomes constrain later ones producing divergent trajectories of well-being; formative (and sometimes fateful) conditions, experiences, or traits in early life that have enduring direct or indirect constraints on later ones; mutually influential processes whose causal relationships are confounded (and confounding) over time (especially the relationship between education and health); deflections or redirections from earlier trajectories as a result of encounters with major life-course redirections stemming from exogenous or agentic interventions; underlying (latent) processes that may become manifest long after their origination—and that are often observed only through smaller surface manifestations of the deeper generative process.

These are inherently stratification processes that lead to the differentiation over time of cohort members whose fortunes in wealth and health diverge as a result of their successive encounters with stratified and stratifying institutions, including families, schools, health care systems, workplaces, neighborhoods, communities, and others, and with life-course risks that disrupt or derail lives, such as illness, job loss, family dissolution, and similar life events. The differentiation process is traceable to observations of the status attainment models of the 1970s that examined the intergenerational transmission of social status and the critical period of adolescence to young adulthood (the transition to adulthood differentiated principally by educational attainment) that had lifelong consequences for SES attainment. Status attainment models were refined by the 1980s—in part because of the maturing of longitudinal databases initiated in the 1960s (e.g., the Panel Study of Income Dynamics; panels of the National Longitudinal Studies; the Wisconsin Longitudinal Study)—to address the significance of variability in the timing and sequencing of life transitions for well-being and their importance in differentiating later outcomes. At the same time, new approaches to incorporate the structural effects of race, gender, class, and state and market institutions extended the prevailing stratification model. Some of these surveys and newer ones (the National Survey of Families & Households; the Health and Retirement Study) continue and have been enriched by linkages to administrative records (e.g., Medicare and Social Security), geographic information systems, and clinical and genomic data collections. The large-scale shift to add prospective data on health to these surveys and to initiate new studies with fine-grained attention to health indicators as focal concerns has been a primary thrust over the last three decades that has provided the empirical bases for studying the societal–health nexus in aging, which is now a core concern.

The continuousness of the manifold aging process raises many challenges for theory. These include the *causal priority* of elements of the process (e.g., genes, environments, and individual agency); *selection–causation* conundra among mutually influential co-occurring processes over time (e.g., SES ↔ health); the *complex multifactorial etiologies* of health conditions; seemingly *uninterpretable N-way interactions* among multiple factors; *comparability* of data sources across populations (e.g., sampling, harmonization of measures) to afford rigorous comparisons for theory building; and *unmeasured (unobserved) heterogeneity* that biases observations, among others. These challenges deserve separate treatment in their own right. For purposes of this general review, I define them briefly here:

- Causal priority: what comes first or before the others. Genes? Environments? Individual propensities and behaviors? Because theory is about causation or contingency, causal priority over time is a fundamental challenge. Genes, environments, and individual agency interact over time in ways that we are only beginning to understand. How do we disentangle cause and effect?
- Selection–causation: related to the earlier challenge is the question of whether prior factors related to social inequality and/or health select individuals into subsequent circumstances and with how much relative effect. How do subsequent conditions mediate or moderate these earlier conditions and why?
- Etiologies of disease refer to the complex (and usually deep) bases of diseases and health conditions and the extent to which they are vulnerable to variations in social environments: what are the relative influences of genes and environments on the onsets and progressions of illnesses?
- Uninterpretable n-way interactions refer to how much sense can be made of the interactions among many factors to produce specific outcomes.
- Data comparability confronts the problem of how, across different samples and data sources, the same "issue" or "problem" is treated equivalently or similarly enough to be a basis of comparison across studies. Is disease or social inequality measured equivalently across studies to contribute to an empirical generalization?
- Unmeasured heterogeneity is the incapacity to have all the data necessary in a single study to capture all the information we probably need to specify the process of interest. What is "out of sight" in the study and how can we ameliorate this with linked data from other sources or with statistical controls that manage the errors in our observations?

Observation of these general empirical components of aging necessarily requires repeated measurements drawn over extended periods and, ideally, from several sources that may include social surveys, administrative records from institutional sources, clinical data collections (biomarker and genomic data), geographic information systems, experiments, and on-the-ground direct observational methods. They also require analytical methods that capture the temporal features of aging (i.e., timing, sequence, duration, and trajectories of continuity, accentuation, and deflection) and that estimate potential causal pathways along the life course.

The normal science of aging—and generally of most sociologically interesting phenomena—pursues explanations by following what Goldthorpe (2001) refers to as "causation as robust dependence." This is a correlational approach to examine multiple covariate effects on an outcome of interest using regression-based techniques. In this approach, efforts to move from association to causation (i.e., that X is a genuine cause of Y) are guided by statistical criteria that the dependence of Y on X is robust, or cannot be eliminated through other variables (some unobserved) or sampling biases (e.g., nonrepresentative samples or selective attrition) by detecting and eliminating spurious causal significance. Causation is defined by the predictive power or explained variation in Y. However, aging researchers are calling for more than statistical predictability. Predictability must be guided by theory, some examples of which follow. And, predictability is not equivalent to causality, which requires what Goldthorpe (2001) refers to as "consequential manipulation" (CM), which will be considered at the end of this section.

Three theoretical projects focused on life-course (aging) inequality are reviewed subsequently. They are successively more encompassing, beginning with the education–health project followed by the fundamental causes of health inequalities theory and ending with cumulative inequality (CI) theory. The large share of publications associated with these theories overwhelmingly follow the causation by robust dependence heuristics. However, some research departs from this in ways that will be briefly summarized.

Education, Health, and Aging

The robust dependence of health on educational attainment is now well established across hundreds of publications over 20 years (e.g., Mirowsky & Ross, 2003; Ross & Mirowsky, 2010; Ross & Wu, 1995). Educational attainment decreases age-specific rates of morbidity, disability, and mortality and increases aspects of mental and physical health functioning and self-assessed health in adult populations, after controlling for numerous earlier and subsequent life-course conditions. The theoretical challenge has been to explain the robust correlation that persists across controls for mediating and moderating factors by situating it in a more generalized theory of action. Human capital theory has been adopted to serve this purpose by leading medical sociologists in this area. The argument is that educational attainment represents accumulated knowledge, skills, values, and behaviors learned at school (Mirowsky & Ross, 2005). These specifically include literacy, numeracy, problem solving, analytical flexibility, observation, and experimentation, among other forms of cognitive capital. Importantly, these forms of (cognitive) capital are purported to spill over into health-related behavior by promoting health literacy to benefit of health over the life course; hence, the mechanism of social action and rational choice within the boundaries of knowledge.

In this research program, the human capital framework has spawned spin-off hypotheses that elaborate the general theory. For example, the gender gap in physical impairment that places women at greater risk for chronic disabilities provides an opportunity to examine gender differences in health and the role of education in their emergence. Because women are in disadvantaged positions relative to men—with fewer opportunities for economic gain, workplace authority, and wider community social status—education assumes a distinctive importance for women in the absence of alternative resources. Lower levels of education will result in higher levels of impairment among women than among men. Mirowsky and Ross (2010) label this hypothesis the "resource substitution" hypothesis; they label the competing hypothesis, the "reinforcement of advantage" hypothesis. Their results support a resource substitution process in which education matters more on average for women's physical impairment than men's, although the gender gap disappears among men and women with college degrees.

Noncognitive factors receive less attention in this work so far, although these variables are receiving more and more attention in the developmental psychology and economics literatures. In developmental psychology, a long tradition of interest has focused on the long-term effects of persistent personality traits and levels of social competence and effectiveness such as self-control, ambition, and self-efficacy, and pointed to a broad domain of noncognitive factors that probably operate jointly with cognitive skills acquired in-school and out-of-school. Researchers with explicit aging interests have linked such noncognitive factors as self-control (Moffitt et al., 2011) and conscientiousness (Israel et al., 2014) in childhood to later outcomes in health, wealth, and well-being in adulthood. The persistent and self-amplifying features of such personality traits into adulthood are expressed in the conduct of adult roles and health behaviors and hence result in socioeconomic and health inequalities.

Economists, who are most closely identified with cognitively centered human capital approaches, have turned to noncognitive factors not only to strengthen the prediction of educational achievement and later related outcomes such as adult earnings, but to establish causal effects of these factors (a point to which I return later in this chapter). Heckman and Kautz (2012) link cognitive and personality factors to predict educational attainment. Cognition is measured as fluid and crystallized intelligence; the former is measured as novel problem solving that implicates both inductive and deductive reasoning, and the latter is the measured use of general knowledge and accumulated skills developed over a lifetime. Noncognitive factors are composed of the "big five" personality traits (and related factors) identified by personality theorists: 1—conscientiousness (the tendency to be organized, responsible, and hardworking); 2—openness to experience (the tendency to be open to new aesthetic, cultural, or intellectual experiences); 3—extraversion (sociability and the orientation toward the outer world of people and things rather than the inner world of subjective experience); 4—agreeableness (the tendency to be cooperative and unselfish); and 5—emotional stability/neuroticism (consistency in emotional reactions, frequency of mood changes, proneness to psychological distress).

The researchers draw data from longitudinal surveys and review experimental studies to establish that personality is a *cause* of achievement after controlling for cognitive abilities. One study compares high school dropouts, general equivalency diploma (GED) completers, and high school graduates. The key finding is that dropouts and GED completers are distinguishable from high school graduates as a result of personality differences more than cognitive differences. They also review random assignment experiments in preschool and kindergarten (e.g., the Perry Preschool Study and Project STAR) settings in which children were assigned to treatment groups purposely to change personality traits or to provide classroom settings (smaller class sizes) in which more attention could be directed to individual student behaviors. Treatment effects were demonstrated to be causal of later higher performance levels.

In short, educational achievement and the cognitive and noncognitive factors that propel it at the individual level appear to constitute a pervasive component of the aging process and life-course inequality. Adult health and wealth inequalities appear to be robustly dependent on education. Ross and Mirowsky (2010) refer to it as a "fundamental cause" of aging, following the theory that Link and Phelan (1995) initially proposed regarding the robust dependence of health on the pervasiveness and underlying generative force of a broader conception of socioeconomic inequality than educational attainment. The latter is a more ambitious theoretical effort to which I turn now.

Fundamental Causes of Health Inequalities

The persistent associations between SES, however measured, and mortality, multiple diseases and overall health, respectively, motivated Link and Phelan (1995) to propose the theory of fundamental causes of health inequalities. That argued that SES was not a simple gradient easily represented by stratified access to a fixed set of resources (knowledge, money, power, prestige, social ties, etc.) that serve as mechanisms through which it operated. Rather, SES was a "basic cause" (following Lieberson, 1985) of health and mortality because of complex and dynamic shifts in the mechanisms linking the two via multiple pathways and their "flexible use" to protect against or to ameliorate poor health. This persistent association could not be explained away by conventional methods associated with robust dependence in which surface indicators of SES could be mediated or moderated. The underlying and pervasive effects of SES were reproduced over time because the mechanisms of their reproduction themselves varied and changed.

A test of the falsifiability of the basic cause is the situation in which causes and cures of fatal diseases are not known (Phelan, Link, & Tehranifar, 2010). Under these circumstances, the resources that can be deployed are not clear, hence SES should then differentiate outcomes much more weakly. Flexible resources can be deployed to highly preventable diseases (e.g., lung cancer), but less so to unpreventable diseases (e.g., brain cancer). As new knowledge is gained regarding formerly unpreventable diseases, new mechanisms for their prevention or amelioration become new resources that advantage those with access to them.

The theory is built on a narrative of social action similar to rational choice, but more specifically tied to identifying specific changing pathways to health outcomes. How does health come about as a function of SES? It comes about with the flexible deployment of unequally distributed resources that are specifically and temporally suited to diverse health outcomes. This implicates both individual and contextual resources, but deals more explicitly with individuals. Resources "must come from somewhere" (Phelan et al., 2010, p. S30). Meso- and macro-contexts include families, neighborhoods, workplaces, community networks, but any single indicator or set of indicators of context(s) can only partially represent complex and pervasive SES.

Luftey and Freese (2005) apply fundamental cause theory in an ethnographic study of two routine endocrinology clinics for diabetics to capture the dynamics of resource use and context. The two clinics treated patients from different socioeconomic backgrounds (Park Clinic—upper middle class; County Clinic—lower middle and lower class); they also differed organizationally in the access to treatment by physicians versus residents, continuity of care by the same practitioner, and resources for in-clinic diabetes education (all privileging Park Clinic patients). The analytical framework links these three in-clinic characteristics with the resources patients bring with them from the outside (financial limitations; occupational constraints; and social support networks) and patients' dispositions in two areas: apparent motivations (the cost of compliance and the magnitude of lifestyle adjustment) and apparent cognitive abilities (interactional differences and capacities as practical achievements).

They observed the multiple ways that SES operates in these contexts through "regimen design" and "enacted regimen" that emerge in the interactions between patients and clinics. The control of long-term glucose level through patient self-management is the objective of diabetes treatment. Yet, this regimen emerges quite differently on a day-to-day basis as organizational resources and practices interact with patient resources and dispositions. The investigators discerned mutual attribution processes in which patients and practitioners appeared to make judgments regarding each other's capacities, intentions, and behaviors. These interactions produced biases among practitioners and resistance among patients to regiment design, especially in the Counter Clinic context. The ultimate consequence was an SES-driven pattern of lower self-management success among poorer patients at both clinics.

The rich complexity portrayed in this project makes a strong case for the fundamental cause argument that SES is so pervasive across levels that its manifestations, taken singly, weakly represent and may obscure its action. SES is a generative process. Following Goldthorpe (2001), SES as a phenomenon exists at a deeper observational level than immediate data afford; it generates the surface causal effects observed that, by themselves, underrepresent the deeper phenomenon.

Cumulative Advantage/Disadvantage and Inequality

Life-course theory throughout the 1970s and early 1980s was driven by an emphasis on inter-cohort variation and within-cohort homogeneity until within-cohort heterogeneity and variation across the life span became more and more evident, especially as longitudinal databases initiated in the 1960s and maturing over two decades were revealing more heterogeneity and inequality within cohorts with age. The aging research community had conceptualized cohort aging as a process of convergence, as shared experiences of retirement and health decline leveled the playing field at older ages. By the 1990s, the appearance of convergence was in part attributable to processes of selective mortality. As average life expectancy has continued to increase and the mechanisms for its continuation are now better understood, cohorts can be differentiated by schedules of healthy life expectancy and degrees of chronic frailty.

Dannefer (1987) aptly characterized the actual phenomenon as "divergent," following Robert K. Merton's "Matthew Effect" as a cumulative process of interindividual divergence and increased inequality that resulted from the successive encounters of individual lives with stratifying institutional processes that set them on, and constrained them within, different life paths. The mechanisms driving the divergence were cumulative advantage and cumulative disadvantage (CAD) as path-dependent trajectories in which earlier status and achievement have persistent influence on later status and achievement, not just as a result of individual motivation and capacity, but as the outcome of institutional processes bearing on individual lives. Hence, for example, educational institutions select and sort students in ways that have lifelong consequences on average within a cohort that lead to inequalities in later years based on factors associated with the educational system, which may go unobserved. The experimental studies reported by Heckman and Kautz (2012), summarized earlier, reveal that school contexts (e.g., class sizes, curricula directed at learning skills) can differentiate students above and beyond their individual motivations and capacities.

The CAD model has fit the data well. The simple, falsifiable, generative features of CAD have motivated considerable research. The simplicity is reflected in its parsimonious prediction that the impact of prior events increases over time in stratified systems.

Falsifiability stems from clear prediction of growing inequality with time that increasingly advantages early higher status, which invites competing hypotheses of reversals, crossovers, or compensatory mechanisms. The theory has been formalized to accommodate rigorous analyses of competing hypotheses (DiPrete & Eirich, 2006). Generativity refers to CAD's capacity to motivate new questions that extend or revise its boundaries.

Theory building based on CAD is now focused on deciphering the tempo and critical phases of divergence and on competing hypotheses. Educational achievement and its timing are a robust determinant of later inequality, as we have reviewed. It is identified in the educational–health literature as causal and as a critical phase of the life course with enduring effects. However, childhood conditions are significant precursors to schooling experiences and achievements and apparently exert persistent direct effects, in their own right, on educational attainment and some later life outcomes, particularly in health. The literature on adverse socioeconomic and health conditions in childhood and their enduring effects is vast and cannot be reviewed here. Both prospective and retrospective data have been examined—and although they face specific limitations across data sets, including shorter views of the life course in prospective studies starting in childhood or infancy and errors in memory in retrospective designs—they arrive generally at similar results regarding the robust dependence of some adult health conditions and risks for poverty on adversity in childhood.

The (probably multiple) mechanisms by which these occur are not firmly established. Some are rooted in bio(neuro)developmental factors influenced by in utero and postnatal environments in the family and broader community (e.g., Barker, 1992; Gruevewald, 2013) and some in diverse psychosocial and behavioral responses to these stress-inducing conditions that condition later reactions to stress (e.g., Moffitt et al., 2011). The questions about the tempo of aging now focus on whether the effects of early life conditions reflect "sensitive" or "critical" periods that imprint the biopsychosocial developmental process in ways that cannot be mediated or reversed with later, more enriching conditions, *or* whether these early life conditions establish an initial disadvantage when facing "chains of risk" that sets a path-dependent course of disadvantage, which may even amplify or accentuate the effects of early conditions with time and under new challenging conditions (e.g., dramatic health decline; unemployment; family dissolution). The patterns of cumulative disadvantage and cumulative advantage are also not symmetrical; the former are probably more path dependent and the latter more stochastic (O'Rand, 2009). By this is meant that initial disadvantage has a significant gravitational force on later life outcomes, while initial advantage does not guarantee the successful navigation through later life shocks and turbulence, but affords the resources to confront them although less predictably.

Studies with competing hypotheses are adding to the development of the CAD model in several ways. An exemplary study in the theory-building process uses the Midlife in the United States (MIDUS) study to identify psychosocial compensatory mechanisms that offset the long-term effects of early adversity (Schafer, Ferraro, & Mustillo, 2011). The question is whether "human agency" in the form of optimism or "buoyant expectations" can overcome early adversity's effects on overall reflections by individuals on their past and future lives. Their results suggest that the experiences of the past constrain expectations for the future, but that human agency is fruitful ground for continuing to test CAD propositions.

Ferraro has moved further on this agenda with a recent effort at theory building in aging by linking the CAD model to other processes associated with aging, including human agency. He is also linking CAD to the stress process model widely studied in medical sociology. Ferraro proposes an axiomatic theory of CI to explain how inequality gets under the skin (Ferraro & Shippee, 2009). The linkage of the stress process to the CAD stratification process directly situates health as formative in aging. The axiomatic framework draws from the extensive literature associated with CAD and the empirical generalizations that have emerged from it and links it to the stress model in medical sociology. The five axioms seek to establish the macro-, meso-, and micro-level foundations for 19 macro-, meso-, and micro-level propositions (Ferraro & Shippee, 2009, p. 337), which are probably not intended to be exhaustive but illustrative. The complement of axioms and propositions is found on an even deeper level model of the process: social change can flow in two directions. The micro–meso–macro dynamics of aging encompass demographic processes associated with the aggregation of the day-to-day actions of individuals facing the macro- and meso-level conditions of their lives—aggregate individual actions stemming from human agency may produce macro-level changes.

CI is a program to integrate the long, broad, and deep components of the aging process at all levels of observation. It draws on empirical generalizations from the CAD framework that has developed for two decades to establish fundamental axioms of aging inequality. It then generates propositions from this axiomatic framework with relevance to aging beyond health or medical sociology concerns. It is not possible here to provide specific comments on the propositional derivations of the axioms, especially as this theory is probably still in development as this chapter is being composed. However, a brief look at the axioms reflects the wide reach of the CI theory. The five axioms are listed as follows:

- Axiom I. Social systems generate inequality, which is manifested over the life course through demographic and developmental processes.
- Axiom II. Disadvantage increases exposure to risk, but advantage increases exposure to opportunity.
- Axiom III. Life-course trajectories are shaped by the accumulation of risk, available resources, and human agency.
- Axiom IV. The perception of life trajectories influences subsequent trajectories.
- Axiom V. CI may lead to premature mortality; therefore, nonrandom selection may give the appearance of decreasing inequality in later life.

These axioms apply to aging inequality across the spectrum of the human life course, and are relevant not just to the role of health per se. Family development (including intergenerational processes), work career trajectories and labor market processes, patterns of identity development, and patterns of attitude formation and change, among other sociologically interesting processes, can be investigated using this axiomatic foundation. However, it is nevertheless clear that questions of health over the entire life course have colonized aging theory, especially those associated with inequality.

■ INTEGRATING BIOLOGICAL AND SOCIAL FACTORS IN AGING

Perhaps the most rapidly developing area of aging research is the linkage between the biological and the social. The patterns of inequality in health and mortality traceable to the "health career" and its SES origins have contributed to the emergent importance of monitoring the "pace of aging," or the rate at which underlying and manifest health conditions shorten the length of life, diminish healthy life expectancies, and constrain the quality of life with age. Indeed, it can be argued that aging research has changed most dramatically in the direction of health because of the growing sophistication of biological data collection and analysis.

Arguably, the decades of research on stress and health, which focused increasingly on how deleterious social experiences like those associated with lower social status "get under the skin" (Ferraro & Shippee, 2009), ushered in this line of thinking. The stress process tradition became interested in the role of chronic or acute social stress on "allostatic load" (or multiple dysregulation measured by steroid hormones) or "wear and tear" and the effect of allostatic load, in turn, on health and aging. The idea took fire by the 2000s when more biomarker data were being collected. Although reviews of the literature in this area suggest that the biosocial link is still not well established (Juster, McEwen, & Lupien, 2010; Weinstein, Glei, & Goldman, 2013), the now vast collection of these data promises continued research with perhaps improved methods of analysis to establish causal relationships.

More recently, biosocial research is getting "deeper under the skin" with social genomics as the newest area. This program investigates how social experience regulates gene activity by studying gene transcription or the rate at which DNA is transcribed into messenger RNA, which in turn produces proteins that are integral to biological processes likes those associated with stress (Gruevewald, 2013) and inflammatory responses (Finch & Crimmins, 2004; see Shanahan, 2013 for a good summary of this area). Genetic transcription is an adaptation to changing circumstances in the organism. The theory proposes that levels of transcription differentially accumulate from early childhood throughout the life course leading to adult health disparities and differential rates of mortality. Early adversity can establish a durable program of the stress response system creating a "defensive phenotype."

The genetics of health and aging is not a new interest. However, the new social genomics has moved beyond twin-sibling studies and target genes to genome-wide studies (GWAS) of DNA sequence variations (mutations) called "single-nucleotide polymorphisms" (SNPs) that can provide genetic fingerprints to detect disease susceptibility (e.g., the apolipoprotein E gene [APOE] mutation is associated with a higher risk for Alzheimer's disease) and behavioral vulnerabilities. The collection, data storage, and computational demands of GWAS research are considerable. The logistics of GWAS data collection in national databases are daunting. These are accentuated by the requirements of longitudinal designs, especially those motivated by life-course theories like CAD and the childhood adversity hypothesis of long-term phenotypic vulnerability. Shanahan (2013) outlines challenges of these data for theory building on this question, especially in adjudicating between the "sensitive period" and the "critical period" models of the childhood origins of adult health outcomes. The "sensitive period" hypothesis argues that biological systems are subject to change at specific points of development, while the "critical period" hypothesis denotes the only time biological systems are subject to change. Clearly, fine-grained longitudinal study of childhood with multiple follow-ups into adulthood are a major challenge.

Traversing the biological–social divide is the most ambitious agenda for aging research no matter what the hypothesis of interest is. Longitudinal design, accurate repeated measurements of relevant social and biological variables, and the estimation of cause-and-effect relationships are three major tasks, each requiring interdisciplinary collaboration and considerable resources over time. The interaction of research and theory over two decades, however, has brought aging inequality research to this point.

■ CAUSE AND EFFECT IN AGING RESEARCH

Goldthorpe (2001) has identified a third approach to causation in the social sciences besides robust dependence and generative processes. He refers to it as "CM," identified primarily with experimental and quasi-experimental designs, but also with econometric modeling that is designed to unmask spurious correlations and identify true causal effects, using techniques that are not yet widespread in the robust dependence literature. Often "causal" variables in aging research, like education, are themselves endogenous (i.e., dependent on prior variables that might alter the observed effects of education on an outcome such as health if they are included) or endogenously interdependent (education ↔ health or SES ↔ health). Also, sample selection decisions can bias the estimates in an analysis, as in the case of using samples restricted to older populations (say above age 65 years) that select out younger individuals who have not survived to the age of 65 years, or select only workers to study wage differences and thus miss nonworkers whose characteristics may be relevant to wage differences but are missed in the analysis. Finally, advocates of CM propose that, besides the major problems of endogeneity and sample selectivity in nonexperimental analyses, the real issue is the definition of causation itself. In this vein, causes should be treated as "treatments" that must be manipulated. CM in this sense requires a more counterfactual approach: What would happen to Y if exposed to treatment X or if not exposed to treatment X? This approach to causation requires random assignment to treatment or control groups in a manner not affected by the assignment process and with the assumption that all the theoretically relevant variables are included in the analysis.

CM is considered by some social scientists as the gold standard of causation (e.g., Angrist & Pischke, 2009). Econometric approaches to deal with these problems previously mentioned have spread to sociology and demography with the application of such techniques as sample selection models and instrumental variables (exogenous variables with unique effects on endogenous variables) to the kinds of survey databases that predominate in aging research (see Bollen, 2012; Elwert & Winship, 2014). These applications have introduced new rigor to statistical analyses that seek to establish causal relationships in the aging process, although they face challenges in secondary analyses that limit the identification of strong instrumental variables or lead to the overuse of instrumental variables leading to overidentification.

However, experimental designs per se have not spread as widely outside of medical and epidemiological research and economics of aging for practical and ethical reasons (Goldthorpe, 2001). The practical concerns about experimental designs are numerous and include such limitations as (a) their potential unrepresentedness, especially when clinical populations or volunteer samples are the source of data; (b) the artificial environments that can be associated with the design; and (c) the potentially unobserved effects of the "treatments" on other variables. Another nontrivial concern about the CM approach to causality is its explicit rejection of intrinsic variables or attributes as treatments because they cannot be manipulated: no causation without manipulation (Goldthorpe, 2001). This means that such variables as sex and race cannot be causes. Sociologists especially express concern about this requirement, although they are quick to admit that these variables always require careful theoretical treatment and serve usually as moderating factors between X and Y, whose effects are themselves embedded in social contexts that imbue them with meaning.

However, CM can reveal sociologically causes that can be treatments. Here I refer you back to the Heckman and Kautz (2012) article on soft skills summarized earlier. A key argument in this study was that school environments matter. In the education and health literature, which is dominant in aging inequality research, school characteristics and related curricular and environmental variables are usually absent as potentially causal variables. Theory building in this area will benefit going forward by creative approaches to linking individual characteristics with critical and formative social environments using diverse methods that might include experiments.

■ CAVEAT: GLOBAL RISKS AND AGING INEQUALITY

Missing from this review so far is a consideration of theory building at higher levels of analysis, such as globalization, nation–state, community institutions, and family. The macrosocial dynamics of aging inequality implicate demography, economy, and policy at a global level. I have addressed some of these issues at some length in another essay composed nearly simultaneously with this one (O'Rand & Bostic, 2015). This chapter points to the asynchronies among population aging, migration, global market processes (especially labor market restructuring and financialization), and the retrenchment of national welfare and labor policies that are contributing to growing inequalities between and within aging cohorts across countries. These asynchronies are unraveling what was putatively a more age-related and coherent life course formed by institutional arrangements that characterized the 20th century and they are introducing pervasive new uncertainties and social stresses across age groups and societies.

A compelling argument has been made that we have entered a post-national era (Beckfield, Olafsdottir, & Sosnaud, 2013) in which most institutional arrangements that bear critically on the life-course well-being of families and individuals no longer fall within the boundaries of the nation–state. And if they do fall within these boundaries, as in the case of aging and health care policies, they serve to exacerbate social inequalities rather than to ameliorate them as a consequence of global processes. The ascendance of global institutions, especially the restructuring and financialization of markets, has superceded national policies and introduced new risks to labor security, health, retirement, and the private accumulation of resources to protect against life-course risks. This occurs through stratified systems of education, income–maintenance, health care services, and more.

The relevance of these macro-trends to the meso- and micro-level agenda of the long–broad–deep program reviewed here is that the forces of inequality are pervasive. If inequality gets under the skin, then the prospect for healthy future populations is problematic.

■ CONCLUSION

Theories develop as they are applied to data and the methods used to collect and analyze them. Methods develop as well, both in response to theoretical demands and in their own right, and thereby serve to develop the theories further. Theory development of aging inequality has followed this pattern for over a half century. Aging research demands longitudinal data and statistical methods suited to these data to estimate causal relationships over time. Data and methods, in turn, make demands of theory to specify causal relationships in ways that they can be falsified and can generate new questions.

Over the last two decades, theory building in aging inequality has focused on defining the role of health in the aging process. Arguably, health is now the core metric of aging; the diverse and complex patterns of disease, disability, and mortality with age have become the central problem for aging researchers, especially those concerned with social inequality and its pervasive and enduring effects. Major theoretical programs have emerged over two decades to address the seemingly inextricable relationships among health, aging, and social inequality across the life span. Four of these programs were considered here: The education–health research program focused on the explanation of the robust relationship between years of schooling and later health; the fundamental cause program that argues that SES is an underlying, pervasive phenomenon that propels the aging process via multiple mechanisms over time that cannot be fully captured by surface indicators alone; the CAD theory that elevated "time" itself through processes of accumulation that generate inequality; and CI that is attempting to expand the CAD project in a broader theory of aging inequality that incorporates health (using the stress process model) and human agency.

The most recent arrival to this active research area is biosocial research (including social genomics) that has enriched the measurement of health and is raising new questions about causal relationships that are forming a new agenda for the future. One example of this is the potential contribution of biosocial research to the understanding of the origins of health inequalities in early life and the subsequent trajectories of health (and the pace of aging) as individuals encounter successive but unequal social risks and resources over their lives. The challenges to this agenda are theoretical and practical, and causal relationships are not well established, but the promise of this research has made it perhaps the most rapidly developing subarea of aging inequality.

Causal relationships defined by theory are the objectives of aging science. And, as a developing research program, aging inequality has followed three different approaches to causation. Robust dependence is the predominant approach concerned with predictive power, the elimination of spurious relationships, and the partialling of focal relationships. The education–health, CAD, and CI literatures overwhelmingly apply diverse statistical methods that fall into the robust dependence category. The fundamental cause project employs robust dependence, but conceptualizes the basic underlying causal impact of SES as a multifaceted generative process that is dynamic over time and difficult to capture with a single variable or small set of repeated variables. This is a strong sociological argument that is moving beyond its epidemiological origins to more structural interests. Finally, CM is the experimental approach focused on counterfactual approaches to causality that make more rigorous demands on design than simple regression-based statistics relied upon in robust dependence. Although practical and ethical concerns constrain the application of experimental designs for some aging inequality research question, efforts in this direction will also contribute to theory development.

The causal processes that concern these theoretical programs do not address the broader macro-level processes that also drive the independent variable(s) of interest, inequality. The aging process and patterns of inequality are being shaped by global forces that affect day-to-day lives. These forces are introducing new risks for individuals and families that bear upon health across the life course through the reorganization or retrenchment of social institutions that once had greater equalizing effects for aging cohorts. The 21st century poses new risks in a post-industrial, post-national era of institution building driven by a market ideology and a financial logic.

REFERENCES

Angrist, J. D., & Pischke, J.-S. (2009). *Mostly harmless econometrics: An empiricist's companion.* Princeton, NJ: Princeton University.

Barker, D. J. P. (Ed.). (1992). *Fetal and infant origins of adult diseases.* London, UK: BMJ Publishing Group.

Beckfield, J., Olafsdottir, S., & Sosnaud, B. (2013). Healthcare systems in comparative perspective: Classification, convergence, inequalities and five missed turns. *Annual Review of Sociology, 39,* 127–146.

Bollen, K. A. (2012). Instrumental variables in sociology and the social sciences. *Annual Review of Sociology, 38,* 37–72.

Dannefer, D. (1987). Aging as intracohort differentiation: Accentuation, the Matthew effect and the life course. *Sociological Forum, 2,* 211–236.

DiPrete, T. H., & Eirich, G. (2006). Cumulative advantage as a mechanism for inequality: A review of theory and evidence. *Annual Review of Sociology, 32,* 271–297.

Elwert, F., & Winship, C. (2014). Endogenous selection bias: The problem of conditioning on a collider variable. *Annual Review of Sociology, 40,* 31–53.

Ferraro, K. F., & Shippee, T. P. (2009). Aging and cumulative inequality: How does inequality get under the skin? *The Gerontologist, 49,* 333–343.

Finch, C. E., & Crimmins, E. M. (2004). Inflammatory exposure and historical changes in human life-spans. *Science, 305,* 1736–1739.

Goldthorpe, J. H. (2001). Causation, statistics and sociology. *European Sociological Review, 17,* 1–20.

Gruevewald, T. L. (2013). Opportunities and challenges in the study of biosocial dynamics in healthy aging. In L. J. Waite & T. J. Plewes (Eds.), *National Research Council's new directions in the sociology of aging* (pp. 217–237). Washington, DC: National Academies Press.

Heckman, J. J., & Kautz, T. D. (2012). Hard evidence for soft skills. *Labour Economics, 19,* 451–464.

Israel, S., Caspi, A., Belsky, D. W., Harrington, H. L., Hogan, S., Houts, R., . . . Moffitt, T. E. (2014). Credit scores, cardiovascular disease and human capital. *Proceedings of the National Academy of Sciences, 111,* 17087–17092.

Juster, R. P., McEwen, B. S., & Lupien, S. J. (2010). Allostatic load of biomarkers of chronic stress and impact of health and cognition. *Neuroscience and Biobehavioral Reviews, 35,* 2–16.

Lieberson, S. (1985). *Making it count.* Berkeley: University of California Press.

Link, B. G., & Phelan, J. C. (1995). Social conditions as fundamental causes of disease. *Journal of Health and Social Behavior, 35*(Extra Issue), 80–94.

Luftey, K., & Freese, J. (2005). Toward some fundamentals of fundamental causality: Socioeconomic status and health in the routine clinic visit for diabetes. *American Journal of Sociology, 110,* 1326–1372.

Mirowsky, J., & Ross, C. E. (2003). *Education, social status and health.* New York, NY: Aldine.

Mirowsky, J., & Ross, C. E. (2005). Education, learned effectiveness, and health. *London Review of Education, 3,* 205–220.

Mirowsky, J., & Ross, C. E. (2010). Gender and the health benefits of education. *The Sociological Quarterly, 51,* 1–19.

Moffitt, T. E., Arseneault, L., Belsky, D. W., Dickson, N., Hancox, R. J., Harrington, H. L.,…Caspi, A. (2011). A gradient of childhood self-control predicts health, wealth and public safety. *Proceedings of the National Academy of Sciences, 108,* 2693–2698.

O'Rand, A. M. (2009). Cumulative processes in the life course. In J. Z. Giele & G. H. Elder, Jr. (Eds.), *The craft of life course research* (pp. 121–140). New York, NY: Guilford Press.

O'Rand, A. M., & Bostic, A. (2015). Lags and leaps: The dynamics of demography, economy and policy and their implications for life course research. In M. Shanahan, J. Mortimer, & M. Johnson (Eds.), *Handbook of the life course* (2nd ed.). New York, NY: Springer Publishing Company.

Phelan, J. C., Link, B. G., & Tehranifar, P. (2010). Social conditions as fundamental causes of health inequalities: Theory, evidence and policy implications. *Journal of Health and Social Behavior, 51,* S28–S40.

Ross, C. E., & Mirowsky, J. (2010). Gender and the health benefits of education. *The Sociological Quarterly, 51,* 1–19.

Ross, C. E., & Wu, C. (1995). The links between education and health. *American Sociological Review, 60,* 719–745.

Schafer, M. H., Ferraro, K. F., & Mustillo, S. A. (2011). Children of misfortune: Early adversity and cumulative inequality in perceived life trajectories. *American Journal of Sociology, 116,* 1053–1091.

Shanahan, M. (2013). Social genomics and the life course: Opportunities and challenges for multilevel population research. In L. J. Waite & T. J. Plewes (Eds.), *National Research Council's new directions in the sociology of aging* (pp. 255–276). Washington, DC: National Academies Press.

Weinstein, M., Glei, D. A., & Goldman, N. (2013). The loyal opposition: A commentary on "opportunities and challenges in the study of biological dynamics in the study of healthy aging." In L. J. Waite & T. J. Plewes (Eds.), *National Research Council's new directions in the sociology of aging* (pp. 243–254). Washington, DC: National Academies Press.

CHAPTER 20

The Interpretive Perspective on Aging
Victor W. Marshall, Anne Martin-Matthews, and Julie Ann McMullin

The interpretive perspective is increasingly being adopted within behavioral and social sciences, and is making important contributions to understanding aging and the life course. "Interpretive perspective" is itself an umbrella term, as there are variations on it, often reflecting its framing within different disciplinary contexts, from sociology and psychology to social work, nursing, and education. In this chapter, we describe the interpretive perspective in all its richness and variability in guiding research and advancing understanding of a wide range of phenomena in aging and life-course research.

We first present a definition of the interpretive perspective and briefly consider both its roots within sociology and its recent wider disciplinary applications. We then contrast the interpretive perspective with other variants of social science theorizing, particularly normative perspectives on aging and life course—placing its development in historical context. We also address the contentious issue of causal explanation, as understood in diverse disciplinary contexts. Next, we present examples of the interpretive perspective as applied in research on selected aging and life-course issues. This includes micro-level research, addressing individuals and their interactions with others, as well as more macro-level research in which individuals engage with or find their lives shaped by more macro-level social structures. And, because scholars theorize phenomena that link macro and micro levels, we consider these applications of the interpretive perspective as well. We conclude by looking to the future and suggesting research questions and policies that would benefit by being considered through an interpretive lens.

■ WHAT IS THE INTERPRETIVE PERSPECTIVE?

The interpretive perspective, rooted primarily in symbolic interactionism within sociology, views individuals not as acting out internalized roles but as "role-taking" and "role-making." Social life in the interpretive view is improvisational, based on "interpretive process in which meanings evolve and change over the course of the interaction" (Wilson, 1970, p. 67). The fundamental tenet of the interpretive perspective is that meanings and definitions of situations are "constituted" (Schutz, 1967), and their "objectivity established through the interpretive processes of interaction rather than by reference to a body of culturally given common definitions" (Wilson, 1970, p. 78). Through the early work of Mead (1934), meaning and the notion of self emerged as key concepts in interpretive research. Indeed, Hendricks (1999) describes Mead's pronouncements on the self as "the lodestar" (p. 190), but notes that the application of interpretive perspectives to the study of aging came much later.

The interpretive perspective has a long and rich history. Weber (1978) defined sociology as "a science concerning itself with the *interpretive understanding* [emphasis added] of social action and thereby with a causal explanation of its course and consequences" (p. 4). Symbolic interactionism, phenomenology, and Weberian approaches in sociology, as well as developments in symbolic anthropology and cultural sociology, together constitute the foundations of the interpretive perspective (Marshall, 1996a, 1996b). The earliest research in social gerontology was quite "descriptive in character," and it was not until around 1961, with the work of Ernest W. Burgess, "that systematic statements of symbolic-interactionist theory [were] applied to the problems of social gerontology" (Rose, 1965, p. 359).

Although sociology is widely recognized as the disciplinary home of the interpretive perspective, there has, in recent decades, been considerable growth in its adoption by researchers in other disciplines. In psychology, for example, the rise and currency of research using qualitative methodology are associated with growing interest in what is called "interpretative phenomenological analysis," whose methodological essence "can be captured in an alliterative three part list: idiographic, inductive, and interrogative" (Smith, 2004, p. 41). This perspective first gained ground in research in health psychology, but also has been utilized in social, clinical, and counseling psychology—and in research on aging. Carol Ryff provided a historical overview of the interpretive perspective in psychology, and much of her work is grounded in the interpretive perspective, as exemplified in her study of the principles guiding the organization and interpretation of life history information (Singer, Ryff, Carr, & Magee, 1998), and in examining macro–micro linkages in the study of psychological well-being (Ryff & Marshall, 1999).

Similarly in social work, constructivism and interpretive paradigms have been central to epistemological debates within the field for some years (Rodwell, 1998). The interpretive perspective has served to advance knowledge and understanding of key issues central to social work research on aging and later life, particularly on topics related to care and caregiving (O'Connor, 2007), dementia and frailty (Grenier, 2012).

Research framed by the interpretive perspective has grown exponentially in health studies, and particularly in nursing, in recent years. As Thorne (2008) has noted, "nursing indelicately straddles the social and biomedical sciences to find its methodological direction" (p. 15). Anderson (2009) attributes nursing's utilization of interpretive approaches as reflecting "increasing attentiveness to the contextual dimension of health and illness" (p. 51) and related behaviors. Similar to other disciplinary applications, nursing's interest in the interpretive perspective lies in its genesis in phenomenological theory, focusing its gaze "on the routine features of everyday life and everyday rationality" (Anderson, 1981, p. 6).

It is important to note, however (and as Anderson, 1981, has acknowledged in relation to nursing research), that the way in which the interpretive perspective is used in other disciplines

> ...may not correspond exactly with how it is used in sociological research....Each addresses problems peculiar to its discipline...[but] there are some fundamental tenets of phenomenological theory which are crucial in interpretive work....[This] approach recognizes that each person brings to an encounter his or her own interpretation of the situation, by which events are evaluated and judged. (p. 8)

The ways in which the interpretive perspective is used across disciplines are further distinguished by disciplinary approaches to the link between theory and methods

(Sandelowski, 2008), and by their divergence on claims to causal explanation. The latter is addressed later in this chapter. For now, we have acknowledged the use of the interpretive perspective in research on aging in psychology, social work, and nursing. For the remainder of this chapter, however, the focus reflects our expertise as sociologists, emphasizing the interpretive perspective in sociological and social gerontological studies of aging and the life course.

Contrasting Interpretive and Normative Perspectives on Aging

We highlight here some prominent normative theoretical approaches in social gerontology, by way of providing a comparative context for our primary consideration of the interpretive perspective. The distinction between normative and interpretive perspectives is perhaps best captured in the different usage of the concept, "role." In the normative approach, widely held views of appropriate behavior for people of different ages are viewed as providing a normative context to guide behavior as people age. Those who employ the normative perspective view people as "internalizing" norms through socialization processes and then following societal norms (which are themselves considered to be widely shared). Research questions in gerontology deal with issues such as the causes and consequences of variability in the clarity of norms for different age-graded stations of life (childhood, adolescence, adulthood, old age, etc.), as well as the causes and consequences of variation in the adoption of norms or in historical changes in the age-based system of norms (see, e.g., Marshall, 1986; Neugarten, 1974; Neugarten & Hagestad, 1976; Rosow, 1974, 1976).

Normative approaches (as originally formulated by the sociologist Talcott Parsons) are exemplified in gerontology by such prominent macro-level theories as modernization theory (Cowgill, 1974; Palmore & Manton, 1974) and the important "age stratification perspective" advanced by Riley (1971, 1976), a student of Parsons. Riley postulated a sense of structure in which roles are components of social structure, rather than viewing actors as creators and navigators of social structure (Dannefer, 2012).

In social gerontology, the normative perspective is also exemplified by Rosow (1974; and see in particular his comprehensive theoretical discussion in 1976). Rosow (1976) argues that aging is associated with major status losses that "start with retirement, widowhood, failing health, and drastically reduced income, and then they spread to other areas as their social contacts and activities dwindle" (p. 466). Furthermore, "the loss of statuses leaves them with few normative expectations, with lives that are unstructured by social guidelines" (1976, pp. 465–466, citing Rosow, 1974, in which he also argues that society makes no attempts to socialize people for the status of old age). Rosow's work is illustrative of a theoretical perspective that links the micro and macro within the context of a normative approach. At the micro level, his important contributions illustrate how society provides inadequate socialization to old age (Rosow, 1974), while he links the macro- and micro-levels of analysis in his chapter on status and role change (Rosow, 1976).

During the 1960s, 1970s, and into the 1980s, the debate between *activity theory* and *disengagement theory* preoccupied many, if not most, social gerontologists. Both approaches were normative and attempted to bridge micro and macro phenomena. Talcott Parsons, the leading exemplar of normative sociology in his era, wrote the Foreword to the book-length presentation of the disengagement theory, Cumming and Henry's *Growing Old: The Process of Disengagement* (1961), which he dubbed as "probably the most serious attempt so far to put forward a general theoretical interpretation of the social and psychological nature of the aging process" (p. v). The "social system" is reified and in the theory, "aging is an inevitable mutual withdrawal or disengagement, resulting in decreased interaction between the aging person and others in the social system he belongs to" (Cumming & Henry, 1961, p. 14); "retirement is society's permission to men to disengage" (Cumming & Henry, 1961, p. 146), and disengagement leads to high life satisfaction.

The counterposition, advocated by Havighurst, Neugarten, and Tobin (1968) at Chicago, Maddox (1965) at Duke, and Rose (1965) at Minnesota, argued that as people age they continue to maintain high levels of life satisfaction by maintaining high levels of activity. Thus, the major theoretical debates of the era dealt with the single problem of understanding how interaction patterns do or do not make older people happy. Rose (1965) best described the differences between the normative and interpretive perspective as applied to gerontology, valorizing the interpretive (which he called "interactionist") perspective that he had seen as important in the early history of the field, but now threatened by the rise of normative theorizing:

> The interactionist perspective . . . seeks to interpret the social facts of aging in terms of the interactions among the aging themselves and between the aging and others in the society. Cultural values and meanings are the most important elements in these interactions, and these are never assumed to be universal or unchanging. The neat, integrated "systems" of the functionalists may appeal to the esthetic sense of readers, but it seems to us that the facts of social life—in this case the social relations of the aging—are too complicated and varied to be encompassed in any notion of equilibrium. Cultural history and human interactions, organizing concepts which have thus far dominated research in gerontology, are better guideposts. (p. 366)

The Contentious Issue of Causal Explanation

More recently, interpretive approaches to understanding social life have been defined as standing in contrast to positivist and normative perspectives that analyze and view the world through ostensibly nonbiased, causal explanations using variables that may or may not be meaningful to social actors (David, 2010). The words "causal explanation" can be applied to both interpretive and normative approaches, but the words seem to be used in contradictory ways. Interpretive understanding in Weber's definition *is* causal explanation, but David (2010) argues that interpretive understanding stands *in contrast* to causal explanation.

To understand this seeming contradiction, one must recognize that the meaning of causality in the discipline of sociology has changed over time. Since the 1960s, particularly in American sociology, causality has come to be associated primarily with quantitative methods. Indeed, in his article "The Causal Devolution," Abbott (1998) goes as far as to say that by the 1960s, "Causality was seen as a property of mathematical and statistical propositions rather than a property of reality" (p. 163). In this sense, causality is about variables predicting other variables and causing outcomes in a manner that is detached from meaning. This view of causality is certainly not one that Weber held, but is consistent with normative approaches to theorizing. For Weber, causal explanation was grounded in observable social action that could then be classified (ideal types) and interpreted within a particular historical context (Weber, 1978).

Today, many interpretive approaches tend to reject the language of causality (Gubrium & Holstein, 1999). Beyond its sociological applications, and within such fields as nursing, the interpretive perspective is seen as limited to the discovery of "associations, relationships and patterns within the phenomenon...described" (Thorne, 2008, p. 50). Indeed, it has been argued that: "Of necessity, interpretive description questions must stop short of formal explanatory pretensions (causation prediction, control, evaluation), for these become the domain of a much different form of enquiry" (Thorne, 2008, p. 51).

The interpretive perspective remains concerned with the meaning that social actors attribute to behavior and the various happenings of everyday life. Studies using the perspective often focus on identity, the social construction of reality, agency, social action, and culture. According to its proponents, it is through these concepts that a deeper and more nuanced understanding of social life takes shape. For some, however, the focus on meaning and a reluctance to discuss causality have also translated into resistance to the use of quantitative methods, to the point where some critics paint all quantitative research with the same positivist, normative brush. The assumption here is that words are better able to reflect the meaning that respondents attribute to social phenomena than are numbers.

We feel that this resistance is misplaced. Words can be a form of measurement (at the nominal level), just as can numbers at the ordinal, interval, or ratio level. The bottom line is that some research questions are better addressed using quantitative research methods. This includes such questions as: What is the mortality rate or the unemployment rate? What percentage of the population retires or anticipates retiring at given ages? Other research questions are better addressed using qualitative research. For example: How do people experience widowhood? How do they experience chronic illness or anticipate their own deaths? What interest groups attempt to influence pension policy, and why?

Still other research questions are best addressed through a mixed quantitative–qualitative approach. Regardless of the research question, explanations of the data can be either normative or interpretive (for more on this point, see McMullin & Cairney, 2004, and for an excellent example and theoretical affirmation of this point, see Clarke's, 2009 mixed-methods study of the experience of stroke). Regardless of approach, qualitative, quantitative, and mixed data can be used to make causal inferences (even though in fact, much gerontological research in both quantitative and qualitative mode, and from both normative and interpretive perspectives, is purely descriptive and makes no specific causal inferences).

■ INTERPRETIVE APPROACHES IN SOCIAL STUDIES OF AGING

A given theoretical perspective in gerontology can focus solely on macro level, structural phenomena (e.g., theories of the behavior of corporations in relation to government pension, health care, or workforce policies), on micro-level behavior and social interaction (e.g., theories to understand life–satisfaction in relation to changes in individual health or marital status; Marshall, 1986, 1995, 1996b), or on understanding of the links between macro and micro phenomena. In any of these categories, theorizing can be grounded in the interpretive or normative traditions, or some combination of both. In this section of the chapter, we consider the characteristics of the interpretive perspective as employed in research focused on micro and macro topics and topics that link the micro and macro levels. We demonstrate the great utility of interpretive approaches in addressing issues of aging and the life course.

Interpretive-Micro Research

Interpretive-micro perspectives place emphasis on individuals, the meaning they attribute to various aspects of social life, and to identity. In gerontology, the interpretive-micro perspective is exemplified in approaches that draw on symbolic interactionism and phenomenology, and that make extensive use of "qualitative data that are typically collected through in-depth interviews, focus groups, or participant observation, which are better able to capture the subjective dynamics of individual experience" (Clarke, 2009, p. 295). Many of these contributions may also be classified as linking micro and macro, because macro can be scaled from small or localized social structures (e.g., kinship, local community, workplace) to large and even global structures such as nation-states.

Breytspraak's (1984) monograph, *The Development of Self in Later Life*, provided an outstanding and comprehensive review of selfhood and aging from several psychological approaches (psychoanalytic, ego, humanistic, and experimental psychology), comparing them to approaches from role theory, symbolic interactionism, and phenomenology. She then focuses on the latter approaches to review the state of the art, at that time, in the social psychology of aging. Her position in the interpretive perspective is well illustrated in her discussion of Gubrium's (1973) important monograph, *The Myth of the Golden Years: A Socio-Environmental Theory of Aging*:

> We are interpretive creatures who are always seeking to find meaning in our situations, perhaps even changing the situations when they do not fit our sense of self. As Gubrium (1973) argues, we live in personal and social contexts that set varying kinds of limits on us, but we also work to reconstruct our everyday world and thereby alter the limits of environmental influence on ourselves. Certainly there are objective conditions that limit our ability to act...But the limits are probably much more flexible than we are sometimes willing to admit. (Breytspraak, 1984, p. 115)

Working from a phenomenological and ethnomethodological perspective, Gubrium (1975) emphasized that social reality is constructed through ongoing, negotiative, and definitional behavior. Not only do theorists construct versions of reality in this way, but people in their everyday lives are seen as doing so. In addition to his study cited previously, his work on aging in a nursing home, on the descriptive organization of Alzheimer's disease, and on family behavior exemplified this approach (Gubrium, 1986; Gubrium & Lynott, 1992).

Career and status passage perspectives were further developed in aging studies by symbolic interactionists such as Marshall (1975a, 1975b, 1978–1979, 1980) and Spence (1986). Marshall made contributions to gerontology using the interpretive perspective through numerous publications that recognized the proactive and often mutual, or social, activities that linked the individual to social structure, or focused on social adaptations at the community level to age-related phenomena such as impending death (Marshall, 1975a, 1975b, 1980). He argued that later life is a unique status passage because it is inevitable, irreversible, and does not lead to any subsequent status (Marshall, 1978–1979).

Interpretive-Macro Research

Interpretive is not just about micro approaches; there are interpretive understandings of social structures as socially constructed and navigated, changed, resisted, and so on. This is well illustrated at a general level by phenomenological sociologists such as

Schutz (1967) and Berger and Luckmann (1967), who emphasize that reality is socially constructed through the collaborative and meaning-sharing activities of people. There is more to social structure than this. Shared meanings become reified, allowing for the development of social structures, taking on a reality independent of their authors and thus setting constraints on individual or collective behavior. For example, an army is more than a collection of soldiers and their weapons; it is politically sanctioned for the exercise of power. A corporation is more than a collection of owners and employees; it is legally sanctioned to conduct its affairs, manage its workforce, and interact with other corporations, as well as the public. Two exemplars of macro interpretive approaches in gerontology are the political economy perspective and European life-course research.

THE POLITICAL ECONOMY OF AGING

Drawing on a rich, sociological history of conflict theory, political economy theorists take issue with normative and highly individualistic theories of aging and instead focus on structural aspects of inequality and, in particular, social class and age-structured social institutions (Marshall & Tindale, 1978). Theorists such as Estes (1979), Guillemard (1982), Myles (1984), Phillipson (1982), and Walker (1981) sought "to explain the relative situation of older individuals by examining the relationship between the economic, political, and ideological structures that these systems of domination construct and reconstruct" (McMullin, 2010, p. 98). Emerging as a reaction to research on aging that explained "the problems of old age" through individuals' inability to adjust to institutions such as retirement, political economy theorists instead focused on macro-level, structural characteristics of institutions such as the state and the economy. This macro focus led theorists to assess social life through a different lens by assessing issues such as how social policies structure dependency on the basis of an arbitrary chronological age, thus creating socially constructed age categories (e.g., old age; Phillipson, 1982; Townsend, 1981; Walker, 1981); how state-led and economy-driven motivations for capital accumulation lead to the commodification of the needs of older adults (Estes, 1979, 1991); how labor market opportunities are limited for older adults, particularly in jurisdictions governed by mandatory retirement (Guillemard, 1982); and how there is an inherent contradiction between two primary goals of most capitalist states—the principles related to social welfare and those related to capitalist accumulation (Myles, 1984).

Through these macro-interpretive approaches, theorists of political economy can imagine a different organization of the social structures and institutions that make up society. Their interpretive perspective allows them to question the very existence of social categories such as old age, and to critically assess the ways in which social institutions and structures are organized and taken for granted. Old age and dependency are thus thought to be social constructions that are perpetuated by the state and the economy (Estes, 1991; Townsend, 1981; Walker, 1981). From this perspective, age is conceptualized in terms of relative age groups and old age is socially constructed as problematic from the point of view of societal institutions.

At the macro level, European scholarship by, or inspired at least in part by, researchers at the University of Bremen, has addressed issues of the political economy in a manner consistent with the interpretive perspective. Thus, as Heinz, Huinink, Swader, and Weymann (2009) have noted:

> Notions of "agency within structures" and "bounded agency" have become crucial
> for a better understanding of how subjects develop meaningful and coherent

biographies in response to objectively contingent life courses....a sophisticated agenda must start with mapping the structural and institutional dimensions as the social contexts of biographical decisions and outcomes. This is most obvious in regard to education and training, employment, family, and social security life domains that individuals have to traverse by actively negotiating contributions, investments, returns, and benefits. (p. 22)

Interpretive-Linking Research

Despite the inherent value in the micro and macro interpretive perspectives as just described, most interpretive scholars theorize not only at macro or micro levels but also theorize phenomena that link macro and micro (Leisering & Leibfried, 1999). Indeed, at least one definition of interpretive sociology explicitly highlights the importance of this link suggesting, "a sociological understanding of behavior must include the meaning that social actors give to what they and others do. When people interact, they interpret what is going on and this is what gives social life its patterned quality" (Crossman, 2014).

In the field of aging research, Kohli (1986, 2007) postulated three models to describe the tensions between the micro and macro levels of analysis: (a) A model focusing exclusively on institutional programs (social structure). A liberal–utilitarian version of this model views actors as complying with institutional programs by their own interests. A social control version sees compliance as based on sanctions. In this model, the actor's biographical perspectives are irrelevant for outcomes. As Kohli notes, this model cannot account for actors who are motivated by more than simple instrumental rationality, or who resist pressures to which they are exposed. (b) A functionalist, Parsonian model that "conceives of institutional programming and biographical construction as parallel processes that complement each other" (Kohli, 1986, p. 292). In this model, socialization is a key mechanism. (c) Kohli's (1986) preferred model is one in which:

> The tension remains alive between the life course as socially ordered reality and biography in terms of individual agency. This requires an approach grounded in a non-normative action theory, such as that set forth by Alfred Schutz or George Herbert Mead. (p. 292; see also Strauss, 1992)

INTERPRETIVE THEORIZING IN THE LIFE-COURSE PERSPECTIVE

Linking approaches are not restricted to, but are most evident in, research and theory framed in terms of the life-course perspective. In the first systematic statement of the life-course perspective, Cain (1964) had included social structure, but also referred to the individual, seen as acting. In this he drew explicitly and at length on the symbolic interactionist Anselm Strauss. Cain also adopted the sociologist Everett C. Hughes's distinction between objective and subjective careers, the latter referring to a "moving perspective in which the person sees his life as a whole and interprets the meaning of his various attributes, actions, and the things which happen to him" (Cain, 1964, p. 298; citing Hughes, 1937).

There are many different versions of the life-course perspective. As noted previously, the first systematic formulation by Leonard Cain, Jr. can be classified as interpretive, while a later form set out by Matilda White Riley, falling centrally within structural functionalism, was not. Shanahan and Elder's (2002) incorporation of the construct of agency as a principle of the life course suggests some sympathy for the interpretive approach, but this approach is more closely tied to developmental psychology, which ignores or downplays the importance of social structure, implying that agency is demonstrated only at transition points or to account for behavior that does not follow convention or comply with social norms (see criticisms in Dannefer, 1989; Marshall & Clarke, 2010; Settersten & Gannon, 2005). However, the most explicit incorporation of the interpretive perspective in life-course research as it seeks to understand micro–macro relationships can be found in two related European research institutions.

The first European group, under the leadership of Walter Heinz, was the Special Research Program, "Status Passages and Risks in the Life Course," at the University of Bremen. The term "status passage" (Heinz, 1991) was taken from the concept originated by symbolic interactionists Glaser and Strauss (1971), sometimes labeling the concept as "career" (drawing on Hughes, 1937, 1971). *Time and Poverty in Western Welfare States* (Leisering & Leibfried, 1999) is a landmark volume from the Bremen center that links macro and micro levels of analysis through constructs such as action and structure, biography and society, and employs the concept of "poverty career", drawing on symbolic interactionists such as Howard Becker (Becker & Strauss, 1956) to theoretically ground the study. Other exemplar overviews and representative research papers of the Bremen research can be found in Marshall and Mueller (2003), Heinz (1991), and Heinz, Huinink, and Weymann (2009).

The LIVES research and doctoral/postdoctoral training program at the University of Lausanne and the University of Geneva (www.lives-nccr.ch) has strong and explicit ties to Bremen. Papers by Swiss, other European scholars (including from Bremen) and from those from the United States, from a launch of PAVIE, the predecessor to LIVES, constitute a volume in *Advances in Life Course Research* (Levy, Ghisletta, Le Goff, Spini, & Widmer, 2005). A representation of this research appears in Levy and Widmer (2013).

These linking interpretive approaches are concerned not only with the meaning of action but also with how the meaning creates a patterned social life course that is reinforced through biography. As Kohli (1988) argues,

> Formally, a biographical conception requires taking into account two levels. The first is to treat the life course as a pattern of sequentially linked positions and experiences…But…the behavioural patterns need to be complemented by a second level, that of biographical perspectives; the biographical anticipations and reminiscences by which people define their place in life, and construct their actions. (p. 379)

As well, linking approaches are concerned with the interplay between meaning and social structures (i.e., social life's patterned quality). Atchley's (1999) formalization of his continuity theory, in which he brings together systems theory and the concept of agency, is one example of this approach in gerontology.

As another example, linking biography to the workplace, McMullin and Marshall (1999) explicitly employ an interpretive approach to agency and structure that is rooted in symbolic interactionism and phenomenology in their examination of the retirement process of Montreal garment workers. They identify agency running through the social lives of the garment workers, but stress how agency is severely constrained and, indeed, constituted, by workers' embeddedness in social structures of age, gender, social class, ethnicity, and family relationships.

Similarly, Martin-Matthews, Tong, Rosenthal, and McDonald (2013) framed their study of elderly Chinese widows in Canada within an interpretive perspective, to examine agency, support, and structural constraints. The circumstances of immigration and of growing old in a foreign land contributed to the complexity and variability of widowhood for these women.

McMullin, Duerden Comeau, and Jovic (2007) bring an interpretive perspective to the examination of the concept of generation in relation to innovations in computing technology, in assessing whether and how it is used to create cultures of difference in the workplace. Their work draws on Mannheim's theorizing about the concept of generation, and examines notions of generation in the context of the culture of successive waves of computer technology. Using discourse analysis, they find that technology has acted as a touchstone for generational bonds among these workers, who prioritize generation over other bases of difference, with a significant articulation of affinities and inequalities through generation.

Linking interpretive perspectives also include critical and humanistic perspectives (see, e.g., two edited collections by Baars, Dannefer, Phillipson, & Walker, 2006; Baars, Dohmen, Grenier, & Phillipson, 2014, and work by Grenier, 2012, and Katz, 2009, as well as cultural gerontology and feminist theory). Critical gerontology has developed in recent decades along two parallel lines—political economy and the humanities—which have occasionally intersected but remained distinct (Holstein & Minkler, 2007; Ray, 2008). We have already considered the political economy perspective. Within the humanities, the essence of critical gerontology is reflexivity of both the researcher and the researched. Critical theory seeks self-awareness and a deconstruction of social gerontological theories and research, casting a critical eye on society and on the field of gerontology itself (Ray, 2008). It often also questions the salience of causation. In recent years, much of the focus of critical theory in social gerontology has been on issues of culture. Here, we examine linking interpretive perspectives through a focus on feminist theory applied to gerontology, and on the emergent subfield of cultural gerontology.

FEMINIST GERONTOLOGY

A body of literature in the field of aging studies emerged in the mid-1990s that explicitly considered gender as a social structure rather than merely an ascribed characteristic of an individual (Arber & Ginn, 1995; Calasanti, 1996; McMullin, 1995). This literature called for a relational understanding of gender as a "deep social structure" (Sewell, 1992), which is typically invisible, taken for granted, and influencing nearly all activities of daily life. At the same time, gender structures are produced and reproduced by individuals in interaction with one another. This recognition that people "do gender" (West & Zimmerman, 1987) and that it is through doing gender that its structure is produced and reproduced, is what classifies most of feminist gerontology as interpretive linking. This same body of literature also called for an intersectional approach to age and gender. Rather than simply adding gender to an analysis that focused on age-based disadvantage or adding age to an analysis that focused on gender-based disadvantage, these scholars believe that both need to be equally considered to garner accurate assessments of social life (Calasanti, 2004; McMullin, 1995, 2000).

Feminist gerontology is distinguishable from other theoretical perspectives in its focus on gender and age relations as they relate to social inequality. The theoretical stance in this perspective is that gender and age relations are power relations and that "disadvantage of certain groups depends on the advantage of others, the oppression that results is relational" (McMullin, 2010, p. 131). Hence, gender and age relations are characterized by power and also by "the meaning that is attributed to these categories of inequality based on relative positioning within social hierarchies" (McMullin, 2010, p. 131).

CULTURAL GERONTOLOGY

The emergence of cultural gerontology reflects shifts in mainstream social sciences often characterized as the "Cultural Turn." Its foundation is the recognition of the unprecedented role of culture in the constitution of social identities and realities (Katz, 2009; Twigg & Martin, 2014). Cultural gerontology thus sits squarely within the interpretive perspective, with its focus on meaning, subjectivity, and identity. Many of the themes or theoretical positions that underlie the Cultural Turn have long been present in the work of classical theorists of society. Through its focus on understanding of aging as a process rather than a state, the lens of cultural gerontology enables "more plural accounts of old age and its boundaries, allowing us to reflect on the ways the definitions of these vary in different cultural fields" (Twigg & Martin, 2014, p. 355).

Cultural gerontology well links micro and macro interpretive perspectives on aging. Some scholars situate its emergence in the effort to escape dominant paradigms that locate aging and old age within social welfare and public policy frameworks emphasizing frailty and burden. The focus of cultural gerontology is instead on presenting a fuller and richer account of old age, encompassing "unproblematic old age" (Twigg & Martin, 2015) and "new aging" (Gilleard & Higgs, 2013, 2015), including the Third Age.

The work of Stephen Katz exemplifies the linking functions of cultural gerontology. *Cultural Aging: Life Course, Lifestyle and Senior Worlds* (2009) is a compendium of his work, spanning such topics as the linguistic shaping of social policy reports on aging, examining how political rationalities become articulated and conveyed to the public, to the commercial "fashioning" of senior worlds in targeting "ageless" consumers, and the intersection of positive aging, anti-ageism, and anti-aging.

Although the examples provided have demonstrated the importance of interpretive perspectives that theorize the link between micro and macro, observations from nursing research identify a challenge. Anderson (2009) notes the problematic aspects of "making the conceptual links between the micro level of experience and macro social structures and addressing the complexity of intersectionalities among the ever-growing list of social determinants and the pathways that mediate relationships" (p. 53). The emergence of research with an explicit intersectionality focus—especially when framed within the interpretive perspective—holds promise here.

■ CONCLUSION: LOOKING TO THE FUTURE

In this chapter, we have situated and considered the interpretive perspective, briefly recounting a long history in social theorizing and its roots in the Weberian, symbolic interactionist and phenomenological traditions within sociology, and their application to a range of applications across disciplines. We have considered interpretive perspectives as a contrast to some "classic" normative approaches to theorizing aging and also considered examples of research that place the application of theory at the macro, micro, and linking levels of analysis.

The chapter on "Constructionist Perspectives on Aging" in the first edition of this handbook concludes with an acknowledgment of the "extraordinarily broad horizon of choices" available to constructionist (and interpretive) researchers in the future, regarding their analytical projects, methodological approaches, and end results (Gubrium & Holstein, 1999). The first 15 years of this millennium have well proven that to be true for interpretive, including constructionist, perspectives. The range of "analytical projects" for interpretive researchers remains not only very broad, but is ever changing.

Hendricks (2010) elegantly forecast many of these issues in his consideration of age, self, and identity in this "global century." The effects of globalization, technological innovation, and public policy, with changes in normative structures, benchmarks, and transitions, and with the spread of consumerism and increasing commodification of experience, all portend a world wherein

> ...constructs that were once taken as foundational for identity are called into question to such an extent they no longer serve as lodestars by which actors can chart their own course. What was once certain becomes contingent and issues of agency, subjectivity, and perception are thrown into flux. (Hendricks, 2010, p. 262)

As Beck, Bonss, and Lau (2003) have argued, and Hendricks (2010) elaborates, "In the face of globalization...meanings change...[and] so too does the significance of individuals and the social construction of ageing" (p. 262).

Although Gilleard and Higgs (2013) frame these changes in terms of a "new ageing" full of the possibilities of active consumerism, travel, and active aging, Hendricks (2010) speaks of the potential of transformation from "the venerable to the vulnerable." Phillipson (2013) similarly notes the "crisis of legitimacy" (p. 81) in societal support of older people, the loosening of institutional supports underpinning the life course, and the general de-standardization of the life course. Although he acknowledges the shift in postmodern society from production to consumption, he (unlike Gilleard & Higgs, 2013) emphasizes new risks and insecurities with the individualization of retirement, and an enlarging of the range of risks facing older people, with a "more fluid and unstable landscape around the end of life course" (p. 81), its increasingly improvisational nature, more discontinuity in key areas of life, individualization and the fragmentation of social institutions, marginalization of social models of care, and the individualization of the transition between systems of care (Phillipson, 2013).

The interpretive perspective has much to contribute to advancing understanding of such issues, heightening the relevance of its foci on micro, macro, and linking approaches, especially in analyses of the link between agency and structure in these widely different scenarios. With its primary focus on self, agency within structure, and meaning, the interpretive perspective is a powerful tool in addressing such issues as perceptions of the Fourth Age as one in which "older people are socially and culturally 'othered'" (Grenier, 2012), or the "highly contingent quality" of later life (Settersten & Trauten, 2009, p. 457) in the context of the risk society, and the transformation of public policies to emphasize individualization.

Methodological advances used within the interpretive perspective hold great promise for future gerontological research. For example, fundamental to the methodology of cultural gerontology is the recognition of the "rise of the Visual, which has to some degree replaced the dominance of the Word central to the earlier modernity" (Twigg & Martin, 2014). With technological advances and the digital age, visual culture is omnipresent. Reflecting this, ways of knowing about aging and old age include auto-photography (Kohon & Carder, 2014) and other visual techniques (Martin, 2015), as well as representations of aging in theater (Bernard & Munro, 2015), film (Swinnen, 2015), popular music (Jennings, 2015), and in social media (Martin-Matthews, 2015).

Digital representations of aging are a particular conundrum for the study of aging, at least in the current era and form of the "digital divide." As Hendricks (1999, citing Hacking, 1992), observes, knowledge is grounded in the intent of the knower, and "how we know what we know becomes self-authenticating" (p. 191). At present, social and digital media as ways of knowing about aging are less populated by older people themselves than they will be in the future, with important methodological and "reflexive" implications.

In the first edition of this handbook, Gubrium and Holstein (1999) predicted "greater free play . . . [stemming] from a radically reflexive openness" (p. 302) in the methodology of constructionist and interpretive perspectives. There has certainly been evidence of this, not only in terms of older people themselves, but in applying the interpretive gaze to our own discipline of social gerontology (Katz, 2009), to subfields within it, such as narrative studies (Laceulle & Baars, 2014), and even to ourselves as social gerontologists (see the *Journal of Aging Studies* [2008], vol. 22, no. 2, special issue on self-reflexivity, including papers by Hendricks, by Phillipson, and by Ray).

The interpretive perspective has much yet to contribute to theorizing about the changing nature of later life itself. Deep old age remains surprisingly understudied in social gerontology, despite the fact that those aged 85 years and older are the fastest growing segment of the population in many parts of the world. Loe's (2011) 3-year ethnographic study of 30 people aged 85 to 102 years is a welcome counterpoint to narratives of decrement and decline among this age group. With a guiding theme of continuity framing the analyses, Loe (2011) finds that continuity requires "real effort and stubborn resilience" (p. 23), as the very old test the waters of inter- and independent living. Research such as this is ever more necessary, elucidating how "growing into oneself" continues into very late in life, as individuals embrace a wide range of resources to achieve self-care, well-being, and comfort in lives characterized by meaning and connection and lived within an "ethos of restraint" (p. 45). The increasing length of our days, and with them, the "co-longevity of different generations" (Phillipson, 2013, p. 112), are rich terrain for theorizing through the interpretive perspective.

What might be some future "end results" for the interpretive perspective, as the first edition of this handbook (Gubrium & Holstein, 1999) asked at the end of the last century (and millennium)? The possibilities are many. We have not been able to address here clinical applications based on narrative approaches. However, for an example, see Clark (2015), who describes the increasing use of narrative approaches with older adults by health professionals in a variety of settings. Certainly, interpretive perspectives are enabling us to transform our scholarship, and assert the relevance of its application.

Whatever the future for aging individuals and aging societies, we assert that varieties of the interpretive perspective now are, and will increasingly be, salient in achieving understanding of what matters to cohorts of people individually and collectively as they age, what happens to social institutions and structures in relation to population aging, and how these changes will influence one another.

REFERENCES

Abbott, A. (1998). The causal devolution. *Sociological Methods & Research, 27*(2), 148–181.

Anderson, J. M. (1981). An interpretive approach to clinical nursing research. *Nursing Papers, 13*(4), 6–11.

Anderson, J. M. (2009). Looking back, looking forward: Conceptual and methodological trends in nursing research in Canada over the past decade. *Canadian Journal of Nursing Research, 41*(1), 47–55.

Arber, S., & Ginn, J. (Eds.). (1995). *Connecting gender and ageing: A sociological approach.* Buckingham, UK: Open University Press.

Atchley, R. C. (1999). Continuity theory, self, and social structure. In C. D. Ryff & V. W. Marshall (Eds.), *The self and society in aging processes* (pp. 94–121). New York, NY: Springer Publishing Company.

Baars, J., Dannefer, D., Phillipson, C., & Walker, A. (Eds.). (2006). *Aging, globalization, and inequality: The new critical gerontology.* Amityville, NY: Baywood Publishing.

Baars, J., Dohmen, J., Grenier, A., & Phillipson, C. (Eds.). (2014). *Ageing, meaning and social structure: Connecting critical and humanistic gerontology.* Bristol, UK: Policy Press.

Beck, U., Bonss, W., & Lau, C. (2003). The theory of reflexive modernization: Problematic, hypotheses and research programme. *Theory, Culture and Society, 20*(2), 1–33.

Becker, H. S., & Strauss, A. (1956). Careers, personality and adult socialization. *American Journal of Sociology, 62*(3), 253–263.

Berger, P. L., & Luckmann, T. (1967). *The social construction of reality: A treatise in the sociology of knowledge.* Garden City, NY: Anchor Books (Doubleday).

Bernard, M., & Munro, L. (2015). Theatre and ageing. In J. W. Twigg & W. Martin (Eds.), *Routledge handbook of cultural gerontology* (pp. 61–68). London, UK: Routledge.

Breytspraak, L. M. (1984). *The development of self in later life.* Boston, MA: Little, Brown.

Cain, L. D. (1964). Life course and social structure. In R. E. L. Faris (Ed.), *Handbook of modern sociology* (pp. 272–309). Chicago, IL: Rand McNally.

Calasanti, T. M. (1996). Incorporating diversity: Meaning, levels of research, and implications for theory. *The Gerontologist, 36*(2), 147–156.

Calasanti, T. M. (2004). Feminist gerontology and old men. *The Journals of Gerontology, Series B, 59*(6), S305–S314.

Clarke, P. (2009). Understanding the experience of stroke: A mixed-methods agenda. *The Gerontologist, 49*(3), 293–302.

Clark, P. G. (2015). Emerging themes in using narrative in geriatric care: Implications for patient-centered practice and interprofessional teamwork. *Journal of Aging Studies, 34*, 177–182.

Cowgill, D. (1974). Aging and modernization: A revision of the theory. In J. F. Gubrium (Ed.), *Late life: Communities and environmental policy* (pp. 123–145). Springfield, IL: Appleton-Century-Crofts.

Crossman, A. (2014). *Interpretive sociology. In About.com.* Retrieved from http:// sociology.about.com/od/I_Index/g/Interpretive-Sociology.htm

Cumming, E., & Henry, W. E. (1961). *Growing old: The process of disengagement.* New York, NY: Basic Books.

Dannefer, D. (1989). Human action and its place in theories of aging. *Journal of Aging Studies, 3*(1), 1–20.

Dannefer, D. (2012). Enriching the tapestry: Expanding the scope of life course concepts. *The Journals of Gerontology, Series B, 67*(2), 221–225.

David, M. (2010). Editor's introduction: Methods of interpretive sociology. In M. David (Ed.), *Methods of interpretive sociology* (pp. xxiiv–xlii). Thousand Oaks, CA: Sage.

Estes, C. L. (1979). *The aging enterprise: A critical examination of social policies and services for the aged.* San Francisco, CA: Jossey-Bass.

Estes, C. L. (1991). The new political economy of aging: Introduction and critique. In M. Minkler & C. Estes (Eds.), *Critical perspectives on aging: The political and moral economy of growing old* (pp. 19–36). Amityville, NY: Baywood.

Gilleard, C., & Higgs, P. (2013). *Ageing, corporeality and embodiment.* London, UK: Anthem Press.

Gilleard, C., & Higgs, P. (2015). The cultural turn in gerontology. In J. W. Twigg & W. Martin (Eds.), *Routledge handbook of cultural gerontology* (pp. 29–36). London, UK: Routledge.

Glaser, B. G., & Strauss, A. L. (1971). *Status passage.* Chicago, IL: Aldine, Atherton.

Grenier, A. (2012). *Transitions and the lifecourse: Contested models of 'growing old.'* Bristol, UK: Policy Press.

Gubrium, J. F. (1973). *The myth of the golden years: A socio-environmental theory of aging.* Springfield, IL: Charles C. Thomas.

Gubrium, J. F. (1975). *Living and dying at Murray Manor.* Charlottesville: University Press of Virginia.

Gubrium, J. F. (1986). *Oldtimers and Alzheimer's: The descriptive organization of senility.* Greenwich, CT: JAI Press.

Gubrium, J. F., & Holstein, J. A. (1999). Constructionist perspectives on aging. In V. L. Bengtson & K. W. Shaie (Eds.), *Handbook of theories of aging* (pp. 287–305). New York, NY: Springer Publishing Company.

Gubrium, J. F., & Lynott, R. J. (1992). Measurement and the interpretation of burden in the Alzheimer's disease experience. In J. F. Gubrium & K. Charmaz (Eds.), *Aging, self, and community: A collection of readings* (pp. 129–149). Greenwich, CT: JAI Press.

Guillemard, A. (1982). Old age, retirement, and the social class structure: Toward an analysis of the structural dynamics of the later stage of life. In T. K. Hareven & K. Adams (Eds.), *Aging and the life course transition: An interdisciplinary perspective* (pp. 221–243). New York, NY: Guilford Press.

Hacking, I. (1992). "Style" for historians and philosophers. *Studies in History and Philosophy of Science Part A, 23*(1), 1–20.

Havighurst, R. J., Neugarten, B. L., & Tobin, S. (1968). Disengagement and patterns of aging. In B. L. Neugarten (Ed.), *Middle age and aging: A reader in social psychology* (pp. 161–177). Chicago, IL: University of Chicago Press.

Heinz, W. R. (1991). Status passages, social risks and the life course: A conceptual framework. In W. R. Heinz (Ed.), *Theoretical advances in life-course research* (pp. 9–21). Weinheim, Germany: Deutscher Studien Verlag.

Heinz, W. R., Huinink, J., Swader, C. S., & Weymann, A. (2009). General introduction. In W. R. Heinz, J. Huinink, & A. Weymann (Eds.), *The life course reader: Individuals and societies across time* (pp. 15–30). New York, NY: Campus Verlag.

Heinz, W. R., Huinink, J., & Weymann, A. (Eds.). (2009). *The life course reader: Individuals and societies across time.* New York, NY: Campus Verlag.

Hendricks, J. (1999). Practical consciousness, social class, and self-concept: A view from sociology. In C. D. Ryff & V. W. Marshall (Eds.), *The self and society in aging processes* (pp. 187–222). New York, NY: Springer Publishing Company.

Hendricks, J. (2010). Age, self, and identity in the global century. In D. Dannefer & C. Phillipson (Eds.), *The SAGE handbook of social gerontology* (pp. 251–264). Thousand Oaks, CA: Sage.

Holstein, M. B., & Minkler, M. (2007). Critical gerontology: Reflections for the 21st century. In M. Bernard & T. Scharf (Eds.), *Critical perspectives on ageing societies* (pp. 13–26). Bristol, UK: Policy Press.

Hughes, E. C. (1937). Institutional office and the person. *American Journal of Sociology, 43*(3), 404–413.

Hughes, E. C. (1971). *The sociological eye: Selected papers.* Chicago, IL: Aldine Atherton.

Jennings, R. (2015). Popular music and ageing. In J. W. Twigg & W. Martin (Eds.), *Routledge handbook of cultural gerontology* (pp. 77–84). London, UK: Routledge.

Katz, S. (2009). *Cultural aging: Life course, lifestyle and senior worlds.* Toronto, Canada: University of Toronto Press.

Kohli, M. (1986). The world we forgot: A historical review of the life course. In V. W. Marshall (Ed.), *Later life: The social psychology of aging* (pp. 271–303). Beverly Hills, CA: Sage.

Kohli, M. (1988). Ageing as a challenge for sociological theory. *Ageing and Society, 8*(4), 367–394.

Kohli, M. (2007). The institutionalization of the life course: Looking back to look ahead. *Research in Human Development, 4*(3–4), 253–271.

Kohon, J., & Carder, P. (2014). Exploring identity and aging: Auto-photography and narratives of low income older adults. *Journal of Aging Studies, 30,* 47–55.

Laceulle, H., & Baars, J. (2014). Self-realization and cultural narratives about later life. *Journal of Aging Studies, 31,* 34–44.

Leisering, L., & Leibfried, S. (1999). *Time and poverty in western welfare states.* Cambridge, UK: Cambridge University Press.

Levy, R., Ghisletta, P., Le Goff, J., Spini, D., & Widmer, E. (Eds.). (2005). *Towards an interdisciplinary perspective on the life course (advances in life course research, volume 10).* Amsterdam, the Netherlands: Elsevier JAI.

Levy, R., & Widmer, E. (Eds.). (2013). *Gendered life courses between standardization and individualization.* Zurich, Switzerland: Lit Verlag.

Loe, M. (2011). *Aging our way: Lessons for living from 85 and beyond.* New York, NY: Oxford University Press.

Maddox, G. L. (1965). Fact and artifact: Evidence bearing on disengagement theory. *Human Development, 8,* 117–130.

Marshall, V. W. (1975a). Organizational features of terminal status passage in residential facilities for the aged. *Journal of Contemporary Ethnography, 4*(3), 349–368.

Marshall, V. W. (1975b). Socialization for impending death in a retirement village. *American Journal of Sociology, 80*(5), 1122–1144.

Marshall, V. W. (1978–1979). No exit: A symbolic interactionist perspective on aging. *International Journal of Aging and Human Development, 9*(4), 345–358.

Marshall, V. W. (1980). *Last chapters: A sociology of aging and dying.* Monterey, CA: Brooks/Cole.

Marshall, V. W. (1986). Dominant and emerging paradigms in the social psychology of aging. In V. W. Marshall (Ed.), *Later life: The social psychology of aging* (pp. 9–31). Beverly Hills, CA: Sage.

Marshall, V. W. (1995). The micro-macro link in the sociology of aging. In C. Hummel & C. Lalive D'Epinay (Eds.), *Images of aging in western societies* (pp. 337–371). Geneva, Switzerland: Centre for Interdisciplinary Gerontology, University of Geneva.

Marshall, V. W. (1996a). Theories of aging. In J. E. Birren (Ed.), *Encyclopedia of gerontology: Age, aging, and the aged* (pp. 569–572). San Diego, CA: Academic Press.

Marshall, V. W. (1996b). The state of theory in aging and the social sciences. In R. H. Binstock & L. George (Eds.), *Handbook of aging and the social sciences, fourth edition* (pp. 12–30). San Diego, CA: Academic Press.

Marshall, V. W., & Clarke, P. J. (2010). Agency and social structure in aging and life-course research. In D. Dannefer & C. Phillipson (Eds.), *The SAGE handbook of social gerontology* (pp. 294–305). Los Angeles, CA: Sage.

Marshall, V. W., & Mueller, M. M. (2003). Theoretical roots of the life course perspective. In W. R. Heinz & V. W. Marshall (Eds.), *Social dynamics of the life course: Transitions, institutions, and interrelations* (pp. 3–32). New York, NY: Aldine de Gruyter.

Marshall, V. W., & Tindale, J. A. (1978). Notes for a radical gerontology. *International Journal of Aging and Human Development, 9*(2), 163–175.

Martin, W. (2015). Visual methods and age. In J. W. Twigg & W. Martin (Eds.), *Routledge handbook of cultural gerontology* (pp. 93–104). London, UK: Routledge.

Martin-Matthews, A. (2015). Widowhood and its cultural representations. In J. W. Twigg & W. Martin (Eds.), *Routledge handbook of cultural gerontology* (pp. 243–251). London, UK: Routledge.

Martin-Matthews, A., Tong, C., Rosenthal, C., & McDonald, L. (2013). Ethno-cultural diversity in the experience of widowhood in later life: Chinese widows in Canada. *Journal of Aging Studies, 27*(4), 507–518.

McMullin, J. A. (1995). Theorizing age and gender relations. In S. Arber & J. Ginn (Eds.), *Connecting gender and ageing: A sociological approach.* Buckingham, UK: Open University Press.

McMullin, J. A. (2000). Diversity and the state of sociological aging theory. *The Gerontologist, 40*(5), 517–530.

McMullin, J. A. (2010). *Understanding social inequality: Intersections of class, age, gender, ethnicity, and race in Canada* (2nd ed.). Toronto, Canada: Oxford University Press.

McMullin, J. A., & Cairney, J. (2004). Self-esteem and the intersection of age, class, and gender. *Journal of Aging Studies, 18*(1), 75–90.

McMullin, J. A., Duerden Comeau, T., & Jovic, E. (2007). Generational affinities and discourses of difference: A case study of highly skilled information technology workers. *British Journal of Sociology, 58*(2), 297–316.

McMullin, J. A., & Marshall, V. W. (1999). Structure and agency in the retirement process: A case study of Montreal garment workers. In C. Ryff & V. W. Marshall (Eds.), *The self and society in aging processes* (pp. 305–338). New York, NY: Springer Publishing Company.

Mead, G. H. (1934). *Mind, self and society*. Chicago, IL: University of Chicago Press.

Myles, J. (1984). *Old age in the welfare state: The political economy of public pensions*. Toronto, Canada: Little, Brown.

Neugarten, B. L. (1974). Age groups in American society and the rise of the young-old. *Annals of the American Academy of Political and Social Science, 415*(1), 187–198.

Neugarten, B. L., & Hagestad, G. (1976). Age and the life course. In R. H. Binstock & E. Shanas (Eds.), *Handbook of aging and the social sciences* (pp. 35–55). New York, NY: Van Nostrand Reinhold.

O'Connor, D. L. (2007). Self-identifying as a caregiver: Exploring the positioning process. *Journal of Aging Studies, 21*(2), 165–174.

Palmore, E., & Manton, K. (1974). Modernization and the status of the aged: International correlations. *Journal of Gerontology, 29*(2), 205–210.

Parsons, T. (1961). Foreword. In E. Cumming & W. E. Henry (Eds.), *Growing old: The process of disengagement* (pp. v–viii). New York, NY: Basic Books.

Phillipson, C. (1982). *Capitalism and the construction of old age*. London, UK: Macmillan.

Phillipson, C. (2013). *Ageing*. London, UK: Polity Press.

Ray, R. E. (2008). Coming of age in critical gerontology. *Journal of Aging Studies, 22*(2), 97–100.

Riley, M. W. (1971). Social gerontology and the age stratification of society. *The Gerontologist, 11*, 79–87.

Riley, M. W. (1976). Age strata in social systems. In R. Binstock & E. Shanas (Eds.), *Handbook of aging and the social sciences* (pp. 187–217). New York, NY: Van Nostrand Reinhold.

Rodwell, M. K. (1998). *Social work, constructivist research*. New York, NY: Garland Publishing.

Rose, A. M. (1965). A current theoretical issue in social gerontology. In A. M. Rose & W. A. Peterson (Eds.), *Older people and their social world* (pp. 359–366). Philadelphia, PA: F. A. Davis.

Rosow, I. (1974). *Socialization to old age*. Berkeley: University of California Press.

Rosow, I. (1976). Status and role change through the life span. In R. H. Binstock & E. Shanas (Eds.), *Handbook of aging and the social sciences* (pp. 457–482). New York, NY: Van Nostrand Reinhold.

Ryff, C. D., & Marshall, V. W. (Eds.). (1999). *The self and society in aging processes.* New York, NY: Springer Publishing Company.

Sandelowski, M. (2008). Foreword. In S. Thorne (Ed.), *Interpretive description* (pp. 11–14). Walnut Creek, CA: Left Coast Press.

Schutz, A. (1967). *The phenomenology of the social world.* Chicago, IL: Northwestern University Press.

Settersten, R. A., & Gannon, L. (2005). Structure, agency, and the space between: On the challenges and contradictions of a blended view of the life course. In R. Levy, P. Ghisletta, J. Le Goff, D. Spini, & E. Widmer (Eds.), *Towards an interdisciplinary perspective on the life course* (pp. 35–55). Amsterdam, the Netherlands: Elsevier JAI.

Settersten, R., & Trauten, M. (2009). The new terrain of old age: Hallmarks, freedoms, and risks. In V. Bengtson, D. Gans, N. Putney, & M. Silverstein (Eds.), *Handbook of theories of aging, second edition* (pp. 455–470). New York, NY: Springer Publishing Company.

Sewell, W. H. J. Jr. (1992). A theory of structure: Duality, agency, and transformation. *American Journal of Sociology, 98,* 1–29.

Shanahan, M. J., & Elder, G. H. Jr. (2002). History, agency, and the life course. In L. J. Crockett (Ed.), *Agency, motivation and the life course. Vol. 48 of the Nebraska Symposium on Motivation* (pp. 145–186). Lincoln: University of Nebraska Press.

Singer, B., Ryff, C. D., Carr, D., & Magee, W. J. (1998). Linking life histories and mental health: A person-centered strategy. *Sociological Methodology, 28,* 1–51.

Smith, J. A. (2004). Reflecting on the development of interpretative phenomenological analysis and its contribution to qualitative research in psychology. *Qualitative Research in Psychology, 1*(1), 39–54.

Spence, D. L. (1986). Some contributions of symbolic interaction to the study of growing old. In V. W. Marshall (Ed.), *Later life: The social psychology of aging* (pp. 107–123). Beverly Hills, CA: Sage.

Strauss, A. L. (1992). *Introduction to the French translation of mirrors and masks.* Paris, France: Editions Metailie.

Swinnen, A. (2015). Ageing in film. In J. W. Twigg & W. Martin (Eds.), *Routledge handbook of cultural gerontology* (pp. 69–76). London, UK: Routledge.

Thorne, S. (2008). *Interpretive description.* Walnut Creek, CA: Left Coast Press.

Townsend, P. (1981). The structured dependency of the elderly: A creation of social policy in the twentieth century. *Ageing and Society, 1*(1), 5–28.

Twigg, J. W., & Martin, W. (2014). The challenge of cultural gerontology. *The Gerontologist, 55*(3), 353–359.

Twigg, J. W., & Martin, W. (Eds.). (2015). *Routledge handbook of cultural gerontology.* London, UK: Routledge.

Walker, A. (1981). Towards a political economy of old age. *Ageing and Society, 1*(1), 74–94.

Weber, M. (1978). *Economy and society: An outline of interpretive sociology*. Berkeley: University of California Press.

West, C., & Zimmerman, D. (1987). Doing gender. *Gender and Society, 1*(2), 125–151.

Wilson, T. P. (1970). Normative and interpretive paradigms in sociology. In J. D. Douglas (Ed.), *Understanding everyday life* (pp. 57–97). Chicago, IL: Aldine.

PART V

Policy, Intervention, and Practice Theories and Concepts

ADVANCES IN THEORY-BASED POLICY AND INTERVENTIONS

Nancy Morrow-Howell

What concepts and theories are driving policy and practice innovations in gerontology? This is an important question, given the profound effects of policy, programs, and services on the everyday lives of older Americans and their families. Income security, family caregiving, long-term care services and supports, supportive neighborhood environments—these issues matter in a real way, at the individual and societal level. We need rigorous applied research to inform the development of our health and social services, and good research goes hand-in-hand with good theory. Yet, too often the demands for action, and for evidence about the outcomes of those actions, leave theoretical explanations as after-thoughts. Although public monies to serve the most vulnerable older adults are shrinking, health and social service agencies are proliferating in response to the growing aging population. This situation demands the development of efficient and effective programs and policies, and this is not possible without understanding and explaining the issues relevant to individual older adults, families, and communities.

In this part of the handbook—Policy, Intervention, and Practice Theories and Concepts—top scholars share concepts and frameworks that guide current practices and suggest future directions for building and testing theory. They focus on critical concerns such as aging in place, long-term care services, caregiving, health promotion programs, health and income policy, and service utilization.

■ NEW PERSPECTIVES ON AGING IN PLACE

National and international efforts have focused on modifying physical and social environments to maximize the chances for older adults to age in place, to "stay put" as long as possible. Programs and organizations are proliferating under this banner, which is usually portrayed as an alternative to nursing home. Yet, in Chapter 21, Andrew

Scharlach and Keith Diaz Moore find current ideas too simplistic and challenge us to develop a more conceptually grounded, nuanced, and useful conceptualization of aging in place. Two ideas stand out. First, we must expand upon Lawton's classic person–environment fit framework to view people as more than a set of competencies, but also possessing intentions, worldviews, and moments in time. Environments also offer resources as well as demands. Second, we must strive to maximize attributes of the person–environment fit, including continuity, compensation, control, connection, contribution, and challenge/comfort.

Scharlach and Diaz Moore illustrate that aging in place is complex and dynamic. It should not be seen as a single, universal goal, but as an adaptive process of continually changing person–place transactions over time. This requires that theory development and subsequent research move beyond homeostatic, cross-sectional frameworks. The authors point to several areas of inquiry that are ripe for theoretical advances: (a) temporal variations in person–environment fit, (b) factors affecting the person–environment fit, (c) the utility of behavioral economic approaches, (d) contextual/cultural variations in residential preferences and behaviors, (e) disparities in the ability to achieve desired person–environment fit, (f) factors associated with actual relocation behaviors, and (g) intervention effectiveness.

■ PERSON-CENTERED APPROACHES

A fundamentally new paradigm is emerging for the provision of services to older adults. In this person-centered approach, older adults are active participants in making decisions about and managing their care. In Chapter 22, Nancy Hooyman, Kevin Mahoney, and Mark Sciegaj describe the programs and policies that have been a part of this paradigm shift as well as evidence that supports its value. New language abounds: consumer-directed care, participant-directed care, person-centered care, self-management, and shared decision making. What all these concepts have in common is the assumption that an individual with a disability knows best about what he or she needs, and that the individual should have maximum decision-making power and control over care arrangements.

Hooyman et al. reflect on relevant psychological and sociological theories, largely focused on individual and small group interactions. They offer a new conceptualization that pulls from all these concepts and guides thinking about consumer-directed care: the Consumer-Directed Theory of Empowerment. They illustrate how individual and family choices about services are affected by psychological, social, and cultural factors. They, therefore, urge future theory development and research to understand this variability, especially the influence of racial/ethnic and socioeconomic factors.

■ THE EVIDENCE-BASED PRACTICE MOVEMENT

The subsequent chapters relate to another movement in aging services: the drive toward the development and use of evidence-based interventions. The evaluation of outcomes associated with interventions often outstrips theoretical development, despite an ever-growing demand for a fully articulated conceptual framework.

In Chapter 23, Rhonda Montgomery, Jung Kwak, and Karl Kosloski review how major theoretical frameworks regarding stress and coping have been adopted to inform basic tenets of caregiving interventions. For example, the authors describe how the theorized mediators of stress (coping and self-efficacy) have been targets of psycho-educational interventions to improve caregiving outcomes. This illustrates the useful application of some of our larger psychosocial theories in guiding gerontological practice innovations. At the same time, theories have been developed specifically to explain processes related to gerontological practice—in this case, the Caregiver Identity Theory. This theory focuses on a caregiver's sense of self in relationship to the care recipient and proposes that identity discrepancy, or the incongruence between a caregiver's behavior and his or her identity standards, is a major source of caregiver stress. It provides a basis for targeting services as the needs of the caregiver change over time, with the goal of reducing incongruence between what the caregiver is doing and what the caregiver believes he or she should be doing.

As Montgomery and colleagues point out, the benefits of these evidence-based programs can be accrued only if programs are used—and a relatively small proportion of caregivers participate in these programs. They emphasize the need to move beyond Andersen's Behavioral Model of Health Services, which offers only limited explanation of the use of formal caregiving support services. They instead point to the practice-oriented framework (Yeatts, Crow, & Folts, 1992), because it includes factors that can be affected by service providers. Montgomery and colleagues illustrate the progress made in understanding the complex process of caregiving, and in developing multicomponent support programs targeted to a diverse range of caregiving needs. The authors advise that theory development should focus on use of these programs—the sustainable uptake, adoption, and implementation of effective caregiver support services in diverse communities.

■ HEALTH PROMOTION AND BEHAVIOR CHANGE THEORIES

In Chapter 24, Susan Hughes, Elske Stolte, and Renae Smith-Ray point out that health promotion programs for older adults have proliferated amid attempts to reduce morbidity and maximize function. There is a drive to produce evidence-based programs, largely around physical activity, weight management, and managing medical conditions. These programs have been developed based on behavior change theories that explain when and how human beings change and maintain behaviors. In their review of behavior change theories, Hughes and colleagues chart theories in relation to phases of behavior change (initiation, maintenance, and relapse) and levels of behavior influenced (individual, relationship, community, and society). They note the historic focus on internal factors of the individual and the more recent appreciation of the plethora of external factors that influence health behavior. Yet, only a small number of intervention development efforts are multilevel, and they advocate for advancing programs that target all levels of the social ecological model.

Hughes and colleagues end with observations about the potential for advances in measurement of health behaviors and the resulting collection of large amounts of data available to test theories of behavior change. The Internet, smartphones, and text messaging all benefit health promotion efforts, including the rapid dissemination of health messages, the collection of real-time assessment data, and instantaneous feedback. In the face of these innovations, the authors call for theory development to understand the way older adults interact with technology as well as differences between younger and older adults with respect to health promotion. They also call for theory development to guide interventions that are multilevel and target multiple behaviors, the use of economic incentives, and the role of genetic testing.

■ CHALLENGES TO POLICY AND PRACTICE

The last two chapters address fundamental issues that underlie the entire aging services network: social policies and service utilization. In Chapter 25, Robert Hudson observes that older adults as a subpopulation are the "the recipients of public benefits that are the envy of every other social policy constituency in the nation." Social Security, Medicare, Medicaid, and the Older Americans Act are all far-reaching policies that touch every older person in the United States. Hudson reviews six theoretical approaches that explain the development and expansion of aging policy in our welfare state: the (a) logic of industrialization and policy development, (b) role of political culture and values, (c) presence (or absence) of working-class mobilization, (d) impact of individual and group participation, (e) weight of state structure, and (f) effects of policy in shaping subsequent events. Although these explanations for the historical development of aging policies have been around a long time, Hudson elucidates how contemporary events tie to these six approaches. For example, technological innovation is the updated version of the industrial revolution; subgroups of immigrants and welfare recipients fare worse than older adults in the resurgence of conservative impulses; and the need for individual and organizational participation has become more important in the current economic and political environment. Hudson explains how older adults have moved from an "advantaged" to a "contender" status, and that, although new old-age initiatives are not likely, the growth of the older population will keep existing aging policies in the forefront of national discussions.

As Dr. Hudson deals with the range of health and social policies aimed at the older population, Drs. Wacker and Roberto point out a fundamental conundrum: the need–use paradox. Many older Americans who appear to have service needs do not come forward to use available services as expected. Underutilization has been documented in many arenas, including meal services, home care, mental health services, and adult day care. Seeking help and using services is a complex process, involving psychological and social factors as well as issues of access and service delivery.

In Chapter 26, Robbyn Wacker and Karen Roberto begin with a historical overview of the Andersen's Behavioral Model of Health Services, the most widely used framework to explain service utilization. The lack of consistency in testing this framework has not produced the knowledge we need. But the framework has elucidated the primary role of *perceived* need in explaining service use and the general pattern of lower levels of formal service use among minority group members. The authors review other theoretical approaches—none explicitly developed to explain service use and not much application to older adults, but all have promising elements to explain the "need–use gap." They show how most ideas have been focused at the intrapersonal level. In fact, Wacker and Roberto find great promise in the Social Ecological Model, which views a person's behavior in the context of complex interpersonal, community, and social factors, and they suggest a research agenda to advance a multilevel approach to understanding service use.

■ CONFRONTING CHALLENGES TO THEORETICAL ADVANCES

The chapters in this section demonstrate the usefulness of theory in the applied realm of gerontological programs and policies. In this realm, the demand for theory development and testing as well as the demand for utilization of theory to support actions is growing—in classroom settings, publications, grant applications, funding decisions, and logic models. Yet in the real world of practice and policy, the resources of time, money, and flexibility are constrained. These constraints challenge the necessity of theory development. The consideration of theory is also limited by a lack of commitment to theoretical explanation by various stakeholders—not just agency partners or consumers themselves, but even editors and reviewers of manuscripts who are inconsistent in the demand for theory. The future of theory building hinges on the expectation for theoretical explication.

It is clear that most theories in these chapters support intervention, program, or policy development. Few directly address the dissemination and implementation (D & I) of these interventions. The gap between development of evidence-based treatments and use of those treatments in real-world settings has been widely noted. An often cited estimate is that there is a 15- to 20-year delay between scientific discovery and use of this knowledge in routine services (Balas & Boren, 2000). Our knowledge of *what* to disseminate and implement outstrips our knowledge about *how* to disseminate and implement these interventions (Brownson, Colditz, & Proctor, 2012).

In response to calls to accelerate the movement of effective interventions into widespread practice, there is an emerging science of D & I aimed at shortening the "translational research gap" (Institute of Medicine, 2001). Theories undergirding this science of D & I seek to explain the components of successful D & I and the factors that influence the execution of these strategies. *Why* and *how* do organizations learn about new practices, commit to trying them, develop plans to introduce them, seek fidelity to the prescribed components, weave new practices into ongoing operations, and maintain new practices over time? And with what results over time and across various populations?

There are a plethora of frameworks and models that currently shape D & I research. Tabak, Khoong, Chambers, and Brownson (2012) identified 61 frameworks designed to guide these activities. This overwhelming number stems from the fact that a complex array of factors and nonlinear iterative processes are involved in the successful uptake, implementation, and maintenance of a new intervention in an organizational setting. Several authors have summarized four major theories that generally inform these frameworks and D & I research activities: (a) diffusion of innovation, (b) stages of change, (c) persuasive communication, and (d) social marketing (Brownson et al., 2012).

Yet the theoretical developments behind the science of D & I seem rather chaotic at the moment, in part due to the newness of this field. Future developments must involve the identification of the most useful theoretical guideposts and a thinning of the possible conceptual models. A body of knowledge about successful D & I will not develop as quickly without a firmer theoretical foundation. Having a theory-based implementation strategy is as important as having a theory-based intervention (Proctor et al., 2009).

It is also clear that theories have become inclusive of multiple levels of influence—from the genetic to the larger socioeconomic contexts. In fact, the Social Ecological Model is probably the most frequently mentioned across all chapters. Yet authors also describe how infrequently this model, with its multiple layers of factors affecting an individual situation, is fully considered in research or practice. Testing a full range of hypotheses derived from such a multilevel framework seems undoable, given the limited nature of data and the available analytic techniques.

Still, new developments in the field of system dynamics (SD) offer promise. SD is a mathematical modeling technique that is used to understand complex issues and problems. SD was originally developed in the corporate sector to understand industrial processes, and it is now spreading throughout the public health, medical, and social sectors to allow more complete analysis of the implications of policy, funding, and behavioral change (Hovmand, 2012). SD models address the issue of reciprocal causation and time lags, which are issues at the heart of gerontology research.

Although SD may be more of a method than a theory, it is an expression of systems theory, and the use of this method signals a clear recognition of the dynamic behavior of complex systems. Modeling involves change over time, time delays between cause-and-effect, nonlinear relationships, interactions, positive and negative feedback loops—as well as the idea that the behavior of the whole cannot be explained by the behavior of the parts. These complexities probably underlie many of the conundrums elucidated by researchers studying age-friendly communities, family caregiving, health promotion, and service utilization. Going forward, theory development in gerontology will require the elucidation of the complex, dynamic nature of the issues that are relevant to older adults and aging societies.

REFERENCES

Balas, E. A., & Boren, S. A. (2000). *Yearbook of medical informatics 2000: Patient-centered systems* (pp. 65–70). Stuttgart, Germany: Schattauer.

Brownson, R., Colditz, G., & Proctor, E. (2012). *Dissemination and implementation research in health: Translating science to practice.* New York, NY: Oxford University Press.

Hovmand, P. (2014). *Community-based system dynamics.* New York, NY: Springer Publishing Company.

Institute of Medicine. (2001). *Crossing the quality chasm: A new health system for the 21st century.* Washington, DC: National Academies Press.

Proctor, E., Landsverk J., Aarons, G., Chambers, D., Glisson C., & Mittman B. (2009). Implementation research in mental health services: An emerging science with conceptual, methodological, and training challenges. *Administration and Policy in Mental Health, 36*, 24–34.

Tabak, R., Khoong, E., Chambers, D., & Brownson, R. (2012). Bridging research and practice: Models for dissemination and implementation research. *American Journal of Preventive Medicine, 43*, 337–350.

Yeatts, D. E., Crow, T., & Folts, E. (1992). Service use among low-income minority elderly: Strategies for overcoming barriers. *The Gerontologist, 32*(1), 24–32. doi: 10.1093/geront/32.1.24

CHAPTER 21

Aging in Place

Andrew E. Scharlach and Keith Diaz Moore

In recent years, there has been substantial attention to aging in place in the empirical literature, as well as in popular media, with the number of published articles on aging in place increasing markedly in the years since 2000 (Vasunilashorn, Steinman, Liebig, & Pynoos, 2012). Interest in aging in place has spurred numerous programs (e.g., Villages and NORC Supportive Services Programs), organizations (e.g., Center for Aging in Place and National Aging in Place Council), and policy initiatives (e.g., Community Innovations for Aging in Place Initiative in the 2006 reauthorization of the Older Americans Act; Geboy, Diaz Moore, & Smith, 2012). As embodied in public policy, aging in place is generally portrayed as a personally and societally desirable alternative to costly nursing home placement, for example, "remaining living in the community, with some level of independence, rather than in residential care" (Davey, de Joux, Nana, & Arcus, 2004, p. 13).

It is widely reported that the vast majority of elderly and near elderly individuals say that they want to "age in place" (AARP, 2005). And yet, what exactly is meant by "aging in place"? What are its theoretical and conceptual roots? Is aging in place inherently beneficial, or even desirable? Is aging in place best understood as a goal, or rather as a process? What factors are associated with the ability to age in place? And, who gets to age where they want, and who doesn't? Motivated by questions such as these, this chapter examines the theoretical and conceptual foundations of the concept of aging in place, as well as implications for future research and theory development.

■ WHAT IS AGING IN PLACE?

Aging in place has been defined as "individuals growing old in their own homes, with an emphasis on using environmental modifications to compensate for limitations and disabilities" (Alley, Liebig, Pynoos, Banerjee, & Choi, 2007, p. 2). Greenfield (2012), similarly, defines aging in place as "being able to remain in one's current residence even when faced with increasing need for support because of life changes, such as declining health, widowhood, or loss of income" (p. 1). A close reading of conceptualizations such as these, however, reveals a number of potentially problematic assumptions regarding the nature of aging in place.

A first assumption is that "aging" within aging in place refers to functional decline, or, perhaps more broadly, to loss. However, assumptions such as this ignore the multifaceted nature of the life course, examined more closely in the following sections of this chapter. Furthermore, the proposition "in" linguistically cues that place is viewed simply as a setting within which aging, or functional decline, occurs; "treating place as a mere 'container' and 'older people' as a homogeneous category" (Wiles et al., 2012, p. 358).

A second assumption is that "place" refers to one's current home or apartment, and that staying within the same physical setting will inevitably have beneficial effects. However, relocation also has benefits (Golant, 2003), prompting many older persons to decide to leave their existing homes, whether to downsize, move close to family, or for amenity destinations. This is apt to be especially true when one's current residence is inadequate to meet one's needs or of poor quality, whether because of deferred maintenance or a less than desirable neighborhood. There is growing evidence that many disabled elders do not receive the most appropriate care within their current residences (Gitlin, 2000), with some estimates that the majority of functionally impaired older persons in the United States have unmet needs for assistance (Shea et al., 2003). Byrnes (2011), for example, found that low-income residents welcomed public housing as better than their long-term residences.

More recently, the concept of "place" in aging in place has been broadened to include the neighborhood or community (e.g., AARP, 2011). However, many of the same characteristics that put older people at risk for disabling chronic conditions (e.g., being poor, 75 years and older, female, living alone because of widowhood, having less than a high school education) also increase the likelihood that their environments will be environmentally deficient (Golant, 2008). Aggregation of these older households may well lead to economic and social instability in neighborhoods. In short, aging in place for these individuals may directly and indirectly exacerbate their lack of safety, comfort, and independence as they age.

Another point of note is the normative assumption that older persons ought to be able to live where and how they wish. The Centers for Disease Control, for example, defines aging in place as "the ability to live in one's own home and community safely, independently, and comfortably, regardless of age, income, or ability level" [http://www.cdc.gov/healthyplaces/terminology.html], a definition which has also been adopted by AARP (2011). Although there is a social justice dimension embedded in definitions such as this, questions arise regarding older adults' unique entitlement to such options. Furthermore, a predominant focus of public policy incentives for aging in place has been as a strategy for reducing public long-term care expenditures associated with residential care, rather than enhancing the well-being of older adults, their families, or their communities.

Based on this brief analysis, it is apparent that there is a need for a more conceptually grounded, nuanced, and useful conceptualization of aging in place. As we have seen, current conceptualizations of aging in place are rooted in the simplistic idea that aging—understood as functional loss—is best addressed within one's long-term residence, "place." However, such conceptualizations ignore the multiple meanings of place, and the possibility that living out one's life in the same home or apartment is neither inherently desirable nor beneficial. Furthermore, the relationship between person and environment is quite dynamic; aging is not homogeneous and place is not simply a static location.

Thus, it is worth reconsidering what is meant by aging in place. For the purposes of this chapter, we conceptualize aging in place as a process rather than a goal; we, therefore, prefer the interconnected term "aging in place," rather than seeing "aging" as something that occurs in a conceptually distinct "place." It seems obvious to us that everyone "ages in place," in that aging (i.e., change over time) occurs in physical and social space. Simply put, we exist in space and time; furthermore, people change over time, as do their physical and social environments. The relevant issue is whether (and how) aging in place results in developmentally salient goals, as individuals, their environments, their goals, and the person–environment (P–E) transactions and processes designed to achieve them, all change over time.

■ THE NATURE OF PLACE

Aging in place as a concept has its theoretical roots within environmental gerontology, which is concerned with "the description, explanation, and modification or optimization of the relation between the elderly person and his or her environment" (Wahl & Weisman, 2003, p. 616). The conceptual cornerstone of environmental gerontology is Lawton and Nahemow's (1973) Ecological Model of Aging, otherwise known as the "competence–press model" of aging (Diaz Moore, 2005; Kendig, 2003). This model is rooted in Kurt Lewin's (1936) field theory equation, $B = f(P,E)$, meaning that observed behavior (B) is a function of both the Person (P) and the Environment (E).

The Ecological Model of Aging theorizes that "behavior is a function of the competence of the individual and the environmental press of the situation" (Lawton, 1982, p. 26). Individuals of a higher competence level are hypothesized to achieve successful behavioral outcomes within a wider range of environmental press than are individuals of diminished capacity. A corollary to this model becomes the environmental docility hypothesis which states: "The less competent the individual, the greater the impact of environmental factors on that individual" (Lawton, 1980, p. 14). Thus, research adopting this perspective typically has focused on the fit between a range of personal competence and environmental press (or "demand quality") as they relate to some desired behavioral, or sometimes affective, outcome. A classic example of a misfit of competence and press is excess disability (Brody, Kleban, Lawton, & Silverman, 1971), wherein elderly residing in a skilled nursing facility may very well be able to make their own meals, for instance, but learn to depend on the meal services provided by the organization. Through the lack of challenge and of doing, the resident may initially experience frustration (a negative affective response) but over time learns to be helpless in this regard, thereby realigning competence and press through lowered competence.

Rubinstein and de Medeiros (2004, p. 64) critique models of P–E fit such as the Ecological Model by arguing that "P–E fit can be altered by the elder's consciousness of the life world, by how the older person experiences the self, by how the person individually interprets cultural meaning, and the importance of place in later life." They go on to suggest two roles of culture in the P–E transaction: first, as an originating frame of reference for a person as to what is expected; second, as an interpretive lens based on past experiences used to assess ongoing transactions and inform subsequent actions. To be fair to Lawton, this may very well be what he was attempting to articulate in extending Lewin's equation to read as $B = f(P,E, P \times E)$, where $P \times E$ is the "combination of subjective experience and external environment (that) may have an effect on behavior that is *in addition to* and *independent of* either the person or the 'objective' environment." However, this was never a core focus of his research. As he stated, "The language of process, temporal state, and development must be supplied by those more gifted than I" (Lawton, 1989a, p. 57).

This recognition of the meaningful aspects of environments led to an "interpretive" turn in environmental gerontology wherein the experience of environments was seen as socially shaped and constructed, as reflected in the classic ethnographic work of Gubrium (1975) and continuing with Rowles (1983), Rubinstein (1989), and Howell (1983). As Gubrium (1978, p. 28) wrote:

> I have found that who or what behavior is spoken of or recorded as senile depends on place.... By place, I mean geographic locations...that are taken for granted to have certain meanings on particular occasions when specific people are gathered there.

In this way, place came to be seen as a sociophysical phenomenon (Wahl & Lang, 2004; Weisman, Chaudhury, & Moore, 2000), encompassing three premises: (a) places combine both a physical–spatial as well as social–cultural dimension; (b) places are socially constructed and socially shaped physical environments; and (c) places are dynamic and show both change and stability over time.

This dynamic understanding of place necessitates a different and more complex conceptualization of aging in place, one that sees people and their environments as inseparable, so that no physical environment can be understood without its social dimensions. Aging in place is better viewed as an ongoing negotiation wherein both the aging experience and the place experience are dynamic and interact with one another. In other words, we age in relationship to the places we inhabit, and our experience of place is affected by our aging experience. Cutchin (2003, p. 1078), for instance, defines aging in place as "a complex set of processes that is part of the universal and ongoing emergence of the person–place whole."

Ecological Framework of Place

The ecological framework of place (EFP; Diaz Moore, 2014) offers a heuristic for considering the negotiation of place within a life-course perspective. Diaz Moore (2014, p. 184) defines place as "a milieu involving people ('place participants'), the physical setting, and the program of the place, all catalyzed by situated human activity and fully acknowledging that all four may change over time." Place as a construct emphasizes the socially constructed, meaningful aspects of our experience and the role those meanings play in the rich tapestry of human variety. People include the individual, but also may be conceptualized at multiple levels of aggregation (group, organizational, and cultural). The physical setting certainly includes objective sensory (e.g., lighting) and spatial (e.g., openness) properties and the systems that shape them (e.g., enclosure and furnishings); however, we must also understand that architecture is purposeful, and thus as much as people bring intentionality to a place, so does the physical setting.

Sometimes the program for which a setting was designed is no longer available as the setting changes over time, or may not be consistent with the changing needs and goals of human inhabitants. Perhaps such incongruence of intentionality is best recognized when settings constrain our ability to further our goals, such as a room proving very small for a group, or a house designed to accommodate the needs of young families that no longer fits the needs of the same post-parental family. The EFP also makes clear that any given setting exists within a system of other settings, which may be conceptualized at different scales (proximate, building/site, neighborhood/community, and settlement). Thus, the framework accommodates the possibility of a home environment perfectly enabling optimal functioning yet situated in a neighborhood whose characteristics may thwart that same functioning beyond the confines of the home environment. For example, one might invest in an award-winning visitable home (Smith,

Rayer, & Smith, 2008)—providing grade-level entry, an entry-level bedroom and bathroom, and the like—but if it is placed in a neighborhood without meaningful destinations within walking distance or well-maintained, accessible sidewalks on both sides of the street, it may well be that independent mobility remains compromised.

The concept of the "program" of place is perhaps the most difficult to understand, yet program is a powerful construct in understanding the negotiation of aging and place. It is a term commonly found within both environmental psychology (Auburn & Barnes, 2006; Barker, 1968; Canter, 1991; Chawla, 2007) and architectural practice (Burry, 2013), in both cases referring to expectations linked with a setting. The concept of program reflects the idea that there are socially shared expectations associated with a place that both inform action and then shape the subsequent interpretation of the resulting transaction. In this way, program captures the influence of culture, which Rubinstein and de Medeiros (2004) suggest has two roles in regard to place: (a) as an originating frame of reference colored by assumptions about space, language, narration, and expectations of self and others; and (b) as a mediating, or interpretive, lens for ongoing transactions, shaped by an individual's past experiences, social status, and the like. This conceptual realm does not exist in Lawton's Ecological Model of Aging, yet there is a wealth of research indicating that the negotiated nature of meaning plays a significant role in the quality of life for older adults (De Medeiros, 2013; Rowles & Bernard, 2013).

Human activity is at the heart of the EFP, for it is through human (trans)action that places become experienced and by which people attribute certain qualities to those place experiences and hence to the places themselves. We find human activity central to numerous theories in developmental science, dating back to the Ecological Systems Theory of Urie Bronfenbrenner (1977, p. 515), wherein he notes, "so that (the) substantive aspect (the nature and purpose of the task) is not overlooked, I use the term activity rather than behavior to identify this essential feature of the microsystem." The EFP also uses activity in the same way, thus reflecting that human agency is an underlying presumption of the model.

Time is a critical if often overlooked factor in shaping meaning and hence one's overall place experience. The other dimensions of place—people, physical setting, program, and activity—all change in relation to time. People's abilities, motivations, assessments, social networks, the organizational structures within which they participate, and cultural norms may all change with time. There are certainly diurnal changes in the physical setting of places (e.g., at night we have lights on) as well as more longitudinal changes associated with entropy and other developmental processes affecting individuals and their environments (e.g., increased maintenance needs). Programs, reflecting our shared expectations, change as well within days and over the span of years as observed in changes in human activity.

This suggests a more nuanced and dynamic meaning for both what is meant by P–E fit as well as for the main topic of this chapter, aging in place. This approach transcends the assumed static nature of place inherent in many definitions of aging in place and the assumed linkage of the aging experience with "loss." In considering the concept of P–E fit, persons must be thought of as not just a set of competencies, but also their intentions, their worldview, their moment in time, and the like must be considered. As to the environment, it cannot be seen as simply offering press, but also resources. Additionally, rethinking environment as place highlights that such press and resources not only stem from the objective characteristics of the physical setting, but also from the socially shared expectations embedded in the program. P–E fit, therefore, must be considered a negotiation between the intentionality of a place and what it is crafted to afford people to do, on the one hand, and the individual projects and underlying goals of its place participants, on the other. These points imply a more robust approach to aging in place, resting on the following three assumptions:

1. The aging experience occurs within worlds of meaning involving an ongoing negotiation between person and place.
2. These worlds of meaning are catalyzed by human activity, which we assume is purposeful if not always successful in achieving its intentions.
3. Time is a critical dimension in calibrating the frames employed for shaping the understanding and subsequent meaning of place.

We share with Cutchin (2003, p. 1077) the recognition that "aging-in-place is a complex geographical process mediated by institutions and other social forces." We also share with Wiles et al. (2012) the idea that the meaningful content of aging in place—which they identify as sense of connection, feelings of security and familiarity, sense of identity furthered by independence, autonomy, caring relationships, and meaningful roles to play—is at the heart of the phenomenon and extends well beyond the home environment. Rather than aging being equated with loss, we view the aging experience as rich with meaning. Rather than place as a "container," we view place as the dynamic, socially constructed and socially shared aspects of experience. Our aging experience is, in part, shaped by the systems of places we have experienced over the life course, and because of the powerful role of expectation, to some degree shaped by those we anticipate to potentially experience in the future. Thus, aging is not simply a phenomenon occurring within a setting nor is place just a container, and both are always impacted by time. Over and through time, there are ongoing transactions occurring amongst aging individuals and the places they experience.

■ THE DEVELOPMENTAL CONTEXT OF AGING IN PLACE

Since the turn of the 21st century, much theorizing within environmental gerontology has attempted to make meaningful linkages with developmental science (Diaz Moore, 2014). At the heart of these advancements are processes (i.e., by what mechanism[s] do people negotiate with place?), outcomes (i.e., what experiential attributes are of interest or the most salient?), and the influence of time (i.e., how do these processes and outcomes change with age?).

Processes

Constructivist theory provides a useful perspective for understanding the processes that guide aging in place, seeing interactions between persons and their environments as intentional, meaningful, and meaning producing. From this perspective, individuals and their environments can be seen as engaging in an ongoing process of mutual adaptation, reflecting the processes of assimilation and accommodation identified by Piaget (1932), who conceived human psychological development as a process of active and intentional engagement with external reality. Assimilation involves the enhancement of existing cognitive schema through syntonic P–E experiences, whereas accommodation involves the development of new cognitive schema through dystonic P–E experiences.

Informed by this perspective, Golant (2011) used the term "assimilation" to refer to individuals' efforts to alter their environments (e.g., by modifying the environment or relocating) in order to preserve internal cognitive structures, and "accommodation" to refer to internally focused strategies such as altering one's aspirations or changing comparison standards (e.g., "others have it worse"). The efficacy of such strategies will be impacted by both personal and physical resources, and the existing opportunity structures associated with each situation.

Objectives

The definition or delimitation of the most salient P–E fit goals for older persons has been a preoccupation of environmental gerontologists and other social scientists for some time (e.g., Calkins & Weisman, 1999; Fleming, 2011; Kader & Diaz Moore, 2015; Lawton et al., 2000). Many of the goals that have been identified can be encapsulated by two fundamental constructs, reflecting underlying dimensions of human behavior: (a) connection and (a) agency. These two constructs have been expressed in a variety of forms, most notably in the efforts of mid-20th-century clinical and social psychologists to conceptualize and measure beneficial aspects of interpersonal relationships: connectedness (warmth) and assertiveness (dominance) (Leary, 1957); affiliation and autonomy (Benjamin, 1974); cohesion and adaptability (Olson et al., 1979).

Interestingly, similar dimensions have been used in conceptualizing social environments and P–E fit. Moos and Otto for example, assessed social environments in terms of relationship and personal growth, virtually identical to the constructs of connection and agency, while also adding a third dimension of system maintenance (Moos & Otto, 1972). Lawton identified the similar dimensions of support, stimulation, and maintenance (Lawton, 1989b). More recently, Wahl, Iwarsson, and Oswald (2012) identified experience-driven belonging and behavior-driven agency as P–E processes that link person, place, and the outcomes of aging well, which are postulated as identity, autonomy, and well-being. Golant's (2011) Theory of Residential Normalcy suggested that two desired experiential states within what he terms "residential normalcy" are comfort and mastery, conceptualized again similar to connection and agency.

Integrated Developmental Model

Drawing upon these various theoretical traditions regarding aging and the environment, Scharlach and his colleagues (e.g., Scharlach, 2009; Scharlach & Lehning, in press) have identified an integrated developmental model of aging friendliness, which incorporates six interrelated attributes of P–E fit: (a) continuity, (b) compensation, (c) control, (d) connection, (e) contribution, and (f) challenge/comfort. These six constructs are hypothesized to represent developmentally salient attributes of P–E interactions in later life that emerge through a constructive process of assimilation and accommodation. We now examine in greater detail the developmental salience of each of these six attributes.

CONTINUITY

Maintaining continuity with regard to personal identity and self-construct is especially relevant in later life, in the face of a variety of forces that threaten to undermine one's sense of self and disconnect a person from much that previously has given life meaning (Hazan, 2011). With age, there is lessened focus on changing one's self (e.g., through the acquisition of new roles and material possessions), and increased focus on maintaining one's existing self-construct (e.g., in the face of potential physical threats and social/environmental barriers; Ouwehand, de Ridder, & Bensing, 2007). The ability to maintain a relatively stable sense of self, supported by self-preserving activities and contexts, is associated with life satisfaction in later life. However, maintaining lifelong interests and activities that support one's sense of self can become more challenging in later life, not only as a result of age-related reductions in functional ability, but also because environments are not well designed to enhance the functioning of older community members. In order to preserve a relatively stable self-construct, individuals may modify their activities, their aspirations, and even their constructions of reality (e.g., Herzog & Markus, 1999).

The concept of place attachment also reflects ways in which environmental continuity can act as a buffer or resource in its own right (Rowles & Bernard, 2013). Rowles and Watkins (2003) suggest four ways in which place may assist continuity: history, habit, heart, and hearth. History refers to maintaining links to the past through environmental interventions such as photographs. Habit captures the rhythms and routines of familiarity, which scaffold the maintenance of function. Heart suggests how we imbue elements in the setting with meaning. Finally, hearth suggests the role home has as anchor for orientation of our social selves through ownership and belonging.

COMPENSATION

Adaptations in self and environment are likely to be required as age-related changes make it more difficult to preserve one's self-concept and achieve meaningful goals. Compensation efforts can include receiving assistance with tasks that can no longer be performed independently, relying on assistive devices, ambient assistive living technologies, environmental modifications, or other sources of support.

Compensation can also involve behavioral changes, including developing new abilities or finding alternative means of achieving goals, as well as adjustments in aspirations and social reference standards to reflect changing circumstances (Romo et al., 2013). In accordance with Paul and Margret Baltes's Selection, Optimization, and Compensation (SOC) model of adaptation (Baltes & Baltes, 1990), compensation is enhanced through a process that includes selection of the domains of functioning that are most important to achieving valued personal goals, and optimization of the capacity for achieving those goals. Utilization of SOC strategies has been associated with a variety of salutary outcomes, including life satisfaction, positive emotions, and psychological well-being, even after controlling for age, health, and personality characteristics (Freund, 2008).

CONTROL

Whereas compensation focuses on the need for support, control focuses on the actual and perceived ability to effect change in one's self and one's environment in order to achieve one's aims, as a fundamental objective in and of itself. Opportunities to exert control over one's self and one's environment as one ages may be especially important in the context of physical and social environments that pervasively undermine autonomy and self-control in later life (Wahl et al., 2012).

Control theory posits that individuals will actively strive to modify their environments and themselves in order to maximize goal achievement and minimize distress (Schulz & Heckhausen, 1996). Two types of control are posited: primary control and secondary control (Heckhausen, Wrosch, & Schulz, 2010). Primary control targets the external world, and involves actively attempting to manipulate physical or social environments in order to attain one's goals. Secondary control involves internal psychological processes, such as adopting more attainable goals, strategic social comparisons, less-demanding comparisons with one's earlier self, and self-protective causal attributions (Heckhausen et al., 2010), in an effort to maintain positive self-esteem in the face of failures in primary control efforts. Secondary control processes tend to increase throughout life, whereas primary control peaks in midlife and declines thereafter, perhaps in response to the lack of adequate external options for resolving complex age-related challenges.

Control can also be expressed through proactive efforts to prevent or alleviate anticipated future threats to P–E fit, as suggested by the Proactivity Model of Successful Aging (Kahana & Kahana, 1996). Age-related preparatory actions (e.g., health promotion, financial planning, skill acquisition, and investing in long-term relationships) are associated with better quality of life years later (Kahana, Kelley-Moore, & Kahana, 2012; Prenda & Lachman, 2001).

CONNECTION

Elders generally strive to remain socially engaged as they grow older, even in the face of substantial personal and contextual barriers. In accordance with socioemotional selectivity theory (Carstensen, 1993), meaningful interpersonal relationships assume increased importance closer to the end of life, especially when those relationships reinforce a positive sense of self. To the extent that older persons believe that future time is limited, they are more likely to manage their time and energy so as to maximize positive interactions with familiar interpersonal contacts rather than seeking potentially stressful new contacts or information (Scheibe & Carstensen, 2010).

Maintaining meaningful social relationships, while more important in later life, also can become more challenging as a result of a variety of factors: health problems and disabling conditions that can restrict mobility and interpersonal communication (Weir, Meisner, & Baker, 2010); a depletion of social networks caused by death, illness, and retirement; ageist and disablist norms that contribute to social isolation by fostering feelings of inadequacy and invisibility; and unsupportive physical environments that can limit mobility and restrict access.

CONTRIBUTION

A "contributory orientation" has been proposed as an important component of aging-related psychosocial development and adaptation (Midlarsky, Kahana, & Belser, 2015).

Prosocial activities support physical and psychological well-being through a number of mechanisms that may be especially salient in later life. At a time when declining personal capacity and dependency-inducing physical and social contexts foster subjective experiences of marginalization, purposelessness, and helplessness, meaningful activities can reinforce a greater sense of mastery, personal control, and self-efficacy, along with a renewed sense of meaning and purpose. At the same time, helping others can promote physical and cognitive stimulation, enhance social bonds, evoke social approval, and increase other social and psychological resources (Gottlieb & Gillespie, 2008). In so doing, contributory activities can help one to sustain a positive self-concept in the face of threats caused by changing capacity, lack of clearly defined role structures, and an ageist society that devalues individuals based on their age and ability.

There is extensive evidence regarding the potential benefits of volunteer participation in later life, including higher levels of life satisfaction, better physical health, better mental health, lower utilization of health services, and decreased mortality risk (Gottlieb & Gillespie, 2008; Luoh & Herzog, 2002; Musick & Wilson, 2003). Beneficial contributions can take a variety of paths: formal volunteer activities through charitable organizations, religious or cultural institutions, and social or athletic clubs; engagement in civil society and formal civic governance structures; informal assistance to friends or neighbors; and care for spouses, partners, and other family members.

CHALLENGE/COMFORT

According to hormesis theory (Rattan, 2008), organisms, from the cellular level to social organizations, require ongoing stimulation in order to grow and flourish, and even just to survive. Whereas high levels of environmental demands or other external threats can have potentially deleterious short-term consequences, smaller intensity demands can stimulate growth, resilience, and coping ability. Through a process of stress conditioning, manageable challenges can foster positive compensatory responses that strengthen an organism's ability to adapt constructively when faced subsequently with more intense stressors. Thus, humans show a strong preference for tasks that extend or challenge their existing abilities, preferring tasks with intermediate levels of difficulty rather than those they can easily accomplish (Nimrod & Kleiber, 2007).

As noted by Golant (2011) and others, comfort and security are fundamental human needs, and situations that are excessively challenging can produce distress and other deleterious outcomes, as hypothesized by the competence–press model developed by Lawton and Nahemow (1973). However, physical and social environments seldom provide the optimum levels of stimulation and growth appropriate for aging bodies and minds, potentially inducing excess dependency and learned helplessness. Disuse, rather than actual disease, appears to be a greater contributor to cardiovascular vulnerability, musculoskeletal fragility, and premature frailty in later life (Bortz, 2009).

■ PUTTING THE PIECES TOGETHER: AGING IN TIME AND SPACE

Let us summarize the basic premises to this point:

1. The concept of aging in place has evolved from the simple homeostatic notion of P–E fit to a more dynamic conceptualization that considers people, places, the programs they embody, constructive selective and accommodative processes, and the goals that motivate the entire enterprise, as they all evolve over time.
2. Aging in place, at its most basic level, could be said to reflect the influence of time (age) on individuals (P), physical and social contexts (E), processes used to negotiate the interface between individuals and contexts ($P \times E$), and the purposes of those negotiations (goals, preferences, priorities, etc.).
3. From this perspective, aging in place is best conceived as an adaptive process rather than as a normative goal. The "goal," if one can be said to exist, is the production of constructive (e.g., developmentally salient) outcomes through transactional processes that transcend simple notions of separable aging and place phenomena.

4. People "construct" physical and social environments (whether by actually physically building them, intentionally selecting them, adapting them, or adapting to them) in a purposeful manner—that is, in order to achieve certain goals. In other words, it is erroneous to assume that places do not have purpose, as that obscures the very real negotiation that occurs between people and place.

5. The six central attributes of the aging experience—continuity, compensation, control, connection, contribution, and challenge—all are impacted by agency, ability, and subsequent activity in relation to the facility of the place or system of places. Places, therefore, may either mediate or moderate where the individual aging experience may fall in relation to these six attributes, with time having a direct effect on both the aging individual and on place.

■ THEORETICAL AND EMPIRICAL IMPLICATIONS

The perspective on aging in place described here suggests a variety of areas for further research and theoretical development regarding the dynamic nature of P–E transactions over time. Lines of research likely to prove especially productive include the following: temporal variations in P × E fit; factors affecting P–E fit; the utility of behavioral economic approaches; contextual variations in residential preferences and behaviors; disparities in the ability to achieve the desired P–E fit; factors associated with actual relocation behaviors; individual and environmental outcomes; and intervention effectiveness.

Temporal Variations in P × E Fit

Based on the integrated developmental model, one can imagine developing a person–place profile, wherein the aging-in-place experience may be assessed from high to low with regard to each of the six attributes at various points in time. Qualitative research designs could help one to develop individual-level salience profiles, specifying the relative importance of each attribute in particular places at particular times. P–E fit could then be assessed based on the extent of fit or misfit between an individual's ratings of salience and actual experience. For instance, it may be that one may be aging in place where five of six constructs are highly supported and achieved, but if the one not supported, such as connection, is most valued and desired, the aging-in-place experience may still be wanting.

For heuristic purposes, Figure 21.1 illustrates the potential relationships among time and the person, place, and attributes of P–E fit. Although presented in two dimensions, the four factors are considered to have mutually reciprocal relationships that change over time.

Findings from in-depth case studies could serve as the basis for cross-sectional research examining individual differences in the relative importance of each attribute in particular places at particular times. Longitudinal and cross-sequential research could examine cohort/age-related variations in P–E fit. For example, which aspects of place, positive as well as negative, become more salient with age, and which aspects become less salient? To what extent do these patterns conform to the predictions of the integrated developmental model presented here? Does negotiating the most appropriate combination of P–E attributes assume greater salience in later life, as suggested by Wahl et al. (2012)?

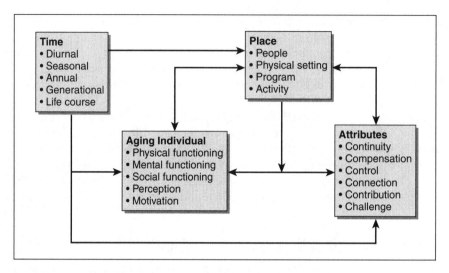

FIGURE 21.1   A heuristic of aging in place.

Factors Affecting P–E Fit

The EFP identifies a variety of factors that are hypothesized to affect P–E fit, including characteristics of individuals (e.g., physical functioning, mental functioning, social functioning, sensory functioning, and motivation), places (e.g., physical setting, people, program, and activity), and time (e.g., diurnal, seasonal, annual, generational, and life course). Utilizing the person–place profile model or a similar framework, research is needed to examine the relative contributions of these various factors to perceptions of P–E fit. Regarding aging-in-place preferences specifically, research is needed regarding the factors that differentiate the 10% to 20% of individuals who do not express a desire to live in the same residence for the rest of their lives, and the considerations that enter into their preferences. Also needed is longitudinal research regarding how desires to relocate or not, and the reasons for wanting to do so, change with age, including how the push and pull factors of places vary over time.

The Utility of Behavioral Economic Approaches

Behavioral economics approaches (e.g., utility theory, production theory, and prospect theory) provide useful frameworks for understanding residential preferences and behaviors in later life. Prospect theory, for example, suggests that people of any age would be reluctant to give up a current residence that was reasonably fulfilling, even for an alternative that had a substantial likelihood of being more fulfilling. In addition to examining actual relocation behavior, residential choices could be examined using "willingness to pay" or other methods that compare the perceived value of various possible scenarios (e.g., the current situation, possible future scenarios in the existing residence, and possible future scenarios in alternative residences). In short, the relatively young field of behavioral economics has intriguing potential contributions to make to gerontology (McConnell, 2013), but we should also not be shy in suggesting that the lifespan perspective and gerontological theories may well prove insightful to behavioral economics.

Contextual Variations in Residential Preferences and Behaviors

It is surprising to note that little is known about ways in which P–E fit, and the associated desire to stay in place, vary by cohort, culture, and other contextual variables. For example, the meanings of "home" are apt to vary across cohorts, across cultures, among immigrant groups, by immigrant generation, and other contextual factors (Diaz Moore & Ekerdt, 2011). Because baby boomers, for example, experienced familial relations that were more fluid and less permanent, with greater incidence of divorce, varied family structures, and a reduced focus on family cohesion, their preferences for achieving the goal of aging in place may be less intense than their elders.

Disparities in the Ability to Achieve the Desired P–E Fit

Further research also is needed regarding structural factors that can affect personal needs and desires, the adequacy of environmental conditions, and the ability to live where one wants. For example, higher socioeconomic status generally is associated with a greater ability to stay put, but also greater options for relocation. It seems likely that some people cannot afford to stay in place, whereas others cannot afford to move. These differences are apt to reflect lifelong patterns of structural inequality that affect available options, and alter the probability that those options will result in constructive or deleterious outcomes.

Relocation Behaviors

Despite extensive research documenting the preferences of middle-aged and older adults to continue to live in their current residences for as long as possible, there is considerably less research examining actual relocation choices, whether from one's existing residence or from one's neighborhood or community. Of particular interest is cross-sectional research regarding age differences in relocation behavior and in reasons for relocating (Smith, 2014). How much of the variance can be explained by individual-level health and functioning factors? Longitudinal research could also help to elucidate the extent to which actual relocation behavior conforms to expressed preferences.

Individual and Environmental Outcomes

Observational and naturalistic research is needed regarding the specific outcomes that are associated with variations in transactions between individuals and their environments, including the extent to which particular aging-in-place scenarios actually help one to achieve particular ends at particular points in time. Particular attention is needed to the contributions of potential mediating and moderating factors, as well as adaptive processes in response to person or environmental changes over time.

Intervention Effectiveness

A final focus concerns the development and testing of interventions designed to promote aging in place. Despite an explosion of programs and organizations promising to promote aging in place (e.g., Villages, NORC Supportive Services Programs, Community Innovations for Aging in Place, Community Partnerships for Older Adults, and AdvantAge Initiative), the evidence base for the effectiveness of such initiatives is meager at best. Considerably more research and theoretical development are needed regarding the actual impact of interventions on individual and environmental well-being, and on the ability of aging individuals and their changing environments to produce developmentally salient attributes. We need to consider what outcomes we are truly seeking, and whether we are adequately measuring intended developmentally salient attributes in relation to specific interventions.

In addition, this approach suggests that there will need to be a diversity of program and architectural interventions to best advance the aging-in-place agenda for the widest spectrum of older adults. With the current rate of growth in the older segment of society, there is great potential for creative entrepreneurialism to promote better aging-in-place outcomes, including facilitating the six developmentally salient attributes identified here. We hope that creative communities may explore the aging-in-place implications of interventions such as the following: accessory dwelling units for fostering a more sustainable economic model of neighborhood residence; elementary schools as sites for older adult services and opportunities for contribution; retrofitting neighborhoods with sidewalks and mid-block cross walks; and innovative destinations such as a café-branch library with a Wi-Fi hotspot.

■ CONCLUSION

In this chapter, we have attempted to illustrate that aging in place is richer and more dynamic than simply understanding aging as loss and place as a static physical environment. Given the diversity of the human life course, aging in place is best understood not as a single, universal goal, but rather as an adaptive process of ongoing person–place transactions over time, as suggested by the EFP. Central to this process are six person–environmental attributes reflected in an integrated developmental approach. Earlier experiences of place and anticipated future experiences together shape our current negotiations with place as well as the attributes that emerge from those experiences.

We believe that the model presented in this chapter has potential to move existing theory and research beyond homeostatic, cross-sectional understandings of P–E fit to a more textured approach that embraces the ongoing negotiation between person and place occurring continuously over the life span. In so doing, this approach may help to deepen our understanding of both human development and of place, in temporal context. In this regard, we share the belief that "Time and place therefore are matters of substance, not error; and to understand human development, one must appreciate how variables associated with person, place and time coalesce" (Lerner, 2007, p. 6).

REFERENCES

AARP. (2005). *Beyond 50.05 survey*. Washington, DC: AARP. Retrieved from http://assets.aarp.org/rgcenter/il/beyond_50_05_survey.pdf

AARP. (2011). *Aging in place: A state survey of livability policies and practices*. Washington, DC: AARP Public Policy Institute. Retrieved from http://assets.aarp.org/rgcenter/ppi/liv-com/aging-in-place-2011-full.pdf

Alley, D., Liebig, P., Pynoos, J., Banerjee, T., & Choi, I. H. (2007). Creating elder-friendly communities: Preparations for an aging society. *Journal of Gerontological Social Work, 49*(1–2), 1–18.

Auburn, T., & Barnes, R. (2006). Producing place: A neo-Schutzian perspective on the 'psychology of place'. *Journal of Environmental Psychology, 26*(1), 38–50.

Baltes, P. B., & Baltes, M. M. (1990). Psychological perspectives on successful aging: The model of selective optimization with compensation. In P. B. Baltes & M. M. Baltes (Eds.), *Successful aging: Perspectives from the behavioral sciences* (pp. 1–34). New York, NY: Cambridge University Press.

Barker, R. G. (1968). *Ecological psychology: Concepts and methods for studying the environment of human behavior.* Stanford, CA: Stanford University Press.

Benjamin, L. S. (1974). Structural analysis of social behavior. *Psychological Review, 81*(5), 392.

Bortz, W. (2009). Understanding frailty. *The Journals of Gerontology, Series A, 65,* 255–256.

Brody, E. M., Kleban, M. H., Lawton, M. P., & Silverman, H. A. (1971). Excess disabilities of mentally impaired aged: Impact of individualized treatment. *The Gerontologist, 11*(2, Pt. 1), 124–133.

Bronfenbrenner, U. (1977). Toward an experimental ecology of human development. *American Psychologist, 32,* 513–531.

Burry, M. (2013). *Scripting cultures: Architectural design and programming.* West Sussex, UK: Wiley.

Byrnes, M. E. (2011). A city within a city: A "snapshot" of aging in a HUD 202 in Detroit, Michigan. *Journal of Aging Studies, 25*(3), 253–262.

Calkins, M., & Weisman, G. D. (1999). Models for environmental assessment. In B. Schwarz & R. Brent (Eds.), *Aging, autonomy and architecture: Advances in assisted living* (pp. 130–142). Baltimore, MD: Johns Hopkins University Press.

Canter, D. (1991). Understanding, assessing, and acting in places: Is an integrative framework possible? In T. Garling & G. Evans (Eds.), *Environment, cognition, and action* (pp. 191–209). New York, NY: Oxford University Press.

Carstensen, L. L. (1993). Motivation for social contact across the life span: A theory of socioemotional selectivity. In J. E. Jacobs (Ed.), *Developmental perspectives on motivation* (Vol. 40, pp. 209–254). Lincoln, NE: University of Nebraska Press.

Chawla, L. (2007). Childhood experiences associated with care for the natural world: A theoretical framework for empirical results. *Children, Youth and Environments, 17*(4), 144–170.

Cutchin, M. P. (2003). The process of mediated aging-in-place: A theoretically and empirically based model. *Social Science and Medicine, 57*(6), 1077–1090.

Davey, J. A., de Joux, V., Nana, G., & Arcus, M. (2004). *Accommodation options for older people in Aotearoa/New Zealand.* Christchurch, NZ: Centre for Housing Research.

De Medeiros, K. (2013). *Narrative gerontology in research and practice.* New York, NY: Springer Publishing Company.

Diaz Moore, K. (2005). Using place rules and affect to understand environmental fit: A theoretical exploration. *Environment and Behavior, 37*(3), 330–363.

Diaz Moore, K. (2014). An ecological framework of place: Situating environmental gerontology within a life course perspective. *International Journal of Aging and Human Development, 79*(3), 183–209.

Diaz Moore, K., & Ekerdt, D. J. (2011). Age and the cultivation of place. *Journal of Aging Studies, 25*(3), 189–192.

Fleming, R. (2011). An environmental audit tool suitable for use in homelike facilities for people with dementia. *Australasian Journal on Ageing, 30*(3), 108–112.

Freund, A. M. (2008). Successful aging as management of resources: The role of selection, optimization, and compensation. *Research in Human Development, 5*(2), 94–106.

Geboy, L., Diaz Moore, K., & Smith, E. K. (2012). Environmental gerontology for the future: Community-based living for the third age. *Journal of Housing for the Elderly, 26*(1–3), 44–61.

Gitlin, L. N. (2000). Adjusting "person–environment systems": Helping older people live the "good life" at home. In R. L. Rubinstein, M. Moss, & M. H. Kleban (Eds.), *The many dimensions of aging* (pp. 41–53). New York, NY: Springer Publishing Company.

Golant, S. M. (2003). Conceptualizing time and behavior in environmental gerontology: A pair of old issues deserving new thought. *The Gerontologist, 43*(5), 638–648.

Golant, S. (2008). Commentary: Irrational exuberance for the aging in place of vulnerable low-income older homeowners. *Journal of Aging and Social Policy, 20*(4), 379–397.

Golant, S. (2011). The quest for residential normalcy by older adults: Relocation but one pathway. *Journal of Aging Studies, 25*(3), 193–205.

Gottlieb, B. H., & Gillespie, A. A. (2008). Volunteerism, health, and civic engagement among older adults. *Canadian Journal on Aging/La Revue Canadienne du Vieillissement, 27*(04), 399–406.

Greenfield, E. A. (2012). Using ecological frameworks to advance a field of research, practice, and policy on aging-in-place initiatives. *The Gerontologist, 52*(1), 1–12.

Gubrium, J. (1975). *Living and dying at Murray Manor.* New York, NY: St. Martin's Press.

Gubrium, J. (1978). Notes on the social organization of senility. *Urban Life, 7*(1), 23–44.

Hazan, H. (2011). From ageless self to selfless age: Toward a theoretical turn in gerontological understanding. In L. W. Poon & J. Cohen-Mansfield (Eds.), *Understanding well-being in the oldest old* (pp. 11–26). New York, NY: Cambridge University Press.

Heckhausen, J., Wrosch, C., & Schulz, R. (2010). A motivational theory of life-span development. *Psychological Review, 117*(1), 32.

Herzog, A. R., & Markus, H. R. (1999). The self-concept in life span and aging research. In H. Gold & J. Libby (Eds.), *Handbook of theories of aging* (pp. 227–252). New York, NY: Springer Publishing Company.

Howell, S. (1983). The meaning of place in old age. In G. D. Rowles & R. J. Ohta (Eds.), *Aging and milieu. Environmental perspectives on growing old* (pp. 97–107). New York, NY: Academic.

Kader, S. & Diaz Moore, K. (2015). Therapeutic goals of hospice care environment: A systematic literature review. In *ARCC Conference Repository 2015.*

Kahana, E., & Kahana, B. (1996). Conceptual and empirical advances in understanding aging well through proactive adaptation. In V. L. Bengtson (Ed.), *Adulthood and aging: Research on continuities and discontinuities* (pp. 18–40). New York, NY: Springer Publishing Company.

Kahana, E., Kelley-Moore, J., & Kahana, B. (2012). Proactive aging: A longitudinal study of stress, resources, agency, and well-being in late life. *Aging and Mental Health, 16*(4), 438–451.

Kendig, H. (2003). Directions in environmental gerontology: A multidisciplinary field. *The Gerontologist, 43*(5), 611–615.

Lawton, M. P. (1980). *Environment and aging.* Albany, NY: Center for the Study of Aging.

Lawton, M. P. (1982). Competence, environmental press, and the adaptation of older people. In M. P. Lawton, P. Windley, & T. Byerts (Eds.), *Aging and the environment: Theoretical approaches* (pp. 33–59). New York, NY: Springer Publishing Company.

Lawton, M. P. (1989a). Behavior-relevant ecological factors. In K. Schaie & K. Schooler (Eds.), *Social structure and aging: Psychological processes* (pp. 57–78). Hillsdale, NJ: LEA Publishers.

Lawton, M. P. (1989b). Three functions of the residential environment. *Journal of Housing for the Elderly, 5*(1), 35–50.

Lawton, M. P. (1998). Environment and aging: Theory revisited. In R. J. Scheidt & P. G. Windley (Eds.), *Environment and aging theory: A focus on housing* (pp. 1–31). Westport, CT: Greenwood Press.

Lawton, M. P., & Nahemow, L. (1973). Ecology and the aging process. In C. Eisdorfer & M. P. Lawton (Eds.), *The psychology of adult development and aging* (pp. 619–674). Washington, DC: American Psychological Association.

Leary, T. (1957). *Interpersonal diagnosis of personality: A functional theory and methodology for personality evaluation.* Oxford, UK: Ronald Press.

Lerner, R. (2007). Developmental science, developmental systems, and contemporary theories of human development. In W. Damon & R. Lerner (Eds.), *Handbook of child psychology* (Vol. 1, pp. 1–17). New York, NY: Wiley.

Lewin, K. (1936). *Principles of topological psychology.* New York, NY: McGraw-Hill.

Luoh, M. C., & Herzog, A. R. (2002). Health and mortality as individual consequences of volunteer and paid work in old age. *Journal of Health and Social Behavior, 43*(4), 490–509.

McConnell, M. (2013). Behavioral economics and aging. *Journal of the Economics of Ageing, 1*, 83–89.

Midlarsky, E., Kahana, E., & Belser, A. (2015). Prosocial behavior in late life. In D. A. Schroeder & W. G. Graziano (Eds.), *The Oxford handbook of prosocial behavior* (pp. 415–432). New York, NY: Oxford University Press.

Moos, R., & Otto, J. (1972). The Community-Oriented Programs Environment Scale: A methodology for the facilitation and evaluation of social change. *Community Mental Health Journal, 8*(1), 28–37.

Musick, M. A., & Wilson, J. (2003). Volunteering and depression: The role of psychological and social resources in different age groups. *Social Science & Medicine, 56*(2), 259–269.

Nimrod, G., & Kleiber, D. A. (2007). Reconsidering change and continuity in later life: Toward an innovation theory of successful aging. *International Journal of Aging and Human Development, 65*(1), 1–22.

Olson, D. H., Sprenkle, D. H., & Russell, C. S. (1979). Circumplex model of marital and family systems: I. Cohesion and adaptability dimensions, family types, and clinical applications. *Family Process, 18*, 3–28.

Ouwehand, C., de Ridder, D. T., & Bensing, J. M. (2007). A review of successful aging models: Proposing proactive coping as an important additional strategy. *Clinical Psychology Review, 27*(8), 873–884.

Piaget, J. (1932/1965). *The moral judgment of the child*. London, UK: Free Press.

Prenda, K. M., & Lachman, M. E. (2001). Planning for the future: A life management strategy for increasing control and life satisfaction in adulthood. *Psychology and Aging, 16*(2), 206.

Rattan, S. I. (2008). Hormesis in aging. *Ageing Research Reviews, 7*(1), 63–78.

Romo, R. D., Wallhagen, M. I., Yourman, L., Yeung, C. C., Eng, C., Micco, G.,…Smith, A. K. (2013). Perceptions of successful aging among diverse elders with late-life disability. *The Gerontologist, 53*(6), 939–949.

Rowles, G. D. (1983). Geographical dimensions of social support in rural Appalachia. In G. Rowles & R. Ohta (Eds.), *Aging and milieu: Environmental perspectives on growing old* (pp. 111–130). New York, NY: Academic.

Rowles, G., & Bernard, M. (2013). The meaning and significance of place in old age. In G. Rowles & M. Bernard (Eds.), *Environmental gerontology: Making meaningful places in old age* (pp. 3–24). New York, NY: Springer Publishing Company.

Rowles, G. D., & Watkins, J. F. (2003). History, habit, heart and hearth: On making spaces into places. In F. Oswald, H. Mollenkopf, H. W. Wahl, & K. Warner Schaie (Eds.), *Aging independently: Living arrangements and mobility* (pp. 77–96). New York, NY: Springer Publishing Company.

Rubinstein, R. (1989). The home environments of older people: A description of the psychosocial processes linking person to place. *Journal of Gerontology, 44*(2), S45–S53.

Rubinstein, R., & de Medeiros, K. (2004). Ecology and the aging self. *Annual Review of Gerontology and Geriatrics, 23*, 59–84.

Scharlach, A. (2009, Summer). Introduction: Why America's cities and towns need to be more aging-friendly. *Generations, 33*(2), 5–11.

Scharlach, A., & Lehning, A. (2016). *Creating aging-friendly communities*. New York, NY: Oxford University Press.

Scheibe, S., & Carstensen, L. L. (2010). Emotional aging: Recent findings and future trends. *The Journals of Gerontology, Series B, 65*, 135–144.

Schulz, R., & Heckhausen, J. (1996). A life-span model of successful aging. *The American Psychologist, 51*, 702–714.

Shea, D., Davey, A., Femia, E. E., Zarit, S. H., Sundström, G., Berg, S., & Smyer, M. A. (2003). Exploring assistance in Sweden and the United States. *The Gerontologist, 43*(5), 712–721.

Smith, E. K. (2014). The impact of residential satisfaction, psychological well-being, and personality on voluntary late-life relocation. *The Gerontologist, 54*, 158.

Smith, S. K., Rayer, S., & Smith, E. A. (2008). Aging and disability: Implications for the housing industry and housing policy in the United States. *Journal of the American Planning Association, 74*(3), 289–306.

Vasunilashorn, S., Steinman, B., Liebig, P., & Pynoos, J. (2012). Aging in place: Evolution of a research topic whose time has come. *Journal of Aging Research, 2012*, 1–6.

Wahl, H.-W., Iwarsson, S., & Oswald, F. (2012). Aging well and the environment: Toward an integrative model and research agenda for the future. *The Gerontologist, 52*, 306–316.

Wahl, H.-W., & Lang, F. (2004). Aging in context across the adult life course: Integrating physical and social environmental research perspectives. *Annual Review of Gerontology and Geriatrics, 23*, 1–33.

Wahl, H.-W., & Weisman, G. D. (2003). Environmental gerontology at the beginning of the new millennium: Reflections on its historical, empirical and theoretical development. *The Gerontologist, 43*(5), 616–627.

Weir, P. L., Meisner, B. A., & Baker, J. (2010). Successful aging across the years: Does one model fit everyone? *Journal of Health Psychology, 15*(5), 680–687.

Weisman, G. D., Chaudhury, H., & Moore, K. D. (2000). Theory and practice of place: Toward an integrative model. In R. Rubenstein, M. Moss, & M. Kleban (Eds.), *The many dimensions of aging: Essays in honor of M. Powell Lawton* (pp. 3–21). New York, NY: Springer Publishing Company.

Wiles, J. L., Leibing, A., Guberman, N., Reeve, J., & Allen, R. E. S. (2012). The meaning of "ageing in place" to older people. *The Gerontologist, 52*(3), 357–366.

CHAPTER 22

Theories That Guide Consumer-Directed/ Person-Centered Initiatives in Policy and Practice

Nancy R. Hooyman, Kevin J. Mahoney, and Mark Sciegaj

This chapter explores a paradigm shift in policy and practice related to the delivery of services and supports to older adults or adults of any age with disabilities—the growth of person-centered (PC) and participant-directed (PD) practice initiatives. The goal of PC and PD care is not agency-based provision of services per se, but rather the individuals' autonomy to decide what supports best promote their quality of life. Demographic and societal trends as well as different theoretical perspectives that explain this shift toward PC and PD care are reviewed. New theoretical approaches are discussed, particularly the Consumer-Directed Theory of Empowerment (CDTE), which are salient to explaining the growth and impact of PC and PD initiatives as an evolving practice model that represents a paradigm shift from past approaches to working with older adults and persons with disabilities. Ways in which these theoretical approaches attend to issues of diversity in the aging experience and shape research and the current knowledge base are described. We conclude with a brief discussion of future directions for research and theory development that are valuable for both analysis and formulation of policies and practices related to PC/PD care.

■ BACKGROUND

If adults with disabilities, regardless of age, need help accessing services or bathing, dressing, or getting out of bed, they typically have had to go to an agency or depend on agency staff to visit them at home. They generally have little say over who or how many people help them, what the help will be or when they meet with these helpers. For example, if an individual needs assistance getting into bed and an agency can send a home care aide only at 4 p.m., the person, even if a night owl, has to get in bed then. Agencies also have numerous restrictions on what their workers can and cannot do. For instance, an agency-based worker cannot drive an individual in his or her car to visit a spouse in a nursing facility or to attend church. Such restrictions are often justified on the basis of minimizing public and private risk. However, as articulated by Koscuilek (2000, 2005), disability when combined with public assistance is not a rationale for others to make decisions about major aspects of a person's life or to presume that they will make risky choices. To his statement, we would add age as not being a rationale for a more traditional hierarchical approach to planning care. Not surprisingly, people with disabilities have for years maintained that, if they had more control over supports, their quality of life would be enhanced without additional cost to providers. Under a PC and PD approach to care, the person in the aforementioned scenario, not a provider, would define goals and "needs." The individual would decide if he or she wanted a helper or preferred other types of supports including household goods, who that helper would be, what the helper would do, and, under more advanced PD initiatives, to manage staff and control the budget to execute these choices.

PC care, first implemented with adults with disabilities but increasingly implemented with older adults, is guided by principles of community inclusion, dignity, and respect or, as the National Center for Self-determination posits, "Freedom, Authority, Support, Responsibility and Confirmation" (Center for Self-Determination, 2014). A PC approach means that the individual is at the center of the planning process and the plan reflects what is most important to that person as well as his or her capacities, strengths, and the supports that individual chooses. The plan focuses on the person's whole life, not just services, and uses informal supports when possible. To embed this approach into the current aging services network, the Administration for Community Living (ACL) has developed a national training program being piloted in eight states with enhanced Aging and Disability Resource Centers (ADRCs). ACL's goal is to have a national certification program for PC, which would be similar to existing certification for information and referral services.

This PC approach is the foundation for PD care, but PD initiatives provide for an extension of decision-making autonomy and authority that goes beyond PC care alone. PD initiatives help people of all ages, across all types of disabilities, maintain their autonomy and determine for themselves what mix of personal assistance supports works best for them. As the individual directs and manages his or her care, PD represents a paradigm shift from traditionally provided services, where the decision-making and managing authority is vested in a professional. Instead, a substantial portion of such decision making, including in many instances employer and budgetary authority, is transferred to the participant; sometimes, if the participant has major cognitive impairments, family members or a representative assists with decisions. *Employer authority* offers participants the ability to employ workers directly, whereas *budget authority* gives them the capacity to manage an individual budget and make purchases related to personal care. The budget authority model of PD services is often called "cash and counseling" (C & C; Brown et al., 2007; Doty et al., 2012).

■ DEMOGRAPHIC AND SOCIETAL TRENDS

Demographic, societal, and policy trends create the larger context for the need for and subsequent growth of PC and PD initiatives. Primary among these trends is the sheer increase in the numbers of older adults with multiple chronic illnesses, functional limitations, and disabilities combined with the increased life expectancy of adults with physical and intellectual disabilities (Anderson & Horvath, 2004). Of all Medicare beneficiaries, 37% have at least four chronic conditions (Center for Medicare and Medicaid Services [CMS], 2012). Of even greater impact on long-term services and supports (LTSS) is that adults aged 85 years and older—the oldest-old with the highest rate of functional limitations and comorbidities—are the fastest growing segment of the population (Administration on Aging, 2014; Gonyea, 2014). Moreover, after years of steady decline, the incidence of disability among adults aged 65 years and older appears to be rising since 2000, with some predicting that baby boomers will face higher disability rates than prior cohorts (Crimmins & Beltran-Sanchez, 2010; Fuller-Thomson, Yu, Nuru-Jeter,

Guralnik, & Minkler, 2009; Martin, Schoeni, & Andreski, 2010). Strikingly, although people are living longer, many are also living sicker and spending a greater proportion of their lifetime with disabilities, particularly individuals from socioeconomically disadvantaged backgrounds who may have experienced health inequities across the life course (Fries, 2003; National Health Interview Survey, 2012).

Approximately 40 million people in the United States have a disability defined by the Institute of Medicine Committee on Disability, as impairments, activity limitations, or participation restrictions (Field & Jette, 2007). Because of medical breakthroughs, these individuals are living longer and thereby contributing to the increased number of older adults with disabilities. With disability rates predicted to grow in the coming decades, the population of people with functional limitations encompasses an 80-year age span from adults in midlife to the oldest-old (Putnam & Frieden, 2014).

Among these rapidly growing populations, their preference for autonomy as central to their identity and life satisfaction has profound implications for the delivery of LTSS. An estimated 70% of adults aged 65 years and older need LTSS during their lifetimes, for an average of 3 years. Moreover, about 40% of people using LTSS are younger than 65 years (Alkema, 2013; O'Shaughnessy et al., 2014). Given the diversity of needs and goals among this heterogeneous population, flexibility within LTSS is needed to promote personal choice in decision making and to address the whole person rather than relying on a stipulated formula for services (Polivka, 2000; Putnam & Frieden, 2014). The medical model that has dominated LTSS, combined with the life circumstances faced by many older adults and people with disabilities, often contribute to a loss of power and inequities across the life course, exacerbating negative health and socioeconomic outcomes later in life (American Psychological Association, 2014; Thompson & Thompson, 2001).

Policy discussions of LTSS have often framed disability as a medical condition and personal deficit that marginalizes and disempowers individuals and assumes that professionals know best the rights, choices, and preferences of the person involved (Putnam & Frieden, 2014, p. 60). The influence of medical models is reflected in the past focus on use of services to perform ADLs and IADLs rather than on active participation in society. Interventions such as care management can convey that the older adult or person with disabilities is someone to be managed; if asked about their preferences, they may feel they do not have meaningful choices nor have been heard and valued. Such disempowering approaches to LTSS are manifestation of the larger societal context of ageism and ableism. Older adults and individuals with disabilities are further marginalized if they face discrimination based on race, gender, sexual orientation, and class.

Even when experiencing loss of power and status, or feeling unable to impact their environments, the vast majority of older adults and adults with disabilities want to participate in the process of setting goals for their lives and to be engaged in their communities (Shearer, 2009). This preference is reflected in the growing demand for community-based LTSS to support individuals in their preferred home settings. The independent living movement, begun in the 1970s, promoted a community-based paradigm for persons with disabilities years before such approaches were advocated by and for older adults. Moreover, the Supreme Court's decision in Olmstead *v.* L.C. (1999) put forth the right of all individuals with disabilities to live in the least restrictive community settings, paving the way for self-determination, control, and choice as best practices in the field of intellectual and developmental disabilities (Putnam & Frieden, 2014; Wehmeyer & Abery, 2013). Although older adults in the past have not been as vocal as disability rights advocates in pressing for decision-making autonomy, this pattern is shifting with boomers' expanded demand for greater choice and control. Such preferences are being codified in policy, such as increased Medicaid funding for Home and Community-Based Services (HCBS) waivers (O'Shaughnessy, 2014) as well as reflected in the growing number of public and private initiatives to support aging in place in the community rather than institutional care.

■ NEW MODELS OF CARE: PC AND PD INITIATIVES

The emergence of social models of LTSS that frame disability as a mismatch of a person's capabilities to an environment's characteristics (e.g., lack of a supportive environment) recognizes this fundamental desire for choice. In this ecological or person-in-environment framework, LTSS are resources to facilitate engagement in life's roles and activities by creating a better balance between a person and his or her environment. In such models, the environment needs to be modified to ensure that the individual is able to be a self-acting agent and that self-determination and decision-making control are viewed as a matter of civil and human rights (Putnam & Frieden, 2014). According to Alkema (2013), the SCAN Foundation has posited a framework for supports to build a PC-integrated system for people with cognitive and functional limitations. Central to this framework are supports that meet consumers' preferences and values and provide choice in providers so that needs can be met in the least restrictive setting.

Two other trends provide an empirical rationale for PC and PD initiatives: (a) increasing research on the social determinants of health and the necessity of caring for the whole person (Robert Wood Johnson Foundation, 2011) and (b) a growing body of evidence on how self-determination and an internal locus of control affect physical well-being and quality of life (Jacobs-Lawson, Waddell, & Webb, 2011; Shearer, 2009).

A number of policy changes support the implementation of PC and PD practices. These include the integration of aging and disability services under the ACL, the development of ADRCs to serve both older adults and persons with disabilities, and a range of community-based initiatives funded under the Patient Protection and Affordable Care Act (ACA).

ADRCs, first authorized by Congress in 2006 and led by ACL and the CMS, aim to improve access to LTSS for older adults, all adults with disabilities, family caregivers, veterans, and LTSS providers. By promoting a concept of a "no wrong door system," they aim to provide one-stop access to information and referral, one-on-one options counseling, and streamlined access to public programs, PC transitions, quality assurance, and continuous improvement (ACL, 2014).

The move toward "no wrong door" and PC care in both public and private health care sectors is congruent with the larger shift of financial incentives for community-based care under the ACA. To illustrate, the State Balancing Incentive Program (BIP) offers higher federal matching payments to states that undertake structural reforms to increase access to HCBS. The Community First Choice option allows consumers choice of either an agency or self-directed model and provides an enhanced match to states that elect to provide PC home and community-based attendant services. The Money Follows the Person Program (MFP) enables people to move out of institutions and into their own homes or other community-based settings (Mahoney, 2011). Moreover, the Older Americans Act has similar goals to promote comprehensive coordinated systems that enable older adults to remain in home and community-based settings responsive to their needs and preferences.

In summary, growing national emphasis on promoting choice and control for a more diverse population in community-based care provides the larger context for PC/PD practice initiatives. In 2013, more than 835,000 individuals of all ages were enrolled in 277 PD programs nationwide (NRCPDS, 2014). Of these programs, 63% reported having budget authority (where participants could decide how much to spend on workers, goods, and services); however, because many of the largest programs did not offer budget authority, 85% of the participants were in programs with only employer authority. California alone had 440,000 individuals with employer authority only in its In-Home Supportive Services (IHSS) program. It is within this macro context that we next discuss the theoretical underpinnings of PC, PD, and the C & C Demonstration model.

■ SALIENT THEORIES AND A PARADIGM SHIFT IN PRACTICE

As noted earlier, the traditional service delivery model vests decision-making and managing authority in the agency provider. As a paradigm shift in service delivery, PD transfers a substantial portion of the decision-making authority to the participant (or instances of severe cognitive impairment, with assistance from family or a representative). For an organization to embrace PD, significant culture change is required— shifting the balance of power to professionals *and* participants; defining the system by its outcomes, not the services it delivers; and focusing on the whole person. It is in this sense that a paradigm shift is occurring in the Aging Network of LTSS.

Empowerment Theory and Locus of Control

PC and PD models of care are informed by theories of empowerment and locus of control. Empowerment theory posits the centrality of promoting self-determination, choice, and control. These basic tenets are exemplified by PD program participant Lillie Brannon's telling words, "I like this program because I'm the boss." At age 88 years, with multiple chronic conditions and severe functional disabilities, Ms. Lillie participated in Arkansas' "Independent Choices" program, one of the three pioneer state programs that made up the original C & C Demonstration and Evaluation. Relying on only the income from Supplemental Security Income (SSI), she lived alone in subsidized senior housing and was confined to her bed or reclining chair. Despite her physical limitations, Ms. Lillie was strong-willed. She thought she could—and ought to—have the right to make decisions about how to live her life, including how to meet her own personal assistance needs. She delighted in telling visitors how she had "escaped" from nursing homes four times. She also made it clear that she had little use for the well meaning, but, in her view, condescending professionals who routinely sought to convince her that she really belonged in a skilled nursing facility.

There are varying definitions of empowerment theory, but human agency, autonomy, and self-determination are central to all frameworks. In the context of PC and PD models of care, individual empowerment encompasses internal/psychological factors, such as a decision-making control, as well as control over the types of assistance and resources given and the organizational ability to manage "getting around in life" (Kosciulek & Merz, 2001).

In implementing PC/PD approaches, individual empowerment is conceptualized as a process of moving from a state of powerlessness and passivity to one of active control (both perceived and actual) over one's life. The empowered individual sees oneself as capable of change, able to use his or her knowledge and skills to solve problems and meet goals, and to work in partnership with professionals. Empowerment potential exists not only in terms of an individual's resources and abilities, but also in terms of agency rules and procedures; in other words, the agency must change in order for the individual to experience real options to act to control of his or her life. Empowerment theory articulates a fundamental difference between inability to act because of lack of choices and lack of ability to act. It informs agency interventions (or "helping") that address asymmetry in power distribution by providing aging adults and persons with disabilities with choices and opportunities to act. When they are able to draw upon their strengths, skills, personal assets, and environmental resources, elders and adults with disabilities move from weak social status and powerless roles to ones in which they themselves as persons of value are competent to bring about change in their lives (Gutierrez, Parsons, & Cox, 1998). So-called clients or patients are then viewed as participants, collaborators, or change agents engaged in self-advocacy and goal attainment to promote their health and well-being.

Closely related to empowerment theory are psychological theories of locus of control, which can be predictive of well-being and help to explain the effectiveness of PC and PD care approaches. Perceived control, which is central to the empowerment process, is found to be related to self-efficacy and, when mediated by social support, can enhance a sense of competence and health (Bisconti & Bergeman, 1999). The extent of locus of control can particularly influence quality of life in long-term care settings. Such settings can be disempowering environments with limited opportunities for choice, which may result in decreased locus of control and self-esteem and increased depression (Hedgpeth, 2012). By contrast, older adults' health locus of control is found to be associated with health self-efficacy (Jacobs-Lawson et al., 2011).

Economic Theory of Utility Maximization

Economic theory explains the "flexibility" rationale behind PD. At its simplest, the traditional delivery system has been a "one size fits all" approach. In some cases, participants, regardless of level of need, received the same circumscribed type and amount of services, for example, predetermined number of hours of care from agency employees. Participant preferences were sometimes considered, but "professionals" made the key decisions and handled the coordination, assessment, and monitoring of services.

Participants' preference for "flexibility" is portrayed by Tammy Svihla, who has multiple sclerosis. Tammy manages her allowance with minimal assistance from a bookkeeper provided by the New Jersey C & C program, known as "Personal Preferences." She can arrange help at the times and amounts she wants. About half of her allowance covers payroll and taxes, whereas the rest is used to buy personal care items and goods for her home, including incontinence pads, an air conditioner, and touch lamps. After purchasing these products, Tammy plans to use her allowance later to give raises to deserving workers.

The economic argument for flexibility is also captured in terms of a comparison between in-kind transfers and a cash benefit (Harvey & Gayer, 2013). Utility theory posits that a fixed dollar amount of a commodity (e.g., in-kind approach) does *not* make a person as well off as the same amount in cash, because the person who receives cash is placed on a higher "indifference curve," that is, (s)he receives a higher level of utility or satisfaction. The in-kind approach "forces a person to consume the full amount of the in-kind benefit" whereas an individual might "prefer to spend the proceeds on other goods" of their choosing (Rosen & Geyer, 2010, p. 27).

Economic theory also posits the centrality of demand and supply that underlies employer authority options. The demand for supports and services in general, and for personal care attendants in particular, is predicted to outpace supply resulting in future worker shortages (Bureau of Labor Statistics, 2014). When demand grows faster than supply, prices typically rise; however, prices in the public sector are controlled. Medicaid rates are constrained and Medicare does not generally cover LTSS, thus limiting wages and benefits for direct-care workers. That being the case, many states are drawn to PD options, because they allow the participant to select and recruit into the workforce family and friends who are already engaged in caregiving largely because of their relationship with the person with a disability. In other words, employer authority options for participants can increase the supply of potential workers to provide personal care.

Socioemotional Selectivity and Exchange Theories

Socioemotional selectivity theory also provides support for "employer authority" models of self-direction in which the participant has the authority to hire, manage, and fire paid workers of his or her choosing and thus to control these interpersonal, often intimate, interactions. It posits that as people age and their perception of future time becomes limited, they focus on interpersonal relationships that are most rewarding and withdraw from those that are not (Carstensen, 1992; Carstensen, Fung, & Charles, 2003). Attaining emotional regulation or control over interpersonal relationships and restoring positive affect can enhance meaning in life (Charles & Carstensen, 2007; Hicks, Trend, Davis, & King, 2012; Kryla-Lighthall & Mather, 2009; Suitor, Gilligan, & Pillemer, 2013); this contrasts with the increased stress and lower well-being that results when support does not meet individuals' expectations (Baumeister et al., 2001; Rook, 1984, 2001; Schuster, Kessler, & Aseltine, 1990). Furthermore, receiving care from those perceived to be empathetic and similar to oneself can be beneficial when it ensures predictability and harmonious relations.

The centrality of emotional selectivity—"receiving care from people you know and love"—is reflected in the story of Janice Maddox. Mrs. Maddox, 75 years old, requires significant help with her personal care needs. She has diabetes and glaucoma, and has had several major operations that have confined her to a wheelchair. Her daughter speaks for her mother by saying "There's just something about having family look after her. She doesn't get nearly as many allergic reactions or bed sores now, and I think that's because when it's your own you're looking after, you pay more attention."

Similarly, social exchange theory has long posited beneficial effects when one can give as well as receive (Dowd, 1980; Lynott & Lynott, 1996). It thus supports the collaborative nonhierarchical nature of the PC/PD relationship between participant and worker, particularly when the worker is a paid family member. Exchange theory is in essence an economic theory in which a person's social status is determined by the ratio of rewards to costs associated with interactions with that person. Interactions that are positively reinforced and create opportunity structures will continue, whereas those that do not yield sufficient benefits will be discontinued (Diggs, 2008). Many caregivers, for instance, welcome the opportunity to be compensated for some portion of their care hours (Foster, Dale, & Brown, 2007). For others, the ability to receive wages for their care allows them to leave other paid work to take on a higher level of caregiving responsibility. For still others, the availability of funds to pay consistent caregivers devoted to their loved one allows them the peace of mind to keep their "day jobs." In all cases, the person receiving the assistance is now able to "pay something back."

The Consumer-Directed Theory of Empowerment

The CDTE, drawing on concepts from the aforementioned social theories, is an attempt to assemble one parsimonious theory on consumer direction that informs PC/PD care. Congruent with empowerment theory, the CDTE emphasizes the need for consumers to have control over practices that affect their lives (Kosciulek & Merz, 2001). Drawing upon utility maximization theory, the CDTE defines consumer direction as the mechanism by which individuals develop the skills necessary to take control of their lives. Finally, similar to what socioemotional selectivity and exchange theories would posit, CDTE maintains that the more an individual is consumer-directed, the more connected the person becomes to his or her community and the more he or she would be able to focus on meaningful relationships.

The CDTE was developed by Kosciulek (1999) and later tested by Kosciulek and Merz (2001) and Kosciulek (2005) to guide the development and evaluation of disability policy and rehabilitation services and to measure service outcomes in terms of community integration and improved quality of life. CDTE maintains that informed consumers, who are the experts on their service needs, should have full access to information and options in LTSS and choice and control over policies and practices that affect their lives (Kosciulek, 2000, 2005). These components of CDTE promote the person's integration in his or her community, increase his or her sense of power and efficacy, and thereby improve his or her quality of life.

Kosciulek and Merz (2001) provided initial evidence that supported the structure of CDTE. Using data from 159 consumers with disabilities who were receiving rehabilitation services, they reported significant path coefficients between consumer direction and community integration, consumer direction and empowerment, and empowerment and quality of life. Kosciulek (2005) later refined the CDTE in a study using a larger sample of 721 consumers from the database of the Longitudinal Study of the Vocational Rehabilitation Services Program. This later study identified positive correlations among consumer direction and community integration, empowerment, and quality of life, as illustrated in Figure 22.1.

Similar findings that decision-making control enhances quality of life are reported in studies such as California's In-Home Supportive Services (IHSS) Program Study (Benjamin & Matthias, 2001) and the C & C Demonstration and Evaluation (Brown et al., 2007).

■ HOW KEY THEORIES AND CONCEPTS SHAPE RESEARCH AND THE CURRENT KNOWLEDGE BASE

The largest study of the employer authority model of PD care focused on California's IHSS program; it compared service experiences and outcomes for consumers in a traditional homecare agency model (PAM) with those in a consumer-directed model (CDM; Benjamin & Matthias, 2001). Consumers and workers were found to differ across models. The CDM consumers had poorer functional status and greater service needs than the PAM clients. Because CDM participants hired their own workers, including family and friends, they were more likely than workers in the traditional agency to be ethnically and linguistically compatible. Consumer-directed participants also reported that their workers had longer tenure and lower turnover. Because of their greater service

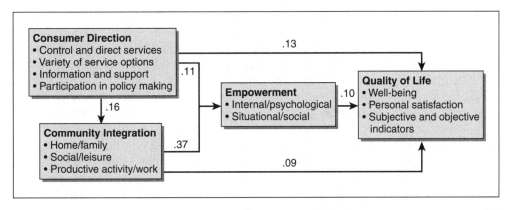

FIGURE 22.1 Tested structural model of Kosciulek's Consumer-Directed Theory of Empowerment, with all coefficients significant at $p < .05$ (Kosciulek, 2005).

needs and latitude to negotiate tasks and hours with their workers free of agency constraints, consumers in the CDM were much more likely than those in a traditional agency to receive unpaid service hours from their providers (Benjamin et al., 2008; Doty, 1998).

The C & C Demonstration and Evaluation has the largest research base and the strongest evidence of efficacy of any budget authority PD model. A large, randomized experiment, the C & C Evaluation was conducted in Arkansas, Florida, and New Jersey (Brown et al., 2007; Shen et al., 2008a, 2008b). This comparative effectiveness study randomly assigned 7,500 applicants into two groups: (a) a treatment group, whose members received a monthly allowance that they could use to hire workers and purchase care-related goods and services, and (b) a control group, whose members could obtain their personal care services only through the traditional agency-based model. The experiment included a broader range of outcome, process, and cost measures than earlier studies. Outcome measures included a sense of empowerment and satisfaction with quality of services and with quality of life; in addition, the study measured access to functional assistance, unmet needs for assistance, and quality of care as indicated by reports of certain adverse health events (e.g., contractures and falls, each of which are often preventable; Brown et al., 2007).

Several significant differences were found. Participants in the treatment group were no more likely to suffer any care-related health problems than their peers receiving traditional agency services. In some cases, self-directing participants even demonstrated a reduced risk of experiencing health problems. In addition, people receiving traditional services were significantly more likely to have an unmet care need than self-directing participants. Treatment group participants also reported significant decreases in family stress and emotional strain from informal caregiving (Brown et al., 2007). The results of the C & C Demonstration and Evaluation have proven influential in bringing about changes in federal law, policy, and regulation that facilitate the inclusion of PD services in publicly funded personal assistance programs.

The advent of the Veteran's-Directed (VD) HCBS Program in 2009 is a noteworthy example of this impact on federal policy. Patterned after the C & C budget authority option, the VD-HCBS as of 2014 had reached approximately 1,500 veterans in 49 veterans' medical centers in 29 states. The 2015 Consolidated and Further Continuing Appropriations Act encourages the expansion of this program and calls for the

Veterans Health Administration (VHA) to report to the Appropriations Committees of both Houses on the cost-effectiveness of expanding the program. The first evaluation of this option, the "sustainability study," examined the VHA coordinators' views (Mahoney & Kayala, 2011). Beyond meeting basic personal care needs, coordinators identified the enhancement and improvement of socialization, dignity, empowerment, mental health, life satisfaction, self-esteem, continuity of care, comfort, and quality of life among participants. In focus groups with veterans, one father noted advantages of the VD approach: "When my son got in the program I was able to quit my job and be his full time caregiver. Before, he was at home by himself and he would be in his chair pretty much all the day." A participant emphasized the benefits, saying, "My caregiver lives just across the street so anytime, day or night, all I have to do is call over there and they see my number and know it is an emergency. To be able to pay her is just phenomenal because I don't feel I am imposing on everybody."

■ LIMITATIONS OF EXISTING THEORIES

A principal constraint of existing theories in explaining and informing PC/PD approaches is that the variability of interactions between individuals, relationships, and social/institutional contexts is often overlooked. Capitman and Sciegaj (1995) addressed this shortcoming in proposing a "contextual autonomy approach" for understanding elder autonomy. A contextual approach acknowledges that the way in which people make choices is determined in part by who they are as distinctive psychological, social, and cultural beings and what their particular relationship is with the LTSS system. The particulars of an individual's situation influence the range of available choices, how the person understands his or her ability to make decisions, and whether and how that person's decision(s) are respected by others. This approach suggests that to adequately assess individual decisions for PD requires examining relationships between the individual, the informal caregiving network, and the formal system of LTSS.

This point is also illustrated by Sciegaj, Capitma, and Kyriacou's (2004) survey of a sample of 731 elders, including 200 African American, 200 Chinese, 131 Latino, and 200 White Western European American older adults. Among their findings, Chinese elders with a greater sense of control in their lives were less likely to select PD service options; from their perspective, receiving culturally competent agency services was sufficient. Latino elders who reported a sense of not being in control of their lives were more likely to choose agency-based services, perhaps needing agency structure to increase their sense of control. These findings of the heterogeneity of preferences for PD care within racial/ethnic groups of older adults point to the need to better understand how individuals, families, and systems interact within the context of LTSS. In contrast, the C & C Demonstration and Evaluation found that non-Caucasians were 2.5 times more likely to be interested in self-direction, although they did not enroll in higher proportions. How ethnic groups used their budgets varied widely (Mahoney, Simon-Rusinowitz, Loughlin, Desmond, & Squillace, 2004; Meiners, Mahoney, Shoop, & Squillace, 2002).

If theoretical frameworks consider race/ethnicity only as a series of dichotomous variables, research findings based on these theories may make simplistic conclusions regarding the effects of race/ethnicity on preferences for PD. Although race/ethnicity gives older individuals a structure through which to view the world, it competes with other factors in determining individual preferences for how elders live, address illness and care, and the kind of help they desire (Angel & Angel, 1997; Mui, Choi, & Monk,

1998). There do not appear to be any published studies on racial/ethnic differences in preferences for PD among persons with disabilities. Overall, there is a critical need for further research on how race/ethnicity interacts with other factors to influence needs and preferences for care of both older individuals and adults with disabilities.

■ FUTURE DEVELOPMENT AND APPLICATION OF THEORY

Research is needed on recent practice and policy changes that have implications for the continued development and examination of theories that support PC and PD care. These include the growth of managed care, the application of PC/PD care to different delivery systems, and the increasing racial/ethnic and socioeconomic diversity of older adults and people with disabilities.

A significant change in the LTSS delivery system is that 31 states have moved, or are moving, from a fee-for-service to a managed care environment. Even before the dramatic growth of managed LTSS, the compatibility of the concepts of *managed care* and *PD* was questioned. Early exploratory studies of staff in managed care organizations identified mixed attitudes toward PD. Although some managed care organizations saw PD as a means to improve service quality and efficiency as well as to increase member independence (Meiners et al., 2002), other organizations expressed concerns over whether participants were up to the task of managing their care (Mahoney, Meiners, Shoop, & Squillace, 2003). Testing the limits of empowerment theory or the CDTE in a managed care service system and evaluating the impact of managed care on PD and, most importantly, on participants are needed.

Another area for future research and theory development is applying what has been learned about PC/PD approaches of care to different types of needs and delivery systems. In addition to the development and evaluation of the VD-HCBS Program, which uses the C & C model, more research is needed on how PC/PD concepts can be applied in different circumstances, such as settings that offer different degrees of flexibility or constraints for participants' decision-making authority. For example, research funded by the Retirement Research Foundation and the Substance Abuse and Mental Health Services Administration (SAMHSA) that reanalyzed the C & C data identified that 18% to 24% of personal care recipients (varying by state) had mental health claims on their Medicaid billings. Further analysis showed that the subgroups of people with behavioral health billings fared better under the self-direction option than under the traditional care system. This led to small controlled experiments in Pennsylvania and Texas that allowed people with serious mental illness to manage budgets to meet their recovery needs as well as to a large multistate effort funded by the Robert Wood Johnson Foundation, SAMHSA, and the New York State Health Foundation to look at system-level effects and cost data (K. J. Mahoney, personal communication, April 14, 2015).

Sciegaj et al. (2004) and Mahoney et al. (2004), as noted previously, suggest the need for further research on racial/ethnic differences. The findings of Blackhall, Murphy, Frank, Michel, and Azen (1995) also illustrate the effect of race/ethnicity on attitudes toward hospital–patient autonomy and the role of family relationships. They report significant racial/ethnic differences, with Korean American and Mexican American elders favoring a more family-centered model of decision making rather than the more traditional individual patient-autonomy model. Using a socioemotional selectivity theory framework to better understand the intersection of race/ethnicity, family, and empowerment/autonomy would be a fruitful area for theory development, given demographic changes and the growing role of family caregivers.

■ CONCLUSION

With both the aging and the increasing diversity of the U.S. population combined with federal policy initiatives related to LTSS, the demand for PC and PD initiatives will continue to grow. To enable individuals to decide the amount, type, and intensity of LTSS that best promotes their quality of life, care delivery systems need to be designed and their employees should be trained on the appropriate competencies to empower older participants and those with disabilities. This entails significant culture change in many of the Aging and Disability Network agencies that provide LTSS. To do so will necessitate better understanding of the different theoretical perspectives that explain this paradigm shift toward PC and PD care and how participant desire for choice and control may vary by race/ethnicity. Similarly, new and robust theoretical development and testing are needed to generate data on the outcomes of PC/PD initiatives for aging persons and those with disabilities.

REFERENCES

Administration for Community Living (ACL). (2014). *Aging and disability resource center*. Retrieved from htpp://acl.gov/NewsRoom/Publications/docs/ADRC_Factsheet.pdf

Administration on Aging. (2014). *A profile of older Americans: 2014*. Retrieved from http://www.aoa.acl.gov/aging_statistics/profile/index.aspx

Alkema, G. (2013). *Current issues and potential solutions for addressing America's long-term care financing crisis*. Long Beach, CA: The SCAN Foundation.

American Psychological Association. (2014). *Disability and socioeconomic status*. Retrieved from http://www.apa.org/pi/ses/resources/publications/factsheet-disability.aspx

Anderson, G., & Horvath, J. (2004). The growing burden of chronic disease in America. *Public Health Reports, 119*, 263–270.

Angel, R., & Angel, J. (1997). *Who will take care of us? Aging and long- term care in multicultural America*. New York, NY: New York University Press.

Baumeister, R. F., Bratslavsky, E., Finkenauer, C., & Vohs, E. (2001). Bad is stronger than good. *Review of General Psychology, 4*, 323–370.

Benjamin, A. E., & Matthias, R. E. (2001). Age, consumer direction and outcomes of supportive services at home. *The Gerontologist, 41*(5), 632–642.

Benjamin, A. E., Matthias, R. E., Kietzman, K., & Furman, W. (2008). Retention of paid related caregivers: Who stays and who leaves home care careers? *The Gerontologist, 48*(Suppl. 1), 104–113.

Bisconti, T. L., & Bergeman, C. S. (1999). Perceived social control as a mediator of the relationships among social support, psychological well-being and perceived health. *The Gerontologist, 39*, 94–103.

Blackhall, L., Murphy, S., Frank, G., Michel, V., & Azen, S. (1995). Ethnicity and attitudes towards patient autonomy. *Journal of the American Medical Association, 274*, 820–829.

Brown, R., Carlson, B., Dale, S., Foster, L., Phillips, B., & Schore, J. (2007). *Cash & Counseling: Improving the lives of Medicaid beneficiaries who need personal care or home and community-based waiver services.* Mathematica Policy Research. Retrieved from http://www.mathematica-mpr.com/~/media/publications/PDFs/ccpersonalcare.pdf

Bureau of Labor Statistics. (2014). *Occupational outlook handbook.* Washington, DC: U.S. Department of Labor. Retrieved from http://www.bls.gov/ooh

Capitman, J., & Sciegaj, M. (1995). A contextual approach for understanding individual autonomy in managed community long-term care. *The Gerontologist, 35*(4), 533–540.

Carstensen, L. L. (1992). Social and emotional patterns in adulthood: Support for socioemotional selectivity theory. *Psychology and Aging, 7*(3), 331–338.

Carstensen, L. L., Fung, H. H., & Charles, S. T. (2003). Socioemotional selectivity theory and the regulation of emotion in the second half of life. *Motivation and Emotion, 27*(2), 103–123.

Center for Medicare and Medicaid Services (CMS). 2012. *Chronic conditions among Medicare beneficiaries, chart book, 2012 edition.* Baltimore, MD: Center for Medicare and Medicaid Services.

Center for Self-Determination. (2014). *Principles of self-determination.* Retrieved from http://www.centerforself-determination.com

Charles, S. T., Carstensen, L. L. (2007). Emotion regulation and aging. In J. J. Gross (Ed.), *Handbook of emotion regulation* (pp. 307–327). New York, NY: Guilford Press.

Crimmins, E. M., & Beltran-Sanchez, H. (2010). Mortality and morbidity trends: Is there compression of morbidity? *The Journals of Gerontology, Series B, 66*(1), 75–86.

Diggs, J. (2008). The exchange theory of aging. In Loue, S., & Sajatovic, M. (Eds), *Encyclopedia of aging and public health* (pp. 340–341). New York, NY: Springer Publishing Company.

Doty, P. (1998). The cash and counseling demonstration: An experiment in consumer-directed personal assistance services. *American Rehabilitation, 24*(3), 27–30.

Doty, P., Mahoney, K., Simon-Rusinowitz, L., Sciegaj, M., Selkow, I., & Loughlin, D. (2012). Cash and Counseling's role in the growth of participant-directed services. *Generations, 36*(1), 28–36.

Dowd, J. J. (1980). *Stratification among the aged.* Monterey, CA: Brooks/Cole.

Field, M. J., & Jette, A. M. (2007). *The future of disability in America.* Washington, DC: Institute of Medicine.

Foster, L., Dale, S., & Brown, R. (2007). How caregivers and workers fared in Cash and Counseling. *Health Services Research, 42*(1), 510–532.

Fries, J. F. (2003). Measuring and monitoring success in compressing morbidity. *New England Journal of Medicine, 303*, 130–135.

Fuller-Thomson, E., Yu, B., Nuru-Jeter, A., Guralnik, J. M., & Minkler, M. (2009). Basic ADL disability and functional limitation rates among older Americans from 2000–2005: The end of the decline? *The Journals of Gerontology, Series A, 64*(12), 1333–1336.

Gonyea, J. (2014). The policy challenges of a larger and more diverse oldest-old population. In R. Hudson (Ed.), *The new politics of old age policy* (3rd ed., pp. 155–182). Baltimore, MD: Johns Hopkins University Press.

Gutierrez, L., Parsons, R., & Cox, E. (1998). *Empowerment in social work practice: A sourcebook.* Pacific Grove, CA: Brooks/Cole.

Harvey, R., & Gayer, T. (2013). *Public finance.* New York, NY: McGraw-Hill Higher Education.

Hedgpeth, J. (2012). *The impact of moving toward a culture of empowerment in the lives of residents of assisted living centers.* Doctoral dissertation, Arizona State University.

Hicks, J. A., Trend, J., Davis, W. E., & King, L. A. (2012). Positive affect, meaning in life and future time perspective: An application of socioemotional selectivity theory. *Psychology and Aging, 27*(1), 181–189.

Jacobs-Lawson, J. M., Waddell, E. L., & Webb, A. K. (2011). Predictors of health locus of control in older adults. *Current Psychology, 30,* 173.

Koscuilek, J. F. (1999). The consumer-directed theory of empowerment. *Rehabilitation Counseling Bulletin, 42,* 196–213.

Koscuilek, J. F. (2000). Implications of consumer direction for disability policy development and rehabilitation service delivery. *Journal of Disability Policy Studies, 65*(2), 82–89.

Koscuilek, J. F. (2005). Structural equation model of the consumer-directed theory of empowerment in a vocational rehabilitation context. *Rehabilitation Counseling Bulletin, 49,* 40–49.

Koscuilek, J. F., & Merz, M. S. (2001). Structural analysis of the Consumer-Directed Theory of Empowerment. *Rehabilitation Counseling Bulletin, 44*(4), 209–216.

Kryla-Lighthall, N., & Mather, M. (2009). The role of cognitive control in older adults' emotional well-being. In V. Bengtson, D. Gans, N. Putney, & M. Silverstein (Eds.), *Handbook of theories of aging* (2nd ed., pp. 323–344). New York, NY: Springer Publishing Company.

Lynott, R. J., & Lynott, P. P. (1996). Tracing the course of theoretical development in the sociology of aging. *The Gerontologist, 36,* 749–760.

Mahoney, E., & Kayala, D. (2011). *The Veterans-Directed HCBS Program evaluation.* Retrieved from https://nrcpds.bc.edu/details.php?entryid=365

Mahoney, K. J. (2011). Person-centered planning and participant decision-making. *Health & Social Work, 36*(3), 233–234.

Mahoney, K. J., Meiners, M., Shoop, D., & Squillace, M. (2003). Cash and counseling and managed long-term care. *Case Management Journal, 4*(1), 18–22.

Mahoney, K. J., Simon-Rusinowitz, L., Loughlin, D. M., Desmond, S. M., & Squillace, M. R. (2004). Determining personal care consumers' preferences for a Consumer Directed Cash and Counseling Option: Survey results from Arkansas, Florida, New Jersey, and New York elders and adults with physical disabilities. *Health Services Research, 39*(3), 643–664.

Martin, L. G., Schoeni, R. F., & Andreski, P. M. (2010). Trends in health of older adults in the United States: Past, present and future. *Demography, 47,* 17–40.

Meiners, M., Mahoney, K., Shoop, D., & Squillace, M. (2002). Consumer direction in managed long-term care: An exploratory survey of practices and perceptions. *The Gerontologist, 42*(1), 32–38.

Mui, A. C., Choi, N. G., & Monk, A. (1998). *Long-term care and ethnicity*. Westport, CT: Auburn House.

National Health Interview Survey. (2012). *Summary health statistics for U.S. adults: 2010*. Washington, DC: U.S. Department of Health and Human Services.

National Resource Center for Participant-Directed Services (NRCPDS). (2013). *The 2013 National Inventory of Participant-Directed Programs*. (Data file). Chestnut Hill, MA: Boston College School of Social Work.

NRCPDS. (2014). *Facts and Figures: 2013 National Inventory Survey on Participant Direction*. Retrieved from https://nrcpds.bc.edu/details.php?entryid=445

Olmstead *v.* L.C., 572 U.S. 581 (1999).

O'Shaughnessy, C. V. (2014). *National spending for long-term services and supports, 2012*. Retrieved from http://www.nhpf.org/library/details.cfm/2783

Polivka, L. (2000). The ethical and empirical basis for consumer-directed care for the frail elderly. *Contemporary Gerontology, 7*(2), 50–52.

Putnam, M., & Frieden, L. (2014). Sharpening the aim of long-term services and supports policy. *Public Policy and Aging Report, 24*, 60–64.

Robert Wood Johnson Foundation. (2011). *Health care's blind side, the overlooked connection between social needs and good health: Summary of findings from a survey of America's physicians*. Retrieved from http://www.rwjf.org/content/dam/farm/reports/surveys_and_polls/2011/rwjf71795

Rook, K. S. (1984). The negative side of social interaction: Impact on psychological well-being. *Journal of Personality and Social Psychology, 46*, 1097–1108.

Rook, K. S. (2001). Emotional health and positive versus negative social exchanges: A daily diary analysis. *Applied Developmental Science, 5*, 87–97.

The Scan Foundation. (2012). *Achieving person-centered care: The five pillars of system transformation (Policy Brief #7)* (pp. 388–396). Long Beach, CA: The SCAN Foundation.

Schuster, T., Kessler, R. C., & Aseltine, R. H. (1990). Supportive interactions, negative interactions and depressed mood. *American Journal of Community Psychology, 18*, 423–438.

Sciegaj, M., Capitman, J. A., & Kyriacou, C. K. (2004). Consumer-directed community care: Race/ethnicity and individual differences in preferences for control. *The Gerontologist, 44*(4), 489–499.

Shearer, N. B. (2009). Health empowerment theory as a guide to practice. *Geriatric Nursing, 30*, 4–10.

Shen, C., Smyer, M. A., Mahoney, K. J., Loughlin, D. M., Simon-Rusinowitz, L., & Mahoney, E. K. (2008a). Does mental illness affect consumer direction of community-based care? Lessons from the Arkansas Cash and Counseling program. *The Gerontologist, 48*(1), 93–104.

Shen, C., Smyer, M. A., Mahoney, K. J., Simon-Rusinowitz, L., Shinogle, J., Norstrand, J.,...Vecchio, P. (2008b). Consumer direction, personal care, and well-being for Medicaid beneficiaries with mental health diagnoses: Lessons from the New Jersey Cash and Counseling Program. *Psychiatric Services, 59*, 1299–1306.

Suitor, J., Gilligan, M., & Pillemer, K. (2013). The role of violated caregiver preferences in psychological well-being when older mothers need assistance. *The Gerontologist, 53*(3), 397–406.

Thompson, N., & Thompson, S. (2001). Empowering older people: Beyond the care model. *Journal of Social Work, 1*(1), 61–76.

Wehmeyer, M. L., & Aberty, B. H. (2013). Self-determination and choice. *Intellectual and Developmental Disabilities, 51*(5), 399–411.

CHAPTER 23

Theories Guiding Support Services
for Family Caregivers

Rhonda J. V. Montgomery, Jung Kwak, and Karl D. Kosloski

Since the publication of the first seminal articles about family caregiver by Ethell Shanas (1979) and Elaine Brody (1985), research about family caregivers has expanded exponentially. Over a period of three decades, research efforts have advanced from conducting descriptive studies of patterns of caregiving and caregiving outcomes to conducting studies with more rigorous methods to assess predictors and outcomes of caregiving and effectiveness of caregiver interventions.

Although caregivers and the caregiving experience have been studied through the lenses of multiple disciplines and theoretical orientations, two theoretical frameworks have most frequently provided the foundation for the design and study of caregiver interventions. The stress process model, first articulated by Pearlin, Mullan, Semple, and Skaff (1990), has been widely used to guide both research and practice related to the caregivers' stress. Variations of the behavioral health model, first introduced by Andersen (1968), have been used by researchers seeking to understand and promote the use of support services by caregivers. Each of these theoretical frameworks and their implications for design and implementation of caregiver support programs are described in the following discussion. Additionally, this chapter includes a discussion of the practice-oriented framework for service use delineated by Yeatts, Crow, and Folts (1992) and the caregiver identity theory articulated by Montgomery and Kosloski (2009, 2013). Both these frameworks have the potential to guide the selection and delivery of caregiver interventions that target the unique needs of, individual caregivers.

■ THE CAREGIVING STRESS PROCESS FRAMEWORK

For more than two decades, the stress process framework articulated by Pearlin et al. (1990) has been a dominant theoretical framework guiding the development and study of interventions to support caregivers. Indeed, our study team recently conducted a review of empirical articles focused on caregiver supports and interventions that have been published since 2000. Notably, more than 25% of the 100 articles were based on, or guided by, a variant of the stress and coping theory. The stress process framework, which is based on earlier work of Pearlin et al. (1981) and the transactional theory of stress and coping by Lazarus and Folkman (1984), was designed to provide a conceptual framework that could advance caregiving research and measurement and account for inconsistent findings from previous research.

Key Components of the Stress Process Framework

A major strength of the stress process framework is that it is a comprehensive framework that organizes a large number of factors into four domains: (a) background characteristics of the caregiver context, (b) stressors, (c) mediators of stress, and (d) the outcomes or manifestations of stress. Each of these major components of the model is described here along with the model's contributions to the caregiving literature.

BACKGROUND AND CONTEXT OF CAREGIVING STRESS

According to the framework, the caregiving context impacts directly and indirectly each of the other sets of factors in the stress process as well as the outcomes for the caregiver. The caregiving context includes key characteristics of the caregiver and the care environment. Variables grouped into this domain include caregiver age, gender, ethnicity, socioeconomic status, educational attainment, employment, family composition, the caregiver's relationship to the care recipient (e.g., spouse or adult child) and the nature of past and current relationships (e.g., amiable or problematic). The caregiving context also includes the availability of support services or resources. Variables included in the care context domain can have significant implications for the types of stressors a caregiver faces, the way in which the caregiver appraises and copes with those stressors, and the outcomes of caregiving.

THE STRESSORS

Stressors are defined by Pearlin et al. (1990) as the "problematic conditions and difficult circumstances experienced by caregivers," and are conceptualized as primary and secondary in nature. *Primary stressors* are challenges or problems that are directly linked to the caregiving situation and the care recipient's illness or disability. Primary stressors are further categorized into primary objective stressors (i.e., care recipient's functional and health status, such as type and severity of the disease, activities of daily living, and behavioral problems) and primary subjective stressors (i.e., caregivers' subjective perception of care demands as stressful such as role overload and relational deprivation). *Secondary stressors* are those that are produced or affected by primary stressors. Secondary stressors include role strains that occur outside of the caregiving arena (e.g., employment, family, and economic strains) and intrapsychic strains related to the caregiver's self-concept, including role captivity, loss of self, competence, and gain.

MEDIATORS OF STRESS

The level of social support and coping skills is identified as mediating factors that influence the stress process both directly and indirectly. The presence of strong social support and coping skills is expected to help sustain the caregiver and lessen the effect of the stressors. Hence, these mediators, in part, account for the fact that caregivers are impacted differently by the same stressors.

OUTCOMES

The stress process affects the caregiver's well-being, physical and mental health, and the ability to continue providing care. Mental health outcomes that have been examined include depression, anxiety, and cognitive disturbances. Physical health outcomes that have been examined include self-rated health, common health problems, injuries and sleep disturbances (Belle et al., 2006; Elliott, Burgio, & DeCoster, 2010; Gaugler, Roth, Haley, & Mittelman, 2008; Lee, Czaja, & Schulz, 2010; Shulz & Maritre, 2004).

PROLIFERATION

"Proliferation" is a key concept that is central to the stress process framework. Proliferation refers to the process whereby stressors in one role or domain of life impact other domains or roles. For example, stress stemming from the caregiving role can impact one's employment role. Stressors rarely occur in isolation from one another, and primary stressors can lead to secondary stressors and can affect global outcomes. Moreover, the model suggests that, at different points along the stress process, coping and social support can potentially intervene as "the mediator to limit the proliferation of secondary stressors" (Pearlin et al., 1990, p. 590). Changes that occur in stressors and changes that occur in mediating factors make the caregiving journey both dynamic and complex (Aneshensel, Pearlin, Mullan, Zarit, & Whitlatch, 1995; Pearlin et al., 1990).

IMPLICATIONS OF THE STRESS PROCESS FRAMEWORK FOR PRACTICE

The stress process framework has not only provided guidance for the study of the caregiving as a dynamic process, but it has also influenced the design of caregiver support programs in two major ways. First, the framework clearly demonstrates that the stress of caregiving involves far more than the burden of providing physical care. Indeed, multiple factors interact to influence the caregiving experience. This understanding of caregiving as a complex experience has helped to explain inconsistent and sometimes enigmatic findings from early intervention studies that focused on a single type of support, such as respite. As the caregiving experience is influenced by factors in multiple domains, it is unlikely that any single intervention will alleviate a caregiver's stress throughout the duration of the caregiving experience.

Perhaps the most significant impact of the stress process framework on caregiver interventions has been the development of a wide range of psychoeducational interventions. Before the introduction of the stress process framework, the major focus of caregiver support programs was to introduce services that would relieve the workload of caregivers, such as respite or chore services. The stress process framework not only provided an explanation for disappointing findings from studies of adult day (e.g., Weissert et al., 1990) and respite programs (Lawton, Brody, & Saperstein, 1991; Montgomery & Borgatta, 1989) that revealed mixed or limited benefits, but it also identified secondary stressors and mediators, such as coping and self-efficacy, that could be targeted by psychoeducation programs. Although results from evaluations of these educational interventions have been mixed (Hepburn, Lewis, Sherman, & Tornatore, 2003; Judge et al., 2011; Savundranayagam, Montgomery, Kosloski, & Little, 2011; Toseland, McCallion, Smith, & Banks, 2004; Tremont, Davis, Bishop, & Fortinsky, 2008), psychoeducation programs have proliferated. Two of the most widely available programs that are guided by stress and coping theory (Lazarus & Folkman, 1984) are Powerful Tools for Caregivers (Cleland et al., 2006) and the Savvy Caregiver Program (Hepburn et al., 2003). Both of these educational programs have been recognized by the U.S. Administration of Community Living as best practice models.

The second way that the stress process framework has influenced the design of caregiver support programs has been to underscore the importance for programs to target multiple domains for intervention. The identification of multiple sources and types of caregiver stress has encouraged the development of multicomponent intervention programs that include components focused on secondary intrapsychic factors, such as mastery and role captivity, and on coping skills and social supports. Notable among such multicomponent interventions that are grounded in the stress and coping models are the caregiver support counseling intervention developed at NYU and the Resources for Enhancing Alzheimer's Caregivers Health (REACH) II interventions. The NYU multicomponent counseling program has three components: individual and family counseling, support group participation, and ad hoc counseling. This intervention has been shown to reduce depressive symptoms and burden, delayed nursing home placement, and also retained the positive effect during caregivers' adaption to bereavement (Gaugler et al., 2008; Haley et al., 2008; Mittelman, Roth, Haley, & Zarit, 2004). However, given the multicomponent nature of the intervention, it is difficult to identify and test specific components of the intervention affecting the caregiver outcomes within the stress process framework.

The REACH program (Belle et al., 2006; Elliott et al., 2010; Lee et al., 2010) has also gained traction in practice settings. The initial evaluation of the REACH program was conducted as a multisite, randomized study that included more than 600 caregivers who self-identified as Black–African American, Hispanic–Latino, or Caucasian–White. The REACH II was designed to be a "tailored" intervention based on individual risk assessment. This intervention, which is based on the stress health framework, targets its multiple components including safety, self-care, social support, emotional well-being, and problem behaviors, making it suitable for testing different components of the stress process model. Several publications of findings from the multisite study of the REACH II program have reported positive outcomes for caregivers, including improved health, sleep, emotional health, and depression. The positive outcomes, however, were not reported for all segments of the study participants. For example, although the older Hispanic and Black caregivers who received the intervention reported a decrease in caregiving burden from baseline to follow-up, there were no significant effects of the intervention on overall Hispanic or White caregivers' depressive symptoms. These findings underscore the importance of caregiver's background characteristics and the care context as factors that may interact with mediators (e.g., family support) or interventions to affect the caregiving outcomes differently across various groups of caregivers. As Pearlin et al. (1990) note, these factors not only influence the stressors and outcomes, but also the mediating factors. Differential impact of these interventions on caregiver outcomes across various groups of caregivers underscores the need for further efforts to efficiently target support services to the specific needs of each individual caregiver.

Finally, more recent studies that have examined the effect of adult day services that include additional components such as care management have found that the inclusion of care management as a component of adult day service is associated with lower depression, increased confidence in managing care receiver behaviors, and enhanced well-being among caregivers in the treatment group (Gitlin et al., 2003; Gitlin, Reever, Dennis, Mathieu, & Hauck, 2006; Kim, Zarit, Femia, & Savla, 2012). These findings provide evidence that the combination of targeting primary stressors by providing respite for family caregivers and targeting secondary stressors by providing additional care management support can improve caregiver outcomes.

■ THEORIES USED TO EXPLAIN USE OF SUPPORT SERVICES

With its emphasis on the caregiving context and secondary strains, the stress process framework has provided insights that help one to explain the diversity of the caregiving experience and guide the development of multicompetent intervention programs. However, the benefits of any intervention can be obtained only if caregivers actually use the support services that are offered to them. Unfortunately, there is substantial evidence that many caregivers do not use services available to them or use them too late to benefit from them. For example, even among caregivers who are aware of the availability of respite programs and who are ostensibly good candidates for them, the programs often go unused (Lawton 1991; Montgomery & Borgatta, 1989; Montgomery, Marquis, Kosloski, Schaefer, & Karner, 2002). In addition to nonuse, there is the problem of brief users. These are caregivers who use the service over a relatively short period of time (e.g., 3 months or less) and then, apparently, never use it again. Brief users have been shown to comprise between 24% and 29% of all respite users (Cox, 1997; Zarit, Stephens, Townsend, Greene, & Leitsch, 1999). These findings have left both researchers and practitioners asking why many caregivers are either nonusers or brief users of supportive services such as respite care. Two frameworks are presented here that have been advanced to explain the use of health and social services in general and have been used to examine service use by family caregivers.

Behavioral Health Model of Service Utilization

The behavioral model of health service utilization (referred to as the "behavioral model" hereafter) is one of the most widely used theoretical frameworks for health services research, and has been applied to a wide range of health, long-term care, and caregiver support services (see Aday & Awe, 1997, for a review of this issue). As initially articulated, the model asserted that use of health services "is dependent on: (1) the predisposition of the individual to use services; (2) his ability to secure services; and (3) his illness level" (Andersen & Newman, 1973, p. 107). Predisposing factors include background and demographic characteristics, such as age, gender, race, and health that make an individual predisposed or susceptible to service use. Enabling factors include family and community resources that can facilitate or hinder service use (e.g., family income, health insurance, availability of health personnel and facilities, and geographic location of the community in which the individual lives). The need component includes the illness level perceived by the individual and the illness evaluated by the delivery system. The model was later modified and expanded to include organizational determinants such as characteristics of the health care system as predictors of service use (Aday & Andersen, 1974; Andersen, 1995; Andersen, Davidson, & Ganz, 1994; Andersen & Newman, 1973). Health care system determinants refer to the arrangements made to provide care to potential consumers and include volume and distribution of resources, access to resources, structure of resource organization, and health policy (Andersen, 1995).

Use of health services is determined directly by individual determinants and indirectly by health care system factors. Health care system factors indirectly influence the use of health services by directly influencing individual determinants (Andersen, 1995). Within the individual determinant components, predisposing factors precede the enabling factors that are followed by need factors (Aday & Andersen, 1974; Andersen & Newman, 1973). Bradley et al. (2002), however, conceptualize psychosocial determinants, which include health beliefs, knowledge, and attitude, to be a separate construct from predisposing factors. Bradley et al. (2002) also suggest that psychosocial factors follow, rather than precede, enabling and need factors and thereby serve as mediating factors that influence health service use and, ultimately, outcomes of service use.

The behavioral model has been applied to a wide range of health services used by older adults including caregiver support services (Bergman, Haley, & Small, 2011; Herrera, Lee, Palos, & Torres-Vigil, 2008; Miller, 2004; Penning, 1995; Radina & Barber, 2004; Scharlach, Giunta, Chun-Chung Chow, & Lehning, 2008; Toseland, McCallion, Gerber, & Banks, 2002). In general, studies guided by the behavioral health model that have examined predictors of formal service use by caregivers have found enabling factors to be significant predictors of caregiver support service use (Herrera et al., 2008; Radina & Barber, 2004; Scharlach et al., 2008; Toseland et al., 2002). The study by Herrera et al. (2008) with Mexican American caregivers of older adults found that enabling factors including knowledge regarding services, health insurance status, and Medicaid insurance status were significant predictors of long-term care service use along with the level of familism among caregivers. Similarly, findings from several other studies that have examined use of formal support services by family caregivers have identified enabling factors as the most dominant predictors of use of services by family caregivers (Radina & Barber, 2004; Scharlach et al., 2008; Toseland et al., 2002). These findings support the view that knowledge of services, social support, and social network are important facilitators of caregiver support use. Other studies examining predictors of bereaved caregiver support services (Bergman et al., 2011), and home health services (Penning, 1995), however, found the need factors to be more important in explaining the use of these services by caregivers.

With the inclusion of some factors that are amenable to change (e.g., public policy, health care beliefs and attitudes, knowledge and sources of health care information) and individual attributes that are immutable, such as predisposing and need factors, the model offers a systematic approach to examine the relative effect of each component of the model. One concern about the various versions of the model (e.g., Aday & Awe, 1997), however, is that predictors may not have been adequately captured because of inconsistent conceptualization and measurement of concepts such as need and illness. The original and modified versions of the model do not specify the relationships between psychosocial variables (e.g., beliefs and knowledge regarding illness), enabling (e.g., social network), need, and service use (Bradley et al., 2002; Kart, 1991). In the case of caregiver support service use, caregivers' beliefs and attitudes toward services that have not been studied extensively include the features or expected outcomes that caregivers associate with the utility of different types of support services (e.g., benefit, usefulness, and convenience) or the specific barriers to the use of such services (Phillipson, Jones, & Magee, 2014). This is an important omission because beliefs are the one predisposing characteristic in the behavioral model (Andersen, 1995) considered to be mutable and potentially an important target area for intervention. The model has also been criticized for giving priority to need as a predictor and for its limited predictive and explanatory capacity (Aday & Awe, 1997; Montoro-Rodriguez, Kosloski, & Montgomery, 2003).

Nevertheless, the flexibility of the behavioral model suggests that the model can be revised or augmented to overcome its limitations. Many researchers have expanded the behavioral model by adding explanatory variables that are relevant and specific to the type of utilization behavior explored in their studies such as several studies of caregivers' use of support as described in this chapter (e.g., Herrera et al., 2008; Radina & Barber,

2004; Toseland et al., 2002). Future studies would benefit further by applying greater specificity in the measurement of the beliefs of caregivers around the use of specific services to better understand the relationship between beliefs and service use behaviors.

Practice-Oriented Service Model

From the perspective of caregiver support programs, which generally operate outside of health care systems, the utility of the behavioral health model has two significant limitations. First, with the exception of health beliefs and knowledge about a disability or disease, the characteristics of individuals included in the model are not amenable to intervention by service providers. Second, most of the organizational characteristics that are included in the revised behavioral health model are attributes of health systems, but not attributes of organizations that provide social services. Consequently, the model is of limited practical use to service providers. In contrast, the practice-oriented framework advanced by Yeatts et al. (1992) has greater potential for influencing service use because it includes "factors specific to areas that can be addressed by social service providers in order to increase service use" (Yeatts et al., 1992, p. 25). The practice-oriented framework shifts the focus from individual characteristics that are mostly immutable to barriers of service use and strategies that can be used by organizations to mitigate the barriers.

Based on an extensive review of the literature focused on barriers to service use among older adults, Yeatts et al. (1992) identified three conditions that must be met for a potential client to use a service. The individual must have "knowledge related to the services, access to the services, and intent to use the service." A deficiency in any of these conditions creates a barrier to use. When Yeatts et al. (1992) articulated the practice-oriented model, they included a catalog of strategies for overcoming barriers that they created using information gained from a case study of strategies used by the 28 Area Agencies on Aging in the state of Texas and a literature review focused on publications that describe strategies that have been used to overcome barriers.

KNOWLEDGE

The knowledge factor as described within the practice-oriented framework includes three types of information that are required for a potential client to use a service. An individual must (a) know or believe he or she has a need, (b) know that a service is available, and (c) know how to obtain the service. For example, if a caregiver is to use a respite program, the individual must self-identity as a caregiver who is in need of help and know that the program exists and know how to enroll in the program. Two major strategies identified to help clients recognize their need for a service are media campaigns and gaining cooperation of significant individuals such as physicians, clergy, or discharge planners to inform potential clients. These two strategies were also included as a means to inform potential clients about service availability and the process for obtaining the service. Dissemination of information at gatherings of community and social groups is another strategy for informing potential clients about services.

ACCESS

The framework includes three types of access barriers: transportation, affordability, and availability. Strategies that organizations can use to overcome access barriers include relocating services to be closer to client populations, increasing the availability of transportation, lowering fares, seeking new sources of funding, and reallocation of existing resources to match organizations' priorities.

INTENT

Intent to use a service is defined as the client's willingness and interest in obtaining service. Three types of barriers to intent are lack of appeal, cultural differences, and negative attitudes toward receiving help. For example, a caregiver will be unlikely to use a respite program if the facility or the food is not appealing, the care recipient speaks a different language from that of staff or other participants, or the caregiver believes he or she is solely responsible for his or her partner's care. Strategies suggested to overcome barriers stemming from cultural differences included the creation of separate programs for different cultural groups that could be offered on different schedules or in different locations. Another strategy is to increase cultural competency of staff. Strategies identified to overcome negative attitudes toward receiving help included enlisting the help of influential and respected community members as advocates and offering incentives to visit a program or use a service on a trial basis.

A limitation of the practice-oriented framework is the absence of evidence to prove the effectiveness of the various strategies that are described. However, there are a number of publications that describe programs that have successfully employed many of these strategies to serve family caregivers of rural and minority communities (e.g., Karner & Hall, 2002; Starns, Karner, & Montgomery, 2002; Sun, Mutlu, & Coon, 2014). Moreover, the framework has frequently been used to explain and interpret study findings that identified measures of knowledge, access, and attitudes toward services as predictors of service use (e.g., Dorfman, Holmes, & Berlin, 1997; Kosloski, Montgomery, & Youngbauer, 2001; Sun et al., 2014). Indeed, the value of the framework for explaining use of services by caregivers was affirmed by Montoro-Rodriguez et al. (2003), who conducted a study of respite use in a sample of 1,158 culturally diverse caregivers. Findings from the study indicated that explanatory models for service use were significantly improved when variables linked to the practice-oriented framework were added to a model that initially included only variables representing factors in the behavioral health model.

Surprisingly, given the very pragmatic implications of the framework for the design and evaluation of caregiver support services, there is little evidence that the framework has intentionally been used for this purpose. It is quite possible that this absence of evidence stems from the fact that organizations that are most likely to use the framework to inform their practice do not regularly engage studies to evaluate their programs or published information about their efforts. In any case, the potential benefits of the practice-oriented model for guiding the development and delivery of caregiver support services remain largely untapped.

Caregiver Identity Theory

Like the stress process model, the Caregiver Identity Theory, as articulated by Montgomery and Kosloski (2009, 2013), was set forth as a conceptual framework that is consistent with findings from extensive research on the caregiving experience, many of which were enigmatic. The theory, which builds on identity theory as articulated by Stryker (1968; Stryker & Burke, 2000; Stryker & Serpe, 1994) and expanded by Burke

(1991; Burke & Reitzes, 1991), conceptualizes caregiving as a series of identity transitions that result from changes in the caregiving context and in personal norms. From this perspective, an identity is a set of meanings applied to the self in a social role or situation that defines an individual's conception of self within that relationship. This set of meanings is tied to a set of personal norms or identity standards that are used as a reference point to guide behavior.

Because individuals have multiple relationships, they also have multiple identities, which together create an individual's conception of self. The caregiver identity theory is focused on a caregiver's sense of self in relationship to the care recipient. A major tenet of the theory is that identity discrepancy, defined as incongruence between a caregiver's behavior and his or her identity standards, is a major source of caregiver stress. The theory is grounded in the fundamental observation that there is no single generic caregiver role and is built around three key premises.

> First, the caregiving role is acquired in a systematic way. Second, caregiving is a dynamic process that changes over time. Third, as caregivers experience change in their role, they also experience a change in their relationship with the care recipient and a change in their identity. (Montgomery & Kosloski, 2013, p. 134)

ACQUISITION OF THE CAREGIVING ROLE AND ACCOMPANYING NORMS

The caregiving role emerges out of another role relationship, usually a familial relationship; and like other social behaviors, the role is governed by norms or social rules. Therefore, to understand the diversity of the caregiving experience in terms of care tasks and differential outcomes, it is important to understand how caregivers acquire the role and the corresponding norms. To a large extent, systematic cultural rules operate to dictate responsibility for care, a fact that is reflected in the prevalence of spouses, adult daughters, and daughters-in-law as primary caregivers (Cantor, 1979). At the same time, there is great variability among caregivers in the extent to which general social norms influence their personal attitudes and behaviors. Caregivers' expectations regarding the types of care tasks that are appropriate and the specific conditions under which it is appropriate to seek assistance from outside the family (e.g., from public or private agencies) are not only influenced by general social norms but are also affected by a caregiver's ethnic and cultural background, unique family ethos, and specific circumstances. Hence, the acquisition of the caregiving role is always an idiosyncratic process and, once assumed, there is no single, generic caregiver role.

CAREGIVING IS A DYNAMIC PROCESS

As the condition and needs of care recipients change, caregivers alter their activities and the responsibilities that they assume. Because caregivers tend to do what needs to be done despite any discomfort with care tasks, they often find themselves engaging in tasks that are inconsistent with their initial familial role (e.g., spouse, daughter, and son). This change in role performance, in turn, leads to a change in the dyadic relationship between the caregiver and the care recipient and ultimately an identity change.

For most caregivers, identity change is a slow process that alternates between periods of relative stability and periods of significant change. The process can best be understood within the Piagetian framework of assimilation and accommodation (Piaget, 1971). Initially, the care needs of the elder may be relatively small and easily met by the caregiver with only minimal change in the original dyadic relationship. For example, a son who is providing support for his elderly mother may begin by assisting his mother with such things as paying bills or driving her to appointments. He is able to *assimilate* these tasks into his lifestyle with minimal distress. As his mother's dementia advances, however, her needs for care increase. The son now finds the personal care tasks that he must perform to be discrepant with his personal norms and identity as a son. Put another way, there is incongruence between the duties the son is now performing and how he views his filial responsibility (i.e., his relationship identity) as a son. This discrepancy creates distress that can manifest as a sense of time compression (i.e., objective burden), strain in the interpersonal relationship (i.e., relationship burden), or anxiety/depression (i.e., stress burden; Savundranayagam & Montgomery, 2010). The son is now motivated to reduce his distress by restoring congruence between his behavior and his personal norms or standards.

How would the son then restore the congruence? If the son is to continue with these tasks, he will have to *accommodate* the care tasks and responsibilities that he has assumed, which require a noticeable shift in identity to allow incorporation of new caregiving activities. The end result is that the identity change process for caregivers is a discontinuous process that proceeds in stops and starts. In situations where the caregiving context is stable, it is easy for an individual to steadily maintain a role identity in relation to the care receiver. As the caregiving context changes, because of increased disability of the care recipient or loss of support, the caregiver is no longer able to "stretch" his or her identity to assimilate the change in caregiving activities. At that point, an identity change is necessary to relieve distress. It is for this reason that two caregivers can be performing the very same activities and for one caregiver the activities are distressing, whereas for the other they are not.

THE IDENTITY MAINTENANCE PROCESS FOR CAREGIVERS

A caregiver's identity cannot always be changing, even though the demands of caregiving may require change from time to time. The identity change process is best understood as an intermittent process that alternates between extended time periods when caregivers experience stability and transition periods marked by high identity discrepancy and distress. An understanding of the identity maintenance process that enables periods of stability provides valuable guidance for intervention during transition periods marked by distress.

Montgomery and Kosloski (2013) describe the caregiver identity maintenance process as a continuous, self-adjusting feedback loop that operates as a homeostatic control system to keep an identity stable. The process involves three key elements: identity standards, behaviors, and self-appraisal. This process begins for a caregiver with the establishment of an *identity standard* or set of internalized norms that a caregiver uses to define the behaviors or actions that are appropriate for interacting with the care recipient. For most caregivers, their initial identity standard is closely linked to a familial role (e.g., wife, husband, son, daughter) and provides guidance for being a "good" spouse, daughter or son. This standard is altered over time to include norms or rules about being a "good" caregiver. Individuals use their identity standards to guide their *behavior*. Individuals also continuously engage in *self-appraisal* to determine the level of congruency between their actions or behaviors and their identity standard. If a caregiver judges his or her actions to be consistent with his or her internalized norms (e.g., identity standards), then there is homeostasis and the current identity is maintained.

If, however, the self-appraisal leads to the conclusion that the caregiver's behavior is incongruent with the identity standard, the caregiver will experience some level of distress because of the discrepancy.

Caregivers experience stability in their identity when the identity maintenance system operates as a closed system wherein the caregiver's behaviors are almost fully governed by the caregiver's identity standard. A significant shift in the care context, however, such as increased disability of the care recipient, can disrupt the identity maintenance process. In this case, a caregiver may engage in behaviors that are not aligned with his or her identity standard, simply because the care recipient needs more help or a different type of help. As a result, the caregiver will experience the distress of identity discrepancy.

When the discrepancy is small, caregivers can often relieve the distress and maintain their current identity by making a small incremental change in behavior. For example, a daughter who in the past had helped mom with shopping on a monthly basis might start doing all of the grocery shopping for her mother on a weekly basis. This small change in behavior is a concession that will allow her to maintain her identity as a daughter and still meet her mother's needs.

In contrast, when a caregiver encounters a situation where he or she is experiencing significant distress, the behavioral change that is required may be too big of a stretch relative to the caregiver's identity standard. In this situation, the identity maintenance process is disrupted, causing the caregiver to experience significant distress. For example, this might occur if a daughter must prepare meals and monitor medications on a daily basis. Large discrepancies create pressure toward identity change.

FIVE PHASES OF CAREGIVING

The pie charts in Figure 23.1 depict the identity change process that occurs as caregivers transition through five phases of caregiving identified by Montgomery and Kosloski (2013). The caregiving journey starts when a family member first engages in tasks or assumes responsibilities that go above and beyond those that she has previously assumed as part of her familial role. An example of phase one is a wife who takes over management of the household finances that in the past had been managed by her husband. During this phase, the salience of the caregiver role is minimal because caregivers tend to view tasks related to this role as an extension of their initial familial role. Caregivers generally enter phase two of their journey when the care tasks and responsibilities that are assumed have increased in quantity or intensity to the extent that the caregiver becomes consciously aware that the tasks are clearly inconsistent with the personal norms that are tied to his or her familial role.

Phase three usually occurs when a caregiver engages in personal care tasks that are clearly inconsistent with the initial family role, such as a wife now assisting with toileting. At this point, caregivers assume an identity within the relationship that is defined equally by their role as a caregiver and their initial family role (e.g., spouse, daughter). A caregiver's identity during phase four of the caregiving journey is dominated by the caregiver role. Caregivers in this phase of the journey are usually providing extensive assistance to a family member who has a high a level of dependency. It is during this phase that a caregiver begins contemplating placement of the care recipient in an alternate care setting, such as a nursing home or assisted living facility. Phase five of the caregiving journey occurs when the caregiver turns the majority of care responsibilities over to a formal care provider by placing the care recipient in an alternate care setting,

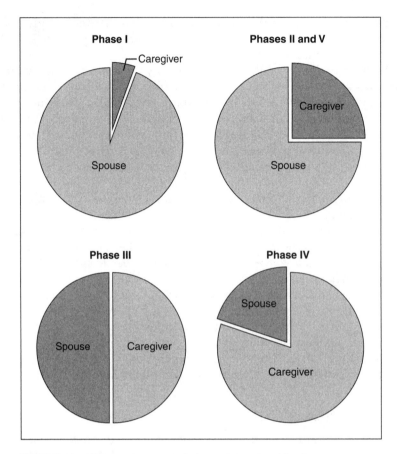

FIGURE 23.1 Phases of accommodation and caregiver identity.

Source: Montgomery and Kosloski (2013, p. 144).

such as a nursing home or assisted-living facility. When this happens, the caregiver can regain an identity that is similar to that of phase two where the familial role again becomes more salient as the caregiver negotiates his or her roles and identity within the relationship.

Although the five phases serve as a useful heuristic, there are great variations in the ways the caregivers progress through the phases. Not all caregivers pass through every phase and sometimes caregivers' paths are not unidirectional. Moreover, duration of time that a caregiver spends in each phase will vary depending on the condition and needs of the care recipient. The uniform aspect of the transition process is that psychological distress in the form of identity discrepancy triggers transitions between phases.

IMPLICATIONS OF CAREGIVER IDENTITY FOR PRACTICE

The caregiver identity theory provides guidance for practice in two ways. At a general level, it offers three insights that can be used to design an effective caregiver support program. At a more specific level, it provides a framework for targeting support services to the specific needs of caregivers as their needs change over the duration of their journey.

With regard to program design, first, the theory fuels the growing consensus that no single intervention can address the needs of the caregiver population. With its emphasis on the diversity of the caregiving experience, the theory provides a framework to explain empirical findings that reveal the most effective caregiver support programs to be those that include multiple support services. Clearly, multicomponent programs are better able to address familial and cultural differences as well as the changing needs of individual caregivers over time. Second, with its emphasis on personal norms as critical factors influencing a caregiver's distress, the theory underscores the limitations of caregiver assessments that focus primarily on care tasks and the need to use reliable measures of a caregiver's psychological well-being to accurately assess a caregiver's needs. Third, the theory highlights the importance for follow-up. One time or limited time interactions with caregivers are likely to be insufficient given the changing nature and duration of the caregiving journey.

At a more specific level, the caregiver identity theory provides very pragmatic guidance for reducing caregiver distress, which is to reduce incongruence between what the caregiver is doing (i.e., caregiving tasks and responsibilities) and what the caregiver believes he or she should be doing (i.e., the caregiver's identity standard). Although this may sound abstract, the theory clearly identifies three strategies for alleviating identity discrepancy. One strategy for reducing identity discrepancy is to help change a caregiver's behaviors to align them with the caregiver's current identity standard. For example, a daughter who is uncomfortable assuming responsibility for her mother's finances might align her behaviors with her identity standard by hiring a financial counselor to assist her mother. A second strategy to reduce identity discrepancy is to change the caregiver's self-appraisal or perception of congruence. It is often the case that caregivers start to "second guess" the appropriateness of their actions when long distance relatives begin giving advice in the absence of a full understanding of the caregiving situation. A counselor or a support group might help a caregiver in this situation by reaffirming the appropriateness of the caregiver's actions. A third strategy for reducing identity discrepancy is to help caregivers change their identity standards to align with their behavior. This strategy can be used when a caregiver inaccurately believes that the care responsibilities that he or she has assumed go above and beyond what is necessary. That is, from the caregiver's perspective, the care recipient is demanding too much help. In cases like this, caregivers often do not have an accurate understanding of the care recipient's true level of disability and need for help. If the caregiver is given an opportunity to learn more about the care recipient's disease process, the caregiver is likely to embrace a larger role as a caregiver and corresponding identity standard. The strength of this model is that a very broad array of services and resources can be aligned with each of the three strategies for intervention. Therefore, a much wider array of services and resources can be drawn on to support caregivers, many of which are not advertised or offered by organizations specifically for caregivers.

TAILORED CAREGIVER ASSESSMENT AND REFERRAL®

To date the caregiver identity theory has most directly impacted the design of the Tailored Caregiver Assessment and Referral (TCARE®) system. TCARE is a care management protocol specifically designed to support family members who are providing care to adults, of any age, with chronic or acute health by connecting them with resources that are most apt to meet their specific needs. As such, TCARE operates as a triaging process to direct caregivers to optimal resources.

The TCARE protocol incorporates three key practice elements that reflect essential elements of the theory. First, the protocol focuses on two major areas as targets for intervention: identity discrepancy, which is viewed as a major source of caregiver burden, and the three types of caregiver burden that can be experienced as a result of identity discrepancy. Second, the protocol includes an assessment tool that not only includes measures of the care recipient's functional level and diagnosis and the caregiver's workload, but also measures of identity discrepancy, caregiver burden, and caregiver depression. Third, the protocol embraces an understanding that caregivers are diverse and that their experiences change over time and is therefore designed to create a care plan tailored to a caregiver's specific needs and preferences as they change over time.

The protocol includes a set of decision algorithms that operate to integrate and interpret extensive information about the caregiver, care receiver, and the care context that is obtained using a standardized assessment tool. The summary information generated by the algorithms enables care managers to create a preliminary care plan tailored to the unique needs of each caregiver. The preliminary plan includes optimal goals, strategies for meeting the goals, and key information about the costs and benefits of the recommended services. Care managers meet with the caregiver to present and discuss this information to enable the caregiver to make informed choices about using services and resources. The protocol also includes a follow-up process at 3-month intervals so that the care plan can be adjusted as appropriate throughout the caregiving journey.

The comprehensive TCARE system includes software, assessment tools, decision algorithms, and training and technical assistance programs. The system is implemented by care managers (usually social workers, nurses, or other human service professionals) who have completed training and been certified as TCARE specialists.

Findings from multiple studies (Lavelle, Mancuso, Huber, & Felver, 2014; Montgomery, Kwak, Kosloski, & Valuch, 2011) provide strong evidence that the use of the TCARE protocol promotes the well-being and mental health of caregivers and can ultimately delay or prevent nursing home placement (Lavelle et al., 2014). It is believed that these positive outcomes can be attributed to more effective assessment of the caregivers' current circumstances and needs and the creation of a care plan that identifies goals, strategies, and resources specifically selected to alleviate or diminish identity discrepancy, depression, and any of three types of burden that a caregiver is experiencing. Currently, the protocol is being used by more than 300 organizations located in 17 states.

■ SUMMARY AND CONCLUSION

Throughout history, family members, most often women, have been the primary providers of care for individuals, young and old, who are in need of assistance. This fact has not changed as the populations of industrialized countries have aged because of improvements in living conditions and health care. What has occurred in the past century is significant growth in the number of family members who are providing care and expansion of the responsibilities that these family caregivers now assume. The steady expansion of family caregiving has been mirrored by the steady expansion of research focused on caregivers and interventions to support them. A large segment of this body of research has been guided by one or more of the four theoretical frameworks reviewed in this chapter.

For more than two decades, the stress process framework advanced by Pearlin et al. (1990) or other variants of the stress and coping theory (Lazarus & Folkman, 1984) have been the dominant theoretical frameworks guiding the development and study of caregiver support interventions. The stress process model provides a comprehensive organizing framework that identifies multiple factors that interact to define the caregiving experience and outcomes of caregiving. With its emphasis on the caregiving context and secondary strains, the stress process framework helps explain the diversity of the caregiving experience and offers insights for the development of multicompetent intervention programs.

The benefits of any intervention, however, can be obtained only if caregivers actually use the support services that are offered to them. In the face of research findings and experience that indicated that a large segment of the caregiver population does not use available supports, researchers have turned to behavioral models of services utilization (Aday & Awe, 1997) and the practice-oriented model by Yeatts et al. (1992). Both models have provided insights for understanding service use and identifying strategies that can be incorporated into service delivery systems to foster use of services. The behavioral model of services utilization has been used to study the use of a wide range of health services by older adults and caregivers. Yet, two aspects of the model have limited its utility as a guide for the delivery of caregiver support services. The model identifies attributes of individual intervention as primary determinants of service and most of these attributes are not amenable to change. Moreover, the organizational characteristics that are included in later versions of the model as secondary factors affecting service use are attributes more closely aligned with health systems than with social service organizations.

The practice-oriented model articulated by Yeatts et al. (1992) addresses these two limitations of the behavioral health model. The three sets of factors included in the model as necessary to promote use of services are all amenable to influence by social service providers. Consequently, the practice-oriented model of service use has very pragmatic implications for strategies that can be used to design and deliver caregiver support services in a manner that will foster service use (Montoro-Rodriguez et al., 2003).

As evidence has mounted affirming the diversity and complexity of the caregiving experience and the merits of multicomponent interventions, providers have been challenged to find ways to effectively tailor and target services and resources to specific needs of a caregiver. The caregiver identity theory articulated by Montgomery and Kosloski (2009, 2013) provides a framework that can be used to target services to caregivers' needs. With its focus on identity discrepancy, which occurs as elements of the care context change, the theory provides guidance for creating support programs that can be tailored to the changing needs of individual caregivers. Indeed, the theory is the foundation for the comprehensive TCARE system that is used by care managers to accurately assess a caregiver's need to create effective care plans.

There is little doubt that the theories presented in this chapter have contributed to the significant progress that has occurred in our understanding of the dynamic and diverse experiences of caregivers. These theories have also contributed to development and delivery of multicomponent support programs and highlighted the need to target services in a way that will maximize benefits for family caregivers.

Although substantial room remains for refining our understanding of the complex process of caregiving, there is also a need for theory that can inform efforts to promote sustainable uptake, adoption, and implementation of effective caregiver support services in various communities. According to a review of the state of translational research on caregiving (Gitlin, 2013), despite increasing efforts to translate effective interventions in various communities (e.g., REACH II and TCARE study) in the last decade, limited data on outcomes of translational research are available, creating a gap in our understanding in terms of best strategies to translate current programs tailored to various communities, to train service providers, and to sustain services after grant funding ends. Building the science of translation and implementation of caregiving remains an important goal for future research.

REFERENCES

Aday, L. A., & Andersen, R. (1974). A framework for the study of access to medical care. *Health Services Research, 9*, 208–220.

Aday, L. A., & Awe, W. C. (1997). Health service utilization models. In D. S. Gochman (Ed.), *Handbook of health behavior research I: Personal and social determinants* (pp. 153–172). New York, NY: Plenum.

Andersen, R. (1968). *A behavioral model of families' use of health services (Research Series 25)*. Chicago, IL: The University of Chicago Center for Health Administration Studies.

Andersen, R. (1995). Revisiting the behavioral model and access to medical care: Does it matter? *Journal of Health and Social Behavior, 36*, 1–10.

Andersen, R. M., Davidson, P., & Ganz, P. (1994). Symbiotic relationships of qualify of life, health services research, and other health research. *Quality of Life Research, 3*, 365–371.

Andersen, R., & Newman, J. F. (1973). Societal and individual determinants of medical care utilization in the United States. *Milbank Memorial Fund Quarterly, 51*, 95–124.

Aneshensel, C. S., Pearlin, L. I., Mullan, J. T., Zarit, S. H., & Whitlatch, C. J. (1995). *Profiles in caregiving; The unexpected career*. San Diego, CA: Academic.

Belle, S. H., Burgio, L., Burns, R., Coon, D., Czaja, S. J., Gallagher-Thompson, D., . . . Zhang, S. (2006). Enhancing the quality of life of dementia caregivers from different ethnic or racial groups: A randomized, controlled trial. *Annals of Internal Medicine, 145*(10), 727–738.

Bergman, E. J., Haley, W. E., & Small, B. J. (2011). Who uses bereavement services? An examination of service use by bereaved dementia caregivers. *Aging and Mental Health, 15*(4), 531–540.

Bradley, E. H., McGraw, S. A., Curry, L., Buckser, A., King, K. L., Kasl, S. V., & Anderson, R. (2002). Expanding the Andersen model: The role of psychosocial factors in long-term care use. *Health Services Research, 37*, 1221–1242.

Brody, E. M. (1985). Parent care as a normative family stress. *The Gerontologist, 25*(1), 19–29.

Burke, P. (1991). Identity processes and social stress. *American Sociological Review, 56*, 836–849.

Burke, P. J., & Reitzes, D. C. (1991). An identity theory approach to commitment. *Social Psychology Quarterly, 54*, 239–251.

Cantor, M. (1979). Social and family relationships of black aged women in New York City. *Journal of Minority Aging, 4*, 50–61.

Cleland, M., Schmall, V. L., Studervant, M., Congleton, L., Kirkbride, K., McFalls, J.,...Turner, H. (2006). *The caregiver helpbook: Powerful tools for caregivers* (2nd ed.). Portland, OR: Legacy Caregiver Services.

Cox, C. (1997). Findings from a statewide program of respite care: A comparison of service users, stoppers, and nonusers. *The Gerontologist, 37*(4), 511–517.

Dorfman, L., Holmes, C. A., & Berlin, K. L. (1997). Service utilization by wife caregivers of frail older veterans. *Social Work in Health Care, 26*(2), 33–52.

Elliott, A. F., Burgio, L. D., & DeCoster, J. (2010). Enhancing caregiver health: Findings from the Resources for Enhancing Alzheimer's Caregiver Health II Intervention. *Journal of the American Geriatrics Society, 58*(1), 30–37.

Gaugler, J. E., Roth, D. L., Haley, W. E., & Mittelman, M. S. (2008). Can counseling and support reduce burden and depressive symptoms in caregivers of people with Alzheimer's disease during the transition to institutionalization? Results from the New York University caregiver intervention study. *Journal of the American Geriatrics Society, 56*(3), 421–428.

Gitlin, L. N. (2013). *Assessing the state of translation work in caregiving: Have we been successful and where do we go from here?* Paper presented at the Gerontological Society of American Annual Conference, New Orleans, LA.

Gitlin, L. N., Belle, S. H., Burgio, L. D., Czaja, S. J., Mahoney, D., Gallagher-Thompson, D.,...Ory, M. G. (2003). Effect of multicomponent interventions on caregiver burden and depression: The REACH multisite initiative at 6-month follow-up. *Psychology and Aging, 18*(3), 361–374.

Gitlin, L. N., Reever, K., Dennis, M. P., Mathieu, E., & Hauck, W. W. (2006). Enhancing quality of life of families who use adult day services: Short- and long-term effects of the adult day services plus program. *The Gerontologist, 46*(5), 630–639.

Haley, W. E., Bergman, E. J., Roth, D. L., McVie, T., Gaugler, J. E., & Mittelman, M. S. (2008). Long-term effects of bereavement and caregiver intervention on dementia: Caregiver depressive symptoms. *The Gerontologist, 48*(6), 732–740.

Hepburn, K. W., Lewis, M., Sherman, C. W., & Tornatore, J. (2003). The Savvy Caregiver Program: Developing and testing a transportable dementia family caregiver training program. *The Gerontologist, 43*(6), 908–915.

Herrera, A. P., Lee, J., Palos, G., & Torres-Vigil, I. (2008). Cultural influences in the patterns of long-term care use among Mexican American family caregivers. *Journal of Applied Gerontology, 27*(2), 141–165.

Judge, K. S., Bass, D. M., Snow, A. L., Wilson, N. L., Morgan, R., Looman, W. J.,...Kunik, M. E. (2011). Partners in dementia care: A care coordination intervention for individuals with dementia and their family caregivers. *The Gerontologist, 51*(2), 261–272.

Karner, T. X., & Hall, L. C. (2002). Successful strategies for serving diverse populations. *Home Health Care Services Quarterly, 21*(3/4), 107–131.

Kart, C. S. (1991). Variation in long-term care services use by aged blacks. *Journal of Aging and Health, 3,* 511–526.

Kosloski, K., Montgomery, R. J. V., & Youngbauer, J. G. (2001). Utilization of respite services: A comparison of users, seekers, and nonseekers. *Journal of Applied Gerontology, 20*(1), 111–132.

Kim, K., Zarit, S. H., Femia, E. E., & Savla, J. (2012). Kin relationship of caregivers and people with dementia: Stress and response to intervention. *International Journal of Geriatric Psychiatry, 27*(1), 59–66.

Lavelle, B., Mancuso, D., Huber, A., & Felver, B. (2014). *Expanding eligibility for the family caregiver support Program in SFY 2012: Updated findings 7.* Retrieved from https://www.dshs.wa.gov/sesa/rda/research-reports/expanding-eligibility-family-caregiver-support-program-sfy-2012

Lawton, M., Brody, E., & Saperstein, A. (1991). *Respite for caregivers of Alzheimer patients: Research and practice.* New York, NY: Springer Publishing Company.

Lazarus, S., & Folkman, S. (1984). *Stress, appraisal and coping.* New York, NY: Springer Publishing Company.

Lee, C. C., Czaja, S. J., & Schulz, R. (2010). The moderating influence of demographic characteristics, social support, and religious coping on the effectiveness of a multicomponent psychosocial caregiver intervention in three racial ethnic groups. *The Journals of Gerontology, Series B, 65*(2), 185–194.

Miller, S. C. (2004). Hospice care in nursing homes: Is site of care associated with visit volume? *Journal of the American Geriatrics Society, 52,* 1331–1336.

Mittelman, M. S., Roth, D. L., Haley, W. E., & Zarit, S. H. (2004). Effects of a caregiver intervention on negative caregiver appraisals of behavior problems in patients with Alzheimer's disease: Results of a randomized trial. *The Journals of Gerontology, Series B, 59*(1), P27–P34.

Montgomery, R. J. V., & Borgatta, E. F. (1989). The effects of alternative support strategies on family caregiving. *The Gerontologist, 29*(4), 457–464.

Montgomery, R. J. V., & Kosloski, K. (2009). Caregiving as a process of changing identity: Implications for caregiver support. *Generations, 33*(1), 47–52.

Montgomery, R. J. V., & Kosloski, K. (2013). Pathways to caregiver identity and implications for support services. In R. C. Talley & R. J. V. Montgomery (Eds.), *Caregiving across the life span: Research practice and policy* (pp. 131–156). New York, NY: Springer Publishing Company.

Montgomery, R. J. V., Kwak, J., Kosloski, K., & Valuch, K. O. (2011). Effects of the TCARE® intervention on caregiver burden and depressive symptoms: Preliminary findings from a randomized controlled study. *The Journals of Gerontology, Series B, 66*(5), 640–647.

Montgomery, R. J. V., Marquis, J., Kosloski, K. D., Schaefer, J. P., & Karner, T. X. (2002). Profiles of respite use. *Home Health Care Services Quarterly, 21*(3/4), 33–64.

Montoro-Rodriguez, J., Kosloski K., & Montgomery, R. J. V. (2003). Evaluating a practice-oriented services model to increase the use of respite services among minorities and rural caregivers. *The Gerontologist, 43*(6), 916–924.

Pearlin, L. I., Lieberman, M. A., Menaghan, E. G., & Mullan, J. T. (1981). The stress process. *Journal of Health and Social Behaviors, 22,* 337–356.

Pearlin, L. I., Mullan, J. T., Semple, S. J., & Skaff, M. M. (1990). Caregiving and the stress process: An overview of concepts and their measures. *The Gerontologist, 30,* 583–594.

Penning, M. J. (1995). Cognitive impairment, caregiver burden, and the utilization of home health services. *Journal of Aging and Health, 7*(2), 233–253.

Phillipson, L., Jones, S. C., & Magee, C. (2014). A review of the factors associated with the non-use of respite services by carers of people with dementia: Implications for policy and practice. *Health & Social Care in the Community, 22*(1), 1–12.

Piaget, J. (1971). *Biology and knowledge*. Chicago, IL: University of Chicago Press.

Radina, M. E., & Barber, C. E. (2004). Utilization of formal support services among Hispanic Americans caring for aging parents. *Journal of Gerontological Social Work, 43*(2–3), 5–23.

Savundranayagam, M. Y., & Montgomery, R. J. V. (2010). Impact of role discrepancies on caregiver burden among spouses. *Research on Aging, 32*, 175–199.

Savundranayagam, M. Y., Montgomery, R. J., Kosloski, K., & Little, T. D. (2011). Impact of a psychoeducational program on three types of caregiver burden among spouses. *International Journal of Geriatric Psychiatry, 26*(4), 388–396.

Scharlach, A. E., Giunta, N., Chun-Chung Chow, J., & Lehning, A. (2008). Racial and ethnic variations in caregiver service use. *Journal of Aging and Health, 20*(3), 326–346.

Schulz, R., & Martire, L. M. (2004). Family caregiving of persons with dementia: Prevalence, health effects, and support strategies. *American Journal of Geriatric Psychiatry, 12*(3), 240–249.

Shanas, E. (1979). The family as a social support system in old age. *The Gerontologist, 19*(2), 169–174.

Starns, M., Karner, T. X., & Montgomery, R. J. V. (2002). Exemplars of successful Alzheimer's demonstration projects. *Home Health Care Services Quarterly, 21*(1/2), 141–175.

Stryker, S. (1968). Identity salience and role performance. *Journal of Marriage and Family, 4*, 558–564.

Stryker, S., & Burke, P. J. (2000). The past, present, and future of an identity theory. *Social Psychology Quarterly, 63*(4), 284–297.

Stryker, S., & Serpe, R. T. (1994). Identity salience and psychological centrality: Equivalent, overlapping, or complementary concepts? *Social Psychology Quarterly, 57*(1), 16–35

Sun, F., Mutlu, A., & Coon, D. (2014). Service barriers faced by Chinese American families with a dementia relative: Perspective from family caregivers and service professionals. *Clinical Gerontologist, 37*(2), 120–138.

Toseland, R. W., McCallion, P., Gerber, T., & Banks, S. (2002). Predictors of health and human services use by persons with dementia and their family caregivers. *Social Science and Medicine, 55*(7), 1255–1266.

Toseland, R. W., McCallion, P., Smith, T., & Banks, S. (2004). Supporting caregivers of frail older adults in an HMO setting. *American Journal of Orthopsychiatry, 74*(3), 349–364.

Tremont, G., Davis, J. D., Bishop, D. S., & Fortinsky, R. H. (2008). Telephone-delivered psychosocial intervention reduces burden in dementia caregivers. *Dementia, 7*(4), 503–520.

Weissert, W., Elston, J., Bolda, E., Zelman, W., Mutran, E., & Mangum, A. (1990). *Adult day care: Findings from a national survey*. Baltimore, MD: Johns Hopkins University Press.

Yeatts, D. E., Crow, T., & Folts, E. (1992). Service use among low-income minority elderly: Strategies for overcoming barriers. *The Gerontologist, 32*(1), 24–32.

Zarit, S. H., Stephens, M. A. P., Townsend, A., Greene, R., & Leitsch, S. A. (1999). Patterns of adult day service use by family caregivers: A comparison of brief versus sustained use. *Family Relations, 48*(4), 355–362.

CHAPTER 24

Theoretical Foundations for Designing and Implementing Health Promotion Programs

Susan L. Hughes, Elske Stolte, and Renae L. Smith-Ray

Although mortality rates across most developed countries have declined over the last century, more people than ever before are living with multiple chronic diseases (Crimmins & Beltrán-Sánchez, 2011). Health promotion efforts will play a powerful role as we work to enhance function and reduce morbidity by intervening on modifiable risk factors such as physical activity (PA), inactivity, social engagement, and nutrition (King & Guralnik, 2010). It is generally agreed that effective behavior change programs should build to the extent possible on theory. Several health behavior change theories have been developed to explain how, why, and under what circumstances persons are more or less likely to change and maintain their behaviors. The last decade has witnessed an explosion of research that seeks to generate "evidence-based" health promotion programs for older adults. This chapter examines the state of the art of theoretical foundations for health behavior change that are used to design and implement health promotion programs for older adults.

We begin by reviewing the most commonly used theories and their constructs and discuss which are currently still in use and how they have been applied to the design and implementation of health promotion interventions. We then turn to an examination of the evidence supporting their utility and discuss new theories that are just now being applied broadly and speculate about their potential to enhance the design of health promotion programs in the future. Next, we review two evidence-based programs that have strong theoretical foundations and discuss how the underlying theoretical constructs were operationalized within the programs and the impact the programs have had on outcomes. Finally, we outline research challenges that still need to be addressed in this area.

A theoretical foundation is recommended as the basis for any effective behavior change program. Health promotion interventionists understand that inducing lasting behavior change is difficult, but most agree that leveraging behavior change interventions on a theoretical foundation is the most effective approach toward evoking change in the desired behavior. Behavior change theories enable us to dissect the cognitive, social, and environmental elements that influence behavior, and to carefully modify these constructs in order to influence behavior.

For the past 40 years, behavior change has been thought of as a phenomenon that occurs at the level of the individual (Golden & Earp, 2012). That is to say that personal volition is the main driving force of behavior change. Recently, critics have argued that this view considerably oversimplifies reality. Our understanding of influences of behavior has grown to understand that volition is influenced by a plethora

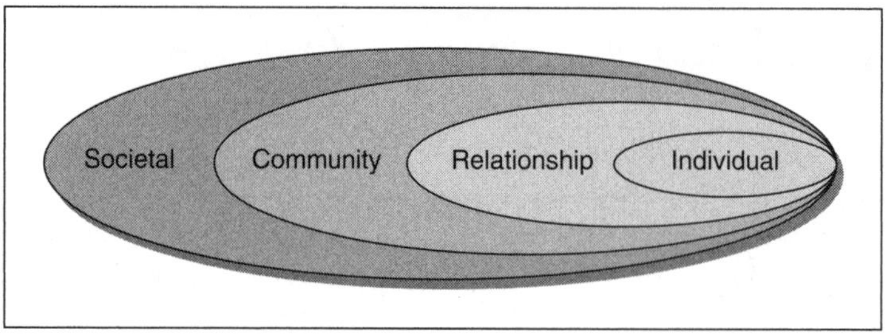

FIGURE 24.1 The Social–Ecological Model.
Adapted from Centers for Disease Control and Prevention (2015).

of external factors that enhance or limit an individual's ability to engage in a desired behavior. In addition to the individual, it is now widely accepted that behavior change is influenced by the behaviors and attitudes of the individual's relationships such as family, the resources available within the community (e.g., are safe trails available for cycling, or well-lit paths for evening walks), as well as policies and norms at the societal level (e.g., Medicare reimbursement for exercise classes). These contextual factors interact with individual-level factors, making vertically integrated projects—that is, those that are inclusive of factors from the individual to societal level—most likely to have the greatest impact. In this chapter, we use the Ecological Model as a guide to describe the level(s) targeted by each theory (Figure 24.1). We present theories targeted at each level and argue for the use of multilevel interventions whenever possible.

■ WHAT DO HEALTH PROMOTION THEORIES TRY TO EXPLAIN?

Health promotion theories try to explain what makes an individual want to adopt a health-promoting behavior (i.e., behavioral intention), the factors that lead to actual behavior change (i.e., behavioral initiation), and the factors that influence habitual performance of that behavior (i.e., maintenance of behavior). Each stage presents unique challenges for the design and implementation of effective health promotion programs. At present, we have a substantial amount of knowledge about the use of theory to promote behavior change at the level of the individual. We know considerably less about how to best apply theory at the community and societal levels, and in particular, how or whether theory at these levels should be tailored for older adults.

■ OVERVIEW OF EXISTING THEORETICAL MODELS

Many health behavior theories exist that can be used to design health promotion programs. For more extensive descriptions of the theories overviewed here and their applications, see Glanz, Rimer, and Viswanath (2008) and Conner and Norman (2005). Here, we briefly describe the historical development of some of the most influential models and view them from the ecological perspective. We then describe how the different models can be used to inform the design of health promotion interventions. Table 24.1 lists the theories covered and indicates both the phase of behavior change and the levels of the Social-Ecological Model that each theory targets.

TABLE 24.1 Theoretical Models by Phase of Change Addressed and Level Influenced

	Phases of Behavior Change			Levels of Behavior Influenced			
	Initiation	Maintenance	Relapse	Individual	Relationship	Community	Society
Health Belief Model	X	X		X			
Social Cognitive Theory	X	X		X	X		
Theory of Planned Behavior	X			X			
Transtheoretical Model	X	X	X	X			
Protection Motivation	X			X			
Diffusion of Innovations	X	X				X	

The Health Belief Model

The Health Belief Model (HBM) is one of the earliest health behavior theories and explains behavior at the level of the individual (Glanz et al., 2008). It originated in the 1950s in the field of preventive medicine when social psychologists in the U.S. Public Health Service were trying to understand why people did or did not use preventive services. As the name implies, HBM posits that a set of beliefs regarding a health problem will influence a person's likelihood to take action. These beliefs include the perceived threat of a specific health problem with respect to both severity and susceptibility; the benefits of avoiding the threat; and factors influencing the ability to act such as barriers, cues to action, and self-efficacy.

Social Cognitive Theory

Social Cognitive Theory (SCT) is based on social learning theory and incorporates determinants at both the individual and relationship levels (Bandura, 1991). The concepts used in SCT include psychological determinants of behavior, observational learning, environmental determinants of behavior, self-regulation, and moral disengagement (Glanz et al., 2008). With respect to psychological determinants, SCT posits that self-efficacy expectancy (perceived confidence that one can perform a specific behavior) and outcome expectancy (anticipated consequences of the same behavior) strongly influence behavior. Environmental determinants are incentives to motivation and include the use of punishment and rewards and facilitation, that is, changing the environment to make it easier to comply with the desired behavior. Observational learning consists of several processes in which people learn new behavior by observing others.

The principles of SCT have been used frequently in health behavior interventions. Interventionists have attempted to improve self-efficacy by including opportunities to demonstrate mastery experience, social modeling, improving physical and emotional states, and verbal persuasion. To achieve mastery experience, participants are encouraged to perform small steps of increasing difficulty toward a health goal, which provide a success experience, which, in turn, boosts participants' confidence in their ability to change. Observational learning has been achieved using peer modeling based on the supposition that people are more likely to identify with peers. Self-regulation provides another set of tools often used in interventions to teach participants how to work toward a health goal. Six self-regulation strategies identified in SCT are self-monitoring, goal setting, feedback, self-reward, self-instruction, and use of social support.

The Transtheoretical Model

The Transtheoretical Model (TTM) or Stages of Change Model originated in the field of psychotherapy and targets the individual level (Prochaska & DiClemente, 1983). This model is based on the experiences of self-changers and distinguishes five phases of change or change processes: precontemplation, contemplation, preparation, action, and maintenance. People do not necessarily proceed through every stage consecutively and relapse is possible. TTM is frequently used to target participants for intervention inclusion who are at specific stages of readiness for change. For example, persons in precontemplation might need more information before starting a PA program. In contrast, persons in contemplation and preparation may be the best group to target for such a program because they are already interested and activated. Furthermore, information can be tailored during the intervention to a participant's stage of change. For example, an online smoking cessation program might use a brief questionnaire every time a participant visits the website to check the participant's current stage. Each stage can then be targeted with a different motivational message to optimize engagement in the intervention and maintenance of the behavior.

The Theory of Planned Behavior/Theory of Reasoned Action

The Theory of Planned Behavior (TPB) is also based on beliefs and works mostly at the individual level, but also includes an element that addresses the relationship level (Ajzen, 1991, 2002). TPB is an extended version of its predecessor, the Theory of Reasoned Action. The Theory of Reasoned Action posits that two dimensions within individuals drive them toward a behavior: attitudes and subjective norms. Attitudes are degrees to which a person has a favorable or unfavorable evaluation of the behavior. Subjective norms are based on beliefs about the expectations that other people hold regarding the behavior. The two dimensions lead to intention, which actually predicts a person's behavior (Ajzen, 1991). TPB adds perceived behavioral control as a third component that influences intention. Perceived behavioral control refers to the person's appraisal of his or her ability to perform a behavior (Ajzen, 2002). In addition, perceived behavioral control can predict behavior directly.

Interventions using the TPB assess which beliefs are most important in the targeted behavior and the specific target group. These beliefs can then be targeted for change so that an individual's intention will increase. For example, designers of a PA intervention might find that older adults think that PA is inappropriate for them and consists only of strenuous sports activities. The intervention can try to change these beliefs by assuring potential enrollees that PA is important for the health of older adults (targeting attitude), giving examples of suitable PA, teaching easy exercises to do at home (self-efficacy), and using success stories of older adults who improved their health by increasing PA (social norm/self-efficacy). Most recently, Ajzen has specified steps that need to be taken when basing an intervention on TPB and how outcomes should be measured (Ajzen, 2014).

Diffusion of Innovations Theory

Diffusion of Innovations operates at the organizational and/or societal level to predict the likelihood that a health promotion program will be implemented and/or sustained (Rogers, 2008). The innovation–decision process categorizes potential adopting organizations into five stages based on organizational readiness to adopt the innovation and, if already adopted, likelihood of sustaining it. The first stage, Knowledge, refers to the early stage of knowledge acquisition and comprehension. This is followed by Persuasion, which takes place when discussions occur at the organization level regarding the positive and negative aspects of the innovation, which may include advocating for or against acceptance of the innovation. The third stage, Decision, encompasses the organization's intention to try the innovation. This is followed by the Implementation stage, which involves organizational use of the innovation. Finally, the Confirmation stage involves evaluating the positive and negative impacts of the innovation and a decision for or against sustained use of the innovation. With regard to health promotion, Diffusion of Innovations theory is most appropriate to apply when an organization or government is considering or has recently adopted a new health promotion intervention.

■ MULTILEVEL APPLICATIONS

Ecological approaches differ from the individual-level models previously discussed. Ecological models assume the presence of multiple levels of influences and assume reciprocal causation between individuals and their environments. We presented the most prominent multilevel approach, the Social–Ecological Model, earlier in the chapter.

Recently, there has been a push toward broader ways of thinking about behavior change using structural approaches that target all levels of the Social–Ecological Model. Several articles in a special issue of *Health Education & Behavior* reviewed the advantages of this approach and described applications of multilevel approaches to behavior change. Allegrante (2015) points out that, despite the need for a broad approach to health promotion in order to increase its impact, of 157 articles published in the journal over the past 20 years, a handful addressed multilevel interventions. Presenting the perspective of the Robert Wood Johnson Foundation, Mockenhaupt and Woodrum (2015) describe a structural approach to achieving a culture of health. They stress that new interventions need to focus on systems and structures as opposed to specific symptoms or diseases and cite policy level changes in tobacco use and adapting food environments to demonstrate how a more systemic way of thinking contributes to broader impact. The development of a resource guide for implementing and evaluating population-level interventions is described in the special issue as well (Lifsey, Cash, Anthony, Mathis, & Silva, 2015).

An inspiring example of a successful multilevel approach can be found in Finland, where policy makers succeeded in radically changing the population's diet resulting in an 80% reduction over a 30-year period in annual population cardiovascular disease mortality rates (Puska & Stahl, 2010). This achievement was the result of a sustained approach involving communities, industry, and the government. It has inspired an even broader new socio-environmental approach called Health in All Policies, which is an ecological view of health that implies health should be embedded in all policies (education, housing), not just the health care sector.

Comprehensive interventions target each social–ecological level, but these expansive intervention designs are not used often because they are challenging to implement. An example of a multilevel ecological intervention that is achievable within small communities can be seen in the Multilevel Intervention for Physical Activity in Retirement Communities (MIPARC) trial (Kerr et al., 2012). The MIPARC trial targeted PA change at each of the four social–ecological levels: pedometer-based monitoring at the *individual* level, group and peer sessions at the *relationship/interpersonal* level, PA promotion signage at the *community* level, and peer-led advocacy and additional PA opportunities at the *societal/policy* level (Kerr et al., 2012). Another example of a multilevel intervention is the CardiACTION trial (Estabrooks et al., 2011). This trial is using a 2 × 2 factorial design to determine whether individual-level, environmental-level, or a combination of individual- and environmental-level components has the greatest impact on PA. The individual-level intervention involves an interactive computer session, automated telephone counseling, and tailored mailings to disseminate PA messages based on protection motivation theory (PMT). The environmental-level intervention entails participants' receiving tailored maps of PA trails, parks, and other resources near two personally meaningful locations (i.e., home and work) as well as a complimentary 1-year voucher to a recreation facility (Estabrooks et al., 2011).

Finally, another issue that is important to discuss is the complexity of the targeted behavior. It is likely that theory selection becomes more complicated as the targeted behavior is more complex. Changing both PA and diet over time, for instance, is a more complex effort than motivating people to participate in a one-time health screening. It is also likely that different theories will need to be applied to different behaviors. For example, people might be motivated by the use of behavioral modeling among peers (SCT) to lose weight or become more active. The same individuals might be more motivated by perceived risk to participate in cancer screening.

■ USING THEORY TO DESIGN INTERVENTIONS

A considerable amount of overlap and a lack of research on the comparative effectiveness of theoretical models make it difficult to decide which theories to use (Noar & Zimmerman, 2005). The PRECEDE/PROCEED approach (Green & Kreuter, 1999), Intervention mapping protocol (Bartholomew, Parcel, Kok, & Gottlieb, 2006; Kok, Schaalma, Ruiter, van Empelen, & Brug, 2004), and the Reach Effectiveness Adoption Implementation Maintenance (RE-AIM) model (Belza, Toobert, & Glasgow, 2007) provide guidelines for the use of theory in different stages of intervention development. Each is briefly described in the following discussion.

PRECEDE–PROCEED Planning Model

This model is essentially a road map that can be used to plan an intervention, its implementation, and its evaluation. Within the roadmap, behavior change theories provide the specific directions to a desired location or outcome.

PRECEDE (Predisposing, Reinforcing, and Enabling Constructs in Educational/ Environmental Diagnosis and Evaluation) was developed in the 1970s based on the premise that diagnosis (needs assessment) should precede treatment (design of a health promotion intervention). In 1991, PROCEED (Policy, Regulatory, and Organizational Constructs in Educational and Environmental Development) was added to the model to underscore the importance of environmental factors as determinants of health behaviors. PROCEED explicitly recognizes that many lifestyle behaviors are influenced by factors outside of the control of the individual including industry, the media, farm policy, and so on. The addition of this component is intended to facilitate the design of interventions that address multiple levels of influence on behavior, in congruence with the Social–Ecological approach.

In 2005, the model was revised again to respond to growing interest in ecological and community participatory approaches to the design of interventions and to incorporate knowledge generated by genetics (Gielen, McDonald, Gary, & Bone, 2008; Glanz et al., 2008). This newer version has four planning phases: Social Assessment; Epidemiologic, Behavioral, and Environmental Assessment; Educational and Ecological Assessment; and Administrative and Policy Assessment and Intervention Alignment. These are followed by the four PROCEED phases of Implementation, Process Evaluation, Impact Evaluation, and Outcome Evaluation. The model is intended to be implemented within a community participatory framework, which posits that at each step in the model the community is an active partner.

Intervention Mapping Framework

This framework is a very detailed approach that builds on the PRECEDE–PROCEED model (Bartholomew et al., 2006; Kok et al., 2004). Complementary to PRECEDE–PROCEED, intervention mapping helps researchers to design interventions by describing the steps needed to select theory-based intervention components and translate theory into program materials. The framework has six steps, which should not be seen as linear. During the design of an intervention, movement back and forth between steps is expected. For example, after identifying the desired proximal outcomes of a PA program and specifying the target behaviors for each outcome, information might be needed from the literature and from the target group. If the intervention seeks to encourage people to track their PA, knowledge is needed about different tracking options (accelerometer? and/or a mobile application? and/or a web-based application?) and what might appeal to the target group (needs assessment). Community participation is included in the framework through the use of a participatory planning group that provides feedback throughout the design process (www.interventionmapping.com).

RE-AIM Model

The RE-AIM Model is an important tool for improving the public health impact of an intervention. First developed in 1999, RE-AIM has gained considerable prominence and is increasingly relied on to facilitate the translation of research into practice (Glasgow, Vogt, & Boles, 1999). The elements of the model include Reach, Effectiveness, Adoption, Implementation, and Maintenance. A key strength of the model is that it is multilevel in nature. The constructs of Reach, Effectiveness, and Maintenance operate at the individual level, whereas Adoption, Implementation, and Maintenance are applied at the setting level. RE-AIM identifies factors that need to be considered early in the intervention design process that are critical for enhancing dissemination and that have largely been ignored by existing theoretical approaches. This model recognizes that, although an intervention may lead to significant improvement in the outcome of interest, ultimately the value of the program rests on the capacity to disseminate it to persons who need it. A highly efficacious program may have little impact if there are setting-level barriers to its adoption (e.g., personnel required to deliver the program are cost prohibitive/in high demand), implementation (e.g., the program has no standardized procedures to ensure consistent delivery), or maintenance (e.g., the program is cost-prohibitive to reproduce broadly.

■ THE EFFECTIVENESS OF THEORY-BASED INTERVENTIONS

Although many sources report that the use of theory is effective, surprisingly, the evidence supporting this contention is mixed (Glanz & Bishop, 2010; Prestwich et al., 2014). A meta-analysis of PA interventions for older adults found that use of theory was not associated with larger effect sizes (Conn, Minor, Burks, Rantz, & Pomeroy, 2003). Theories included in the analysis were SCT, TTM, and TPB. However, the number of studies using each theory was too low to compare effect sizes for specific theories. A second meta-analysis of PA interventions in healthy adults found a smaller effect size for interventions that used TTM ($d = 0.15$) compared with those that did not use TTM ($d = 0.21$; Conn, Hafdahl, & Mehr, 2011). Use of SCT was as effective as TTM with an effect of $d = 0.12$ compared with $d = 0.20$ for studies not using SCT. On the other hand, more extensive use of theory was associated with larger effects in a third study that reviewed Internet interventions promoting health behavior change (Webb, Joseph, Yardley, & Michie, 2010). The use of theory to *select intervention participants* was related to larger effect sizes, whereas other uses of theory were associated with smaller effect sizes. TPB was associated with larger effect sizes whereas TTM and SCT were not. However, these conclusions were based on a small number of studies and, therefore, should be interpreted with caution.

In an attempt to resolve ambiguous results regarding the effectiveness of theory use in interventions, Prestwich et al. 2014 developed a more rigorous method to code theory use (Prestwich et al., 2014). The Theory Coding Scheme is a structured method to report, not only whether theory was used, but also to what extent and for which part of the intervention design and implementation (Michie & Prestwich, 2010). The rationale for this approach is that most evidence to date has used a very crude measure for theory use by reporting a dichotomous measure of theory use when *extent of theory use* might influence its effectiveness. However, a meta-analysis of PA and healthy eating interventions using the Theory Coding Scheme did not find interventions to be more effective when they were explicitly based on theory (Prestwich et al., 2014). The authors did not find better results for interventions using TTM or SCT as opposed to interventions not based on theory. The meta-analysis also found that only half of the reviewed studies used theory to guide their interventions. Taken together, results supporting the use of theory are disappointing but they should be interpreted cautiously. It could be that studies that use TTM and SCT are also more rigorous in their methodology; however, Prestwich et al. controlled the use of more rigorous methodology and still found TTM and SCT to be less effective (Prestwich et al., 2014).

Underreporting of theory use may also explain these results. Currently, page space in most journals is at a premium. Therefore, it is possible that editorial concerns about article length may cause theoretical applications in clinical trials to be underreported. Underreporting theory use makes it difficult to assess the impact of theory on intervention effects and undermines the strength of a rigorous approach such as the Theory Coding Scheme. To move the field of health promotion forward, it is important that the application of theory be reported thoroughly and in a consistent format so that we can better understand its relationship to outcomes (Dombrowski, Sniehotta, Avenell, & Coyne, 2007).

■ THEORETICALLY DRIVEN EVIDENCE-BASED PROGRAMS AND THEIR OUTCOMES

We now turn to the application of theories by interventions that have successfully changed health behaviors among older adults.

One of the most commonly used evidence-based health promotion programs is the Chronic Disease Self-Management Program (CDSMP) developed by Lorig and colleagues at Stanford. In 1990, Lorig and colleagues developed CDSMP to address the self-management of multiple different chronic diseases simultaneously. CDSMP is a group education intervention led by trained lay leaders who, in many cases, also have chronic diseases. The program concentrates on participants' self-defined needs and self-management options for problems such as pain and fatigue that cut across specific conditions. Program components are based on SCT and seek to increase participants' confidence in their ability to manage their conditions. As part of self-management, participants develop skills to enhance communication with physicians, including the ability to monitor and report changes in their conditions and the ability to share concerns, questions, and treatment preferences. CDSMP also helps participants to manage emotional changes associated with disease burden such as anger, uncertainty, and changed expectations. Tools based on SCT that are built into the program include skill mastery, reinterpretation of symptoms, modeling, and social persuasion to enhance personal self-efficacy. Mastery of skills over the 6-week program occurs through the use of action plans and feedback on progress (Sobel, Lorig, & Hobbs, 2002).

CDSMP has been evaluated extensively. The original efficacy trial found that, compared with controls, treatment participants improved at 6 months on exercise participation, cognitive symptom management, communication with physicians, self-reported health, health distress, fatigue, disability, and social/role activity limitations. Treatment participants also had significantly fewer hospitalizations and fewer hospital days (Lorig et al., 1999; Ritter et al., 2001).

A follow-up study that examined outcomes out to 24 months found significant improvements on health distress, self-efficacy, and fewer physician and emergency department visits at 1 and 2 years (Lorig, Ritter, et al., 2001). Cost savings ranged between $70 and $200 per participant. A dissemination study undertaken in 1997 (Lorig, Sobel, Ritter, Laurent, & Hobbs, 2001) found improved health behaviors, self-efficacy, and health status; fewer emergency department and physician visits; and a trend toward fewer hospital days. The savings in utilization per participant, compared with the program implementation cost, yielded a 1:4 cost–savings ratio. Most recently, CDSMP was evaluated nationally using the Triple Aim (better health, better health care, and better value) framework (Ory, Ahn, et al., 2013). The evaluation found that emergency department visits decreased significantly from baseline to 12 months, whereas significant reductions in hospital use were seen between baseline and 6 months. As or more noteworthy than these outcomes, the sample for the study was a subset of an estimated 100,000 persons who participated in CDSMP with funding from the American Recovery and Reinvestment Act of 2009. This remarkable translation effort is described by an editorial in the *Journal of the American Geriatrics Society* that documents this unprecedented national reach of a self-management program (Ory, Smith, et al., 2013).

The other intervention that we will briefly describe is Fit and Strong! (F&S), an exercise/behavior change intervention for older adults with lower extremity arthritis. F&S builds on findings from a longitudinal study of older adults in Chicago who were followed for 4 years to examine risk factors for disability. Because prior work by the same team identified a high prevalence of arthritis among chronically homebound older adults, the team obtained baseline joint impairment measures on all study participants ($N = 484$). Joint impairment measures were divided into upper versus lower body assessments and used in classification tree analyses that found that lower extremity joints were the route through which disability developed (Dunlop, Hughes, & Manheim, 1997).

These findings signaled an urgent need to design a PA intervention to interrupt this disability trajectory. The first step in the design process was a review of the osteoarthritis (OA) literature that found that, in addition to impaired joints, persons with OA had weaker muscle strength and were aerobically deconditioned compared with age-matched controls (Minor, Webel, Kay, Hewett, & Anderson, 1989; Semble, Loeser, & Wise, 1990). Armed with this information, the team worked with physical therapists to design a multicomponent PA intervention that included flexibility exercises, accompanied by sustained aerobics and progressive lower extremity strength training.

Based on the advice of psychologists, the team also included a health education/ behavior change component largely incorporating the concepts of SCT. Thus, the final intervention is an 8-week program that meets three times per week. The first hour of each session is devoted to PA followed by 30 minutes of structured health education/group problem solving that includes peer modeling, reinforcement, brainstorming, and action plans to reinforce behavior change. The program also includes a negotiated adherence contract that participants develop with the instructor during week 6. Participants sign the contract and take it home on the last day of class. The contract is their personalized plan for ongoing PA maintenance.

F&S has also been tested extensively. The efficacy trial found significant treatment group improvements at 2 months in self-efficacy for PA, PA engagement, and decreased joint stiffness. At 6 months, these benefits persisted and were accompanied by improved self-efficacy for adherence to PA over time, and decreased pain. Many of the 6-month findings were maintained at 12 months with strong effect sizes for SE for PA (0.78, 0.80, and 0.91) and PA engagement (0.86, 0.71, and 0.67; Hughes et al., 2006). A follow-up study examined the duration of treatment effects out to 18 months. It found significant benefits on engagement in PA, joint stiffness, pain and function, lower extremity (LE) strength (timed sit–stand) and mobility (6-minute distance walk) as well as depression/anxiety at 2 months that were maintained at 18 months (Hughes et al., 2010). The sustained impact of the program on LE strength and mobility is noteworthy because diminished strength is a risk factor for falls and diminished mobility is both a risk factor for falls and an independent risk factor for mortality (Rubenstein, 2006; Studenski et al., 2011). A dissemination study enabled the program to be totally manualized with standardized instructor training materials, fidelity protocols, and offerings in six states (Hughes, Smith-Ray, Shah, & Huber, 2015). Finally, when the maintenance study was in the field, study participants asked for more help with weight management. As a result, a new version of the program—F&S! Plus—that addresses both PA and weight management has been developed and is being tested in a comparative effectiveness trial (Smith-Ray et al., 2014)

Recently, CDSMP and F&S! along with Enhance Fitness and A Matter of Balance were invited to participate in a congressionally mandated evaluation of the impact of top-tier evidence-based programs for older adults on Medicare expenditures. The evaluation is examining quality-of-life outcomes and Medicare claims data for program participants and comparing these outcomes to those experienced by a matched comparison group. Results will be used to assess the appropriateness of Medicare reimbursement for the programs.

■ FUTURE DEVELOPMENT: EMERGING MEASURES AND MODELS

Emerging interdisciplinary areas of behavioral and social sciences include behavioral economics; the social, behavioral, cognitive, and affective neurosciences; neuroeconomics; behavioral genetics and genomics; and social network analysis.

Measures

One of the new measurement advances that is worth noting concerns patient activation. Hibbard and colleagues have examined the utility of a new Patient Activation Measure (PAM; Hibbard, Stockard, Mahoney, & Tusler, 2004). Developed in 2004, PAM assesses patients' willingness and ability to manage their health. PAM consists of 13 statements about beliefs, confidence in managing health-related tasks, and self-assessed knowledge. Items are scored and respondents are characterized into four levels of activation, ranging from least activated to most activated. The measure has been demonstrated to be reliable and valid across different languages, cultures, demographic groups, and health statuses (Hibbard & Greene, 2013) and has been shown in cross-sectional analyses to be related to 12 of 13 patient outcomes in the expected direction (Greene & Hibbard, 2012).

The predictive power of the PAM was assessed in a longitudinal study, which found that higher PAM scores at baseline predicted better self-management, improved functioning, and lower use of health care services over 4 years. The group also found that when activation measures changed, outcomes changed in the same direction. They concluded that the instrument can be a powerful tool for health plans that seek to identify persons who have high chronic disease burden and low activation levels. This group may be most in need of personal coaching that would enable them to be activated patients in the future. In contrast, persons with equally high disease burden scores but high activation scores might be supported more appropriately with automated reinforcement messages (Hibbard, Greene, Shi, Mittler, & Scanlon, 2015).

Technology

We predict that the increased use of technology in health behavior interventions will have a substantial impact on the development and testing of theories. Health behavior change interventions will benefit from technology in many ways; including, but not limited to, rapid and cost-effective dissemination of health messages, the ability to collect real-time assessment data from participants without asking them to travel to a research lab, automated and tailored treatment delivery, and the ability to provide instantaneous feedback to participants. The Internet, smartphone apps, and text messaging all promise tremendous flexibility in the dissemination of health behavior change interventions while improving treatment fidelity through standardized delivery.

Although 75% of adults aged 65 to 69 years report using the Internet, this rate of use drops to 47% for adults aged 75 to 79 years (Zickuhr & Madden, 2012). However, older adults who use the Internet do so habitually, with 82% of adult Internet users going online at least three times per week (Zickuhr & Madden, 2012). These figures present both challenges and opportunities. Because of lack of familiarity with technology and sometimes greater apprehension about learning to use new technology, implementation challenges may exist with the use of computer or smartphone-driven interventions among adults aged 75 years and older. However, other technology-driven options exist that are suitable for this age group, including interactive voice response (IVR) telephone calls. IVR offers all of the benefits mentioned previously, but its only prerequisite for use is access to a telephone. Of adults that participated in an IVR-based PA intervention, 75% perceived this technology favorably (Estabrooks & Smith-Ray, 2008).

Tremendous opportunities exist for the use of technology among adults who are younger than age 75. Future cohorts of older adults will enter old age with greater familiarity with a range of technological applications. The potential to employ a range of technology-based interventions will expand over the next 15 years as the largely technologically savvy baby boomer generation ages (Zickuhr & Madden, 2012).

As the field moves forward with the application of technology in health promotion programs, three important issues regarding the use of theory must be considered. First, the type and amount of data that will become available using technology-based interventions will make it possible to test how well theories predict behavior change over time. This increase in data warrants the use of more sophisticated statistical approaches to fully assess the complexity of these relationships among variables, including the use of structural equation modeling to understand potential bi-directional relationships and mediational analyses to explicate behavioral mechanisms. Moreover, these data will make it possible to track interactions of concepts over time; for instance, the development of emotions and their influence on motivations. Theories that are able to explain the interaction of multiple concepts over time will be in demand.

Second, the decreased cost of wearable monitors and increased uptake of communication devices with Internet access among older adults make it possible to conduct real-time measurement of people's behavior when faced with a facilitator or a barrier to a new behavior. This development creates the opportunity to intervene in real time in people's normal lives. For example, a recent pilot study by Zenk and colleagues tested the ability of a cell phone app that called participants at random times during the day and night to assess the presence of stressors and PA or dietary responses to them (Zenk et al., 2014). This real-time data collection technique enabled investigators to obtain responses from participants while they were actively engaged in and making decisions regarding food purchases, meal preparation, and watching TV to assess current levels of motivation to adhere to dietary and PA guidelines along with perceived stress and other barriers and facilitators.

Third, the increased use of technology in health promotion interventions brings with it an urgent need to understand the way people interact with technology that promotes health. New models that have emerged regarding the use of technology in health promotion include a behavioral change model for Internet interventions (Ritterband, Thorndike, Cox, Kovatchev, & Gonder-Frederick, 2009), persuasive system design (Oinas-Kukkonen & Harjumaa, 2009), and the BIT model (Mohr, Schueller, Montague, Burns, & Rashidi, 2014).

The Ritterband behavioral change model was designed specifically for Internet interventions (Ritterband et al., 2009). It seeks to describe how behaviors change and symptoms improve through use of Internet interventions, guide program development and facilitate intervention testing, and establish a theoretical foundation for Internet interventions. The model builds on several theories and incorporates nine components that form steps in a nonlinear change process involving the user, the environment, the website and its characteristics, change mechanisms, problem specific outcomes, and maintenance to the intervention. The website component alone describes eight areas that can influence the experience of the user such as appearance and content. This model provides a comprehensive overview of the concepts that have to be considered when developing and evaluating a website but does not specify how the components should be used to design specific website features to achieve intervention goals.

That same year, the Persuasive System Design framework was also described (Oinas-Kukkonen & Harjumaa, 2009). This framework describes three steps in the development of a persuasive system as well as some basic assumptions underlying persuasive technology. The framework further specifies four system principles of support: primary task, dialogue, system credibility, and social support. An example of primary task support is tailoring, and praise is an example for dialogue support.

An even newer framework includes elements of both the Ritterband model for website intervention development and Persuasive System Design among others. The Behavior Intervention Technology (BIT) model specifies why, what, how, and when BIT should occur (Mohr et al., 2014). The framework clearly specifies the aim of each intervention technique and uses behavioral intervention strategies to translate theory into specific applications. It also specifies technical elements in a workflow that makes it clearer how BITs can work over time. Currently, the application of the framework quickly becomes complicated and it does not integrate design processes. However, BIT can be viewed as an important starting point that needs to be tested empirically and modified as needed.

■ CURRENT STATE AND FUTURE CHALLENGES FOR HEALTH PROMOTION THEORIES

Differences in Older Populations

Well-defined theories that explain the adoption of health-promoting behaviors have been tested extensively with younger populations. However, we know that older adults are cognitively different from younger adults (Salthouse, 2010). Older adults perceive threats differently and are less likely to be swayed by negative images and/or health consequences (Isaacowitz, Wadlinger, Goren, & Wilson, 2006; Peters, Dieckmann, & Weller, 2011). When presented with negatively framed health messages, compared with younger adults, older adults are better at rationalizing the threat and instead focus on positive attributes (Buschkuehl et al., 2008; Peters et al., 2011). The way older adults evaluate outcome expectations may also differ from those taken up by younger adults. For example, if older adults know that they have a shorter time period in which to enjoy the benefits of a given behavior, do they weigh the outcome differently?

These cognitive differences between young and old adults may have important implications for the application of theory across age groups. As most theoretical development has been tested within cohorts of young-to-middle age adults, it may be inappropriate to assume that these findings can be generalized to older adults. Consider Protection Motivation Theory, for example. This theory posits that adults who are faced with a health threat are motivated to change behavior to alleviate that threat (Plotnikoff & Trinh, 2010). Accordingly, an adult will be motivated to engage in PA by the following message: "Lack of regular physical exercise increases your risk of developing coronary heart disease." However, a growing body of evidence suggests that this message may be effective for young adults, but older adults are less likely to be motivated by the threat. Positive messages are more effective at motivating older adults to change (Peters et al., 2011). A positive health message might state: "Participation in regular PA will make it easier for you to keep up with your grandchildren." As research on health behavior theories moves forward, it is critical to evaluate a theory's impact among older and younger adults alike in order to determine which theories are moderated not only by behavioral stage but also by the age of the target population.

Multiple Levels

We believe that we have consistently made the case throughout this chapter regarding the need for multilevel interventions that include but go beyond the level of the individual to simultaneously address family, community, and societal policies and norms that serve as critical barriers and facilitators to the initiation and maintenance of behavior change. This is definitely the direction in which behavior change research is headed.

Multiple Behaviors

In addition to the recognized importance of multilevel interventions, there is increasing awareness of the need for multiple behavioral interventions. Multiple chronic conditions among older adults are now the norm (Barnett et al., 2012). On average, adults aged 65 years and older have 2.6 morbidities. To improve public health impact and target the two thirds of older adults living with more than one chronic condition, interventions should target more than one health behavior when possible (Barnett et al., 2012).

Effectiveness of Theoretical Applications

Considerable work remains to be done testing the contribution of theories to intervention outcomes. Journal editors may need to require that authors provide systematic information on the foundational use of theories and their operationalization within interventions. This type of information would be considerably more useful than the dichotomous yes/no responses currently used in meta-analyses of theoretical applications. Similarly, substantial work remains to be done with respect to analyses of the causal role of theories in predicting interim, proximal, and distal outcomes using structural equation modeling that quantifies the role of theories as mediators of intervention outcomes.

Similarly, the availability of functional MRI (fMRI) for direct imaging in the brain to test the impact of reinforcement or other mechanisms on differential receptors in the brain has tremendous promise in both bolstering the validity of a given theory and explicating its physiological pathway. Research in this area has the potential to be truly transformative.

Economic Incentives

We are beginning to examine the role of economic incentives as adjuncts to theoretical inducements of behavior change. The role of reduced premiums, deductibles, or co-payments for Medicare beneficiaries who enroll in evidence-based programs and the role of reduced insurance premiums for older workers who participate in worksite wellness programs are topics that also beg for systematic evaluation in the future.

Activation

Another important issue for future research is delineating the role of patient activation. The phases of behavior change that we display in Table 24.1 begin with initiation. It could be that all behavior change models should instead begin with activation based on the theory that activated persons will have the capacity to initiate self-management and related behavior changes. If activation is a foundational threshold that persons must cross before initiating behavior change, this means that concerted policy level initiatives are needed to reach precontemplators. In other words, activation among precontemplators might require wholesale change in the culture surrounding a given behavior like healthy eating/weight management. If, in fact, activation is a necessary precursor to behavioral initiation, then a stepped care approach for health promotion may be needed that would enable persons with low activation levels to reach the point where they are more likely to participate in theory-driven interventions.

Finally, new scientific discoveries might turn the whole field of health promotion upside down. One realistic expectation is that the field of behavioral genetics and genomics will expand (McBride, Koehly, Sanderson, & Kaphingst, 2010). This expansion could create the possibility of screening people to create risk profiles not only for disease but also for addiction and overeating, sedentary behavior, and so forth. Based on these genetic profiles, behavioral interventions might be prescribed to very specific target groups at high risk of disease and high likelihood of changing the given behavior successfully.

As readers can hopefully see from this brief review, the current and future fields of theoretical foundations for health behavior interventions are anything but static. Rather, they are evolving rapidly, with the promise of assisting to deliver increasingly targeted, efficient, and effective interventions in the future.

REFERENCES

Ajzen, I. (1991). The theory of planned behavior. *Organizational Behavior and Human Decision Processes, 50*(2), 179–211.

Ajzen, I. (2002). Perceived behavioral control, self-efficacy, locus of control, and the theory. *International Journal of Entrepreneurship Behaviour and Research, 4*(1), 28–50.

Ajzen, I. (2014). The theory of planned behaviour is alive and well, and not ready to retire: A commentary on Sniehotta, Presseau, and Araújo-Soares. *Health Psychology Review, 9*(2), 1–7.

Allegrante, J. (2015). Policy and environmental approaches in health promotion: What is the state of the evidence? *Health Education and Behavior, 42*(1), 55–75.

Bandura, A. (1991). Social cognitive theory of self-regulation. *Organizational Behavior and Human Decision Processes, 50*(2), 248–287.

Barnett, K., Mercer, S. W., Norbury, M., Watt, G., Wyke, S., & Guthrie, B. (2012). Epidemiology of multimorbidity and implications for health care, research, and medical education: A cross-sectional study. *The Lancet, 380*(9836), 37–43.

Bartholomew, L., Parcel, G., Kok, G., & Gottlieb, N. (2006). *Planning health promotion programs. An intervention mapping approach; 2006.* Mountain View, CA: Mayfield.

Belza, B., Toobert, D. J., & Glasgow, R. E. (2007). *RE-AIM for program planning: Overview and applications.* Washington, DC: National Council on Aging.

Buschkuehl, M., Jaeggi, S. M., Hutchison, S., Perrig-Chiello, P., Däpp, C., Müller, M., ... Perrig, W. J. (2008). Impact of working memory training on memory performance in old–old adults. *Psychology and Aging, 23*(4), 743–753.

Centers for Disease Control and Prevention. (2015). *The Social–Ecological Model: A framework for prevention.* Retrieved from http://www.cdc.gov/violenceprevention/overview/social-ecologicalmodel.html

Conn, V. S., Hafdahl, A. R., & Mehr, D. R. (2011). Interventions to increase physical activity among healthy adults: Meta-analysis of outcomes. *American Journal of Public Health, 101*(4), 751–758.

Conn, V. S., Minor, M. A., Burks, K. J., Rantz, M. J., & Pomeroy, S. H. (2003). Integrative review of physical activity intervention research with aging adults. *Journal of the American Geriatrics Society, 51*(8), 1159–1168.

Conner, M., & Norman, P. (2005). *Predicting health behaviour.* New York, NY: McGraw-Hill International.

Crimmins, E. M., & Beltrán-Sánchez, H. (2011). Mortality and morbidity trends: Is there compression of morbidity? *The Journals of Gerontology, Series B, 66*(1), 75–86.

Dombrowski, S. U., Sniehotta, F. F., Avenell, A., & Coyne, J. C. (2007). Current issues and future directions in *Psychology and Health*: Towards a cumulative science of behaviour change: Do current conduct and reporting of behavioural interventions fall short of best practice? *Psychology and Health, 22*(8), 869–874.

Dunlop, D. D., Hughes, S. L., & Manheim, L. (1997). Disability in activities of daily living: Patterns of change and a hierarchy of disability. *American Journal of Public Health, 87*(3), 378–383.

Estabrooks, P. A., Glasgow, R. E., Xu, S., Dzewaltowski, D. A., Lee, R. E., Thomas, D.,…Smith-Ray, R. L. (2011). Building a multiple modality, theory-based physical activity intervention: The development of CardiACTION! *Psychology of Sport and Exercise, 12*(1), 46–53.

Estabrooks, P. A., & Smith-Ray, R. L. (2008). Piloting a behavioral intervention delivered through interactive voice response telephone messages to promote weight loss in a pre-diabetic population. *Patient Education and Counseling, 72*(1), 34–41.

Gielen, A. C., McDonald, E. M., Gary, T. L., & Bone, L. R. (2008). Using the precede–proceed model to apply health behavior theories. *Health Behavior and Health Education: Theory, Research, and Practice, 4*, 407–433.

Glanz, K., & Bishop, D. B. (2010). The role of behavioral science theory in development and implementation of public health Interventions. *Annual Review of Public Health, 31*(1), 399–418.

Glanz, K., Rimer, B. K., & Viswanath, K. (2008). *Health behavior and health education: theory, research, and practice.* San Francisco, CA: Jossey-Bass.

Glasgow, R. E., Vogt, T. M., & Boles, S. M. (1999). Evaluating the public health impact of health promotion interventions: The RE-AIM framework. *American Journal of Public Health, 89*(9), 1322–1327.

Golden, S. D., & Earp, J. A. L. (2012). Social ecological approaches to individuals and their contexts: Twenty years of health education & behavior health promotion interventions. *Health Education and Behavior, 39*(3), 364–372.

Green, L., & Kreuter, M. (1999). *The precede–proceed model. Health promotion planning: An educational approach* (pp. 32–43). Mountain View, CA: Mayfield Publishing Company.

Greene, J., & Hibbard, J. (2012). Why does patient activation matter? An examination of the relationships between patient activation and health-related outcomes. *Journal of General Internal Medicine, 27*(5), 520–526.

Hibbard, J. H., & Greene, J. (2013). What the evidence shows about patient activation: Better health outcomes and care experiences; fewer data on costs. *Health Affairs (Millwood), 32*(2), 207–214.

Hibbard, J. H., Greene, J., Shi, Y., Mittler, J., & Scanlon, D. (2015). Taking the long view: How well do patient activation scores predict outcomes four years later? *Medical Care Research and Review, 72*, 324–337.

Hibbard, J. H., Stockard, J., Mahoney, E. R., & Tusler, M. (2004). Development of the patient activation measure (PAM): Conceptualizing and measuring activation in patients and consumers. *Health Services Research, 39*(4p1), 1005–1026.

Hughes, S. L., Seymour, R. B., Campbell, R. T., Desai, P., Huber, G., & Chang, H. J. (2010). Fit and Strong!: Bolstering maintenance of physical activity among older adults with lower-extremity osteoarthritis. *American Journal of Health Behavior, 34*(6), 750.

Hughes, S. L., Seymour, R. B., Campbell, R. T., Huber, G., Pollak, N., Sharma, L., & Desai, P. (2006). Long-term impact of Fit and Strong! on older adults with osteoarthritis. *The Gerontologist, 46*(6), 801–814.

Hughes, S. L., Smith-Ray, R. L., Shah, A., & Huber, G. (2015). Translating Fit and Strong!: Lessons learned and next steps [opinion]. *Frontiers in Public Health, 3*, 131.

Isaacowitz, D. M., Wadlinger, H. A., Goren, D., & Wilson, H. R. (2006). Selective preference in visual fixation away from negative images in old age? An eye-tracking study. *Psychology and Aging, 21*(1), 40–48.

Kerr, J., Rosenberg, D. E., Nathan, A., Millstein, R. A., Carlson, J. A., Crist, K.,...Marshall, S. J. (2012). Applying the ecological model of behavior change to a physical activity trial in retirement communities: Description of the study protocol. *Contemporary Clinical Trials, 33*(6), 1180–1188.

King, A. C., & Guralnik, J. M. (2010). Maximizing the potential of an aging population. *Journal of the American Medical Association, 304*(17), 1944–1945.

Kok, G., Schaalma, H., Ruiter, R. A., van Empelen, P., & Brug, J. (2004). Intervention mapping: Protocol for applying health psychology theory to prevention programmes. *Journal of Health Psychology, 9*(1), 85–98.

Lifsey, S., Cash, A., Anthony, J., Mathis, S., & Silva, S. (2015). Building the evidence base for population-level interventions: Barriers and opportunities. *Health Education & Behavior, 42*(1, Suppl.), 133s–140s.

Lorig, K. R., Ritter, P., Stewart, A. L., Sobel, D. S., William Brown, B. J., Bandura, A.,...Holman, H. R. (2001). Chronic disease self-management program: 2-year health status and health care utilization outcomes. *Medical Care, 39*(11), 1217–1223.

Lorig, K. R., Sobel, D. S., Ritter, P. L., Laurent, D., & Hobbs, M. (2001). Effect of a self-management program on patients with chronic disease. *Effective Clinical Practice: ECP, 4*(6), 256–262.

Lorig, K. R., Sobel, D. S., Stewart, A. L., Brown, B. W. J., Bandura, A., Ritter, P.,...Holman, H. R. (1999). Evidence suggesting that a chronic disease self-management program can improve health status while reducing hospitalization: A randomized trial. *Medical Care, 37*(1), 5–14.

McBride, C. M., Koehly, L. M., Sanderson, S. C., & Kaphingst, K. A. (2010). The behavioral response to personalized genetic information: Will genetic risk profiles motivate individuals and families to choose more healthful behaviors? *Annual Review of Public Health, 31*, 89–103.

Michie, S., & Prestwich, A. (2010). Are interventions theory-based? Development of a theory coding scheme. *Health Psychology, 29*(1), 1–8.

Minor, M. A., Webel, R. R., Kay, D. R., Hewett, J. E., & Anderson, S. K. (1989). Efficacy of physical conditioning exercise in patients with rheumatoid arthritis and osteoarthritis. *Arthritis & Rheumatism, 32*(11), 1396–1405.

Mockenhaupt, R., & Woodrum, A. (2015). Developing evidence for structural approaches to build a culture of health: A perspective from the Robert Wood Johnson Foundation. *Health Education & Behavior, 42*(1, Suppl.), 15s–19s.

Mohr, D. C., Schueller, S. M., Montague, E., Burns, M. N., & Rashidi, P. (2014). The behavioral intervention technology model: An integrated conceptual and technological framework for eHealth and mHealth interventions. *Journal of Medical Internet Research, 16*(6), e146.

Noar, S. M., & Zimmerman, R. S. (2005). Health Behavior Theory and cumulative knowledge regarding health behaviors: Are we moving in the right direction? *Health Education Research, 20*(3), 275–290.

Oinas-Kukkonen, H., & Harjumaa, M. (2009). Persuasive systems design: Key issues, process model, and system features. *Communications of the Association for Information Systems, 24*(1), 28.

Ory, M. G., Ahn, S., Jiang, L., Smith, M. L., Ritter, P. L., Whitelaw, N., & Lorig, K. (2013). Successes of a national study of the Chronic Disease Self-Management Program: Meeting the triple aim of health care reform. *Medical Care, 51*(11), 992–998.

Ory, M. G., Smith, M. L., Patton, K., Lorig, K., Zenker, W., & Whitelaw, N. (2013). Self-management at the tipping point: Reaching 100,000 Americans with evidence-based programs. *Journal of the American Geriatrics Society, 61*(5), 821–823.

Peters, E., Dieckmann, N. F., & Weller, J. (2011). Age differences in complex decision making. *Handbook of the Psychology of Aging, 7*, 133–148.

Plotnikoff, R. C., & Trinh, L. (2010). Protection motivation theory: Is this a worthwhile theory for physical activity promotion? *Exercise and Sport Sciences Review, 38*(2), 91–98.

Prestwich, A., Sniehotta, F. F., Whittington, C., Dombrowski, S. U., Rogers, L., & Michie, S. (2014). Does theory influence the effectiveness of health behavior interventions? Meta-analysis. *Health Psychology, 33*(5), 465–474.

Prochaska, J. O., & DiClemente, C. C. (1983). Stages and processes of self-change of smoking: Toward an integrative model of change. *Journal of Consulting and Clinical Psychology, 51*(3), 390–395.

Puska, P., & Stahl, T. (2010). Health in all policies—The Finnish initiative: Background, principles, and current issues. *Annual Review of Public Health, 31*, 315–328.

Ritter, P. L., Stewart, A. L., Kaymaz, H., Sobel, D. S., Block, D. A., & Lorig, K. R. (2001). Self-reports of health care utilization compared to provider records. *Journal of Clinical Epidemiology, 54*(2), 136–141.

Ritterband, L. M., Thorndike, F. P., Cox, D. J., Kovatchev, B. P., & Gonder-Frederick, L. A. (2009). A behavior change model for internet interventions. *Annals of Behavioral Medicine, 38*(1), 18–27.

Rogers, E. (2008) *Diffusion of innovations* New York, NY: Free Press.

Rubenstein, L. Z. (2006). Falls in older people: Epidemiology, risk factors and strategies for prevention. *Age and Ageing, 35*(Suppl. 2), ii37–ii41.

Salthouse, T. A. (2010). Selective review of cognitive aging. *Journal of the International Neuropsychological Society: JINS, 16*(5), 754–760.

Semble, E. L., Loeser, R. F., & Wise, C. M. (1990). Therapeutic exercise for rheumatoid arthritis and osteoarthritis. *Seminars in Arthritis and Rheumatism, 20*(1), 32–40.

Smith-Ray, R. L., Fitzgibbon, M. L., Tussing-Humphreys, L., Schiffer, L., Shah, A., Huber, G. M.,...Hughes, S. L. (2014). Fit and Strong! Plus: Design of a comparative effectiveness evaluation of a weight management program for older adults with osteoarthritis. *Contemporary Clinical Trials, 37*, 178–188.

Sobel, D. S., Lorig, K. R., & Hobbs, M. (2002). Chronic disease self-management program: From development to dissemination. *The Permanente Journal, 6*(2), 15–22.

Studenski, S., Perera, S., Patel, K., Rosano, C., Faulkner, K., Inzitari, M.,...Guralnik, J. (2011). Gait speed and survival in older adults. *Journal of the American Medical Association, 305*(1), 50–58.

Webb, T. L., Joseph, J., Yardley, L., & Michie, S. (2010). Using the internet to promote health behavior change: A systematic review and meta-analysis of the impact of theoretical basis, use of behavior change techniques, and mode of delivery on efficacy. *Journal of Medical Internet Research, 12*(1), e4.

Zenk, S. N., Horoi, I., McDonald, A., Corte, C., Riley, B., & Odoms-Young, A. M. (2014). Ecological momentary assessment of environmental and personal factors and snack food intake in African American women. *Appetite, 83*(0), 333–341.

Zickuhr, K., & Madden, M. (2012). Older adults and internet use. *Pew Internet & American Life Project, 6*, n.p.

CHAPTER 25

Theories of the Politics and Policies of Aging
Robert B. Hudson

There can be little doubt that older people have today assumed a special place in the American social policy and political landscape. They constitute a large and growing population, they are increasingly well organized, and they are the recipients of public benefits that are the envy of every other social policy constituency in the nation.

This chapter reviews and assesses different theoretical approaches that may help account—in all or in part—for these fairly recent and remarkable developments. Although there is some variety in how welfare state analysts have organized and distinguished between these approaches (Amenta, Bonastia, & Caren, 2001; Garfinkel, Smeeding, & Rainwater, 2010; Myles & Quadagno, 2002; Pampel & Williamson, 1992), they have each identified a fairly common set of alternatives. The organization here centers on six distinct (though potentially reinforcing) theoretical avenues for better understanding these political and policy developments: the logic of industrialization and policy development, the role of political culture and values, the presence (or absence) of working-class mobilization, the impact of individual and group participation, the weight of state structure, and the effects of policy in shaping subsequent events.

The logic of industrialization, emphasizing the emergence of demographic aging, is principally of historical importance (though globalization and digitization may represent contemporary analogs). The lens of political culture and values has relevance for American social policy development because of its focus on the country's allegedly "exceptionalist" view of the role and power of government in national life, a belief set frequently depicted as accounting for a pattern of welfare state development notably different from that found among other industrialized nations. Of particular relevance for purposes here is how such values may have found elders to be a rather unique beneficiary group, one which could be indulged, whereas most others are being denied.

The working-class mobilization approach to welfare state development centers around the ability of workers to use their numbers and the ability to withhold labor as a means of forcing political parties and other actors to press for benefits workers are unable to gain from owners through the unfettered private economy. Older people are found to gain (or lose) relative advantage depending on the success of these forays by labor into politics. Democratic and group participation centers on individuals and organized interests being able to identify with or organize around mutual concerns in a manner more particularistic than that associated with working class or other social movements. In the United States, where working-class cohesion was never firmly established, multiple demands organized along these lines have long been prominent. By the 1980s, the aged in the United States could very surely be identified as one such interest.

The final two theoretical approaches to aging politics and policy are "state-centered," directing attention to the autonomy and cohesion of public and quasi-public institutions. These institutional elements include formal constitutional conditions, such as federalism and governmental structure; quasi-public entities, such as political parties; and, importantly, the product of those structures, that is, *public* policy. It is worth distinguishing between two variants of state-centered theory, one focused on the state itself and the second on the policy outcomes. How the state is structured, and in particular, how much autonomy its incumbents—both political and administrative—enjoy is critical to the first of these. The second understands the policies generated by the state to have critical effects in shaping and constraining subsequent political activity. Put differently, policy is understood here as an independent rather than as a dependent variable in explaining welfare state developments. A rich literature focusing on age-related policy has in recent years come to serve virtually as Exhibit #1 in pushing this perspective to the theoretical fore.

The following pages review these six theoretical understandings. Each discussion frames the particular approach, places it in both the American and comparative contexts, and finally finds the place of the aged in these understandings. As will be seen, there exists a rich literature on the first two of these three elements; the principal value-added of this presentation finds itself in the aging-related material, the old—until quite recently—having been often treated more in passing than as central players in social policy development.

■ THE LOGIC OF INDUSTRIALIZATION

The birth of the modern welfare state in Western nations occurred in the wake of the process of industrialization and urbanization in the 19th century. Analysts vary on how dominant was the role of industrialization alone, but none questions its essential contribution. It is also the case that older people—through both their emerging plight and their growing numbers—provide a key link between the forces of industrialization and early welfare state development.

At the most basic level, industrialization made possible the accumulation of resources not possible in pre-industrial society. Industrial organization and technological advances grew symbiotically and make investment, not only consumption, possible. By so doing, surpluses could accumulate, allowing for social welfare expenditures among other uses. It is over the use of these surpluses that capitalist and anticapitalist ideologues have struggled since the dawning of industrialization. These twin processes of industrialization and urbanization disrupted traditional economic, social, familial, and geographic relationships. The status which older people enjoyed in agricultural economies, where farmers have considerable control over their own employment and where "landed property is power" (Gratton, 1986), waned with the onset of industrialization. Over time, workers became disabled or exhausted, and owners demanded ever higher levels of productivity, especially during "the industrial efficiency" movements of the late 19th and early 20th centuries. For their part, families found the economic utility of children lessened in urban settings, abetted by small and squalid living arrangements. "At this point, all of the things that happen to old people become much more tragic" (Wilensky & Lebeaux, 1958, p. 77). In this "resources plus needs" formulation, the old come to hold a relatively unique, if very unfortunate, place. Their family supports have been undermined (fewer children, higher divorce, and disabled kin), and their economic value has been diminished (physically weak and technologically backward).

It is here that the state steps in, performing something of a regulatory function by instituting programs to provide for those necessarily (and appropriately) forced from the productive economy. The proximate factors that might make this so—sympathy, assuring work for the young, responding to pressures from adult children—are not specified by this approach; however, cross-national analyses covering welfare state expansion from inception through the 1970s find the aged to be a strong correlate if not an established engine of public social expenditure growth. In Wilensky's (1975) words, "As economic level climbs, the percentage of aged climbs, which shapes spending directly; with economic growth the percentage of aged goes up, which makes for an early start and swift spread of social security programs" (p. 27).

At one level, this approach is hard to fault: it would be hard to account for welfare state growth absent the effects of economic growth and population aging (Myles & Quadagno, 2002). Importantly, these forces are at work today as well as they were yesterday. Numerous analysts have posited economic growth as the absolutely essential (if not sole) factor behind the explosion in post–World War II social welfare expenditures (Cameron, 1978). Indeed, the potentially dominant role of economic growth (today associated more with technology than industrialization)—played down in the 1980s and 1990s by those emphasizing political factors in accounting for welfare state expansion—has received renewed attention in explaining assaults on the welfare state since the mid-1970s. That is, if economic growth fuels expansion, why would economic stagnation not contribute to program contraction? Yet, although welfare state cutbacks have been observed in numerous national settings over the period (Beland, Howard, & Morgan, 2014; Stephens, Huber, & Ray, 1999)—and amid alarming increases in inequality (Piketty, 2014)—there remains disagreement about whether the economics and politics of austerity are the mirror image of the economics and politics of expansion (Pierson, 1994).

A stronger version of the economic development approach is more contested. Cross-nationally, there is great variation between levels of economic growth on the one hand, and the growth and size of welfare states on the other, a divergence that strongly suggests that forces other than the narrowly economic must be at work. Perhaps most notable is the United States, where industrial growth was early and fierce yet where social welfare spending has long lagged behind (Skocpol, 1992). A critique of this approach holds that it does not account for the proximate activities that generate change For example, it does not take a terribly advanced understanding of human behavior to intuit that it is relatively easy to raise public revenue when gross domestic product (GDP) is expanding, but countries have done so at far different rates nonetheless.

These larger debates about welfare state growth aside, the place of the aged in the industrialism approach is notable. In historical context, population aging appears as a driver of pension and (later) health care spending, and today analysts on both sides of the "coming crisis in age-related spending" debate employ a GDP/aging expenditure ratio to make their points—based on very different assumptions (Gist, 2014; Teles, 2007). There is some irony in this concern being driven by population aging (a.k.a., the aging of the baby boomers) in that the causal arrows are again up for grabs: whereas population aging presumably helped drive welfare state development 100 years ago, it is also the case today that the enormity of welfare state expenditures has centrally contributed to the imposing presence represented by this generation of seniors. Whether this growth in age-related spending will drive out "new social risks" associated with immigration, globalization, and labor force shifts—or be driven out by them—is a topic of great current interest in cross-national welfare state studies (Lynch & Myrskyla, 2009; Tepe & Vanhuysse, 2010).

■ POLITICAL CULTURE AND VALUES

An "exceptionalist" and reinforcing set of national values served as the predominant theme in post–World War II writings about the unique place the United States appeared to occupy in comparative welfare state development (Orloff, 1988). Americans' historical attachments to individualism, self-reliance, voluntarism, free markets, and a Protestant-based moralism were seen as instrumental in both understanding the etiology of poverty and ill health and in limiting the role government should play in their amelioration (Lipset, 1997; Rimlinger, 1971). Poverty and ill health were attributed largely to individual failings and immoral behavior, a diagnosis which left little room or justification for government involvement (Rosenberg, 1962). In early New England, the "old and the disabled were proper objects of relief, but not the able-bodied poor, who received harsher treatment" (Quadagno, 1988, p. 25). During this period, Americans warmed to Herbert Spencer's juxtaposing Charles Darwin and Protestantism, "a philosophy of liberation from the trammels of government" (Fleming, 1963, p. 127).

This value set poses a direct challenge to the logic of the industrialization approach, since the country underwent massive economic dislocations in the almost complete absence of public intervention on behalf of those dislocated. Although other countries were instituting unemployment, health care, and pension policies, social policy efforts in the United States were largely limited to the regulatory and "good government" initiatives of the progressives. Moreover, even these followed the more substantive European developments by over a decade. Skocpol's work highlighting early Civil War pensions and state-level mothers' pensions has served as a partial correction to these earlier understandings of how delayed American developments were and, as such, adds a cautionary note about the national values argument. Nonetheless, these benefits being confined to veterans, women, and children was in sharp contrast to the European experience where the needs, grievances, and demands of the working class were the essential ingredient.

Differences in national value structures also inform conceptual understandings of different welfare regimes. Under one formulation, the exceptionalism of the United States takes on particular salience. In a series of lectures delivered at Oxford in 1949, British sociologist T. H. Marshall (1964) delineated three types of citizenship—civil, political, and social—that have marked the evolution of modern societies and contrasted their pattern of development cross-nationally. Civil citizenship encompassed a basic set of rights necessary to freedom in the modern world: the right to liberty, the right to property, and the right to the even-handed administration of justice. A second set of rights were political ones: the right to vote, to organize, and to hold office. The third stage was social rights, referring to economic security and the right to enjoy a reasonable level of well-being understood not only in terms of absolute well-being but in relationship to one's fellow citizens.

Marshall's and others' analyses clearly find the United States as having succeeded at the civil and political stages, both sets of rights—if only for White men—being firmly established before anywhere else, including Britain. Yet, the third stage has never developed as fully as elsewhere. The "right" to health care, to decent housing, to employment, to a decent standard of living has never been codified here in a manner to seriously approach most other nations. There may be more than one way to account for this relative failing, but an entrenched set of deeply rooted exceptional values is certainly high on the list.

Value salience can also help account for rationales associated with American social policy interventions when they did ultimately occur. Franklin Roosevelt and his advisors were nearly obsessed with the work disincentives that might be associated with New Deal initiatives. Writing of that and subsequent periods, long-time Social Security Commissioner Robert Ball (2000) repeatedly emphasized how important the idea of work was to all discussions:

> Private pensions, group insurance, and social insurance all belong, along with wages and salaries, to the group of work-connected payments, and it is this work connection, the fact that it is earned, which gives social insurance its basic character. (p. 43)

Indeed, the controversy that sprung up about extending Old Age Insurance to cover survivors in 1939 centered on the absence of any work history among those individuals.

The values perspective can also help account for what many observers see as major gaps in American social policy. Most notable is the absence of any kind of inclusive family policy, acknowledging the individual costs and societal benefits of child rearing in the modern world. American policy toward young families, especially low-income ones, has been viewed as exclusionary (Ryan, 1971), residual (Wilensky & Lebeaux, 1958), and behaviorist (Marmor, Mashaw, & Harvey, 1990), most recently associated with welfare reform and the Temporary Assistance to Needy Families program. Historical beliefs around the obligation to work and the primacy of the nuclear family have unquestionably slowed the expansion of social policy to the benefit of younger and especially middle-aged individuals.

Critical to this discussion, the national values perspective has much to say about the relatively privileged position seniors have enjoyed in the United States. This is perhaps best captured through an emerging literature focused on the "target populations" of public policy, in particular how different groups are socially constructed and how politically powerful they might be. At the time of Schneider and Ingram's (1993) path-breaking contribution to this literature, elders were seen as "advantaged," that is, positively constructed and politically strong. However, in an historical vein, Hudson and Gonyea (2012) employ Schneider and Ingram's framework to see elders having evolved politically through three stages. In social policy's early years, they were seen as having been "dependent" (positive construction, weak power), emerging as advantaged in the late 20th century but, most recently, having been recast, at least by some elite-level actors, as "contenders" (negative construction, strong power), an understanding seeing them as being "greedy" (Samuelson, 2013), generationally favored (Kotlikoff & Burns, 2004), and the principal contributor to the nation's presumed "entitlement crisis" (Gerson, 2010). Important to say, seniors—unlike several other social welfare constituencies—have never been viewed as "deviant" (negative construction, weak political power).

Yet, older people's positive construction during the first two periods can substantially account for the impressive series of "aging only" (or largely) policies that have come to constitute the heart of the American welfare state: Old Age Assistance, Old Age Insurance, Disability Insurance (initially only for those older than 50 years), Medicare (only for the old until 1972), and Supplemental Security Income (a latter day replacement to Old Age Assistance, Aid to the Blind, and Aid to the Totally and Permanently

Disabled). Because in the early years, elders were assumed to be poor and frail, they alone could pass the American values litmus test around work and self-sufficiency. This also made the aged a favored group among social policy reformers who wished to institute benefits that would ultimately extend beyond the aged to other population groups.

■ WORKING-CLASS MOBILIZATION

This approach to understanding welfare state development has the organized presence of industrial workers at center stage. Unlike the logic of industrialization model, here there is "agency" in that industrial workers use their numbers and organizations to impact the political system. The strike is the workers' economic weapon, and the vote is the workers' political one. Because in free-market economies, workers will always outnumber owners, the political realm is a fertile one, especially when political parties organize to mobilize and channel worker concerns. The organizational element is critical; the extension of political democracy absent effective organization is not sufficient to generate needed pressures on the existing system. Early on in the European experience, expansion of the franchise largely through the efforts of left-wing parties (and by conservative parties trying to co-opt workers) created political opportunities propitious for welfare state development.

There is a well-established empirical literature supporting the positive relationship between left-wing legislative presence and welfare state growth (Cameron, 1978; Esping-Andersen, 1985). The logic of the theory is, obviously enough, that social democratic parties will prevail, form governments, and enact expansive programs. That, of course, happened, but one also finds that the approach can be operative even when rightist parties are in power. This occurred most famously in the case of Bismarck's creation of the German welfare state in the 1880s. Antecedent to this, but related, would be Conservative Prime Minister Benjamin Disraeli extending the franchise to workers in 1860s Britain; in both cases, a co-optation hypothesis—paternalistic privilege of the right—indulges the emerging working class in order to forestall the further organization of the left.

Not surprisingly, very little is said of the American experience in these discussions. As has been well documented, in comparative perspective the United States failed to generate permanent, sizeable, or cohesive left-wing political movements. On the economic side, there were periodic appearances—the Industrial Workers of the World, the Knights of Labor—but these were mercurial and fleeting. When mainstream labor did organize, it was the more skilled craft unions that first emerged, ultimately to form the American Federation of Labor (AFL). Far from an orthodox leftist union leader, the AFL's founder Samuel Gompers opposed federal unemployment insurance well into the early years of the Depression. In the political domain, an American socialist party emerged around the turn of the century—Eugene Debs won nearly 7% of the vote in the 1912 election—but the Democratic Party has served as the closest approximation of a leftist party in the United States for over a century.

A vast literature exists on why "socialism failed in America" (Greenstone, 1970; Lipset & Marks, 2001). Most obviously at work are the exceptionalist values discussed earlier. Geography and the frontier have long been argued to have played a role in dispersing the disgruntled and defusing tensions. Much has been laid to race and ethnic animosities, whereby "blood being thicker than class" vitiates attempts to bring workers of different backgrounds together. And, of course, employers vehemently opposed organizing efforts on behalf of workers and attacked workers and their leaders who attempted organization. As a result of these various factors, it is widely agreed that the United States failed to generate a viable and cohesive working class–based political movement.

There are interesting ramifications of this failure for the emerging older population. On the one hand, an effective working-class movement would appear to benefit the aged, if only because current workers would become old, and pension benefits were almost included as one of a package of worker demands. Indeed, pensions can be seen as a way for workers to press for (future) benefits in a manner that was less threatening to employers than were demands for improvements in current wages and working conditions. Because public pensions have come to constitute a comparatively enormous portion of American welfare state expenditures and because pension and health benefits were the lion's share of fringe benefits negotiated for by workers, the aged in the United States can be seen as both conceptually and economically advantaged through leftist (or at least progressive) efforts at benefit expansion. The passage of Medicare in the 1960s serves as further evidence of this advantage. Its passage has been partially attributed to organized labor trying to push union-funded retiree health care costs—another form of deferred income—off onto the public sector in order that those energies and resources could be channeled into efforts on behalf of current workers (Quadagno, 2005).

On the other hand, as Pampel and Williamson (1992) observe, the workings of this theory could be seen as inimical to the concerns of the aged. Organized labor's political action efforts might work to exclude other groups, including women and populations of color, who might have been workers but not unionized ones. Certainly, the historical segregationist impulses of mainstream American labor would serve to substantiate such a concern.

Moving to a more contemporary concern, Pampel and Williamson (1992) note that intergenerational tension might emerge for unions (and, conceivably, the Democratic Party) in a situation in which there was a call for higher dues or taxes to be imposed to support pension benefits for current retirees. Pension obligations were central issues in Detroit's bankruptcy proceedings and pension burdens lie at the heart of several states' precarious fiscal outlooks.

Despite these possibilities and events, the dangers of such a split are reduced in the American case by, once again, the limited impact of purely working-class political movements. The recent erosion of union membership, the spread of "right to work" laws across the industrial Midwest in recent years, to say nothing of an influx of hard-to-unionize low-wage immigrant workers, makes this potential working-class "threat" to the old a marginal possibility at best (Davey, 2015). More broadly, Levine (2015) finds lower income groups demonstrably concerned with three social policy issues—involuntary job loss, health care costs, and college costs—largely unable to mobilize around them, whereas older people have been able to organize effectively around the issue of retirement insecurity.

■ DEMOCRATIC AND GROUP PARTICIPATION

Perhaps the most commonly presented construct of "how a (social policy) bill becomes a law" in the United States centers on how interests are articulated, aggregated, and realized. In the classic democratic participation model, citizens express their views through voting, letter writing, campaigning, and contributing; interest groups are organized around clusters of citizen concerns and carried by them to political parties and directly into the halls of government; and political parties join separate demands into coherent platforms as a means of structuring political debate (Easton, 1957).

Associated very much with pluralist theories of the political system (Polsby, 1963), this model has both empirical and normative dimensions. Mainstream political science saw these pluralistic impulses as marking how American government worked from World War II through the 1960s, but it was widely held that the pluralists often conflated depictions of how the system worked with how they preferred it to work. Voter, group, and party competition functioned not unlike the workings of the free economic market, with myriad demands being muted and compromises being forged. In all of this, the government served as something of a referee, ratifying the winners and losers and lending formal recognition to the balance of political powers at any given point in time. A growing tide of criticism (Lowi, 1967; Parenti, 1970) and events of the 1960s and 1970s led to the model's fall from grace. Nonetheless, the pluralists' desire to document and defend democratically stable political systems in light of the widespread failure of democratic governments earlier in the century was more than understandable.

There can be no question that the basic ingredients of the model were (and are) very much in evidence in the United States. Long seen as a nation of joiners, the United States has more interest groups, many of them highly particularistic, than found elsewhere. Whereas political parties in other nations do, in fact, perform critical aggregating functions around candidate selection and policy formulation, in the United States it is said to be K Street—home to hundreds of special interests, many of them generously funded—where disproportionate influence on these key functions is effectively exercised (Gilens & Page, 2014). The logical basis for this reality derives in part from what we saw as the United States not possessing a strong working class. As a result, in the pluralist model, the critical unit of analysis becomes particularistic groups, whereas in the worker mobilization model it was social class. In 2010 to 2012, the Occupy Wall Street Movement aimed at creation of a class-based movement, but, as have many earlier such movements, it faded from the scene (Levine, 2015).

Older people present a fascinating case study of the potential validity of the interest group model and its limitations, both empirical and normative. They are a large and growing population, they are very active politically, they are extremely well organized, they have particularistic policy concerns, and roughly one third of the federal budget is devoted to their interests. As they say, that is a very potent political cocktail. However, it need be kept in mind that correlation is not causation and, as we will see subsequently, exactly how the cocktail is mixed may make all the difference.

It is first important to note that seniors' organized presence in Washington is reinforced by its imposing electoral standing. Not only a large population, seniors now participate at higher rates than any other age group (U.S. Bureau of the Census, 2012). In off-year and primary elections, that disproportionate presence is even more pronounced. Yet, it is equally important to observe that older people vote much like younger ones in general elections (Binstock, 2009), suggesting that their population-specific interests do not necessarily determine their voting decisions. Of course, because no candidate campaigns on an anti-aging platform, this "nonevent" becomes a potent illustration of how elders exercise a "second face of power" (Bachrach & Baratz, 1962; Gaventa, 1980), that is, keeping unwanted alternatives off the political agenda altogether. There is little evidence that voting patterns of older people directly shape aging-related policy results, but a fair summation of older voters' place in the policy process may simply be that "they are there, and they are aware."

Seniors' interest group presence in Washington is formidable, and it is here that the potential exercise of "the first face of power" is in full view. Organizations ranging from the AARP (with 34 million members) to the National Academy of Elder Care Attorneys and the American Society of Consulting Pharmacists are among 62 organizations that constitute the Leadership Council of Aging Organizations (LCAO, 2014), that is, an organization of aging organizations. A few of the members, such as AARP, are mass-membership organizations, but the majority of the groups represent professionals and other providers with interests in Washington and the states serving older Americans.

Although these organizations' significant presence is beyond dispute, their exact role in securing the enormous benefits today's elders enjoy is a matter of some controversy. Certainly, there has been much commentary in both popular (Peterson, 1999; Samuelson, 2005) and scholarly circles (Pratt, 1976; Price, 1997) pointing—usually with alarm—at the influence the organized aged have in Washington. AARP has been portrayed as the capital's most powerful group, and its support of President Bush's Medicare Part D prescription drug program is widely believed to have been critical to the legislation's passage (Iglehart, 2004).

In many other legislative episodes, however, it has been difficult to isolate a determinative role that the groups have played. As the groups themselves have been organized only quite recently—AARP and National Council of Senior Citizens (NCSC) were the first, both dating back only to the late 1950s—they played no role in the formative years of aging policy. And accounts of particular legislative episodes report mixed results as well. In each of the following cases, the organized aged and their allies were engaged, but evidence of their role in determining ultimate policy outcomes is more mixed: Social Security (Derthick, 1979; Light, 1985), Medicare (Marmor, 1970), Supplemental Security Income (Burke & Burke, 1974), repeal of Medicare Catastrophic Coverage Act (Himelfarb, 1995), and private pension benefit protection (Madland, 2007).

Nonetheless, recent events and significant changes in the aging policy environment have necessitated involvement of voters and groups in ways that was not earlier necessary. In the cases of resisting President G. W. Bush's efforts to privatize Social Security in 2005 and more recent attempts by congressional Republicans to change the Social Security cost-of-living adjustment formula and to transform Medicare into a partially privatized voucher program, direct political involvement was called for to defend measures that were already in place. Moreover, older people may not only promote their own direct interests but may also oppose others whose concerns they see as inimical to their own. Thus, evidence finds elders disproportionately in opposition to the Affordable Care Act (ACA) as manifested in both public opinion data (Ashok, Kuziemko, & Washington, 2015) and in voting during the 2010 congressional elections (Binstock, 2012) because of concern that cuts in the Medicare program were being used to fund the ACA.

■ THE ROLE OF THE STATE: STRUCTURE

The role of the state in aging-related welfare state developments would seem to be self-evident in that it is, of course, the state that formally enacts and funds policies of all sorts. Yet, in the approaches reviewed thus far, the role of governmental institutions and incumbents is remarkably marginal. Industrialization theory sees it as responding in some quasi-automatic and unspecified way to an emerging combination of technological innovation and human suffering; the working-class approach sees the state as the prize that one or the other of two class-based interests will control; and the pluralism inherent in the political interest model finds state actions as largely a ratification of the balance of organized group influence within the polity.

The 1980s saw the re-emergence of the state as a central analytical ingredient in accounting for welfare state developments. The center of attention in political science's very early years—Woodrow Wilson wrote famously about it while at Princeton (Robertson, 1993)—the role of the state lost standing to the aforementioned alternative approaches, especially in the post–World War II years. Two scholars in particular are associated with this reemergence of interest in the state. Theodore Lowi (1964) suggested that what the state does critically affects the subsequent political process, not simply the reverse as suggested by social democratic and democratic process approaches. At the 1981 American Political Science Association, Lowi and his co-chair Sydney Tarrow, argued: "We do not reject the perspective that focuses on the political process, or on political behavior—even when it is *mass* behavior—but we argue that processes and behavior can best be studied within the context of institutions" (quoted in Robertson, 1993, p. 20). Skocpol and colleagues have produced a significant literature over the past 20 years under the rubric of "bringing the state back in," the essential argument being: "States conceived as organizations claiming control over territories and people may formulate and pursue goals that are not simply reflective of the demands or interests of social groups, classes, or society" (Skocpol, 1985, p. 9).

The essence of the argument is that state structures play an independent role in shaping political activity and political outcomes. These structures include all significant elements of the state—formal constitutional structures and quasi-public institutions such as political parties. Robertson (1993) sees measures of both *political capacity* and *political coherence* as being critical in state-centered analysis. Three key measures of capacity are the boundaries of legitimate governmental intervention, fiscal capacity, and expertise of legislators and administrators. Coherence involves two dimensions: the extent to which authority within a level of government is unified or fragmented and the autonomy possessed by different levels of government.

If not once again exceptional, the American experience is at least notable if we briefly examine it against these five items. In comparative perspective, the boundaries of legitimate governmental action in the social policy realm are noticeably narrow. The exceptionalism of the national values perspective weighs in heavily here as does the Marshall formulation noting how far social citizenship trails behind the civic and political in the United States. A famous passage from Tom Paine (1791) captures Americans' historical disdain for the state: "the more perfect civilization is, the less occasion it has for government, because the more does it regulate its own affairs and govern itself."

Fiscal capacity of the national government was historically weak, one of many examples being that the budget of the U.S. State Department was drawn exclusively from consular fees until just before World War I. While slowing the gap modestly, the United States continues to spend considerably less on social welfare functions than do other advanced nations (Organization for Economic Cooperation and Development [OECD], 2014).

The United States also trails other nations in critical aspects of administrative expertise. For myriad reasons, the civil service in the United States has never enjoyed the autonomy and prestige of its counterparts in other nations. The traditions about the administrative sphere of government differ sharply on either side of the Atlantic. In Europe, the autonomy of the state is long established and taken as an institutional reality across a range of critical social activities (Nettl, 1968). This is in direct contrast to the

U.S. experience where "the civil administration of the early twentieth-century American state was quite weak, given the lack of an established state bureaucracy and the dispersion of authority inherent in U.S. federalism and the division of powers" (Orloff, 1988, p. 59).

The lack of cohesiveness of America's political structures is known, if not fully appreciated, by generations of students. Cohesion was intentionally attenuated from the beginning: a federal restructure with divided areas of sovereignty, separated branches of government, checks and balances, bicameral legislature (with the Senate embodying overt state-level representation), and staggered elections within and between the legislative and executive branches. Samuel Huntington (1966) argues that, among American governmental institutions, "sovereignty was divided, power was separated, and functions were combined in many different institutions" (p. 392). In Huntington's analysis, it is America's consensual society that makes this institutional chaos possible: "In America, the ease of modernization within society precluded the modernization of the political system. The United States thus combines the world's most modern society with the world's most antique politics" (p. 406). Why this state of institutional events would impede social policy development is not hard to deduce. In the bastardized words of a popular advertisement: "You expect less of the American government, and you get it." Limited capacity and coherence—especially when intended—do not bode well for reformers' agendas.

As well, for purposes here, weak political institutions also can be used to account for how older people have fared in the United States. The most interesting application comes in Skocpol's widely heralded rethinking of when America's version of the welfare state actually began. In her work highlighting the importance of Civil War pensions and so-called mothers' pensions, Skocpol (1992) argues that, however selectively, the United States preceded what famously occurred elsewhere. By the late 19th century, these payments were roughly equal to any expenditure category in the federal budget, and in 1910, about 28% of men older than 65 years—more than one-half million—were receiving these benefits.

More interesting than their size, however, is their theoretical relevance: These pensions were awarded in great numbers to farmers and townspeople not central to industrialization, and they were not demanded by industrial workers or principally extended to them (Skocpol, 1992). Instead, pension expenditures expanded greatly until the end of the century, caught up in a uniquely American political process whereby they moved from "relatively straightforward compensation for wartime disabilities into fuel for patronage politics" (p. 120). In her words, the Civil War pension "evolved from a generous partially utilized program of compensation for combat injuries and deaths into an even more generous system of disability and old-age benefits which were taken up by 90 percent of the union veterans surviving in 1910" (pp. 109–110).

A second application of this perspective to old-age policy in the United States centers on the role of government civil servants in the welfare state enterprise. That such individuals were central to European developments has been well established (Beer, 1966). In perhaps the first of the state-centered monographs, Heclo (1974) reviews and downplays the roles of industrialization, elections, political parties, and interest groups: "At no time did organizations of the aged or pensioners themselves play any prominent part" (p. 156). Rather, he concludes that "the bureaucracies of Britain and Sweden loom predominant in the policies studied" (p. 301).

Despite the institutional shortcomings in the United States, there are important instances of public officials making a critical difference in social policy developments.

And many of these involved older adults. Most notable in this regard is Franklin Roosevelt's Committee on Economic Security, which fashioned the original Social Security Act (Witte, 1963). As Ikenberry and Skocpol (1987, p. 405) bluntly conclude, "the policy process through which Social Security was planned and drafted in the mid-1930s was strikingly closed." Derthick has chronicled how closed was Social Security policymaking from the beginning through the mid-1970s, concluding:

> Program specialists in executive bureaus are one of the principal sources of supply for politicians who are looking for ideas for things to do. In the case of social security, for several decades they were almost the only source of supply. (p. 210)

Policy elites inside government were critical to later successes, again disproportionately involving the aged. Wilbur Cohen, Oscar Ewing, and two key congressional figures—Senator Patrick McNamara of Michigan and Representative Aime Forand of Rhode Island—centrally fashioned Medicare strategy from the mid-1950s until its enactment in 1965 (Marmor, 1970). John Veneman, Undersecretary of the Department of Health, Education, and Welfare, was the central actor in the phoenix-like transformation of President Nixon's failed Family Assistance Plan for Aid to Families with Dependent Children into the Supplemental Security Income program (Burke & Burke, 1974). These key actors, working in an admittedly semi-incoherent political system, seized critical moments and were able to strike when the policy moment was hot. And, in these efforts, they often seized on the plight of older people and the sympathy they engendered in the American context. In this manner, the aged served as something of an "ideological loss-leader" for these reformers, eager not only to help the aged but to use them in hopefully advancing policy agendas to other groups as well (Hudson, 1978).

However, as recent politics have become more contested, a new set of elite actors opposing expansion of old-age policy benefits has moved to the fore. In addition, they give agency to anti-government attitudes of the post-Reagan years—marked by the rhetoric of "getting government off your back," "bring government closer to the people," and "promoting traditional family values"—each speaking to enduring beliefs designed to limit state authority in the United States. The tension between small-government advocates and the political potency of age-based policies is seen in Tea Party adherents' positive views toward Social Security (Williams, Skocpol, & Coggin, 2011) and as well in a dilemma facing the Republican party's primary field leading to the 2016 election, namely, that "(t)he party's base of White—often older—voters includes many blue-collar conservatives who mistrust the government but depend on its programs for older Americans" (Haberman, 2015).

■ THE ROLE OF THE STATE: POLICY

In various ways, each of the aforementioned perspectives addresses factors and actors that may be seen responsible for the timing and shape of aging-related welfare state policies. This last perspective reverses the causal arrows by asking, instead, to what degree do the policies themselves shape subsequent political activity. Here, policy becomes an independent variable affecting politics and, in turn, future policy. This hypothesis derives directly from the state-centered perspective in that policies, being formal product of states, both contribute to and derive from state autonomy and capacity. Policies can serve as a powerful mechanism in attaching citizens to the political world by clearly demonstrating what government can do for them or what it may do to them. Moreover, because levels of political participation have been declining and Americans' civic engagement has been called into question (Putnam, 1995), the role of public policy in fostering citizen involvement has normative as well as empirical ramifications.

Schattschneider (1935) was the first to identify and examine the phenomenon of how "policy causes politics" in his early discussion of tariff policy. Later investigations of "policy types" (Lowi, 1964; Wilson, 1973) demonstrated how the scope and distributive consequences of various enactments shaped subsequent activity. One of the most prominent examples of policy drawing individuals into the political system is found in the case of the G. I. Bill, where Mettler (2005) has shown how its enactment following World War II both contributed to broad-based economic gains and "also prompted higher levels of subsequent involvement in civic and political activities" (p. 196). However, policies can have alienating political effects as well, as in the cases of public assistance, where requirements and decisions around means-testing can lead to cynicism and mistrust (Soss, 1999). The "policy feedback" connection is surely suggestive, but its application is tied to particular population and problem constructions (Campbell, 2012).

Within this policy → politics template, the political place and policies of older people find a very compatible home. In part, this is because the programs—Social Security, Medicare, a large part of Medicaid, and numerous lesser ones—dominate the federal domestic social policy landscape (Gist, 2014). However, the connection and timing between the growth in policies and the subsequent actions of older citizens and their interest groups are yet more remarkable.

Walker (1983) was the first to document the role of policy in stimulating political activity, contrasting the timing of interest group formation against existing policies central to the concerns of those groups. His study determined that more than one half of the 43 aging-related interest groups examined came into being after 1965, the breakthrough year that saw the enactment of Medicare, Medicaid, and the Older Americans Act. In Walker's words:

> In all of these cases, the formation of new groups was one of the *consequences* of major new legislation, not one of the *causes* of its passage. A pressure model of the policymaking process in which an essentially passive legislature responds to petitions from groups of citizens who have spontaneously organized because of common social or economic concerns must yield to a model in which influences for change come as much from inside the government as from beyond its institutional boundaries. (p. 403)

Actions subsequent to passage of the Older Americans Act—a program funding an array of social and in-home services to people aged 60 years and older—provide a concrete example of this process at work. The state agencies charged with administering the program formalized their trade association, the National Association of State Units on Aging, in the years after 1965; the substate agencies, brought into existence through amendments in 1972, created their trade association, the National Association of Area Agencies on Aging, in the wake of that authorization (Hudson, 1994). Groups of nutrition, transportation, and legal service providers were also formed subsequent to these amendments.

Yet more compelling evidence of the policy-generating politics chain is seen in the creation of seniors themselves as a self-identified political constituency. Campbell (2003) documents how the growing presence of older Americans in the political process owes much of its existence to the expansion of Social Security. In carefully crafted research juxtaposing public opinion and voting data with Social Security program expansion, Campbell shows how levels of political consciousness, participation, and salience followed in the wake of Social Security's growth. Seniors are the only group whose electoral participation in presidential elections over the past 40 years has actually increased, whereas the participation rates of voters aged 18 to 24, 25 to 44, and 45 to 64 years have each declined. In relative terms, a higher proportion of seniors now vote than does any other age group; in 1964, they exceeded only the youngest group. Campbell shows, as well, that participation rates of seniors in other forms of political activity—letter writing, campaigning, contributing—have also increased in both relative and absolute terms.

In assessing these findings, Campbell concludes that Social Security, in dramatically improving the economic well-being of older people, created both time and interest—what Pierson (2007) calls "material and cognitive incentives"—for seniors to involve themselves in political matters more heavily than had ever been the case:

> Senior mass membership groups did not create Social Security policy. Rather, the policy helped create the groups. Social Security's effects on individuals—the increases in income, free time due to retirement, and political interest—enhance the likelihood of group membership. Social Security created a constituency for interest group entrepreneurs to organize, just as it defined a group for political parties to mobilize. (Campbell, 2003, p. 77)

Although the causal role of policy is the principal contribution of this analysis, the secondary effects of policy's role is equally important. Thus, at "Time 1" public policy may have been critical in the creation and institutionalization of the organized aging, but at "Time 2" the groups become critical in efforts to expand or—more recently—to defend the policies against outside encroachment. Put differently, the Walker/Campbell argument does not dismiss the role of interest groups; rather, it helps explain both their origins and the dynamic—that is, benefit protection—that keeps formal members or informal adherents tuned in to their messages. In short, although "AARP may be the biggest lobby in Washington," it would not be where it is if (a) Social Security had not helped galvanize the elderly and if (b) Social Security and other programs were not there as a policy fulcrum around which AARP could rally the membership.

■ CONCLUSION

Whether viewed separately or in combination, these six theoretical approaches go a very long way in accounting for the birth and expansion of aging policy within the American welfare state. Industrialization created a "resources plus needs" scenario allowing and necessitating state intervention on behalf of elders. Prevailing political values contributed to development of social policy in the United States being "late, low, and slow," but the deservingness of seniors opened policy doors that had long been shut. Similarly, the absence of a cohesive working-class movement found the United States, unlike other industrial nations, inaugurating policies where populations other than workers were the principal beneficiaries, principally elders. Weak state capacity of the American government did not allow for the passage of broad-based inclusionary welfare policy; instead, it left policy doors open to particularistic constituencies—of whom elders were clearly one—working through decentralized legislative and administrative bodies. Finally, as such time that policies did arrive and bureaucracies were established to administer them, the policies served to activate individuals and groups to promote their expansion or guard against retrenchment, Social Security being most notable.

In conclusion, it is instructive to examine contemporary events surrounding aging policy through these complementary theoretical lenses. These explanatory approaches remain relevant even as constituent elements are being transformed by contemporary events. The principal events that inform these approaches are economic constraints, ideological tensions, demographic transformations, and technological advances.

An updated version of industrialization theory centers on technological innovation and its impact on longevity, health, mobility, and inequality. A growing older population, and the oldest-old within it, is having major political and policy consequences. Longer lives and increased chronicity are creating a need—if not a demand (Levitsky, 2014)—for a massive infusion of long-term care services; high- and low-level technological devices are providing greater autonomy for impaired elders and may—for better or worse—substitute for personal care provision. Increasing numbers of elders of color—burdened by lifetimes of limited opportunity and discrimination—will bring new disparities and policy claims with the passage of time. The logic of industrialization profoundly affected 19th-century older adults and necessitated the development of social programs; the technology revolution we are experiencing today will also transform the aging population; whether it will generate needed policy interventions is less clear.

Resurgent views about the centrality of individualism, family, markets, and the primacy of work and the private sector are shaping much of today's social policy debate. More muted during the prosperity of the 1950s and the Great Society of the 1960s, these cultural mainstays have been a formidable presence in the post-Reagan years. They have had a depressing effect on social policy initiative across the board, but especially among those populations seen as deviating from this set of norms. Compared with these, elders have been largely spared the policy consequences generated by these conservative impulses. Initiatives directed at welfare recipients, the unemployed, and immigrants have been far more restrictive than those addressed to elders (Palmer & Sawhill, 1984). This being the case reintroduces the importance of the Schneider and Ingram (1993) typology, viewed through which seniors have been variously positively viewed and/or able to take care of themselves, whereas populations deemed "dependent" or "deviant" have not. There is more continuity here than change.

From one vantage point, the historical weakness of the American labor movement continues, with the percentage of unionized workers continuing to decline and both public and private sector unions facing an organized assault across much of the nation. Yet, to the extent that this model speaks to ideological divisions more broadly, the emerging picture is less clear. On the political front, partisanship and gridlock have become new hallmarks in Washington and are actively threatening the type of consensus that Huntington (1966) earlier heralded.

For seniors, the emerging tension revolves around conservatives' efforts to forestall aging-related policy initiatives (repeal of the CLASS Act addressing long-term care [Caldwell & Bedlin, 2014]; further privatization of Medicare through "premium support" initiatives [Morgan, 2014]) and progressives' attempts to expand such initiatives (increase Social Security benefits [Sargent, 2013]; limit cost sharing in Medicare and Medicaid [Center for Medicare Advocacy, 2013]). Again, the ideological dimension is somewhat more muted in aging-related policy than elsewhere, but it is more prominent today than it has ever been.

The place of individual and organized political participation in aging politics has taken on unprecedented importance in the nation's current economic and political environment. The earlier era in which, politically, "you couldn't do enough for the elderly," and, economically, where resources were seen as being more readily available, has yielded to a period in which elders face major economic/budgetary and political challenges. Under these circumstances, elders and their advocates have been forced to play their political hand in a manner not previously required. During earlier years, the combination of elders' positive political construction and the *presumption* that they could wield political power—what Binstock (2005) termed the "electoral bluff"—was all that was required. Today, ranged against resurgent small-government proponents and well-funded conservative think tanks, the bluff is being called. Yet, as evidenced in policy battles such as repeal of the Medicare Catastrophic Coverage Act, passage of the Medicare Part D prescription drug program, and the failure of G. W. Bush's Social Security privatization plan, elders' political standing today is more than a bluff. In elders' new "contender" stage, we cannot know how future battles will play out, but seniors are well positioned to engage in any forthcoming battles.

A major reason that they are well positioned centers on the *political* contributions that continue to be made by *policy* enactments and implementation. The relative weakness of American state capacity inhibited welfare state growth, yet key reformers and government incumbents initially created what was essentially an "old-age welfare state," one that both benefited and used older Americans through its creation. The putative phrase "workers, no; elders, yes" speaks to what was finally possible and which today remains a prominent feature of American social policy, with aging-oriented Social Security, Medicare, and Medicaid dominating the social policy landscape.

The final theoretical perspective—"path dependency," featuring the independent role of policy in shaping politics—now shifts into gear. Before the passage and growth of these major aging policies, older Americans had at best a marginal political standing, voting less than others and being politically unorganized until some time in the 1960s. Largely through Social Security, the argument goes, elders emerged as a self-identified political constituency, one with a common calling and with the material, temporal, and psychological resources to play in the political theatre. In turn, advocates, providers, and researchers seized on elders' new political prominence to promote both elders' interests and their own.

The result has been a powerful symbiotic relationship between old age policy and politics, with each reinforcing the other. The political potency is seen in seniors today voting at a higher rate than any other age group and there being so many aging-oriented interest groups in Washington that they had to form their own confederate organization. The policy potency is seen in the relative place of old-age expenditures in the federal budget, with Social Security standing at Number Two, Medicare at Number Three, and Medicaid at Number Five.

Given the tenor of the times, there is little reason to think that major new old age initiatives are in the offing, but the natural growth of those already in place assures elders—for better or worse—a prominent place in policy discussions for the foreseeable future. On the one hand, there are looming needs associated with growing numbers of very old people (Applebaum & Bardo, 2014) and the inadequate retirement preparation underway among today's middle aged (Rix, 2014). Yet, on the other hand, aging programs are unquestionably expensive and the nation still contends with an accumulated $17 trillion debt to which critics want to tie the "voracious appetite" of America's senior citizens. In Schneider and Ingram's words, elders have unquestionably moved from "advantaged" to "contender" status (Hudson & Gonyea, 2012).

REFERENCES

Amenta, E., Bonastia, C., & Caren, N. (2001). U.S. social policy in comparative and historical perspective: Concepts, images, arguments, and research strategies. *Annual Review of Sociology, 27*, 213–234.

Applebaum, R., & Bardo, A. (2014). Will you still need me, will you still feed me, when I'm 84? Long-term care challenges for an aging America. In R. B. Hudson (Ed.), *The new politics of old age policy* (3rd ed., pp. 221–235). Baltimore, MD: Johns Hopkins University Press.

Ashok, V., Kuziemko, I., & Washington, E. (2015). Support for redistribution in an age of rising inequality: New stylized facts and some tentative explanations. *Brookings papers on economic activity*. Washington, DC: Brookings Institution.

Bachrach, P., & Baratz, M. (1962). The two faces of power. *American Political Science Review, 56*, 947–952.

Ball, R. (2000). *Insuring the essentials: Bob Ball on Social Security*. New York, NY: Century Foundation Press.

Beer, S. H. (1966). *British politics in the collectivist age*. New York, NY: Alfred A. Knopf.

Beland, D., Howard, C., & Morgan, K. J. (Eds.). (2014). *The Oxford handbook of U.S. social policy*. New York, NY: Oxford University Press.

Binstock, R. H. (2005). The contemporary politics of old age policies. In R. B. Hudson (Ed.), *The new politics of old age policy* (pp. 265–293). Baltimore, MD: Johns Hopkins University Press.

Binstock, R. H. (2009). Older voters and the 2008 election. *The Gerontologist, 49*, 697–701.

Binstock, R. H. (2012). Older voters and the 2010 U.S. election: Implications for 2012 and beyond? *The Gerontologist, 52*(3), 408–417.

Burke, V. J., & Burke, V. (1974). *Nixon's good deed*. New York, NY: Columbia University Press.

Caldwell, J., & Bedlin, H. (2014). Beyond the CLASS Act: The future of long-term care financing reform. *Public Policy and Aging Report, 24*(2), 46–49.

Cameron, D. R. (1978). The expansion of the public economy: A comparative analysis. *American Political Science Review, 72*, 1243–1261.

Campbell, A. L. (2003). *How policies make citizens: Senior political activism and the American welfare state*. Princeton, NJ: Princeton University Press.

Campbell, A. L. (2012). Policy makes mass politics. 2012. *Annual Review of Political Science, 15*, 333–351.

Center for Medicare Advocacy. (2013). *Study shows high cost-sharing significantly harms family health and finances*. Washington, DC: Center for Medicare Advocacy.

Davey, M. (2015). Scott Walker is set to deliver new blow to labor in Wisconsin. *New York Times*, p. A14.

Derthick, M. (1979). *Policymaking for Social Security*. Washington, DC: Brookings Institution.

Easton, D. (1957). An approach to the analysis of political systems. *World Politics, 9*, 383–400.

Esping-Anderson, G. (1985). *Politics against markets: The social democratic road to power*. Princeton, NJ: Princeton University Press.

Fleming, D. (1963). Social Darwinism. In A. Schlesinger (Ed.), *Paths of American thought* (pp. 123–145). New York, NY: Houghton-Mifflin.

Garfinkel, I., Rainwater, L., & Smeeding, T. (2010). *Wealth and welfare*. New York, NY: Oxford University Press.

Gaventa, J. (1980). Power and participation. In J. Gaventa, *Power and powerlessness: Quiescence and rebellion in an Appalachian valley* (pp. 3–32). Urbana, IL: University of Illinois Press.

Gerson, M. (2010, December 28). Face social security. *Washington Post*, p. A13.

Gilens, M., & Page, B. (2014). Testing theories of American politics: Elites, interest groups, and average citizens. *Perspectives on Politics, 12*(3), 564–581.

Gist, J. (2014). Fiscal effects of population aging in the United States. In R. B. Hudson (Ed.), *The new politics of old age policy* (3rd ed., pp. 29–68). Baltimore, MD: Johns Hopkins University Press.

Gratton, B. (1986). The new history of the aged: A critique. In D. Van Tassel & P. N. Stearns, (Eds.), *Old age in a bureaucratic society* (pp. 3–29). Westport, CT: Greenwood Press.

Greenstone, J. D. (1970). *Labor in American politics*. New York, NY: Vintage Books.

Haberman, M. (2015). Mike Huckabee seems to be going his own way on social programs. *New York Times*, p. A19.

Heclo, H. (1974). *Modern social politics in Britain and Sweden*. New Haven, CT: Yale University Press.

Himelfarb, R. (1995). *Catastrophic politics: The rise and fall of the Medicare Catastrophic Coverage Act*. University Park, PA: Pennsylvania University Press.

Hudson, R. B. (1978). The graying of the federal budget and its consequences for old-age policy. *The Gerontologist, 18*, 428–440.

Hudson, R. B. (1994). The Older Americans Act and the defederalization of community-based care. In P. Kim (Ed.), *Services to the aged: Public policies and programs*. New York, NY: Garland.

Hudson, R. B., & Gonyea, J. G. (2012). Baby boomers and the shifting political construction of old age. *The Gerontologist, 52*(2), 273–282.

Huntington, S. (1966). Political modernization: America vs. Europe. *World Politics, 18*, 378–414.

Iglehart, J. (2004). The new Medicare prescription drug benefit: A pure power play. *New England Journal of Medicine, 350*, 826–833.

Ikenberry, J., & Skocpol, T. (1987). Expanding social benefits: The role of Social Security. *Political Science Quarterly, 102*(3), 389–416.

Kotlikoff, L., & Burns, S. (2004). *The coming generational storm: What you need to know about America's economic future*. Cambridge, MA: MIT Press.

Leadership Council of Aging Organizations (LCAO). (2014). Retrieved from lcao.org

Levine, A. S. (2015). *American insecurity: Why our economic fears lead to political inaction*. Princeton, NJ: Princeton University Press.

Levitsky, S. (2014). *Caring for our own: Why there is no political demand for new American social welfare rights*. New York, NY: Oxford University Press.

Light, P. (1985). *Artful work: The politics of Social Security reform*. New York, NY: Random House.

Lipset, S. M. (1997). *American exceptionalism: A double-edged sword*. New York, NY: W. W. Norton.

Lipset, S. M., & Marks, G. (2001). *It didn't happen here: Why socialism failed in the United States*. New York, NY: W. W. Norton.

Lowi, T. J. (1964). American business, public policy, case-studies, and political theory. *World Politics, 16*, 677–715.

Lowi, T. J. (1967). The public philosophy: Interest group liberalism. *American Political Science Review, 61*(1), 5–24.

Lynch, J., & Myrskyla, M. (2009). Always the third rail? Pension income and policy in preferences in European democracies. *Comparative Political Studies, 42*(8), 1068–1097.

Madland, D. (2007). The politics of pension cuts. In T. Ghilarducci & C. E. Weller (Eds.), *Employee pensions: Policies, problems, and possibilities* (pp. 187–214). Champaign, IL: Labor and Employment Relations Association.

Marmor, T. (1970). *The politics of Medicare*. Chicago, IL: Aldine.

Marmor, T., Mashaw, J., & Harvey, P. (1990). *America's misunderstood welfare state*. New York, NY: Basic Books.

Marshall, T. H. (1964). *Class, citizenship and social development*. Garden City, NY: Doubleday.

Mettler, S. (2005). *Soldiers to citizens: The G. I. Bill and the making of the greatest generation*. New York, NY: Oxford University Press.

Morgan, K. J. (2014). The Medicare challenge: Clients, cost controls, and Congress. In R. B. Hudson (Ed.), *The new politics of old age policy* (3rd ed., pp. 201–220). Baltimore, MD: Johns Hopkins University Press.

Myles, J., & Quadagno, J. (2002). Political theories of the welfare state. *Social Service Review, 76*(1), 34–57.

Nettl, J. P. (1968). The state as a conceptual variable. *World Politics, 20*(4), 559–592.

Organization for Economic Cooperation and Development (OECD). (2014). *Public social expenditure as a percent of GDP, 2007 and 2014*. Retrieved from http://www .oecd.org/social/expenditure.htm

Orloff, A. S. (1988). The political origins of America's belated welfare state. In M. Weir, A. S. Orloff, & T. Skocpol (Eds.), *The politics of social policy in the United States* (pp. 37–80). Princeton, NJ: Princeton University Press.

Paine, T. (1791). *The rights of man*. Philadelphia, PA.

Palmer, J. L., & Sawhill, I. V. (1984). *The Reagan record*. Cambridge, MA: Ballinger.

Pampel, F., & Williamson, J. (1992). *Age, class, politics, and the welfare state*. New York, NY: Cambridge University Press.

Parenti, M. (1970). Power and pluralism: A view from the bottom. *Journal of Politics, 32*, 501–530.

Peterson, P. G. (1999). *Gray dawn: How the coming age wave will transform America—and the world*. New York, NY: Times Books.

Pierson, P. (1994). *Dismantling the welfare state? Reagan, Thatcher, and the politics of retrenchment*. New York, NY: Cambridge University Press.

Pierson, P. (2007). The rise and reconfiguration of activist government. In P. Pierson & T. Skocpol (Eds.), *The transformation of American politics* (pp. 19–38). Princeton, NJ: Princeton University Press.

Piketty, T. (2014). *Capital in the 21st century*. Cambridge, MA: Belknap Press.

Polsby, N. (1963). *Community power and political theory*. New Haven, CT: Yale University Press.

Pratt, H. (1976). *The gray lobby*. Chicago, IL: University of Chicago Press.

Price, M. C. (1997). *Justice between generations: The growing power of the elderly in America*. Westport, CT: Greenwood.

Putnam, R. (1995). Bowling alone: America's declining social capital. *Journal of Democracy, 6*(1), 65–78.

Quadagno, J. (1988). *The transformation of old age security*. Chicago, IL: University of Chicago Press.

Quadagno, J. (2005). *One nation, uninsured*. New York, NY: Oxford University Press.

Rimlinger, G. (1971). *Welfare policy and industrialization in Europe, America, and Russia*. New York, NY: Wiley.

Rix, S. (2014). Working, retiring, and the new old age. In R. B. Hudson (Ed.), *The new politics of old age policy* (3rd ed., pp. 117–137). Baltimore, MD: Johns Hopkins University Press.

Robertson, D. B. (1993). The return to history and the new institutionalism in American political science. *Social Science History, 17*(1), 1–36.

Rosenberg, C. (1962). *The cholera years*. Chicago, IL: University of Chicago Press.

Ryan, W. (1971). *Blaming the victim*. New York, NY: Knopf.

Samuelson, R. J. (2005). AARP's America is a mirage. *Washington Post*.

Samuelson, R. J. (2013). We need to stop coddling the elderly. *Washington Post*. Retrieved from http://www.washingtonpost.com/opinions/robert-j-samuelson-we-need-to-stop-coddling-the-elderly/2013/11/03/4063ebc0–430f-11e3-a624–41d661b0bb78_story.html

Sargent, G. (2013). Elizabeth Warren: Don't cut Social Security. Expand it. *Washington Post*.

Schattschneider, E. E. (1935). *Politics, pressures, and the tariff*. New York, NY: Prentice-Hall.

Schneider, A., & Ingram, H. (1993). Social construction of target populations. *American Political Science Review, 87*, 333–347.

Skocpol, T. (1985). Bringing the state back in: Strategies of analysis and current research. In P. Evans, D. Rueschemeyer, & T. Skocpol (Eds.), *Bringing the state back in* (pp. 3–37). New York, NY: Cambridge University Press.

Skocpol, T. (1992). *Protecting soldiers and mothers*. Cambridge, MA: Belknap Press.

Soss, J. (1999). Lessons of welfare: Policy design, political learning, and political action. *American Political Science Review, 93*, 363–380.

Stephens, J. D., Huber, E., Ray, L., Kitschelt, H., Lange, P., & Marks, G. (1999). *Continuity and change in contemporary capitalism*. Cambridge, UK: Cambridge University Press.

Teles, S. (2007. Conservative mobilization against entrenched liberalism. In P. Pierson & T. Skocpol (Eds.), *The transformation of American politics* (pp. 160–188). Princeton, NJ: Princeton University Press.

Tepe, M., & Vanhuysse, P. (2010). Elderly bias, new social risks and social spending: Change and timing in eight programmes across four worlds of welfare, 1980–2003. *Journal of European Social Policy, 20*, 217–234.

U.S. Bureau of the Census. (2012). *Current Population Survey*. Reported voting and registration, by age, sex, and educational attainment. Retrieved from http://www.census.gov/hhes/www/socdemo/voting/publications/p20/2012/tables.html

Walker, J. (1983). The origins and maintenance of interest groups in America. *American Political Science Review, 77*, 390–406.

Wilensky, H. (1975). *The welfare state and equality*. Berkeley: University of California Press.

Wilensky, H., & Lebeaux, C. (1958). *Industrial society and social welfare*. New York, NY: Free Press.

Williams, V., Skocpol, T., & Coggin, J. (2011). The Tea Party and the remaking of Republican conservatism. *Perspectives on Politics, 9*(1), 2–43.

Wilson, J. Q. (1973). *Political organizations*. New York, NY: Basic Books.

Witte, E. E. (1963). *The development of the Social Security Act*. Madison, WI: University of Wisconsin Press.

CHAPTER 26

Theories of Help-Seeking Behavio. Understanding Community Service Use by Older Adults

Robbyn R. Wacker and N   A. Roberto

The act of seeking help involves a complex, multifaceted, and iterative interplay of psychological and sociological factors (Cornally & McCarthy, 2011; Pescosolido, 1992). The initiation of help-seeking behavior begins with an awareness and self-acknowledgment that a specific need exists that presents a challenge to personal abilities and cannot be solved alone (see Figure 26.1). With awareness and self-acknowledgment comes contemplation about the assignment of either internal or external reasons why the unmet need exists and consideration of any perceived psychological costs of publicly seeking help. If the contemplation process leads to an openness to seeking help, the next task is to explore the existence and viability of available informal support, and possibly, formal services that can resolve the unmet need. If formal services are available and deemed appropriate to resolving the unmet need, resources that enable access must exist to connect the individual to the service. The culmination of the contemplation and exploration steps leads to the act of service use.

With the rapid growth of the older population, both in the United States and across the globe, understanding how older adults traverse this path from awareness of need to service use is paramount for researchers, practitioners, and policy makers alike. Older adults' unmet need for assistance with activities of daily living (ADL) has been linked to negative physical outcomes such as hunger, weight loss, dehydration, falls and burns (LaPlante, Kaye, Kang, & Harrington, 2004), high rates of hospital or nursing home admission (Gaugler, Kane, Kane, & Newcomer, 2005; Sands et al., 2006), high mortality rates (Blazer, Sachs-Ericsson, & Hybels, 2005; Gaugler et al., 2005), and caregiver stress and burden (Stirling et al., 2010; Yates, Tennstedt, & Change, 1999).

An additional catalyst for considering the utilization of formal services in late life is the strong preference of older adults for aging in place (Keenan, 2010). Older adults' desire to maintain their independence within their homes and communities for as long as is reasonably possible often means that older adults turn to family, friends, and other people or resources in their communities, either readily or reluctantly, for information and periodic help with minor personal or household tasks. If their need for assistance escalates or they experience changes in their physical, cognitive, or emotional status that require more frequent or greater levels of care with instrumental activities of daily living (IADL; e.g., managing finances, preparing meals, and managing medications) and personal care (ADL; e.g., feeding, bathing, and dressing), most older adults rely on family

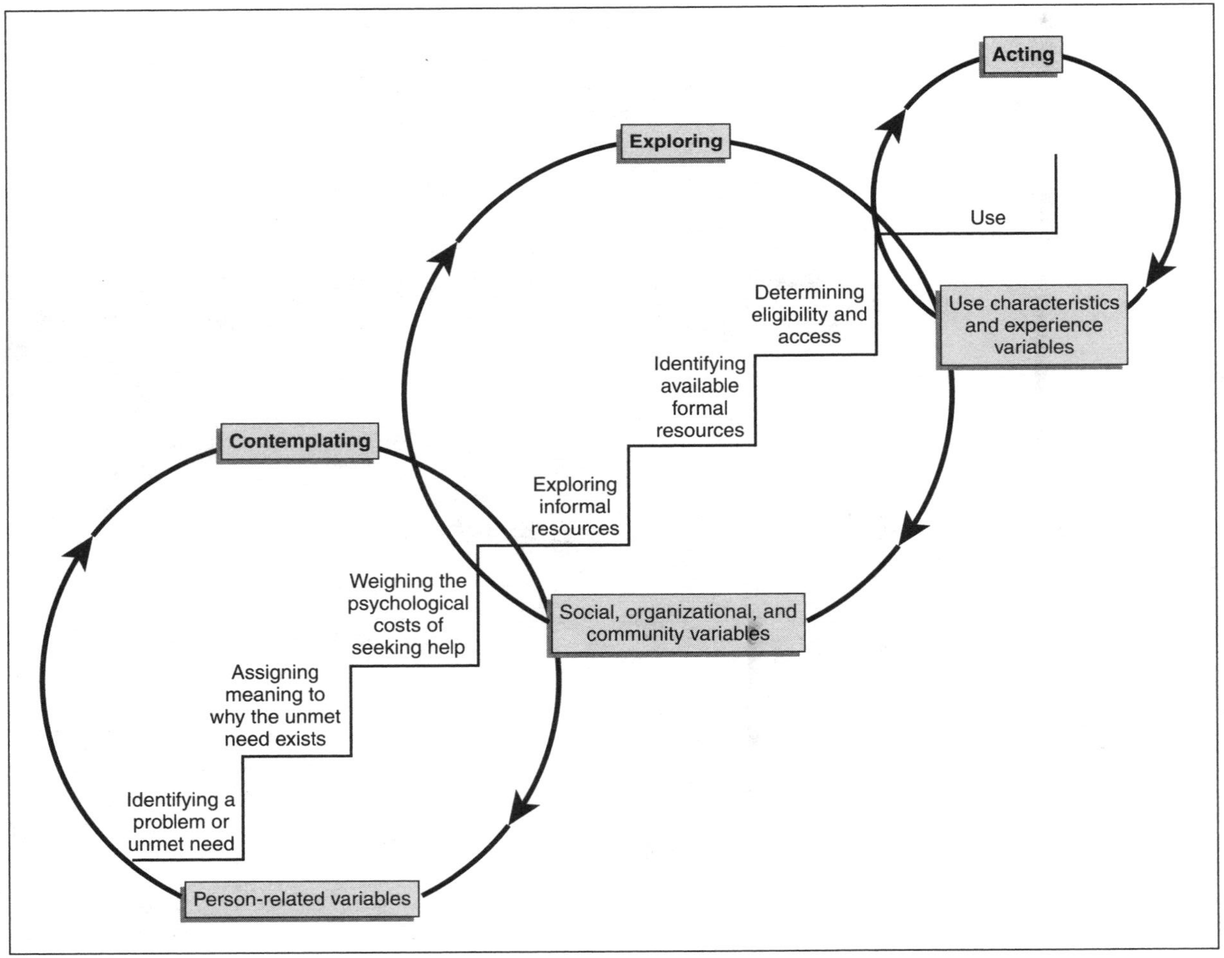

FIGURE 26.1 The process of help-seeking behavior.

members to provide the help and care needed to allow them to remain in their homes (Spillman, Wolff, Freedman, & Kasper, 2014).

In nearly all communities across the United States, there also exists a portfolio of federal, state, and local programs and services that stand ready to offer help and support to older adults and their family care providers. These formal programs and services are designed to support and assist older adults in a variety of ways. They benefit older adults with low levels of dependency (e.g., information, referral, and assistance; senior centers) to older adults who need assistance in maintaining and enhancing their current level of functioning (e.g., meal programs, transportation, and mental health services) to individuals with high dependency needs (e.g., care management and home care services; Roberto, Weaver, & Wacker, 2014). However, availability of a wide variety of programs and services does not automatically result in their use by older adults. Both empirical and anecdotal evidence reveals a "need–use paradox"—that is, in spite of an apparent unmet need, service utilization by older adults often does not occur (Casado, van Vulpen, & Davis, 2011; Cohen-Mansfield & Frank, 2008; Krout, 1983; Mitchell, 1995; Spense, 1992; Sun, 2011). The need–use gap has been documented in use of mental health services (Lee & Dugan, 2015), home and community-based services (HCBS) among non-Whites (Clark & Gibson, 1997; Li, 2004; Schure, Conte, & Goins, 2014), among caregivers of older adults (Brown, Friedemann, & Mauro, 2014), and in the use of adult day care, respite care, personal care, meals, and transportation services (Casado et al., 2011; Li, Chadiha, & Morrow-Howell, 2005).

In 2011, the Government Accounting Office undertook a nationwide study using data from the Current Population Survey, the Health Retirement Study, and a random sample of 125 local Area Agencies on Aging to determine what is known about the need for HCBS and the potential unmet need for these services (U.S. General Accounting Office, 2011). The results indicated that many older adults who were in need of congregate and home-delivered meals did not receive meal services. For example, it was estimated that 90% of the 19% of low-income older adults who were classified as being food insecure did not receive any meal services and 83% of the 17% of older adults with low incomes and at least two difficulties with ADL did not receive meal services. Results also indicated that 66% of older adults from all income levels who reported problems with one or more ADL did not receive home-based help or services from any source. Of the 34% of older adults who did receive some help, only 4% received some help from professionals or organizations. Although research over the past 20 years has confirmed that community services often have low utilization rates among older adults who have unmet needs, it has failed to provide a consistent explanation for why older adults in need do not readily engage community services.

To effectively meet the needs of older adults who can benefit from using community services requires strong, theoretically grounded knowledge of the social and psychological dynamics of help-seeking behavior of older adults and their family care providers as they consider reaching out to the formal service network. This chapter focuses on the prominent psychosocial theories and models used to predict service utilization. We begin with a discussion of Andersen's Behavioral Model of Health Services (Andersen, 1968, 1995), the most commonly used framework for predicting formal service use among older adults. We then turn our attention to other help-seeking behavior models that were not necessarily developed for or frequently used with older populations, but have the potential for enhancing the study of service use in late life. Within the presentation of each of the models, we provide the most up-to-date research available on service utilization. Although some of the research was conducted decades ago, the findings remain relevant and continue to influence current thinking about service use in late life today. We conclude with recommendations for strategic directions for further development of service utilization theory.

■ THE BEHAVIORAL MODEL OF HEALTH SERVICES USE

The Behavioral Model of Health Services (Andersen, 1995; Andersen & Newman, 1973) is based on Andersen's (1968) original model of medical service use, which proposed that the use of services was a function of an individual's predisposing characteristics, enabling resources, and perceived or evaluated need. Although Andersen and his colleagues revised the model over a two-decade period by adding measures of health services use, consumer satisfaction, characteristics of the external environment, personal health practices, and health status outcomes (Andersen, 1995), the most frequently used version of the Behavioral Model reflects the tenets of the original model (see Figure 26.2). Based on our review, it is the most widely used framework in gerontological research to study formal help and service use in late life.

According to Andersen (1995), *predisposing* characteristics include four subcomponents: (a) demographic factors such as age, sex, marital status, race, and ethnicity; (b) social structure factors thought to determine status in the community, including education and occupation; (c) ability to cope with the problem at hand and the resources available to deal with the problem; and (d) personal belief or attitude factors about the use of formal support services. *Enabling* characteristics that facilitate the use of services include personal and community characteristics. Personal characteristics include such variables as income level, insurance coverage, access to transportation, and awareness of service. Community-level enabling characteristics include the availability of the service, cost of services, eligibility, and the distance to the service. Finally, *need* includes both an individual's perceived need for assistance and evaluated need provided by a professional.

Andersen's model has been used to explore the use of a wide variety of community services (e.g., home care, mental health services, nutrition services, respite care, and transportation services) as well as the degree of unmet need and willingness to use community services. A review of the gerontology literature reveals some consistency across studies with regard to characteristics related to service use. For example, predisposing characteristics of being older, female, unmarried, more highly educated, and having a positive attitude toward service use (Blieszner, Roberto, & Singh, 2001; Krout, 1983; Sun, 2011) have been positively correlated with service use, as have enabling

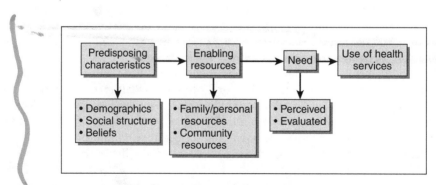

FIGURE 26.2 Behavioral model of health services use.

characteristics of income, access to transportation, a lack of an informal network, and awareness (Krout, 1983; Lai & Chau, 2007; Peterson, 1989; Sun, 2011). However, these univariate relationships often do not hold up in multivariate analyses of predisposing, enabling, and need predictors of service use where perceived need has consistently been found to be the strongest predictor for both discretionary and nondiscretionary service use (Chappell & Blandford, 1987; Krout, 1984; McAuley, Spector, & Van Nostrand, 2009; Mitchell & Krout, 1998; Shen, Feld, Dunkle, Schroepfer, & Lehning, 2015; Wolinsky et al., 1983).

After decades of use, the Behavior Model has not been able to provide theoretical clarity about what other factors trigger service use beyond perceived need. The lack of a definitive conclusion about which characteristics and defining variables best explain service use has resulted partly from the variation in dependent variables. In addition to the use of health services in late life (Kiyak, 1987; Nemet & Bailey, 2000; Surood & Lai, 2010; Wolinsky, 1994), researchers have attempted to identify predictors of specific community services (e.g., Nelms, Johnson, Teshuva, Foreman, & Stanley, 2009) as well as community services used more broadly. For example, Chen and Berkowitz (2012) categorized services as discretionary or nondiscretionary, whereas others used a summative measure of community service utilization that combined a number of different community-based services into a single use variable (e.g., Blieszner et al., 2001; Kuo & Torres-Gil, 2001; Sun, 2011). The different ways in which service use has been operationalized make it difficult to achieve consistency or clarity about which aspect of the Behavioral Model predicts use.

There is also wide variation in the operationalization of the model's independent variables or constructs. Researchers have included measures of housing quality, ability to access healthy food, proportion of White residents as a measure of neighborhood segregation (Ferris, Glicksman, & Kleban, 2016), duration of residence in the community (Calsyn & Winter, 2001), social interaction (Nelms et al., 2009), perceived discrimination (Calsyn & Winter, 2001), eligibility for both Medicaid and Medicare or private insurance coverage (Laditka, Laditka, & Drake, 2006), household size (Chen & Berkowitz, 2012), and social support (Nelms et al., 2009; Sun, 2011) as enabling factors. Need has also been operationalized as perceived overall health (Ferris et al., 2016; Moon, Lubben, & Villa, 1998), ADL and IADL limitations (Chen & Berkowitz, 2012; Laditka et al., 2006), perceived loneliness, and poor mental health days (Calsyn & Winter, 2001).

To improve on the Behavior Model's ability to predict community service utilization, the addition of new elements has been considered. For example, Blieszner et al. (2001) proposed that psychosocial barriers or costs, including the value placed on independence and self-reliance and attitudes toward formal service use, would mediate the effects of predisposing and enabling factors on service use by rural older adults. They found that the intrapersonal variables such as perceptions of personal autonomy and self-esteem did not contribute to the explanation of service use, but rather that formal care use was directly related to an attitudinal preference toward using community services. Demaerschalk et al. (Demaerschalk, Vanden Boer, Bronselaer, Molenberghs, & Declercq, 2013) also added a focus on place (i.e., municipality characteristics) as a contextual influence on individual predisposing, enabling, and need characteristics ability to predict services use. Informal and formal home care use were related to two predisposing variables, the mean income per inhabitant and number of inhabitants/100 km, and one enabling variable, the number of people aged 80 years and older in relation to the number of residents aged 50 to 59 years respectively, but none of the selected predisposing, enabling, or need municipal characteristics were related to health service use.

Finally, a review of studies using the Behavior Model to examine service use between minority group members (e.g., older adults of color and lesbian, gay, bisexual, and transgender [LGBT] older adults) and dominant group members (e.g., non-Hispanic Whites) has found a general pattern of lower community and health service use among subordinate group members (Gardner, de Vries, & Mockus, 2014; Heck, Sell, & Gorin, 2006; Kirby & Lau, 2010; Moon et al., 1998; Tjepkema, 2008; White-Means, 2000). In order to better understand variables related to service use among older adults of different race and ethnic groups as well as LGBT older adults, the Behavior Model must be expanded to include variables that capture the process of contemplating and exploring service use from the perspective of older adults who are members of less predominant groups. Key determinants of service utilization among older adults of minority groups may be linked to past and current experiences of discrimination, lack of perceived culturally sensitive services or staff, and prior negative experiences with services (King, 2009; Kuo & Torres-Gil, 2001; Moon et al., 1998; National Resource Center on LGBT Aging, 2010; Scharlach et al., 2006; White-Means & Rubin, 2004).

■ THEORY OF PLANNED BEHAVIOR

The Theory of Planned Behavior (see Figure 26.3; Madden, Ellen, & Ajzen, 1992), which emerged from the Theory of Reasoned Action, purports that behavior is directly related to the intention to perform a behavior. Intention is the function of three independent determinants: attitude toward the behavior, subjective norms about performing that behavior, and perceived behavioral control (Ajzen, 1985; Madden et al., 1992). *Attitude* (either positive or negative) toward a behavior is based on beliefs about the expected outcomes of performing a behavior and the evaluation of the value of the outcomes. *Subjective norms* include perceived normative beliefs (whether referent others believe one should perform the behavior) and motivation to comply (the importance one places

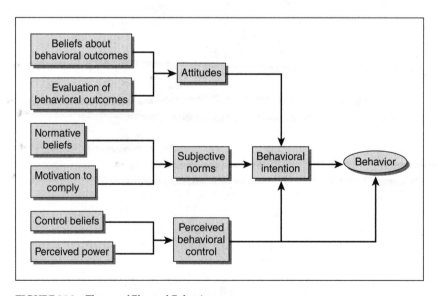

FIGURE 26.3 Theory of Planned Behavior.

Adapted from Montaño and Kasprzyk (2008).

on the reaction of significant others if the behavior is performed). *Perceived behavioral control* is the extent to which the person believes the behavior is under volitional control and the required resources and opportunities for performing a given behavior exist. Perceived behavioral control has both an indirect effect on behavior through intention and a direct effect on behavior, and demographic variables such as age and gender are viewed as external variables and indirectly influence attitudes, subjective norms, and perceived behavioral control (Madden et al., 1992). The Theory of Planned Behavior posits that, when a person has a more favorable attitude toward a behavior, perceives social pressure exists to perform the behavior, and has volitional control over the behavior, there is a likelihood that the intention to perform the behavior will be stronger and the behavior will occur (Madden et al., 1992). Researchers have found significant correlations between intention and attitudes, intention and subjective norms, and intention and perceived behavioral control (Armitage & Conner, 2001; McEachan, Conner, Taylor, & Lawton, 2011).

Over the past 30 years, the Theory of Planned Behavior has been widely used to predict both behaviors and intentions associated with behavior change. Studies guided by this theory typically have included young and middle-aged adult samples and have been successful in explaining 40% to 49% of the variance in intention and 19% to 36% of the variance in behaviors (Ajzen, 1991; McEachan et al., 2011; Schulze & Whittmann, 2003; Trafimow, Sheeran, Conner, & Finlay, 2002). Specific investigations have focused on individual health behaviors such as diet (Armitage, 2004; Conner, Norman, & Bell, 2002), exercise (Bozionelos & Bennett, 1999), safe sex practices (Albarracín, Kumkale, & Johnson, 2004), and smoking cessation (Godin, Valois, Lepage & Desharnais, 1992; Hanson, 2006), as well as service utilization including preventive health screenings (DeVellis, Blalock, & Sandler, 1990; Drossaert, Boer & Seydel, 2003; Michie, Dormandy, French, & Marteau, 2004), transportation (Heath & Gifford, 2002), and psychological services (Smith, Tran, & Thompson, 2008).

Although markedly fewer in number, the Theory of Planned Behavior also provided the framework for studies of older adults' health behaviors such as exercise (Courneya, Nigg, & Estabrooks, 1998) and physical activity (Gretebeck et al., 2007) as well as their use of preventative health services (Gallagher & Povey, 2006) and mental health services (Westerhof, Maessen, de Bruijn & Smets, 2008). Gallagher and Povey (2006) found that Irish older adults' attitudes and subjective norms and two additional variables of anticipated regret and past behavior predicted intention to obtain the influenza vaccine. Westerhof et al. (2008) found in their study of Dutch older adults that the intention to use preventive and professional mental health services was related to two components of attitude: a propensity to seek help, and an openness toward seeking help.

The Theory of Planned Behavior is a model that has been used to identify predictors of behavior change across a wide variety of behaviors and has been successfully used to guide behavior change interventions, particularly related to exercise and diet (McEachan et al., 2011). Its use, however, has been primarily limited to health-related intentions and behaviors and limited to samples of young and middle-aged adults. Given the theory's wide adoption and relative success in predicting intention and behaviors, testing its utility with older adults could help illuminate reasons related to a lack of community service use.

■ REACTANCE THEORY

Reactance Theory states that individuals value personal freedoms—that is, behaviors believed to be under their control and free to be engaged in at any moment or in the future (Brehm, 1966; Brehm & Brehm, 1981). When one's perceived or actual freedom is threatened, reduced, or eliminated, a negative psychological state (reactance) occurs and individuals respond attitudinally or behaviorally in an attempt to reestablish their freedom. The degree of reactance experienced depends on the significance of the freedom, the number of freedoms already believed to be or anticipated to be lost or threatened, implications for future freedom of choice, and the strength of the threat (Brehm, 1966; Brehm & Brehm, 1981; Kirmayer, 1990). Reactance can emerge when one feels threatened in interactions with known individuals, in interactions with institutions and their employees, and when witnessing another person's freedom being threatened or eliminated (Chadee, 2011; Miron & Brehm, 2006; Morrissette, 1998). Whether reactance is a situation-specific response and differs by context or is an individual trait is still under debate (Miron & Brehm, 2006; Woller, Buboltz, & Loveland, 2007). Finally, reactance can occur when individuals observe that they are perceived by others as having a particular trait that is associated with a stereotyped pattern of expected behavior and is linked to members belonging to a particular social category (Miron & Brehm, 2006). In these instances, individuals seek to distance themselves from the imposed social category and reassert their threatened identity.

An extensive literature review uncovered only two studies drawing upon Reactance Theory that included older adults. Woller et al. (2007) examined the relationship between age, ethnic background, gender, and psychological reactance among persons aged 18 to 62 years. They found a curvilinear relationship between reactance and age, with higher reactance scores among the youngest (aged 18–24 years) and oldest groups (aged 55+ years). The authors suggested that higher reactance among older adults may be because of a decrease in perceived control of life outcomes with age. Miron and Brehm (2006) used the Reactance Theory concept of autonomy to examine how rural older adults balanced the need to maintain autonomy and receive assistance. Although the older adults perceived control over their lives to be slipping away, they developed strategies to maintain power and autonomy. Some older adults viewed the act of giving control to others as a way to maintain power and control, particularly in situations where a choice or freedom was surrendered before it was taken away by others. Findings suggest that when older adults voluntarily give up or lose a freedom, reactance may be experienced initially, but soon dissipates because the loss is perceived to be under their control and no longer elicits a reactance response.

Although Reactance Theory has not been used to explain utilization of community service use among older adults, its constructs of freedom, autonomy, and choice are valued by older adults (Bell & Menec, 2015; Fine & Glendinning, 2005; Lloyd, Calnan, Cameron, Seymour, & Smith, 2014) and may be associated with seeking help. As one ages, physical, social, and personal losses are associated with an increased need for assistance. Seeking help may be viewed as immediate loss of independence as well as a harbinger of a future with little or no freedom, autonomy, or choice. Therefore, reactance behaviors may emerge to protect autonomy and choice and be expressed through a reluctance to engage in formal service use.

■ THEORY OF EXTERNAL ATTRIBUTION

The Theory of External Attribution states that individuals seek to explain why certain events occur based on either internal (personal) or external (situational or environmental) characteristics (Kelley, 1967). This assessment also includes considerations about the *distinctiveness* of the behavior (is the behavior unique?), *consensus* (are others responding similarly?), and *consistency* (how often does the behavior occur?) (Fiske & Taylor, 1991). An internal attribution of behavior occurs when the cause is perceived to have low distinctiveness (it is not unique and distinct to the situation), low consensus (nobody else responds similarly), and high consistency (the individual always behaves this way in this situation). An external attribution of behavior occurs when the cause is perceived to have high distinctiveness (it is unique and distinct to the situation), high consensus (everyone else responds similarly), and high consistency (the individual always behaves this way in this situation). If an individual who is pondering the question "Why do I need help?" concludes that it is because of an internal attribution, help-seeking will be less likely to occur as he or she will be hesitant to admit to and to expose his or her inadequacies (see Figure 26.4; Fisher, Nadler, & Whitcher-Alagna, 1982). Conversely, if the conclusion leads to an external attribution and is not attributed to an internal disposition, help-seeking behavior is more likely to occur.

Attribution Theory has been used in studies that examined older adults' causal beliefs related to fall prevention (Feuering, Vered, Kushnir, Jette, & Melzer, 2014), exercise (Sarkisian, Prohaska, Davis, & Weiner, 2007), management of urinary incontinence (Locher, Burgio, Goode, Roth, & Rodriguez, 2002), and social participation and loneliness (Newall et al., 2009). Although Attribution Theory has not been used to examine community service use, this theoretical framework has the potential to further understanding of community service use. For example, based on the constructs of the theory, as older adults become aware of an unmet need, the decision to use formal services may be influenced by their attributions about why they need assistance. If older adults reflect on their need for assistance and view it as something with which others have difficulties (high consensus), unique with regard to the particular circumstance (high distinctiveness), and unusual (low consistency), then chances are that they will be less hesitant about seeking assistance from a formal source (Gerber, 1969; Tessler & Schwartz, 1972). The difficulty with this theory, as with the others, is how to ensure that key elements of the theory are operationalized consistently across studies and with different types of service use.

■ THE THREATS TO SELF-ESTEEM MODEL

The Threats to Self-Esteem Model (Fisher et al., 1982) is based on the premise that most help-seeking situations contain a mixture of both positive (supportive) and negative (self-threatening) elements (see Figure 26.5). Receiving help can be interpreted as either a positive or negative experience related to the salient nature of the quality of help provided (Nadler, 2012). For example, the individual may experience feelings of gratitude and support as a result of receiving needed help or have negative perceptions of himself or herself, the helper, and the act of receiving helping (Nadler, 2012). Whether the helping situation is perceived as supportive or self-threatening depends on (a) the characteristics of the helper, (b) characteristics of the help, and (c) characteristics of the recipient.

If helper characteristics are similar to the recipient characteristics and the help provided is viewed as an expression of helper superiority, the aid will be viewed as self-threatening (Nadler, Sheinberg, & Jaffe, 1981). When the characteristics of help are such that they highlight inferiority or inadequacy, thus making the recipient's dependency explicit (e.g., conspicuous, dependency oriented, or the recipient is identifiable), help will be viewed as self-threatening. Recipient characteristics are also thought to influence how the help-giving episode is perceived. Misalignment of personality

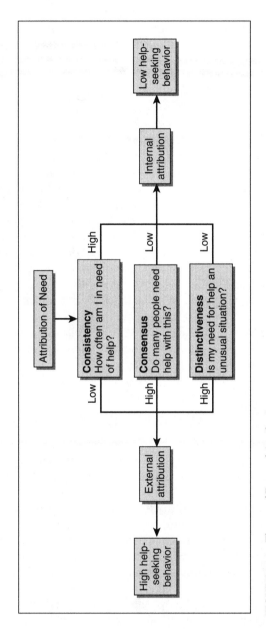

FIGURE 26.4 Theory of External Attribution.

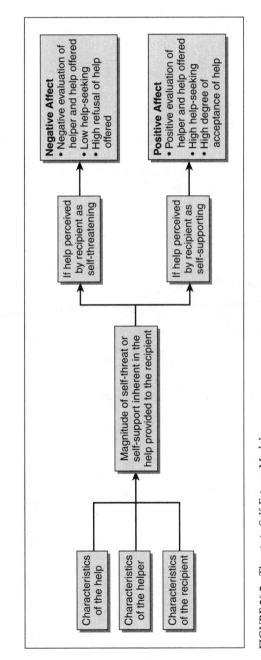

FIGURE 26.5 Threats to Self-Esteem Model.

Adapted from Fisher et al. (1983).

dispositions or self-image with the need for help are thought to be related to characterizing the help as self-threatening. For example, seeking or receiving help may be viewed as self-threatening for individuals whose dependency is inconsistent with self-image, who have a high need for achievement, and who have high levels of self-esteem and the help episode is ego-relevant (Bornstein, 1992; Nadler, 1986, 1991, 1998). In addition, individuals with high self-esteem may be more defensive when help is offered and reluctant to seek help because it denotes dependence, rather than independence and competency, and is seen as self-threatening and the result may be preference for hardship rather than risk self-threatening dependency (Nadler, 2012).

The Threats to Self-Esteem Model, although underused in research involving older adults, suggests that feelings and beliefs about oneself may come under threat when the need for help arises in late life. Findings regarding the relationship between self-esteem and receiving help are mixed. Adults with high self-esteem were more reluctant to accept help than those with low self-esteem (Nadler & Mayseless, 1983) and adults who were ego-involved in the task and who valued autonomy were more threatened by receiving assistance (DePaulo & Fisher, 1980; Nadler et al., 1981). In contrast, older adult care recipients with lower self-esteem were more likely to respond negatively to receiving care received (Newsom & Schulz, 1998) and reported lower satisfaction with support (Hobfoll, Nadler, & Leiberman, 1986; Lakey, Tardiff, & Drew, 1994) than older persons with high self-esteem.

■ THE SOCIAL ECOLOGICAL MODEL

The Social Ecological Model (SEM) has its historical roots from a variety of disciplines including the fields of social ecology (Alihan, 1964), psychology (Binder, 1972), human development (Bronfenbrenner, 1979), sociology (Pescosolido, 1992), and public health (Stokols, 1996). The SEM highlights individuals' behaviors over the life course within the context of multiple interlocking settings within their social environment (Chard & Stuart, 2012). Behaviors are influenced by intrapersonal factors as well as the interactions among and between interpersonal characteristics in the formal and informal social networks, institutional and organizational program characteristics, community level characteristics, and structural characteristics (see Figure 26.6).

A number of scholars have touted the SEM as an important advancement in understanding individual behaviors because it shifts the focus from an individual or intrapersonal analysis to one that stresses the importance of the influence of the broader community, it is interdisciplinary in nature, and it allows for multilevel analyses (Stokols, 1996). The SEM is emerging as a theoretical framework useful in investigating older adults' participation in health promotion programs (Richard, Gauvin, Ducharme, Leblanc, & Trudel, 2012), physical activity and exercise (Carlson et al., 2012; Chard & Stuart, 2012; Satariano & McAuley, 2003) and healthy aging practices (Waites, 2012). The results of these studies, particularly those investigating health promotion, are promising for the study of help-seeking behaviors and formal service utilization as results indicate that there are synergistic interactions between the environment and psychosocial factors that can positively influence behaviors (Brownson, Baker, Housemann, Brennan, & Bacak 2001; King, Stokols, Talen, Brassington, & Killingsworth, 2002). This area of research is in its infancy and further work is needed that addresses measurement of factors across all domains (Cunningham & Michael, 2004).

Elements from Continuity Theory (Atchley, 1989) may provide insights for further operationalizing intrapersonal variables within the SEM. Continuity Theory posits that,

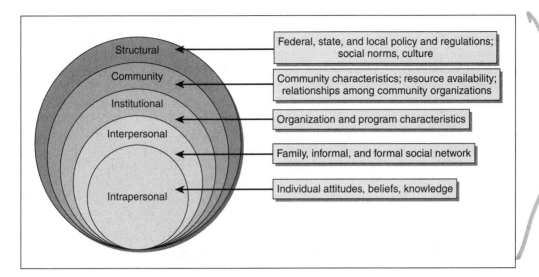

FIGURE 26.6 Social Ecological Model.

in making adaptive choices, older adults attempt to preserve and maintain existing internal and external structures and they prefer to accomplish this objective by using strategies tied to their past experiences of themselves and their social world. Change is linked to the person's perceived past, producing continuity in inner psychological characteristics as well as in social behavior and in social circumstances. The concept of continuity helps explain the need–use paradox as older adults may wish to maintain routines and patterns of daily living, as well as use lifelong patterns of decision-making and problem-solving strategies (Atchley, 1989, p. 183).

■ THEORETICAL INFLUENCES ON THE DESIGN AND IMPLEMENTATION OF SERVICES

The focus on community-based care began at the turn of the 21st century with the design of a broad range of services and supports provided in the home to help older adults with chronic illness and disabilities remain as functionally independent as possible (Stone, 2011). Although initially organizations typically took a one-size-fits-all approach to service delivery, the current trend is for significant involvement of older adults in managing their needs by selecting and directing services as they deem necessary (Coffey, 2008). Although not explicitly theory driven, this shift in service provision from traditional agency-based services to consumer-directed care was supported by service use research pointing to older individuals' desire to maintain a sense of agency and choice in late life (Wacker & Roberto, 2014).

Theories and models of help-seeking behavior and service use have tremendous potential in informing how programs can more effectively and intentionally address unmet need. However, in our review of help-seeking behavior literature, we were unable to identify any research that analyzed service use that was based on a theoretical framework to increase formal service use among older adults. There is, however, precedent for utilizing theory as a framework to inform and develop public health campaigns and programs designed to change personal behaviors (see Glanz & Bishop, 2010). For example, the Theory of Planned Behavior has been used to structure outreach programs designed to change personal behaviors related to physical activity, preventive health checkups, and HIV/STD prevention (Albada, Ausems, Bensing, & van Dulmen, 2009; Kalichman, 2007; Sarkisian et al., 2007). A similar approach whereby the implementation and evaluation of HCBS, programs, or policies based on theoretical understandings about the need–use paradox would be a significant contribution for practitioners as well as researchers. Individually and in concert with one another, the theories reviewed in this chapter provide practitioners with insights about when, how, and why older adults seek help from formal services. Understanding the key explanatory variables in these theories of service use will allow providers to unpack the complex relationship between individual and situational context and in turn, better align outreach and service delivery with these characteristics. Moreover, linking theoretical constructs with use will provide for a more direct evaluation of service use and nonuse.

■ FUTURE DIRECTIONS FOR THEORY DEVELOPMENT

Our review of key theories and models used to examine help-seeking behavior in general, and community service utilization in particular, points to the need for future theory development. First, current theories and models are primarily, and in some cases exclusively, focused on intrapersonal characteristics (see Figure 26.7). As discussed earlier in this chapter, three of the theories reviewed, Reactance Theory, External Attribution, and Threats to Self-Esteem, all have a singular focus on intrapersonal characteristics posited to be linked with help-seeking behavior. The Theory of Planned Behavior also takes an intrapersonal perspective, but does include a construct of social pressure from members of one's social network that is thought to influence behavior. The Behavioral Model also goes beyond the intrapersonal framework by its inclusion of the enabling resources

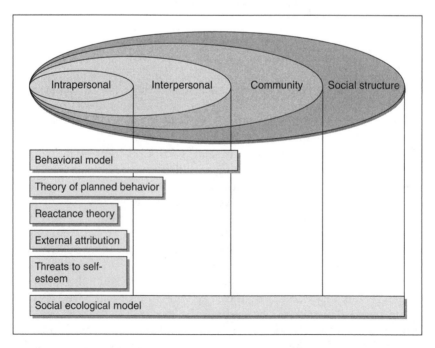

FIGURE 26.7 Scope of theories and models of help-seeking behaviors and service.

construct, which researchers frequently operationalize as social network support variables, and on rare occasion, include other variables such as availability of services and transportation in the community. As a whole, the research informed by these intrapersonal theories has established that help-seeking behaviors are explained, in part, by relevant psychological characteristics. Individuals contemplate and apply attributions as to why an unmet need exists and whether the act of seeking help, formally or informally, poses a threat to self-esteem, self-image, and valued states such as independence, competence, autonomy, and choice.

Although intrapersonal theories make a significant contribution to understanding how individuals reason their way through the help-seeking process and is the "engine of action" (Pescosolido, 1992), their focus on one aspect of the help-seeking process results in an incomplete analytic framework. The inclusion of interpersonal, organizational, community, and social structure characteristics offers the possibility of a more complete framework by providing new insights into HCBS use. The SEM is the only model that includes elements from intra-, interpersonal, community, and social structure domains. Because the SEM has a more comprehensive and systemic perspective, it has great potential of addressing the gaps in our understanding of community service use; however, as the theory is in its early stages of development, it requires further empirical evidence to establish its utility in predicting service use.

A second limitation we identified is that many of the intrapersonal theories discussed in this chapter are focused on help-seeking behavior between an individual and another person in his or her informal network (e.g., a friend, peer, or supervisor) rather than an individual seeking assistance from formal resources. In addition, the research framed by these theories has paid relatively little attention to older adults in need of assistance. This is unfortunate as many of the intrapersonal factors explored in these theories have great promise and relevance in examining the help-seeking process of older adults.

We contend that systemically identifying and testing factors that influence help-seeking behaviors is the next great challenge to theory development and research focused on community service use of older adults. Knowing that the decision to seek services is influenced by intrapersonal, interpersonal, community, and social structure characteristics, future models must reflect this complexity in order to advance knowledge and understanding of service utilization in late life.

Intrapersonal Characteristics

Researchers must expand on the intrapersonal characteristics relevant to how older adults navigate the challenges that occur in later life and intersections of aging and ageism. This would include exploring the following:

- Age-group discussions in order to investigate if a reluctance to engage in help-seeking behaviors is associated with avoidance of negative attributes currently assigned to old age (Weiss & Freund, 2012; Weiss & Lang, 2012).
- Intersections of gender, race, ethnicity, socioeconomics, and sexual orientation on service use. Because older people are often stigmatized, the intersection of ageism with multiple forms of oppression often leave the most vulnerable or at-risk older adults wary of health and service systems. Further research is required to identify and assess perceived and actual biases within the service sector and the necessary systemic changes needed to the service delivery system (Meyer, 2011; Musa, Schulz, Harris, Silverman, & Thomas, 2009).

- Perceptions and beliefs of seeking help as a forced reliance on others, becoming a burden to others, and a loss of autonomy, or as a means of maintaining independence (Cohen, 2013). We need to better understand how older adults weigh potential benefits of obtaining help with potential compromises to self-image, independence, and control in the current circumstance as well as in the future.
- Goal(s) older adults hold relative to desired level of health and activity and service use.
- Tipping points with respect to various types and levels of unmet need that precipitates older adults' help-seeking behaviors and use of formal community services.

Interpersonal Characteristics

Interpersonal characteristics need to be explored further by researchers to understand how help-seeking behavior is influenced by the interactions that are a part of the "stream of social life" (Pescosolido, 1992). This would include research that would further our understanding about:

- The role of strong and weak ties within the formal network (Fingerman, 2009)
- How peers, partners, and family actors in the social network engage, disengage, and reengage during help-seeking episodes that serve to facilitate or impede help-seeking behavior for community services (Carpentier & Bernard, 2011)

Organizational and Community Characteristics

The implications of organizational and community characteristics are probably the least understood of all of the variables associated with service use and help-seeking behavior. Organizational characteristics to be explored further by researchers include:

- Factors related to service use, such as visibility and outreach efforts to increase awareness of available services
- Convenience related to geographic location, hours of operation, degree of flexibility, and accommodation of individual differences in need
- Eligibility and cost
- Interactions with staff and demonstrated cultural competencies in how services are offered and delivered (Moon et al., 1998)

Community characteristics to be explored include:

- Number of community-based services
- Availability of public transportation
- Neighborhood characteristics
- Demographics, including race, ethnicity, and age
- Community economic characteristics (e.g., percent of persons living below poverty level, unemployment rate, and per capita income)
- Number of age-friendly characteristics

■ METHODOLOGICAL NEEDS

The majority of research on service utilization by older adults is cross-sectional and as a result does not capture the iterative process of help-seeking behaviors (e.g., moving from contemplation of help-seeking to actively seeking out help or the timing that occurs between contemplation, exploration, and use). To develop new theories of service utilization will require the use of more sophisticated methodologies and statistical approaches to model both intrapersonal and interpersonal influences on help-seeking behavior. Carpentier and Bernard (2011) suggested that the study of the sequence of events would allow for a better understanding of the cumulative effect of decisions and how actors with either strong or weak ties engage and disengage in the act of influencing help-seeking behavior. Similarly, Dearing and Twaragowski (2010) suggest that help-seeking behavior is an outcome of the interplay between the person and environmental context; help-seeking is not limited to the moment or one act, but a help-seeking episode influences future actions as well. At the same time, rigorous qualitative investigations are needed to provide insight about the dynamics surrounding formal service use, including the influence of age, gender, race, and cultural variations in self-perceptions, relationship expectations, and help-seeking behaviors.

Researchers also must expand their efforts to understand how different types and levels of unmet needs present a unique set of characteristics that in turn influence intrapersonal and interpersonal considerations for seeking formal assistance. For example, it may be possible that the decision to attend a congregate lunch program is perceived and processed differently if the alternative is to depend on someone to shop and prepare meals. One approach to disentangling the multiple influences on help-seeking behavior and service utilization is to focus on one type of service to investigate and align the intrapersonal and interpersonal variables most likely to influence service use. Once key variables have been established and findings replicated across studies, the model can be advanced to study different service types.

■ CONCLUSION

In closing, there is a tremendous opportunity for gerontological researchers to address the paucity of theories and models needed to explain community service use by older adults. Moreover, advances in the use of Big Data and statistical modeling can now accommodate greater methodological complexities and account for multiple levels of interaction that is more interdisciplinary, complex, and comprehensive in scope. Unfortunately, service utilization research frequently goes unpublished in scientific journals, appearing more often in evaluation reports about localized programs or government initiatives, which have limited circulation. The more explicit use of theory will strengthen research on service use in late life and deepen the interpretation of results (Roberto, Blieszner, & Allen, 2006). In addition, greater availability of theorized research about services utilization is necessary to inform practitioners in their quest to link older adults in need of help with available services and to support older adults in maintaining some degree of independence as they age. Developing new theories and further elaborating and testing existing models are essential for unraveling the use–need paradox and helping reduce the barriers to programs and services that, when accessed, can contribute to increased well-being of older adults.

REFERENCES

Ajzen, I. (1985). From intentions to actions: A theory of planned behavior. In J. Kuhl & J. Beckmann (Eds.), *Action control: From cognition to behavior* (pp. 11–39). Heidelberg, Berlin: Springer-Verlag.

Ajzen, I. (1991). The theory of planned behavior. *Organizational Behavior and Human Decision Processes, 50,* 179–211.

Albada, A., Ausems, M. G., Bensing, J. M., & van Dulmen, S. 2009. Tailored information about cancer risk and screening: A systematic review. *Patient Education and Counseling, 75,* 155–71.

Albarracín, D., Kumkale, G. T., & Johnson, B. T. (2004). Influences of social power and normative support on condom use decisions: A research synthesis. *AIDS Care, 16*(6), 700–723.

Alihan, M. A. (1964). *Social ecology: A critical analysis.* New York, NY: Cooper Square Publishers.

Andersen, R. (1968). *Behavioral model of families' use of health services* (Research Series No. 25). Chicago, IL: Center for Health Administration Studies, University of Chicago.

Andersen, R. M. (1995). Revisiting the behavioral model and access to medical care: Does it matter? *Journal of Health and Social Behavior, 36*(1), 1–10.

Andersen, R., & Newman, J. (1973). Societal and individual determinants of medical care utilization in the United States. *Milbank Memorial Fund Quarterly, 51,* 95–124.

Armitage, C. J. (2004). Evidence that implementation intentions reduce dietary fat intake: A randomized trial. *Health Psychology, 23,* 319–323.

Armitage, C. J., & Conner, M. (2001). Efficacy of the theory of planned behaviour: A meta-analytic review. *British Journal of Social Psychology, 40*(4), 471–499.

Atchley, R. C. (1989). A continuity theory of normal aging. *The Gerontologist, 29*(2), 183–190.

Bell, S., & Menec, V. (2015). "You don't want to ask for the help." The imperative of independence: Is it related to social exclusion? *Journal of Applied Gerontology, 34*(3), 1–21.

Binder, A. (1972). A new context for psychology: Social ecology. *The American Psychologist, 27,* 903–908.

Blazer, D. G., Sachs-Ericsson, N., & Hybels, C. F. (2005). Perception of unmet basic needs as a predictor of mortality among community-dwelling older adults. *American Journal of Public Health, 95*(2), 299–304.

Blieszner, R., Roberto, K. A., & Singh, K. (2001). The helping networks of rural elders: Demographic and social psychological influences on service use. *Ageing International, 27,* 89–119.

Bornstein, R. F. (1992). The dependent personality: Developmental, social, and clinical perspectives. *Psychological Bulletin, 112,* 3–23.

Bozionelos, G., & Bennett, P. (1999). The theory of planned behaviour as predictor of exercise: The moderating influence of beliefs and personality variables. *Journal of Health Psychology, 4*(4), 517–529.

Brehm, J. W. (1966). *A theory of psychological reactance.* New York, NY: Academic Press.

Brehm, S. S., & Brehm, J. W. (1981). *Psychological reactance: A theory of freedom and control.* New York, NY: Academic Press.

Bronfenbrenner, U. (1979). *The ecology of human development: Experiments by nature and design*. Cambridge, MA: Harvard University Press.

Brown, E. L., Friedemann, M., & Mauro, A. (2014). Use of adult day care service centers in an ethnically diverse sample of older adults. *Journal of Applied Gerontology, 33*(2), 189–206.

Brownson, R. C., Baker, E. A., Housemann, R. A., Brennan, L. K., & Bacak, S. J. (2001). Environmental and policy determinants of physical activity in the United States. *American Journal of Public Health, 91*(12), 1995–2003.

Calsyn, R. J., & Winter, J. P. (2001). Predicting four types of service needs in older adults. *Evaluation and Program Planning, 24*(2), 157–166.

Carlson, J. A., Sallis, J. F., Conway, T. L., Saelens, B. E., Frank, L. D., Kerr, J.,… King, A. C. (2012). Interactions between psychosocial and built environment factors in explaining older adults' physical activity. *Preventive Medicine, 54*(1), 68–73.

Carpentier, N. & Bernard, P. (2011). The complexities of help-seeking: Exploring challenges through a social network perspective. In B. A. Pescolido, J. K. Martin, J. D. McLeod, & A. Rogers (Eds.), *Handbook of the sociology of health, illness, and healing: A blueprint for the 21st century* (pp. 465–479). New York, NY: Springer.

Casado, B. L., van Vulpen, K. S., & Davis, S. L. (2011). Unmet needs for home and community-based services among frail older Americans and their caregivers. *Journal of Aging and Health, 23*(3), 529–553.

Chadee, D. (2011). Toward freedom: Reactance theory revisited. In D. Chadee (Ed.), *Theories in social psychology* (1st ed., pp. 13–43). New York, NY: Blackwell.

Chappell, N. L., & Blandford, A. A. (1987). Health service utilization by elderly persons. *Canadian Journal of Sociology, 11*, 195–215.

Chard, S. E., & Stuart, M. (2012). An ecological perspective on the community translation of exercise research for older adults. *Journal of Applied Gerontology, 31*, 28–51.

Chen, Y.-M., & Berkowitz, B. (2012). Older adults' home- and community-based service use and residential transitions: A longitudinal study. *BMC Geriatrics, 12*(44), 1–12.

Clark, D. O., & Gibson, R. C. (1997). Race, age, chronic disease, and disability. In K. Markides & M. Miranda (Eds.), *Minorities, aging, and health* (pp. 107–128). Thousand Oaks, CA: Sage.

Coffey, G. (2008). *The Administration on Aging's Nursing Home Diversion program*. Washington, DC: National Senior Citizen's Law Center. Retrieved from http://www.globalaging.org/elderrights/us/2008/diversion.pdf

Cohen, A. L. (2013). Family assistance and autonomy in the lives of rural elders. *Marriage and Family Review, 49*(6), 491–503.

Cohen-Mansfield, J., & Frank, J. (2008). Relationship between perceived needs and assessed needs for services in community-dwelling older persons. *The Gerontologist, 48*(4), 505–516.

Conner, M., Norman, P., & Bell, R. (2002). The theory of planned behavior and healthy eating. *Health Psychology, 21*(2), 194–201.

Cornally, N., & McCarthy, G. (2011). Help-seeking behaviour: A concept analysis. *International Journal of Nursing Practice, 17*(3), 280–288.

Courneya, K. S., Nigg, C. R., & Estabrooks, P. A. (1998). Relationships among the theory of planned behavior, stages of change, and exercise behavior in older persons over a three year period. *Psychology and Health, 13*(2), 355–367.

Cunningham, G., & Michael, Y. L. (2004). Concepts guiding the study of the impact of the built environment on physical activity for older adults: A review of the literature. *American Journal of Health Promotion, 18*(6), 435–443.

Dearing, R. L., & Twaragowski, C. (2010). The social psychology of help seeking. In J. E. Maddux & J. P. Tangney (Eds.), *Social psychological foundations of clinical psychology* (pp. 395–415). New York, NY: Guilford Press.

Demaerschalk, M. F., Vanden Boer, L. E., Bronselaer, J. L., Molenberghs, G., & Declercq, A. G. (2013). The influence of municipal characteristics on the use of informal home care and home care services by the elderly Flemish. *European Journal of Public Health, 23*(2), 241–246.

DePaulo, B. M., & Fisher, J. D. (1980). The costs of asking for help. *Basic and Applied Social Psychology, 1,* 23–35.

DeVellis, B. M., Blalock, S. J., & Sandler, R. S. (1990). Predicting participation in cancer screening: The role of perceived behavioral control. *Journal of Applied Social Psychology, 20*(8), 639–660.

Drossaert, C. H. C., Boer, H., & Seydel, E. R. (2003). Prospective study on the determinants of repeat attendance and attendance patterns in breast cancer screening using the theory of planned behaviour. *Psychology and Health, 18,* 551–565.

Ferris, R. E., Glicksman, A., & Kleban, M. H. (2016). Environmental predictors of unmet home- and community-based service needs of older adults. *Journal of Applied Gerontology, 35,* 179–208.

Feuering, R., Vered, E., Kushnir, T., Jette, A. M., & Melzer, I. (2014). Differences between self-reported and observed physical functioning in independent older adults. *Disability and Rehabilitation, 36*(17), 1395–1401.

Fine, M., & Glendinning, C. (2005). Dependence, independence or interdependence? Revisiting the concepts of "care" and "dependency." *Ageing and Society, 25*(04), 601–621.

Fingerman, K. L. (2009). Consequential strangers and peripheral ties: The importance of unimportant relationships. *Journal of Family Theory and Review, 1*(2), 69–86.

Fisher, J. D., Nadler, A., & Whitcher-Alagna, S. (1982). Recipient reactions to aid. *Psychological Bulletin, 91*(1), 27–54.

Fisher, J. D., Nadler, A., & Whitcher-Alagna, S. (1983). Four conceptualizations of reactions to aid. In J. D. Fisher, A. Nadler, & B. M. DePaulo (Eds.), *New directions in helping* (Vol. 1, pp. 51–84). New York, NY: Academic Press.

Fiske, S. T., & Taylor, S. E. (1991). *Social cognition* (2nd ed.). New York, NY: McGraw-Hill.

Gallagher, S., & Povey, R. (2006). Determinants of older adults' intentions to vaccinate against influenza: A theoretical application. *Journal of Public Health, 28*(2), 139–144.

Gardner, A. T., de Vries, B., & Mockus, D. S. (2014). Aging out in the desert: Disclosure, acceptance, and service use among midlife and older lesbians and gay men. *Journal of Homosexuality, 61*(1), 129–144.

Gaugler, J. E., Kane, R. L., Kane, R. A., & Newcomer, R. (2005). Unmet care needs and key outcomes in dementia. *Journal of the American Geriatrics Society, 53*(12), 2098–2105.

Gerber, I. (1969). Bereavement and the acceptance of professional service. *Community Mental Health Journal, 5*, 487–495.

Glanz, K., & Bishop, D. B. (2010). The role of behavioral science theory in development and implementation of public health interventions. *Annual Review of Public Health, 31*, 399–418.

Godin, G., Valois, P., Lepage, L., & Desharnais, R. (1992). Predictors of smoking behaviour: An application of Ajzen's theory of planned behaviour. *British Journal of Addiction, 87*(9), 1335–1343.

Gretebeck, K. A., Black, D. R., Blue, C. L., Glickman, L. T., Huston, S. A., & Gretebeck, R. J. (2007). Physical activity and function in older adults: Theory of planned behavior. *American Journal of Health Behavior, 31*(2), 203–214.

Hanson, M. J. S. (2006). Predicting smoking behavior in college students. *American Journal for Nurse Practitioners, 10*, 26–35.

Heath, Y., & Gifford, R. (2002). Extending the theory of planned behavior: Predicting the use of public transportation. *Journal of Applied Social Psychology, 32*(10), 2154–2189.

Heck, J. E., Sell, R. L., & Gorin, S. S. (2006). Health care access among individuals involved in same-sex relationships. *American Journal of Public Health, 96*(6), 1111–1118.

Hobfoll, S. E., Nadler, A., & Leiberman, J. (1986). Satisfaction with social support during crisis: Intimacy and self-esteem as critical determinants. *Journal of Personality and Social Psychology, 51*(2), 296–304.

Kalichman, S. C. (2007). The theory of reasoned action and advances in HIV/AIDS prevention. In I. Ajzen, D. Albarracín, & R. Hornik (Eds.), *Prediction and change of health behavior: Applying the reasoned action approach* (pp. 265–272). Mahwah, NJ: Lawrence Erlbaum.

Keenan, T. A. (2010). *Home and community preferences of the 45+ population.* Retrieved from http://assets.aarp.org/rgcenter/general/home-community-services-10.pdf

Kelley, H. H. (1967). Attribution theory in social psychology. *Nebraska Symposium on Motivation, 15*, 192–238.

King, A., Stokols, D., Talen, E., Brassington, G., & Killingsworth, R. (2002). Theoretical approaches to the promotion of physical activity. Forging a transdisciplinary paradigm. *American Journal of Preventive Medicine, 23*(Suppl. 2), 15–25.

King, S. D. (2009). *Midlife and older gay men and their use of physical and mental health services: Exploring the effects of health enablers, health need, psychosocial stress and individual health coping* (Doctoral Dissertation). Retrieved from http://etd.ohiolink.edu/view.cgi?acc_num=osu1257437705

Kirby, J. B., & Lau, D. T. (2010). Community and individual race/ethnicity and home health care use among elderly persons in the United States. *Health Services Research, 45*(5), 1251–1267.

Kirmayer, L. J. (1990). Resistance, reactance and reluctance to change: A cognitive attributional approach to strategic interventions. *Journal of Cognitive Psychotherapy, 4*(2), 83–104.

Kiyak, H. A. (1987). An explanatory model of older persons' use of dental services: Implications for health policy. *Medical Care, 25*(10), 936–952.

Krout, J. (1983). Knowledge and use of services by the elderly: A critical review of the literature. *International Journal of Aging and Human Development, 17*, 153–167.

Krout, J. (1984). Knowledge of senior center activities among the elderly. *Journal of Applied Gerontology, 3*, 71–81.

Kuo, T., & Torres-Gil, F. M. (2001). Factors affecting utilization of health services and home- and community-based care programs by older Taiwanese in the United States. *Research on Aging, 23*(1), 14–36.

Laditka, S. B., Laditka, J. N., & Drake, B. F. (2006). Home- and community-based service use by older African American, Hispanic, and Non-Hispanic White women and men. *Home Health Care Services Quarterly, 25*(3–4), 129–153.

Lai, D. W. L., & Chau, S. B. Y. (2007). Predictors of health service barriers for older Chinese immigrants in Canada. *Health and Social Work, 32*(1), 57–65.

Lakey, B., Tardiff, T. A., & Drew, J. B. (1994). Negative social interactions: Assessment and relations to social support, cognition, and psychological distress. *Journal of Social and Clinical Psychology, 13*(1), 42–62.

LaPlante, M. P., Kaye, H. S., Kang, T., & Harrington, C. (2004). Unmet need for personal assistance services: Estimating the shortfall in hours of help and adverse consequences. *The Journals of Gerontology, Series B, 59*(2), 98–108.

Lee, H. J., & Dugan, E. (2015). How large is the gap between self-report and assessed mental health and does it impact older adult mental health service utilization? *Journal of Gerontological Social Work, 58*(1), 3–19.

Li, H. (2004). Barriers to and unmet needs for supportive services: Experiences of Asian-American caregivers. *Journal of Cross-Cultural Gerontology, 19*(3), 241–260.

Li, H., Chadiha, L. A., & Morrow-Howell, N. (2005). Association between unmet needs for community services and caregiving strain. *Families in Society, 86*(1), 55–62.

Lloyd, L., Calnan, M., Cameron, A., Seymour, J., & Smith, R. (2014). Identity in the fourth age: Perseverance, adaptation and maintaining dignity. *Ageing and Society, 34*(01), 1–19.

Locher, J. L., Burgio, K. L., Goode, P. S., Roth, D. L., & Rodriguez, E. (2002). Effects of age and causal attribution to aging on health-related behaviors associated with urinary incontinence in older women. *The Gerontologist, 42*(4), 515–521.

Madden, T. J., Ellen, P. S., & Ajzen, I. (1992). A comparison of the theory of planned behavior and the theory of reasoned action. *Personality and Social Psychology Bulletin, 18*(1), 3–9.

McAuley, W. J., Spector, W., & Van Nostrand, J. (2009). Formal home care utilization patterns by rural–urban community residence. *The Journals of Gerontology, Series B, 64*, 258–268.

McEachan, R. R. C., Conner, M., Taylor, N. J., & Lawton, R. J. (2011). Prospective prediction of health-related behaviours with the theory of planned behaviour: A meta-analysis. *Health Psychology Review, 5*(2), 97–144.

Meyer, H. (2011). Safe spaces? The need for LGBT cultural competency in aging services. *Public Policy and Aging Report, 21*(3), 24–27.

Michie, S., Dormandy, E., French, D. P., & Marteau, T. M. (2004). Using the theory of planned behaviour to predict screening uptake in two contexts. *Psychology and Health, 19*(6), 705–718.

Miron, A. M., & Brehm, J. W. (2006). Reactance theory—40 years later. *Zeitschrift für Sozialpsychologie, 37*(1), 3–12.

Mitchell, J. (1995). Service awareness and use among older North Carolinians. *Journal of Applied Gerontology, 14*(2), 193–209.

Mitchell, J., & Krout, J. A. (1998). Discretion and service use among older adults: The behavioral model revisited. *The Gerontologist, 38*, 159–168.

Montaño, D. E., & Kasprzyk, D. (2008). Theory of reasoned action, theory of planned behavior, and the integrated behavioral model. In K. Glanz, B. L. Rimer, & K. Viswanath (Eds.), *Health behavior and health education: Theory, research, and practice* (4th ed., pp. 67–96). San Francisco, CA: Jossey-Bass.

Moon, A., Lubben, J. E., & Villa, V. (1998). Awareness and utilization of community long-term care services by elderly Korean and non-Hispanic White Americans. *The Gerontologist, 38*, 309–316.

Morrissette, P. J. (1998). Reconceptualizing perceived client resistance: Inroads for counseling and human service interns. *Human Service Education: A Journal of the National Organization for Human Service Education, 18*(1), 15–25.

Musa, D., Schulz, R., Harris, R., Silverman, M., & Thomas, S. B. (2009). Trust in the health care system and the use of preventive health services by older Black and White adults. *American Journal of Public Health, 99*(7), 1293–1299.

Nadler, A. (1986). Self-esteem and the seeking and receiving of help: Theoretical and empirical perspectives. *Progress in Experimental Personality Research, 14*, 115–163.

Nadler, A. (1991). Help-seeking behavior, psychological costs and instrumental benefits. In M. S. Clark (Ed.), *Review of personality and social psychology* (Vol. 12, pp. 290–312). New York, NY: Sage.

Nadler, A. (1998). Relationship, esteem, and achievement perspectives on autonomous and dependent help seeking. In S. A. Karabenick (Ed.), *Strategic help seeking: Implications for learning and teaching* (pp. 61–93). Mahwah, NJ: Erlbaum.

Nadler, A. (2012). From help-giving to helping relations: Belongingness and independence in social interaction. In K. Deaux & M. Snyder (Eds.), *The Oxford handbook of personality and social psychology* (pp. 394–417). New York, NY: Oxford University Press.

Nadler, A., & Mayseless, O. (1983). Recipient self-esteem and reactions to help. In J. D. Fisher, A. Nadler, & B. M. DePaulo (Eds.), *New directions in helping* (Vol. 1, pp. 167–188). New York, NY: Academic Press.

Nadler, A., Sheinberg, L., & Jaffe, Y. (1981). Coping with stress by help seeking: Help seeking and receiving behaviors in male paraplegics. *Stress and Anxiety, 8,* 375–386.

National Resource Center on LGBT Aging. (2010). *LGBT older adults and exclusion from aging services and programs.* New York, NY: Sage. Retrieved from http://www.lgbtagingcenter.org/resources/pdfs/LGBTOlderAdultsand ExclusionfromAgingPrograms.pdf

Nelms, L., Johnson, V., Teshuva, K., Foreman, P., & Stanley, J. (2009). Social and health factors affecting community service use by vulnerable older people. *Australian Social Work, 62*(4), 507–524.

Nemet, G. F., & Bailey, A. J. (2000). Distance and health care utilization among the rural elderly. *Social Science and Medicine, 50*(9), 1197–1208.

Newall, N. E., Chipperfield, J. G., Clifton, R. A., Perry, R. P., Swift, A. U., & Ruthig, J. C. (2009). Causal beliefs, social participation, and loneliness among older adults: A longitudinal study. *Journal of Social and Personal Relationships, 26*(2–3), 273–290.

Newsom, J. T., & Schulz, R. (1998). Caregiving from the recipient's perspective: Negative reactions to being helped. *Health Psychology, 17*(2), 172–181.

Pescosolido, B. A. (1992). Beyond rational choice: The social dynamics of how people seek help. *American Journal of Sociology, 97*(4), 1096–1138.

Peterson, S. A. (1989). Elderly women and program encounters: A rural study. *Journal of Women and Aging, 1*(4), 41–56.

Richard, L., Gauvin, L., Ducharme, F., Leblanc, M.-E., & Trudel, M. (2012). Integrating the ecological approach in disease prevention and health promotion programs for older adults: An exercise in navigating the headwinds. *Journal of Applied Gerontology, 31*(1), 101–125.

Roberto, K. A., Blieszner, R., & Allen, K. R. (2006). Theorizing in family gerontology: New opportunities for research and practice. *Family Relations, 55,* 513–525.

Roberto, K. A., Weaver, R., & Wacker, R. R. (2014). Delivering aging services: Stability and change in policies and programs. *Generations, 38*(2), 14–21.

Sands, L. P., Wang, Y., McCabe, G. P., Jennings, K., Eng, C., & Covinsky, K. E. (2006). Rates of acute care admissions for frail older people living with met versus unmet activity of daily living needs. *Journal of the American Geriatrics Society, 54,* 339–344.

Sarkisian, C. A., Prohaska, T. R., Davis, C., & Weiner, B. (2007). Pilot test of an attribution retraining intervention to raise walking levels in sedentary older adults. *Journal of the American Geriatrics Society, 55*(11), 1842–1846.

Satariano, W. A., & McAuley, E. (2003). Promoting physical activity among older adults: From ecology to the individual. *American Journal of Preventive Medicine, 25*(Suppl. 2), 184–192.

Scharlach, A. E., Kellam, R., Ong, N., Baskin, A., Goldstein, C., & Fox, P. J. (2006). Cultural attitudes and caregiver service use. *Journal of Gerontological Social Work, 47*(1–2), 133–156.

Schulze, R., & Whittmann, W. W. (2003). A meta-analysis of the theory of reasoned action and the theory of planned behaviour: The principle of compatibility and multidimensionality of beliefs as moderators. In R. Schulze, H. Holling, &

D. Bohning (Eds.), *Meta-analysis: New developments and applications in medical and social sciences* (pp. 219–250). Ashland, OH: Hogrefe & Huber.

Schure, M. B., Conte, K. P., & Goins, R. T. (2014). Unmet assistance need among older American Indians: The Native Elder Care Study. *The Gerontologist, 55*(6), 920–928. doi:10.1093/geront/gnt211

Shen, H. W., Feld, S., Dunkle, R. E., Schroepfer, T., & Lehning, A. (2015). The prevalence of older couples with ADL limitations and factors associated with ADL help receipt. *Journal of Gerontological Social Work, 58*, 171–189.

Smith, J. P., Tran, G. Q., & Thompson, R. D. (2008). Can the theory of planned behavior help explain men's psychological help-seeking? Evidence for a mediation effect and clinical implications. *Psychology of Men & Masculinity, 9*(3), 179–192.

Spense, S. A. (1992). Use of community-based social services by older rural and urban Blacks: An exploratory study. *Human Services in the Rural Environment, 15*(4), 16–19.

Spillman, B. C., Wolff, J., Freedman, V. A., & Kasper, J. D. (2014). *Informal caregiving for older Americans: An analysis of the 2011 National Health and Aging Trends Study.* Retrieved from http://aspe.hhs.gov/daltcp/reports/2014/NHATS-IC.cfm#execsum

Stirling, C., Andrews, S., Croft, T., Vickers, J., Turner, P., & Robinson, A. (2010). Measuring dementia carers' unmet need for services—An exploratory mixed method study. *BMC Health Services Research, 13*(10), 122.

Stokols, D. (1996). Translating social ecological theory into guidelines for community health promotion. *American Journal of Health Promotion, 10*(4), 282–298.

Stone, R. (2011). *Long-term care for the elderly.* Washington, DC: Urban Institute Press.

Sun, F. (2011). Community service use by older adults: The roles of sociocultural factors in rural–urban differences. *Journal of Social Service Research, 37*(2), 124–135.

Surood, S., & Lai, D. W. (2010). Impact of culture on use of Western health services by older South Asian Canadians. *Canadian Journal of Public Health, 101*(2), 176–180.

Tessler, R. C., & Schwartz, S. H. (1972). Help seeking, self-esteem, and achievement motivation: An attributional analysis. *Journal of Personality and Social Psychology, 21*, 318–326.

Tjepkema, M. (2008). Health care use among gay, lesbian and bisexual Canadians. *Health Reports, 19*(1), 53–64.

Trafimow, D., Sheeran, P., Conner, M., & Finlay, K. A. (2002). Evidence that perceived behavioural control is a multidimensional construct: Perceived control and perceived difficulty. *British Journal of Social Psychology, 41*, 101–121.

U.S. General Accounting Office. (2011). *Older Americans Act: More should be done to measure the extent of unmet need for services (GAO-11-237).* Retrieved from http://www.gao.gov/products/GAO-11-237

Wacker, R. R., & Roberto, K. A. (2014). *Community resources for older adults: Programs and services in an era of change.* Thousand Oak, CA: Sage.

Waites, C. (2012). Examining the perceptions, preferences, and practices that influence healthy aging for African American older adults: An ecological perspective. *Journal of Applied Gerontology, 32*(7), 855–875.

Weiss, D., & Freund, A. M. (2012). Still young at heart: Negative age-related information motivates distancing from same-aged people. *Psychology and Aging, 27*(1), 173–180.

Weiss, D., & Lang, F. R. (2012). "They" are old but "I" feel younger: Age-group dissociation as a self-protective strategy in old age. *Psychology and Aging, 27*(1), 153–163.

Westerhof, G. J., Maessen, M., de Bruijn, R., & Smets, B. (2008). Intentions to seek (preventive) psychological help among older adults: An application of the theory of planned behaviour. *Aging and Mental Health, 12*(3), 317–322.

White-Means, S. I. (2000). Racial patterns in disabled elderly persons' use of medical services. *The Journals of Gerontology, Series B, 55*(2), S76–S89.

White-Means, S. I., & Rubin, R. M. (2004). Is there equity in the home health care market? Understanding racial patterns in the use of formal home health care. *The Journals of Gerontology, Series B, 59*(4), S220–S229.

Wolinsky, F. D. (1994). Health services utilization among older adults: Conceptual, measurement, and modeling issues in secondary analysis. *The Gerontologist, 34*, 470–475.

Wolinsky, F. D., Coe, R. M., Miller, D. K., Prendergast, J. M., Creel, M. J., & Chavez, M. N. (1983). Health services utilization among the noninstitutionalized elderly. *Journal of Health and Social Behavior, 24*, 325–337.

Woller, K. M. P., Buboltz, W. C., & Loveland, J. M. (2007). Psychological reactance: Examination across age, ethnicity, and gender. *The American Journal of Psychology, 120*(1), 15–24.

Yates, M. E., Tennstedt, S., & Change, B. H. (1999). Contributors to and mediators of psychological well-being for informal caregivers. *The Journals of Gerontology, Series B, 54*(1), 12–22.

PART VI

Transdisciplinary Perspectives on Theory Development in Aging

ADVANCES IN TRANSDISCIPLINARY THEORIES OF AGING
Vern L. Bengtson

In this section, we examine recent developments in theory building across disciplinary boundaries. In the previous edition of this handbook, we noted that a striking theoretical trend during the prior decade had been the advancement of cross-disciplinary theories of aging. Despite the challenges in bridging disciplines, and despite the challenges of working with different research paradigms and methods, we could see significant breakthroughs in explanations of aging phenomena that actively integrate perspectives from multiple disciplines. Eight years later, these commitments continue—especially across biology, psychology, and sociology—and we are able to see the fruits of cross-pollination in many substantive areas of research.

■ THE "SUCCESSFUL AGING" MODEL AND ITS CRITICS

In Chapter 27, Jack Rowe and Theodore Cosco review recent developments in the "successful aging" model. This term has itself been a monumentally successful concept. As the authors note, research based on this concept generated 180 peer-reviewed articles in 2014 alone. Yet critics examining this literature have asked: Where is the theory in the successful aging movement? Is the concept so wide, encompassing so many issues and variables, as to be of limited theoretical value? Moreover, there are difficulties related to empirical measurement. If, as noted in Chapter 27, a review of studies employing the model finds that between 0.4% and 97% of elders are "aging successfully" (with a median value of 23%), how useful is it?

The lead author, Jack Rowe, whose work has been most responsible for the widespread adoption of the "successful aging" paradigm, and coauthor Theodore Cosco describe the origin and evolution of the model and address some of the criticisms pertaining to it. They first note that the term has variously been used as a model, a theory, a paradigm, an intervention program, or simply a goal. Their now-classic definition involves three basic components: (a) low risk of disease and disease-related disability; (b) maintenance of high mental and physical function; and (c) active engagement with life, including active relations with others and productivity in paid work or volunteering.

Rowe and Cosco address three major criticisms of the model. The first is that the original successful aging formulation overemphasizes personal choice to the neglect of social and environmental factors, as well as life circumstances, that serve to constrain an individual's choices and thus the capacity to age successfully. A second criticism is that the model is overly objective, lacking subjective components such as what people value and what success means to them. And third, the model is too focused on those who are privileged, discounting individuals with limitations or disabilities as well as populations that are disadvantaged.

Rowe and Cosco respond to these criticisms by indicating that the model is being modified. Furthermore, they address large-scale implications of the model by discussing successful aging in the context of an aging society. They suggest that, in light of the demographic imperatives of an increasingly aging population, societies must: (a) reengineer core societal institutions, such as education and work; (b) reengineer the life course, such as redistributing education and work across the entire life span; and (c) focus on human capital and consider risks alongside benefits.

Important questions remain for the future development of this model. Conceptually, what is "successful"? What is the outcome, the criteria for success, and how can it best be measured? Theoretically, *why* and *how* is successful aging created and maintained? What are the strongest explanations of it?

■ COPING, OPTIMAL AGING, AND RESILIENCE

A sister topic to successful aging—"Optimal Aging"—is presented by Carolyn Aldwin and Heidi Igarashi in Chapter 28. The authors note that coping and resilience are central to the aging process, and they advocate for rigorous theoretical and empirical investigation of these processes. In particular, prior definitions do not adequately address the dynamic and reciprocal transactions that occur between individuals and the social contexts in which they are embedded.

Current theories of coping and aging fall into two categories. First, there are those that deal with changes in adaptive styles, such as the selection, optimization, and compensation (SOC) theory developed by Paul Baltes. SOC states that, in the face of declining resources, older people must select on which goals or activities to focus, optimize their performance of these activities, and compensate for any limitations. Second, there are those that deal with changes in coping processes, such as Socioemotional Selectivity Theory (SST) originated by Laura Carstensen. In SST, the awareness of a limited amount of time to live prompts unconscious shifts in motivation, creating a positivity bias— avoiding paying attention to negative or unpleasant situations—and a gradual focusing on meaningful relationships rather than attempting to enlarge social networks.

Aldwin and Igarashi propose a new definition of resilient aging to address these limitations: "Resilience is a strength-based approach to understanding positive development within a context of diversity." Resilience is thus the ability to recognize, use, and develop or modify resources for three goal-related processes: (a) effective coping in the service of functional health, (b) the development of a comfortable life structure, and (c) a sense of meaning and purpose in life. Outcomes of resilience include the recovery from stressors, the capacity to move forward and sustain positive meaning, and "gerotranscendence."

Aldwin and Igarashi conclude by presenting a new theory of the coping and resilience process, which they term Coping, Optimal Aging, and Resilience in Society (COARS). In this "transactional" model, coping with specific stressors can prompt post-traumatic growth and/or stress-related growth, which can in turn facilitate resilience and adaptive styles. Resources in the sociocultural context not only shape how individuals cope, but how individuals cope also shapes the sociocultural context.

■ RELIGIOUS AND SPIRITUAL ASPECTS OF AGING

In Chapter 29, Peter Coleman, Elisabeth Schröder-Butterfill, and John Spreadbury focus attention on three areas of research concerning religion and spirituality in older peoples' lives: (a) age contrasts in religious belief and practice, (b) health benefits to older people who engage in spiritual activities, and (c) influences on social and intergenerational relationships that result from membership in a faith-based group.

Regarding age differences in religion and spirituality, Coleman and colleagues discuss the tension between cohort and maturation effects. First, it is necessary to take into account cohort and historical differences in religiosity. Religious decline has occurred throughout the 20th century, with studies of successive cohorts showing lower church membership and attendance. However, surveys that demonstrate such decline have focused only on religious participation and church membership, not other important dimensions of religiosity. Second, there are developmental (i.e., aging- or maturation-based) changes in religiosity. The few existing longitudinal studies of religion show remarkable stability in religious and spiritual belief and practice over the bulk of adult life, but an increase in "spiritual seeking" (i.e., a surge in religious and spiritual exploration) in later life.

An accumulation of evidence shows that religion and spirituality bring benefits for physical and mental health (e.g., increased longevity, lower depression, increased quality of life). The authors note, however, that aging research in this area rarely employs explicit theory, instead pointing to explanatory mechanisms—such as how religion and religious institutions encourage healthy lifestyles, or how they provide opportunities for social interaction and support. But the mechanisms that appear to have the greatest influence in accounting for the positive relationship between religion and health are cognitive—stemming from the sense of meaning that is derived from religion. In cognitive and stress models, religious beliefs are used in appraising and interpreting distressing life events in manageable ways, which reduce their harmful physiological effects.

The authors also review literature on religious transmission and identity in intergenerational relationships. These emphasize that (a) warm and affirming parenting styles are central to explaining successful transmission; (b) religion is an important dimension of intergenerational solidarity and conflict; and (c) religious children are more supportive of aging parents.

In addition, religious communities are sources of support, and older people who belong to congregations are more likely to receive support than those who do not. Several theories have been used to explain this. Social network theory builds on the fact that congregations are social networks that connect people on the basis of shared religion and on values centered on altruism and human welfare. This nurtures the development of trust or "social capital" within religious networks, something easily translated into availability of support to older members in need. Another perspective, social identity theory, posits that intense social interaction creates stronger identification with the group and greater trust and willingness to cooperate within the group. This translates into both latent and manifest social support in times of need.

In pointing to a number of theoretical and conceptual contributions to religion and aging, Coleman and his colleagues conclude that research on spirituality and health not only represents an exciting area for theory development, but also has far-reaching applied implications. However, there is still a dearth of theorizing about how religion and spirituality influence such outcomes as cognitive functioning and dementia. It is clear, though, that religion and spirituality have a beneficial influence by encouraging regular cognitive stimulation, thus stimulating and reinforcing neural networks.

■ THEORIZING WISDOM AND AGING

What is wisdom, and does it increase with age? In Chapter 30, Monika Ardelt and Hunhui Oh begin with a review of the many definitions of wisdom proposed by scholars past and present. All of these dimensions, they say, have a common theme: Wisdom is multidimensional, consisting of cognitive, reflective, and benevolent components that benefit the person and others. They outline two main explanatory frameworks: (a) expert wisdom theories, which emphasize cognition and analytic abilities; and (b) implicit wisdom theories, which are based on the assumption that individuals know implicitly who and what is wise, as revealed in studies of how laypeople define wisdom.

As a means of advancing beyond these two conceptualizations, Ardelt summarizes her culturally inclusive wisdom theory, the Three-Dimensional Wisdom Model. Its components are (a) cognitive wisdom, which entails a desire to know the truth and a deep understanding of life, particularly relationship with others; (b) reflective wisdom, which highlights the ability to perceive phenomena (including the self) from multiple dimensions; and (c) compassionate wisdom, which reflects the motivation to foster the well-being of others.

Knowing something about the life curve of wisdom is an important point of theory development. One possibility is that it is linear (as suggested by Erik Erikson's theory); another is that it is curvilinear (an inverted-U shape), upward through midlife and falling thereafter. The field of wisdom is also plagued by questions about the effects of cohort versus aging (or maturation), and about discrepancies between cross-sectional versus longitudinal evidence, much like those reviewed in the previous chapter on religion. These areas are ripe for theory.

What factors might promote or inhibit an increase in wisdom with age? This is another area ripe for theory. Some possibilities include the presence of other wise individuals, close intergenerational relations and friendships, and having a "wise" role model. What about religion being a factor promoting wisdom? On one hand, it may be that religious groups constitute subcultures that encourage wise behaviors. On the other hand, there may be negative influences: a religion that stresses unquestioning faith in teachings of the Bible and Church might impede growth in cognitive and reflective wisdom. Nevertheless, early interest in religion might lead individuals on a spiritual quest resulting in greater wisdom in later life—but as Ardelt and Oh note, deeply religious older people are not necessarily wise.

Ardelt and Oh close by suggesting new directions for integrating psychological and sociological perspectives. Wisdom can be a psychosocial developmental resource that becomes most relevant during times of hardship by helping people to feel greater control of their lives; social environments may be the source of hardship, offer social supports for coping with it, and condition the development of wisdom.

■ AGING PERSONS AND THEIR ENVIRONMENTS

The aim of environmental gerontology, which Hans-Werner Wahl and Frank Oswald discuss in Chapter 31, is to describe, explain, and optimize the relationship between the aging person and his or her environment. Such an aim places a premium on theory. "Environment" is a term that has a wide variety of meanings across research traditions. But regardless of discipline, environmental gerontology rests on three major principles that emphasize the importance of (a) person–environment (P–E) transactions (e.g., in Bronfenbrenner's model, life-span development is a never-ending sequence of ecological transitions); (b) the physical–spatial environment; and (c) achieving ecological validity in research, such as defining what "feeling at home" means.

Wahl and Oswald propose a new model of P–E aging that focuses on the interplay between two fundamental processes: *P–E belonging* (having a sense of positive connections with the environment) and *P–E agency* (becoming a change agent through intentional behaviors imposed on the environment). Their model follows these processes to developmental outcomes such as identity, well-being, and autonomy. They also discuss new environments that pose opportunities for theory development, especially the implications of new technology on the environments of older people (e.g., Internet, automation, and robots).

■ BIODEMOGRAPHY AND AGING

The biodemography of aging represents an effort to integrate biological and demographic methods so as to address questions about the mechanisms of aging and longevity, and of variability among populations in aging and health. In Chapter 32, Leonid Gavrilov and Natalia Gavrilova address recent developments in this area, particularly problems in biodemography having to do with heritability and variability of lifetimes, sex differences in lifetimes, and the changing life span of organisms in the process of evolution.

Gavrilov and Gavrilova note that the study of biomarkers in population-based surveys is one of the most rapidly developing areas of biodemographic research, particularly as predictors of health and longevity. Some of the theories that address the "*Why* do we age?" question are evolutionary theories that explain aging as a result of declining forces of natural selection. Three major evolutionary theories are mutation accumulation theory, antagonistic pleiotropy theory, and disposal soma theory. What these evolutionary theories have in common is that they take aging to be programmed, and that the programmed death of the old is ultimately meant to free up resources to ensure the welfare of younger people. One interesting transdisciplinary conclusion from the disposable soma theory is that having daughters promotes the life span of mothers—presumably because of the lower physiological costs of daughters, and the fact that daughters more often become caregivers to older parents. Another is the "grandmother hypothesis": in human evolution, postmenopausal life (and being a grandmother) promotes an increase in life span. As a result, the growth and survival of descendants have been enhanced, which in turn has promoted selection for postre-productive survival.

Other theories address the question *"How* do we age?" Among these are free radical theory, cell membranes theory, oxidative stress/mitochondria theory, and immunological theory. These theories focus on specific chemical processes that damage organs and tissues, and which are triggered by environmental factors. For example, one application of the neuroendocrine theory of aging is that declining old-age mortality is caused by the decreasing burden of infection and inflammatory causes that are rooted in the external environment. Another group of theories focuses on the life course and life events as influences of aging and disease. Examples here are cumulative risk theory and the cumulative disadvantage/advantage theory.

Gavrilov and Gavrilova conclude by discussing the reliability theory of aging, which they have helped to develop. This theory, which they suggest answers both the "why" and "how" questions of aging, explains the leveling off of mortality in advanced age as being caused by the exhaustion of the organism's reserves, or redundancy, at extremely old ages. Thus, a process of redundancy loss largely drives aging.

■ MULTIPLE PROCESSES AND TIME FRAMES OF AGING

In Chapter 33, Dario Spini, Daniela Jopp, Stéphanie Pin, and Silvia Stringhini suggest that the complexity of aging processes requires accounting for (a) multiple time frames, (b) multidirectionality, (c) multidimensionality, and (d) multilevel influences. Fortunately, after decades of relying on cross-sectional studies in which age-related changes could only be inferred from age-group comparisons, longitudinal studies are now available to enable a better understanding of the changes within and between people.

The first concept, "multiple time frames," refers to the fact that aging is development, which happens over different time scales: some observed over a long time course, others as lagged effects with short duration. Three models are particularly helpful here: (a) the critical period model, (b) the accumulation model, and (c) the pathway model. These are, however, not competing models; they may be integrated into a general theory of aging in which the pathway model represents the general social process that drives life course trajectories, and in which the critical period and accumulation models represent the biological processes of disease causation.

Second, the concept of "multidirectionality" refers to the fact that aging is character-ized by several trajectories, resulting in heterogeneity because of interindividual differ-ences in change that lead to variations in the direction of development across individuals or groups. Although most individuals show decrement with age, some individuals do not. This is because of the fact that differences in function between individuals of the same age may be greater than differences between individuals of very different ages.

Third, "multidimensionality" is important in considering the interplay of determi-nants of aging. Having positive emotions, for example, is different from having the absence of negative emotions, and there is a difference between objective and subjective dimensions of health. Finally, "multilevel influences" refer to the fact that individuals are simultaneously embedded in many different social contexts, which virtually affect all aspects of aging in independent and interactive ways. For example, social capital is a resource that is shaped by factors that exist across many social contexts, and persistent and pervasive social inequalities in health have made more visible the role of social contexts in determining health.

■ CONCLUSION

What do we learn from these chapters about the state of theory and directions for theory development in aging? Despite the formidable challenges faced by bridging disciplinary boundaries, we see major leaps in transdisciplinary theories and research over the past decade, a trend that reflects aggressive efforts in research, training, publishing, and funding in this direction. These leaps are also made possible by new models of team science, stronger methods, and more comprehensive longitudinal data. The chapters in this section provide many excellent examples of how to continue advancing transdisciplinary theory and research in the years ahead.

CHAPTER 27

Successful Aging

John W. Rowe and Theodore D. Cosco

The general topic of successful aging (SA) has long been a major theme in gerontology and has been an especially prominent and growing aspect of gerontological research and program development over the past 25 years. Although the phrase "successful aging" was introduced by Robert Havighurst in 1961 in the first issue of *The Gerontologist*, the concept of aging well has existed for centuries and was, for example, discussed by Cicero in his *Discourse on Old Age* (Franklin, 1778). When Havighurst wrote *Successful Aging*, Cumming and Henry's "Disengagement Theory" (1961) was a popular (albeit inevitably discredited) perspective on the aging process. Disengagement theory posited that aging naturally involved an inevitable, ubiquitous, and progressive withdrawal from social institutions and loss of the individual (Cumming & Henry, 1961). In contrast to this largely negative perspective on the aging process, Havighurst posited his Activity Theory, suggesting that aging involves maintenance and replacement of the activities and attitudes of middle age. Rather than withdrawing from activities, Havighurst (1961) advocated for engagement in new social roles, for example grandparenting. Activity theory principles have been further articulated through empirical study, notably by Lemon, Bengtson and Peterson (1972), Longino and Kart (1982), and Knapp (1977).

It is important to be aware that, as currently used, the term "Successful Aging" has many uses and is variously treated as a theory, a paradigm or model, a process, a clinical program, or a goal. Although much of the work in the field is at the level of theory, which is the focus of this chapter, there has also been substantial empirical research that builds on the general concept of SA to inform theory evolution and various forms of program development at the individual and community level. This very broad use of the term is reflected in the substantial progressive increase in academic interest in this area over the past two decades (Figure 27.1).

■ LIFE-COURSE AND LIFE-SPAN PERSPECTIVES ON AGING

There has been very substantial theoretical work, over several decades, on the interrelated but differentiated dual approaches of the life-course and life-span perspectives on aging. Although these are discussed in detail elsewhere in this volume, a brief summary will set the stage for a more detailed consideration of current treatments of SA. Briefly, life-course theories can be seen to focus on events at the macro level, studying the effects of groups, organizations, and institutions on the lives of the individuals who populate them and the social pathways that are deterministic of sequential events. Principal considerations in this area include age stratification, cohort and historical time periods, and the accumulation of advantage and disadvantage over time. Not surprisingly, many proponents of a life-course perspective are sociologists.

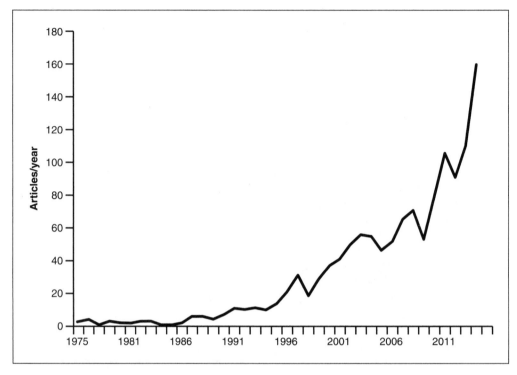

FIGURE 27.1 Peer-reviewed articles per year on successful aging (MEDLINE).

On the other hand, traditional life-span theorists, many of whom are psychologists, focus primarily on the endogenous processes within a given individual. This approach, which includes focus on interindividual differences and intraindividual plasticity, attempts to describe the patterns of change in individuals over the life course.

Although the "life spanners" and the "life coursers" have traditionally been on separate tracks and often do not hesitate to point out the deficiencies of the alternate approach, the seemingly inevitable convergence of the two approaches is well underway, driven in part by the evolution of the strategies of leaders in the field, such as Elder and Kohli, to develop approaches that meld features of each approach as well as the increasing importance of large comprehensive data sets, such as the Health and Retirement Study (HRS) and the Survey of Health, Ageing and Retirement (SHARE), which include information relevant to both approaches, thus facilitating a comprehensive analysis that includes components from each perspective.

■ CURRENT MODELS OF SA

In the context of the life-span versus life-course theoretical frameworks discussed earlier, the models of SA that have been the major focus of work in this area over the past two decades might generally be considered to be in the life-span camp, given their focus on heterogeneity across older individuals and the inherent importance of plasticity and within-individual change. The most prominent models, which will be discussed here, are the MacArthur model (also referred to by some as the Rowe–Kahn model), which is primarily a bio-psycho-social approach, and two psychologically based models, the Berlin or Baltes model of selective optimization and compensation (SOC) and Carstensen's Socioemotional Selectivity Theory (SST; Carstensen et al., 1999).

■ THE MACARTHUR MODEL OF SA

In 1984, the MacArthur Foundation assembled a Research Network on Successful Aging, an interdisciplinary group of 16 scholars to address concerns that the field of gerontology lacked a sufficiently comprehensive interdisciplinary framework.

This group saw the field, including both scholars and funders, as preoccupied with the negative aspects of aging, with disease and disability to the neglect of the positive aspects. Additional concerns included a belief that there was insufficient emphasis on interdisciplinary research, that success was too often identified simply as lack of failure, that function late in life was largely genetically determined, and that functional status could not be enhanced late in life. As reflected in the general perspective of lifespan gerontologists, this group focused on the interindividual differences that dominate physiology in old age and on the innate plasticity and self-regulation within individuals that implied potential for improvement.

The group's early conceptual work was based on the observation that, with respect to many physiological variables, the older people became the less like each other they became. This age-related increase in heterogeneity in advanced age was found for many functions including cardiac, immune, pulmonary, kidney, lung, glucose homeostasis, and the like.

It became apparent that the heterogeneity was not solely because of the contamination of "normal" aging with individuals who had specific pathological abnormalities (diseases) in the organ system being studied. Indeed, elimination of diseased individuals left substantial variability, which increased with age.

This observation led to the view that "normal," that is nonpathological, aging can and should be divided into two forms (Rowe & Kahn, 1987). The first, "usual aging," was viewed as, at least in part, preventable and demonstrated the effects of various external and lifestyle factors (smoking, sedentary lifestyle, overeating, alcohol excess, exposure to pollutants, etc.). Usual aging was seen as laden with risk of disease and disability mediated by lifestyle-related increased lipids, glucose, and blood pressure, and decreased renal, pulmonary, cardiac, immune, and central nervous system (CNS) function. The second form was "successful aging" in which one observed something akin to a "pure aging syndrome."

Two large research projects to identify the predictors of SA and to quantify the proportion of SA that was heritable informed the further development of the MacArthur paradigm. In a longitudinal study of an initially rather homogeneous group of high-functioning elders, it was observed that there was wide variation over time. Although many lost function, one quarter of the respondents actually improved with advancing age, whereas there was no change in half!

Major predictors of improved or stable performance included the close relation between mental and physical function, emotional (not instrumental) support, moderate or strenuous physical activity, pulmonary function, and self-esteem (Albert et al., 1995; Berkman et al., 1993; Seeman et al., 1994).

In a study of a large cohort of twins drawn from the Swedish National Twin Registry, twins reared apart were matched with same gender, zygosity, and age twins reared together. An analysis of the relative contributions of heredity and nonheritable factors (i.e., environment and life experience) to the apparent effect of age showed that only about 30%

of most physiologic changes in most organ systems, and 50% of cognitive and psychological changes, were heritable (Rowe & Kahn, 1997). These findings, which have since been confirmed by several studies, provided a rationale for the general view that a person can have a major influence on his or her "aging" through changes in lifestyle factors.

Based on these empirical studies, the network formulated the concept of SA of an individual as including the possibility that a substantial proportion of older persons, but by no means all, had the potential to age successfully, which was defined as having three principal components (Rowe & Kahn, 1997, 1998): low risk of disease and disease-related disability; maintenance of high mental and physical function; and active engagement with life, including active relations with others and productivity, either in paid work or volunteering.

■ APPLICATIONS AND MODIFICATIONS OF THE MACARTHUR MODEL OF SA

The MacArthur model of SA has found application into theory, empirical research, and practice in a wide variety of fields (Bulow & Soderqvist, 2014; Depp & Jeste, 2006; Dillaway & Byrnes, 2009; Jeste & Depp, 2010; Katz & Calasanti, 2015; Martin et al., 2015; Martinson & Berridge, 2015; Rubinstein & de Medeiros, 2015). More than 100 variations of the model, with specific modifications including additions, deletions, or changes in emphasis, have been published and the original model has been applied to a very large number of groups of various racial, ethnic, and national origins, as well as specific subgroups such as those with HIV/AIDS (Kahana & Kahana, 2001), disabilities, the lesbian, gay, bisexual, and transgender (LGBT) community, and many racial and ethnic groups.

To provide perspective on the voluminous commentary, it is useful to have an understanding of the relative prevalence of the various opinions. For this, we rely on an analysis of 103 studies with 105 unique variations of the MacArthur model (Cosco, Prina, Perales, Stephan, & Brayne, 2014) and the work of Martinson and Berridge (2015), who published a critique of the critiques of the MacArthur model.

There have been three major areas in which scholars have urged modifications of the original MacArthur SA model. These include calls for more consideration of social factors and the life course, greater emphasis on subjective considerations of older persons, and a definition that is less exclusive and considers SA from a broader portion of the population. Each modification will be reviewed briefly.

■ CALLS FOR GREATER EMPHASIS ON SOCIAL FACTORS AND A LIFE-COURSE PERSPECTIVE

As can be predicted from the prior discussion regarding the dual pathways of life-course and life-span analysis in aging, soon after the original MacArthur model was proposed, a number of social scientists, including the distinguished Matilda White Riley, raised the objection that the model was too narrowly focused on the individual to the neglect of the important influence of external factors including structural and social and socioeconomic factors in the environment that were necessary to achieve success (Pruchno, Wilson-Genderson, Rose, & Cartwright, 2010; Riley, 1998). There was concern that the model overemphasized personal choice to the neglect of the various social and environmental factors and life situations that either limited or facilitated choice and the capacity to age successfully (Kahn 1998, 2002). In this regard, Kahana, Kelley-Moore, and Kahana (2012) proposed a broader "proactivity" model. Similar concerns were also raised regarding the life-span-oriented psychological theories discussed earlier. It is apparent that the important influences of social factors, including the structure and function of a variety of social factors and institutions, were not sufficiently explicitly considered in the initial formulation of the MacArthur model. The broad range of these important externalities includes, among other elements, social networks; family structure and function; economic conditions; opportunities for productive engagement in work or volunteering; access to high-quality affordable health care; and the impacts of housing, urban design, and transportation.

The same holds for the value of a life-course perspective and identification of antecedents of SA. Exploiting the richness of data sets such as birth cohort studies (e.g., MRC National Survey of Health and Development; Kuh et al., 2011) will be invaluable in unpacking aspects of individuals' lives that affect their SA both proximally and distally. Through the elucidation of aspects of early life that foster SA throughout the life course, positive aging trajectories can be facilitated. For example, researchers at the University of Cambridge have employed longitudinal latent variable modeling techniques to identify heterogeneous trajectories of SA in longitudinal population-based cohort studies. Furthermore, by comparing individuals' memberships in these trajectories with their educational attainments, they were able to identify a strong independent relationship between higher educational attainment and SA trajectories later in life.

Consistent with the gradual tendency toward blurring of the distinctions between these two perspectives, these considerations figure prominently in our view of the future directions for evolution of the SA model, as discussed in the following discussion in some detail.

■ CALLS FOR A SUBJECTIVE COMPONENT

The MacArthur model was seen by many to be overly objective and lacking a sufficient subjective model; it also lacked components of the things older people value (Glass, 2003), their experiences over the life course (Schulz & Heckhausen, 1996), and what success means to them, which is often more multidimensional than classical theory (Jopp et al., 2015; Katz & Calasanti, 2015). The MacArthur Network did not completely neglect subjective measures, and self-esteem was a strong predictor of SA in the initial studies, but it is certainly a fair criticism that the model initially offered did not include subjective measures as central to aging successfully.

This has led to valuable additional empirical research and a recent report reviewed 26 published studies that included surveys asking, "What is your definition of successful aging?" All studies included psychosocial components, 76% (n = 20 studies) included biomedical components, and 58% (n = 15 studies) included external components. These findings can provide a useful basis for supplementation of the model with a subjective component.

■ CALLS FOR LESS EXCLUSIVITY

Strawbridge, Wallhagen, and Cohen (2002) and others felt that the defining criteria in the original model would categorize a very small portion of the elderly as aging successfully, which is inconsistent with numerous surveys that showed that a fairly large proportion of older persons consider themselves to be aging successfully. They and others felt that this tended to create an elite subset of "winners," thus relegating all other elders to being "losers," a point of view that inevitably led to the accusation that the career-long group of gerontologists who formulated the model were "ageist"! Related to this concern regarding exclusivity, a group described as "critical scholars," notably Meredith Minkler and her colleagues (Holstein & Minkler, 2003), expressed concern that the model excluded individuals with disabilities from the possibilities of aging success-fully, thus providing a "blame the victim" perspective. This objection is not surprising as pointed out by Martinson and Berridge (2015) that a normative model such as the models offered for SA is by definition exclusionary. The model is not meant to apply to everyone, but to those who do not have limitations of whatever type that make the objective goals of the model unattainable.

Regarding the actual proportion of the older population that meets the criteria of SA, Cosco et al. (2014) found great variability depending on the application of the rather ill-defined general criteria. In a review of the literature, the proportion of elders identi-fied as aging successfully varied from 0.4% to 91.7% (median: 23.1%, unweighted mean: 28.3% [SD: 20.1%; 95% CI [24.6%–32.0%]]). Furthermore, researcher-defined measures identified an average of 26.0% (SD: 21.0%; 95% CI [22.1%–29.9%]) of study participants as successfully aging, while self-reports identified an average of 71.3% (SD: 18.6%; 95% CI [56.4%–86.2%]).

■ PSYCHOLOGICAL MODELS OF SA

With respect to psychological theories of SA, no overview would be complete without a discussion of the important contributions of Paul and Margaret Baltes (1990) and their colleagues who worked at the Max Plank Institute for Human Development and the Berlin Aging Study and Laura Carstensen (1992) at Stanford. Paul Baltes and his col-leagues made major contributions in defining the life-span approach to aging, with an emphasis on three core components: communalities, interindividual differences, and intraindividual plasticity.

Baltes and Baltes (1990) edited the book *Successful Aging: Perspectives from the Behavioral Sciences* and wrote several articles (Baltes & Baltes, 1989, 1990; Baltes & Carstensen, 1991; Baltes & Smith, 2003; Baltes, Smith, & Staudinger, 1991), based on their well-recognized theory of Selection (S), Optimization (O), and Compensation (C) throughout the life course. The SOC model included consideration of antecedent conditions; the interme-diary processes of S, O, and C; and outcomes, such as functional status. Feedback was inherent through the life course and outcomes became antecedent conditions for the next phase of life.

The SOC model of SA triggered interest and critiques from many psychologists, who expressed varying degrees of agreement or disagreement and proposed modifications and applications (Abraham & Hansson, 1995; Baltes & Carstensen, 1996; Garfein & Herzog, 1995; Lang & Tesch-Romer, 1993; Schulz & Heckhausen, 1996).

A second notable advancement regarding psychological aspects of SA that has con-tinued to attract interest and support came with Carstensen's (Carstensen, Isaacowitz, & Charles, 1999) SST, which was consistent with the SOC model and articulated the strategies individuals use with advancing age to enhance their experiences through modifications of their emotional and social goals and interactions.

The psychological models and the MacArthur model are generally not considered to be inconsistent with each other as much as they are just seen as dealing with different issues. In general, Paul and Margret Baltes, Laura Carstensen, and other psychologists cautioned against an overemphasis on structural factors and definitive criteria and presented models that urged a more dynamic approach that emphasized the "how" (psychological processes) rather than the "what" (strict definition of end result) of the MacArthur model. For psychologists, the key to thinking about SA was not so much in establishing rigid objective criteria but in understanding the psychological processes by which individuals navigate their life course, develop strategies, and make choices to compensate for losses. In addition, although Paul Baltes agreed with Rowe and Kahn regarding the heterogeneity of aging and the utility of separating usual from SA, he felt that age-related decrements were often age determined and unavoidable (reaction time, muscle strength, etc.).

Opinions have varied as to whether the model should be revised or replaced, but the continued presence of it in the literature supports the view recently expressed by Stowe and Cooney (2015) that "the popularity of the model in the mainstream literature and extensive use in scientific inquiry warrants modifications over disposal" and by the editors of *The Journals of Gerontology, Series B:* "While the original successful aging model generated many empirical assessments, critiques, and calls for revision, the core concepts have remained intact" (Call for papers, *The Journals of Gerontology, Series B,* May 2015).

■ DIRECTIONS FOR THE FUTURE

Going forward it seems clear that SA will continue to be an important theme in gerontology. The psychological theories discussed here briefly, and in more detail elsewhere in this volume, continue to attract interest and facilitate valuable empirical research. The biosocial model proposed by the MacArthur Network is under evolution with several important components being added to the initial rather spare and rigidly defined core. In addition to the issues of inclusion of more social factors and greater subjectivity, discussed previously, some of the additions and elucidations are consistent with the initial focus of the model on the individual (life-span perspective) and reflect new approaches and developments that have emerged since the initial theory was proposed in 1987. Specifically, these include the role of new developments in basic biology, especially genetics, in identifying factors that may predict, facilitate, or impede SA; technological developments in facilitating physical and cognitive function; engagement productivity; and social interaction of individuals.

Beyond the individual, there is growing interest in application of the concept of SA to the level of society as it also "ages," including not only the reengineering that must occur in the society's core institutions but also the policies that are needed to be put in place to facilitate these adaptations. Thus, SA of societies is emerging as an area of theoretical effort and empirical work that complements the work of SA at the level of an individual. The clear relationship between the impact of the function of the society and its institutions on the capacity of an individual to age successfully, and the growing availability of comprehensive interdisciplinary data sets that permit elucidation of the early and midlife antecedents of SA in late life, provides the long-called-for synthesis of the individualistic life-span perspective of the initial MacArthur model with a more comprehensive life-course perspective. The importance of these new areas in the evolution of the theory of SA can be seen in the fact that *The Journals of Gerontology* plans a theme issue on these topics for mid-2016.

Basic Biological Considerations in SA

Recently, Silverstein (2015) has called for increased recognition by social and behavioral scientists of the potential value of information on biomarkers and genetics as useful predictors of SA. This contrasts with the concerns of some early critics who, in the late 1980s, felt that the model was too biomedical. As Silverstein has emphasized, it is important to understand that this orientation toward basic biology should not be to the exclusion or marginalization of social and psychological dimensions of SA, but rather toward a full understanding of the relative contributions of biology and experience. The goal is to use the biological information to inform the development of theory and empirical research in this area. This emphasis is consistent with a major rapidly developing movement in medicine and biomedical research toward "personalized medicine" or "precision medicine," which aims to take advantage of new and powerful biological tools to assess the genetic and physiological as well as social and behavioral risk of individuals to develop disease and disability. This effort aims to provide sufficient person-specific as well as population-based information to permit the application of tailored approaches to behavioral or medical interventions toward risk reduction and early detection of disease.

Technology

Research is emerging on the impact of the continuing technological revolution on the capacity of individuals to function well in late life. The relevant issues that deserve study here vary from the use of assistive devices such as hearing aids and glasses to the impact of the Internet on engagement and well-being, and to the changes in job content and its physical demands, including dexterity, mobility, and strength. Will the new technologies foster SA and break down the societal barriers of age segregation, or will age-related differences in ability to adapt to technologies and utilize them effectively broaden the gaps between generations and further isolate older persons? These issues present challenges to employers and policy makers as they struggle to use technology to unleash the valuable human capital in the growing elderly population.

SA in the Context of an Aging Society

Since the introduction of the modern era theory of SA, the United States has become an aging society reaching a point in the demographic transformation where the number of individuals younger than age 15 years is less than the number older than age 65 years. This dramatic and rapid change poses great challenges and opportunities for our society and adds a new and critically important dimension to the consideration of the aforementioned effects of social structures and functions on the capacity of an individual to age successfully. As scholarship on SA advances, there is a growing and already rich literature urging that the concept of SA of a person be supplemented with theory and research regarding the effects on individuals of the degree of success a society has attained as it ages (Rowe, 2015).

Theoretical and empirical work on an aging America must transcend the current preoccupation with the solvency of the Medicare and Social Security Trust Funds and focus on other critically important issues. More importantly, almost no acknowledgment of the substantial positive aspects and potential of an aging society is occurring.

A successfully aging society can be seen as one that is productive, cohesive, secure, and equitable. We need policies that facilitate continued engagement of older persons in society, whether it be in work for pay or through volunteering; policies that provide support for evolving families to continue to provide their traditional role, safety net role, and policies that reduce disparities and inequalities and the tensions they bring that tear at the fabric of our society.

Key considerations in this work on SA of society include the following.

REENGINEER CORE SOCIETAL INSTITUTIONS

Our society's core institutions were not engineered to support a population with the age distribution we will soon have. For our future society to be productive and produce the goods and services needed by our future population, a primary focus should be on adjusting and adapting an array of core institutions, including education, work and retirement, health care, *and* the design and function of housing and cities, and transportation.

REENGINEER THE LIFE COURSE

Aging societies need to adopt a perspective that urges redistribution of life's activities (e.g., education, work, retirement, childrearing, leisure) across individuals' lives. The approach must identify opportunities for creating new roles and responsibilities for older adults in an aging society that lead to win-wins for all generations (Duflo & Saez, 2003).

FOCUS ON HUMAN CAPITAL AND CONSIDER BENEFITS AS WELL AS RISKS

Too little attention is paid to the potential upside (the longevity dividend) including the availability of previously unimagined older individuals, many fully capable of participating productively in society either through the workforce or via civic engagement. Older people have much to offer, including their accrued knowledge, stability, unique creative capacities for synthetic problem solving, and increased ability to both manage conflicts and take the perspectives of other age groups into account.

The focus should be on strategies that use all the talent in the population, employ social norms based on ability rather than chronological age, and transition from an emphasis on investment early in life to recognition that investments can pay off across the full life span.

■ CONCLUSION

The concept of SA, either as a process or as an outcome, has a sustained presence in the gerontological literature and has been an important catalyst for empirical research and theoretical inquiry. Regrettably, the theoretical work sometimes seems to be outstripping the empirical research base.

Although the prevalent biosocial and psychological models of SA, which are largely based on a life-span approach, have attracted important and valuable additions and modifications, the core concepts have remained intact. These include a focus on the positive aspects of aging; a distinction within normal aging between usual and successful;

an emphasis on engagement rather than on disengagement in late life; and a focus on cognitive and physiological plasticity in late life and the maintenance or enhancement in function that it implies.

As we strive to provide insight, and perhaps even reach consensus, on what it means to age successfully in the 21st century, theoretical and empirical research efforts must increasingly rely on a melding of life-course and life-span perspectives. The core concepts listed earlier should be weaved into a rich social and life-course perspective. Individuals should be placed in the context of a society that is undergoing both dramatic demographic and technologic transformations that may have dramatic impacts on the capacity of individuals to age successfully.

REFERENCES

Abraham, J. D., & Hansson, R. O. (1995). Successful aging at work: An applied study of selection, optimization, and compensation through impression management. *The Journals of Gerontology, Series B, 50*(2), P94–P103.

Albert, M. S., Jones, K., Savage, C. R., Berkman, L., Seeman, T., Blazer, D., & Rowe, J. W. (1995). Predictors of cognitive change in older persons: MacArthur studies of successful aging. *Psychology and Aging, 10*(4), 578–589.

Baltes, M. M., & Carstensen, L. (1991). Possible selves across the life span. *Human Development, 34*(4), 256–260.

Baltes, M. M., & Carstensen, L. (1996). Aging well: Thoughts about a process-oriented metamodel of successful aging. *Psychologische Rundschau, 47*(4), 199–215.

Baltes, P. B., & Baltes, M. M. (1989). Selective optimization with compensation—A psychological model of successful aging. *Zeitschrift Fur Padagogik, 35*(1), 85–105.

Baltes, P. B., & Baltes, M. M. (1990). *Successful aging: Perspectives from the behavioral sciences.* New York, NY: Cambridge University Press.

Baltes, P. B., & Smith, J. (2003). New frontiers in the future of aging: From successful aging of the young old to the dilemmas of the fourth age. *Gerontology, 49*(2), 123–135.

Baltes, P. B., Smith, J., & Staudinger, U. M. (1991). Wisdom and successful aging. *Nebraska Symposium on Motivation, 39*, 123–167.

Berkman, L. F., Seeman, T. E., Albert, M., Blazer, D., Kahn, R., Mohs, R.,...McClearn, G. (1993). High, usual and impaired functioning in community-dwelling older men and women: Findings from the MacArthur Foundation Research Network on Successful Aging. *Journal of Clinical Epidemiology, 46*(10), 1129–1140.

Bulow, M. H., & Soderqvist, T. (2014). Successful ageing: A historical overview and critical analysis of a successful concept. *Journal of Aging Studies, 31*, 139–149.

Carstensen, L. (1992). Motivation for social contact across the life span: A theory of socioemotional selectivity. *Nebraska Symposium on Motivation, 40*, 209–254.

Carstensen, L. L., Isaacowitz, D. M., & Charles, S. T. (1999). Taking time seriously: A theory of socioemotional selectivity. *American Psychologist, 54*(3), 165.

Cosco, T. D., Prina, A. M., Perales, J., Stephan, B., & Brayne, C. (2014). Operational definitions of successful aging: A systematic review. *International Psychogeriatrics, 26*(3), 373–381.

Cumming, E., & Henry, W. (1961). *Growing old*. New York, NY: Basic Books.

Depp, C. A., & Jeste, D. V. (2006). Definitions and predictors of successful aging: A comprehensive review of larger quantitative studies. *American Journal of Geriatric Psychiatry, 14*(1), 6–20.

Dillaway, H. E., & Byrnes, M. (2009). Reconsidering successful aging: A call for renewed and expanded academic critiques and conceptualizations. *Journal of Applied Gerontology, 28*(6), 702–722.

Duflo, E., & Saez, E. (2003). *Implications of information and social interactions for retirement saving decisions*. Pension Research Council Working Paper. Philadelphia, PA: Pension Research Council.

Franklin, B. J. T. (1778). *M. T. Cicero's Cato Major*. London, UK: Fielding and Walker.

Garfein, A. J., & Herzog, A. (1995). Robust aging among the young-old, old-old, and oldest-old. *The Journals of Gerontology, Series B, 50*(2), S77–S87.

Glass, T. A. (2003). Assessing the success of successful aging. *Annals of Internal Medicine, 139*(5, Pt. 1), 382–383.

Havighurst, R. J. (1961). Successful aging. *The Gerontologist, 1*(1), 8–13.

Holstein, M. B., & Minkler, M. (2003). Self, society, and the "new gerontology." *The Gerontologist, 43*(6), 787–796.

Jeste, D., & Depp, C. (2010). Positive mental aging. *American Journal of Geriatric Psychiatry, 18*(1), 1–3.

Jopp, D. S., Wozniak, D., Damarin, A. K., De Feo, M., Jung, S., & Jeswani, S. (2015). How could lay perspectives on successful aging complement scientific theory? Findings from a U.S. and a German life-span sample. *The Gerontologist, 55*(1), 91–106.

Kahana, E., & Kahana, B. (2001). Successful aging among people with HIV/AIDS. *Journal of Clinical Epidemiology, 54*(Suppl. 1), S53–S56.

Kahana, E., Kelley-Moore, J., & Kahana, B. (2012). Proactive aging: A longitudinal study of stress, resources, agency, and well-being in late life. *Aging and Mental Health, 16*(4), 438–451.

Kahn, R. L. (1998). Successful aging—Dr. Rowe and Dr. Kan reply. *The Gerontologist, 38*(2), 151.

Kahn, R. L. (2002). On "Successful aging and well-being: Self-rated compared with Rowe and Kahn." *The Gerontologist, 42*(6), 725–726.

Katz, S., & Calasanti, T. (2015). Critical perspectives on successful aging: Does it "Appeal More Than It Illuminates"? *The Gerontologist, 55*(1), 26–33.

Knapp, M. R. (1977). The activity theory of aging: An examination in the English context. *The Gerontologist, 17*(6), 553–559.

Kuh, D., Pierce, M., Adams, J., Deanfield, J., Ekelund, U., Friberg, P., . . . Hardy, R. (2011). Cohort profile: Updating the cohort profile for the MRC National Survey of Health and Development: A new clinic-based data collection for ageing research. *International Journal of Epidemiology, 40*(1), e1–e9.

Lang, F. R., & Tesch-Romer, C. (1993). Successful aging and social relations: Selection and compensation in social contact behavior. *Zeitschrift fur Gerontologie, 26*(5), 321–329.

Lemon, B. W., Bengtson, V. L., & Peterson, J. A. (1972). An exploration of the activity theory of aging: Activity types and life satisfaction among in-movers to a retirement community. *Journal of Gerontology, 27*(4), 511–523.

Longino, C. F., Jr., & Kart, C. S. (1982). Explicating activity theory: A formal replication. *Journal of Gerontology, 37*(6), 713–722.

Martin, P., Kelly, N., Kahana, B., Kahana, E., Willcox, B. J., Willcox, D. C., & Poon, L. W. (2015). Defining successful aging: A tangible or elusive concept? *The Gerontologist, 55*(1), 14–25.

Martinson, M., & Berridge, C. (2015). Successful aging and its discontents: A systematic review of the social gerontology literature. *The Gerontologist, 55*(1), 58–69.

Pruchno, R. A., Wilson-Genderson, M., Rose, M., & Cartwright, F. (2010). Successful aging: Early influences and contemporary characteristics. *The Gerontologist, 50*(6), 821–833.

Riley, M. W. (1998). Successful aging. *The Gerontologist, 38*(2), 151.

Rowe, J. W. (2015). Successful aging of societies. *Daedalus, Spring 2015,* 5–11.

Rowe, J. W., & Kahn, R. L. (1987). Human aging: Usual and successful. *Science, 237*(4811), 143–149.

Rowe, J. W., & Kahn, R. L. (1997). Successful aging. *The Gerontologist, 37*(4), 433–440.

Rowe, J. W., & Kahn, R. L. (1998). *Successful aging.* New York, NY: Pantheon Books.

Rubinstein, R. L., & de Medeiros, K. (2015). "Successful Aging," gerontological theory and neoliberalism: A qualitative critique. *The Gerontologist, 55*(1), 34–42.

Schulz, R., & Heckhausen, J. (1996). A life span model of successful aging. *The American Psychologist, 51*(7), 702–714.

Seeman, T. E., Charpentier, P. A., Berkman, L. F., Tinetti, M. E., Guralnik, J. M., Albert, M., . . . Rowe, J. W. (1994). Predicting changes in physical performance in a high-functioning elderly cohort: MacArthur studies of successful aging. *Journal of Gerontology, 49*(3), M97–M108.

Silverstein, M. (2015). Foreword (and Farewell). *The Journals of Gerontology, Series B, 70*(1), 85–86.

Stowe, J. D., & Cooney, T. M. (2015). Examining Rowe and Kahn's concept of successful aging: Importance of taking a life course perspective. *The Gerontologist, 55*(1), 43–50.

Strawbridge, W. J., Wallhagen, M. I., & Cohen, R. D. (2002). Successful aging and well-being: Self-rated compared with Rowe and Kahn. *The Gerontologist, 42*(6), 727–733.

CHAPTER 28

Coping, Optimal Aging, and Resilience in a Sociocultural Context

Carolyn M. Aldwin and Heidi Igarashi

How individuals cope with stressors is central to the aging process, both in terms of adaptation to aging and in mitigating the adverse effects of stress on health. With old age comes a variety of challenges, both physical and psychosocial, to which individuals need to adapt and even surmount. However, studies have consistently found that simple exposure to stressors is less important in affecting health outcomes than how individuals cope with the stressor (Aldwin, 2007; Ursano, Wheatley, Sledge, Rahe, & Carlson, 1986). Given that coping is integral to stress resilience, it is possible that coping is an even more important factor in the human aging process than stress, and may be one of the factors involved in the well-known divergence in health trajectories with age.

In this chapter, we provide a brief introduction to approaches to coping theory—from its early roots in psychodynamic *defense mechanisms*, through cognitive and personality approaches to *coping styles*, to more current work on *coping and adaptive processes*. In general, we focus on key controversies rather than attempt an exhaustive review of the coping literature. For example, in reviewing classical theories of coping and aging, the major controversy was whether older adults were better or worse copers, while more modern theories address more nuanced arguments on whether and how coping changes with age. Developmental scientists who study adulthood have applied constructs from the child developmentalists, including self-regulation and resilience. Indeed, researchers dissatisfied with the strictures of the traditional definitions of successful aging, for example, Rowe and Kahn's (1997) emphasis on the absence of chronic illnesses as a *sine qua non* of successful aging (despite the wide prevalence of these conditions in late life), have turned toward resilience as a way of better characterizing positive functioning in aging.

However, the current definitions of resilience in adulthood are overly broad, and a major goal of this chapter is to create a new definition of resilient aging, one which is broad enough to encompass the possibility of both multiple patterns of successful aging and equifinality, but specific enough to address the transactions between individuals and their contexts, which are critical to understanding resilience (Lerner et al., 2012). Briefly, we develop a definition *of* "resilience" as the ability to recognize, utilize, and develop or modify resources at the individual, community, and sociocultural levels in the service of three goal-related processes: maintenance of optimal functioning, given current limitations; development of a comfortable life structure; and development of a sense of purpose in life. We then address the larger issue of resilience and aging with an eye toward the importance of diversity in understanding the process of resilience. Finally, we identify issues that should be addressed in future research.

■ COPING AND AGING

A Brief Introduction to Coping

The construct of coping has its roots in the recognition that there are individual differences in response to stress, which may either exacerbate or mitigate its adverse effects. For some individuals, stressors may represent enjoyable challenges; for others, stressors are sources of unrelenting distress. The approach taken to the study of coping—as individual differences in response to stress—has varied by academic discipline. In psychology, coping has its roots in several subdisciplines, including psychodynamic theory (*defense mechanisms*); cognitive/information processing and personality theory (*coping styles*); and cognitive behavior theory (*coping processes*).

DEFENSE MECHANISMS

The earliest studies of individual differences in response to stress were conducted by psychoanalysts. Freud (1966) developed the theory of "defense mechanisms," which are defined as largely unconscious attempts to deal with anxiety generated by the ego to reconcile conflict between the id and the superego. These included mechanisms such as denial, projection, introjection, sublimation, and the like. By definition, defense mechanisms distort reality. Vaillant (1977) developed a hierarchy based on the degree to which reality was distorted, ranging from the gross distortions of the more psychotic defense mechanisms such as delusional projection and denial to theoretically more adaptive mechanisms such as altruism and sublimation.

However, it is clear that individuals use defense mechanisms not just to deal with internal conflicts, but to negotiate external situations as well. For example, individuals who are being violently assaulted, such as rape or torture victims, often can use only dissociation—detaching or dissociating from what is happening to one's own body. Indeed, anyone who has interacted with individuals undergoing extreme stress has seen examples of defense mechanisms in action, from the father who simply cannot recognize that the dead teenager in the morgue is his child (denial) to the mother who becomes very involved with Mothers Against Drunk Driving to cope with the death of her child (sublimation). Nonetheless, the use of self-report measures to assess unconscious processes is highly problematic (Cramer, 2000), and most current studies rely more on coding of defenses (Cramer, 2015). However, many researchers prefer to focus on strategies that individuals consciously use to deal with stressors.

COPING STYLES

These are strategies that individuals are thought to use on a habitual basis, and are rooted in cognitive/information process approaches, which focus on (usually dichotomous) attentional processes, generally types of approach/avoidance processes (Roth & Cohen, 1986). These include repression–sensitization (Byrne, 1964) and blunting/monitoring (Miller, 1980). Repressors and blunters avoid information, whereas sensitizers and monitors seek information. It has long been argued that such simple dichotomies are inadequate to deal with the complexities of coping cognitions and behavior, and, indeed, most people use both approaches in stressful situations, either contextually (e.g., ignoring some aspects and focusing on others), or sequentially (e.g., many individuals gather in as much information as possible but then withdraw when the stress becomes too much; see Aldwin, 2007 for a review).

Coping style measures that are based more on personality characteristics focus on identifying patterns of coping that individuals usually use. These are usually more complex than the simple approach/avoidance theories and may index a variety of different types of behaviors and cognitions (e.g., Carver, Scheier, & Weintraub, 1989). Carver and Connor-Smith (2010) recently attempted to map out coping styles onto the Big 5 personality theory. Alternatively, coping styles measures may focus on one in particular strategy, such as rumination (Nolen-Hoeksema, 2000) or religious coping (Pargament, Koenig, Tarakeshwar, & Hahn, 2004), without denying the possibility that multiple strategies may be used.

A conceptual problem with the coping styles approach is that, if there are consistent patterns that are tightly linked to personality, then why not simply assess personality? Especially given that personality indices usually have much better psychometric properties than coping measures, which often have rather poor psychometrics (see Skinner, Edge, Altwood, & Sherwin, 2003). However, adult developmentalists sometimes take an adaptive styles approach to examining how individuals cope with the aging process, which will be reviewed below.

In contrast, *coping process* approaches (Lazarus & Folkman, 1984) focus on the actual strategies that individuals use in particular stressful situations. This stems from the cognitive revolution in psychology, in which individuals' experiences became the central focus. Individuals are thought to appraise a situation as stressful, depending on the fit between the environmental demands and the individuals' resources. If the magnitude or type of problem is greater than an individual's resources, that situation is perceived as stressful. Thus, stress appraisals—and the coping that stems from them—are a function of the transaction between the individual and the environment.

The coping process approach recognizes that coping strategies are influenced not only by person characteristics such as personality, values, and developmental history but also by environmental demands and resources. Coping strategies are thought to be plastic—people can and do modify their strategies based on situational demands. How one copes with a crying infant, for example, is different from how one deals with a deadline at work. Thus, a coping process approach lends itself more readily both to interventions and also to a developmental perspective, in that it recognizes that individuals learn how to cope through trial and error, modeling and socialization in childhood and adolescence (Kliewer, Sandler, & Wolchik, 1994; Skinner & Edge, 2002), and through self-reflection processes in adulthood (Levenson, Aldwin, & Cupertino, 2001). However, they may be better suited to predicting proximal outcomes in particular situations, rather than long-term health outcomes (Aldwin, 2007).

The distinction between coping styles and coping processes can become blurred, in part because measures such as the COPE (Carver et al., 1989) can be used either as style measures (e.g., how do you usually cope?) or as process measures (how did you cope with this particular situation?). However, coping style measures have little relationship to the actual strategies used in a particular situation (Aldwin, 2007). For example, Ptacek, Pierce, and Thompson (2006) assessed coping processes daily for 30 days, and the coping styles measure did not significantly correlate with coping strategies on any particular day. However, when aggregated across situations, coping styles did have a modest correlation with average coping strategies. Thus, individuals may prefer some types of strategies over others, but in general can tailor which strategies they use to the requirements of the particular problem.

As we shall see, these distinctions—between defense mechanisms, coping styles, and coping process—play an important role in studies examining whether and how coping may change with age.

Classical Theories of Coping and Aging

In general, classical theories approach to the question of coping and aging focused on determining whether older adults were better or worse copers than younger adults, or whether there were few or no age differences (see Aldwin & Yancura, 2011, for a review). For example, the psychodynamic school was divided. An early study by Gutmann (1974) assessed age differences in coping styles in a Druze sample by using Thematic Apperception Test (TAT) cards, in which individuals are shown ambiguous pictures and asked to tell stories. He argued that the stories told by young adults were characterized by "active" mastery; those told by the middle-aged adults by "passive" mastery: and those by older adults by "magical" mastery, and concluded the older adults were poorer copers. In contrast, Vaillant (1977) coded longitudinal interviews from young–adulthood to midlife, and found that older adults were better copers—individuals who had used neurotic or immature defense mechanisms as college students were likely to transition into more mature defense mechanisms such as sublimation or altruism by midlife. However, Vaillant was unable to replicate his results in two other longitudinal studies (Vaillant, 1993; Vaillant, Bond, & Vaillant, 1986), although he did confirm a positive association between the use of mature defense mechanisms and well-being. More recently, Diehl et al. (2014) found longitudinal evidence for a nonlinear effect, with decrease in less adaptive defense mechanisms and an increase in more adaptive mechanisms from young adulthood through midlife, which may reverse, though, in later life.

The coping styles school was somewhat more consistent. McCrae's (1989) review found that older adults were less likely to use avoidant strategies. Although approach strategies also appeared to decrease, McCrae argued that this was more likely because of changes in the types of problems faced in late life. He argued that approach strategies with problems such as bereavement are less appropriate, and thus the decrease in approach strategies with age is more of a function of changes in context (e.g., increases in less controllable stressors) rather than developmental processes per se.

Coping process studies explicitly focused on differences in the level of effort with age, with some finding that older adults used fewer problem-focused strategies (Folkman, Lazarus, Pimley, & Novacek, 1987), with the implication that they may be more passive copers, but others finding no age differences (Aldwin, 1991). However, Aldwin, Sutton, Chiara, and Spiro (1996) distinguished between coping effort and coping efficacy, arguing that older adults conserve their resources when by using fewer strategies when coping with stress (see also Baltes, Lindberger, & Staudinger, 2006; Hobfoll, 2004), but that they may rate the coping as equally efficacious as younger adults. For example, a middle-aged man, when confronted with a flooded cellar, is likely to try to figure out the problem and solve it, often necessitating several hours of labor and multiple trips to the hardware store. An 80-year-old man, on the other hand, will wisely avoid wading into the cellar, and is more likely to call his son to come fix it. Both strategies are efficacious, but the latter conserves effort.

However, not all studies find that older adults are just as efficacious as younger adults. Although Newth and DeLongis (2004) supported the Aldwin et al. study, others found that older adults reported lower levels of efficacy (Logan, Pelletier-Hibbert, & Hodgins, 2006). However, these studies examined efficacy in individuals coping with painful chronic illnesses, which may be less amenable to coping strategies. Zautra and Wrabetz (1991) controlled for various stressor characteristics, and confirmed that age was unrelated to coping efficacy, which implies the continuity of coping efficacy into late life.

Thus, early theories of coping and aging focused on somewhat simple questions of whether older adults were "better" or "worse" copers, or whether they were more "active" or "passive." They were limited by relatively simplistic constructs of coping and by the conflation of coping effort with coping efficacy. Further, by reliance on cross-sectional studies, they confounded age and cohort differences, as well as stressor characteristics. In contrast, more current coping theories examine the process through which age can affect the stress and coping process, and examine more specific, nuanced coping strategies, and, more rarely, the longitudinal changes in coping processes and outcomes as well.

Current Theories of Coping and Aging

Current theories addressing how older individuals cope with stress have broadened into several different types. Perhaps the most common are theories that deal with adaptive styles. As we shall see, they have grown out of developmental theory rather than stress and coping theory, and thus use somewhat different terminology, but do examine age differences and sometimes changes in adaptation with age. Current coping process approaches, on the other hand, try to examine *why* and *how* specific coping strategies change with age, and are more likely to be focused on positive age-related changes. As we shall see, however, the field is growing toward a greater emphasis on self-regulation and resilience processes, which may or may not take place within a stressful situation.

COPING/ADAPTIVE STYLES

A common assumption of life-span developmental theories is that the increasing physical and sometimes cognitive limitations with age necessitate changes in adaptive processes. There are four major theories in this category: selection, optimization, and compensation (SOC) theory (Baltes & Staudinger, 2000); the related socioemotional selectivity theory (SST; Charles & Carstensen, 2014); primary and secondary control theory (Schulz & Heckhausen, 1999); and assimilation/accommodation theory (Rothermund & Brandtstädter, 2003).

SOC THEORY

SOC theory argues that, in the face of declining resources, older individuals must select which goals or activities to focus on, optimize their performance of these activities, and compensate for any limitations. The oft-used example is Vladimir Horowitz, the famous pianist known for his fiery playing who kept performing into his 90s. Horowitz is reported to have done so by decreasing his repertoire (i.e., *selecting* his best pieces) and focusing on practicing (*optimizing*) those pieces. To compensate for age-related slowing, Horowitz would slow the pace right before a particularly fiery episode, with the contrast enhancing the apparent speed (*compensating*).

For a very influential theory, there have been surprisingly few explicit empirical tests of SOC, and the ones that exist sometimes provide only partial support. Lang, Rohr, and Williger (2011) divided this literature into cognitive and psychosocial studies. They interpreted the results of cognitive multitasking studies as showing support for selection—older adults are much more likely to focus on one of the tasks than younger adults, who are better able to divide their attention. However, children also are more likely to focus on just one of the tasks.

Psychosocial studies make it clear that SOC is not just a theory of adaptation in late life, but describes strategies that are used throughout the life span and are associated with positive outcomes at many stages. For example, it makes good sense that younger adults who are able to focus (select) and optimize career-related strategies are more successful and report higher job satisfaction (Abele & Wiese, 2008). However, Freund and Baltes (1998) found that age correlated negatively with both selection and optimization, but positively with compensation, a finding replicated by other studies (see Freund, 2008). If older adults were being forced to select among activities caused by decreased resources, selection should be positively related to age. However, Freund argues that selection decreases as a strategy because all resources decrease. But if that were the case, then compensation should also decline.

Although it is intuitively appealing that older adults decrease in their activities and are forced to select, optimize, and compensate, Aldag (1997) did not find evidence for decreased activity levels. She interviewed older adults (aged 70+ years) in a subsidized housing community, examining self-reported change and stability over 5 years in five domains: house maintenance, social, physical, cognitive, and passive leisure. She found that housekeeping was the only domain in which there was a consistent decrease in activities. In other areas, there was often stability and sometime increases in activity levels, for example, when the older adults would join a new social group or take up a new hobby. However, partial evidence for SOC theory was found. Consistent with Freund's (2008) emphasis on the importance of resources, individuals with higher resources were more likely to use selection, while those with lower resources were more likely to drop activities, but they also were more likely to use both compensatory and optimization strategies. Thus, clearly more work is needed on when and if older adults use these types of adaptive strategies, which may vary by resource level and possibility of control.

Charles and Carstensen (2014) argued that socioemotional selectivity is the fundamental hallmark of adaptation in late life. The basic tenet of SST is that the recognition of a limited amount of time to live prompts unconscious shifts in motivation. For example, the positivity bias in late life is fairly well established, with numerous studies showing that older adults tend to avoid paying attention to negative or unpleasant situations and focus more on positive ones. Further, emotional salience of relationships takes center stage, with individuals focusing more on meaningful relationships with close significant others rather than attempting to enlarge their social networks. Thus, older adults may selectively deploy their attention and resources in social situations to enhance self-regulation and control.

PRIMARY AND SECONDARY CONTROL THEORY

Primary and secondary control theory (Schulz & Heckhausen, 1999) also assumes that resources decrease with age, and argues that younger adults are more likely to use primary control to exert influence over the environment, but that older adults are faced more with losses and thus use secondary control to manage their emotions. However, as Skaff (2007) pointed out, there are both global and domain-specific control beliefs that may change differentially with age. There are undoubtedly individual differences in that change, as well as clear sociohistorical context and cohort effects. Further, she argued that one must distinguish between control beliefs and efforts used to exert control, and cited Baltes and Smith (1999), who argued that internally direct efforts may be more adaptive in later life. Skaff suggested that, with age, individuals may simply become more realistic about what is actually controllable in the environment.

From a stress and coping point of view, we have known for decades that individuals use both problem- and emotion-focused strategies in the vast majority of situations (Folkman & Lazarus, 1980). Furthermore, in the child development literature, researchers often emphasize that self-control is a prerequisite for effective environmental control (e.g., Diaz & Eisenberg, 2015). Most difficulties have multiple dimensions that can evoke problem-focused strategies even in the face of uncontrollable losses. For example, the first author conducted a series of interviews on coping strategies in older men (Aldwin et al., 1996), and was surprised to find reports of problem-focused coping with seemingly uncontrollable stressors such as bereavement. Inspection of the interviews showed that these men were focused on funeral arrangements, dealing with wills, the disposition of assets, and other aspects of the situation which were amenable to control and thus problem-focused coping. Similarly, Aldwin (1991) found that health problems evoked both problem-focused strategies and a sense of efficacy in older adults. As any caregiver knows, even if a health problem is unavoidable, it still may create a host of other problems (medication management, doctors' appointments, etc.) that require problem-focused skills and management. Thus, both primary and secondary control are processes necessary for adaptation across the life span.

ASSIMILATION AND ACCOMMODATION THEORY

Assimilation and accommodation theory (Rothermund & Brandstädter, 2003) addresses the interplay between different types of control processes, and argues that a sense of control can be maintained in late life through focusing on those roles in which control can be executed. "Assimilation" refers to goal-oriented activities aimed at shaping one's environment and personal development. "Accommodation," on the other hand, refers to changing one's goals when efforts to achieve the original goals prove not to be feasible. They argued that accommodative processes increase in later life, and present evidence suggesting that individuals who do this developmental shift have higher levels of well-being in late life. Dockendorff (2014) also found that accommodative processes were most effective with stressors involving losses.

More recent work, however, recognized that these adaptive modes may be complementary rather than antagonistic. Brandtstädter, Rothermund, Kranz, and Kühn (2010) conducted a series of studies showing a shift toward "value-rational," or intrinsic, self-transcendent goals in late life. Indeed, Staudinger and Bowen (2010) presented cogent arguments for the difference between adjustment versus growth in later life, with adjustment reflecting the effects of problem-focused coping and hedonic well-being, but growth relating to more intrinsic processes related to the meaning of life. Clearly, older adults use adaptive strategies in complex ways, depending on their resource levels and the types of problems they face.

COPING PROCESSES

In general, coping process studies have shown that older adults use more adaptive strategies and are better at emotion regulation. They are less likely to ruminate, use escape/avoidant strategies, express hostility, use wishful thinking and emotional numbing, and are more likely to use positive reappraisal (for a review, see Aldwin, 2011). In interpersonal situations, they may be particularly effective, as they are less likely to become angry (Blanchard-Fields & Coates, 2008; Coats & Blanchard-Fields, 2008). They may be more likely to use dyadic coping strategies than younger adults, especially when confronted by chronic illnesses (Berg & Upchurch, 2007). Of course, their ability to problem solve effectively is affected by cognitive status—individuals with mild cognitive impairment may also have impaired problem-solving abilities (Diehl et al., 2005).

One important issue being addressed is whether older adults are more vulnerable to psychosocial stress. We know that older individuals are more vulnerable to physical stressors—the thousands of older adults who died in Europe in a heat wave a few years ago is a good example. Older adults have chronic illnesses such as heart disease and diabetes, which may make it more difficult for them to regulate stress and be more vulnerable to the adverse effects of physical stressors. However, the evidence for vulnerability to psychosocial stress is extremely mixed, with some suggesting that older adults are more vulnerable, and others that they are less (for reviews, see Aldwin, Park, & Spiro, 2007; Charles, 2010).

Both Charles's (2010) Strength and Vulnerability Integration (SAVI) model and Aldwin et al.'s (2007) model, which we now are calling the "Coping, Appraisal, and Resilience in Aging" (CARA) model, suggest similar solutions to this dilemma. The basic idea is that older adults recognize their heightened vulnerability to stress of all sorts, so they take steps to either prevent the occurrence of stress or to minimize its impact through both appraisal and coping processes. The SAVI model focuses on coping. Older adults use a variety of proactive coping strategies to avoid stressors such as making extensive preparations for any activity that could potentially result in problems. For example, Johnson and Barrer (1993) found that 80-year-olds who were still driving in San Francisco would carefully plot out routes that avoided making left-hand turns.

Although acknowledging the importance of coping, the CARA model focuses more on appraisal processes. Older adults may also be less likely than younger or middle-aged adults to appraise situations as a problem, and, if a problem is acknowledged, it may be rated as less stressful (Boeninger, Shiraishi, Aldwin, & Spiro, 2009; Park, Aldwin, Fenster, & Snyder, 2008). For example, one man in an earlier study mentioned that he used to get upset about a lot of things, but he developed high blood pressure, so he learned how just not to get bothered so much (Aldwin et al., 1996). Not becoming stressed in the first place is a more efficient strategy than having to cope with the distress caused by appraising a situation as problematic.

In general, the study of coping and aging is gradually shifting toward a self-regulation perspective, with the recognition that people not only actively respond to an immediate stressor but also seek to arrange their lives in ways that minimize stressors and maximize positive affect and perhaps meaning as well.

Summary

In summary, the field of coping and aging has come a long way in the past few decades: from early studies suggesting that older adults are more passive and "worse" copers, to the current recognition that coping processes and adaptive styles in later life are flexible, develop through experience, and result in complex patterns of changes in appraisal and self-regulation processes that vary by resource level and environmental demands. Older adults, barring cognitive impairment or long-standing mental illness, have learned self-regulation skills that minimize distress, and cope in ways that make the most efficient use of changing resources. They can become more adept at regulating their emotions, and focus on maintenance of meaningful close relationships. These skills may form the basis of resilience in late life.

■ RESILIENCE AND OPTIMAL AGING

The concept of resilience grew out of a recognition that even children who have experienced extreme trauma grow up to lead mostly relatively normal lives (Masten & Wright, 2010; Werner & Smith, 2001). Thus, resilience focuses on the strengths that individuals, families, and communities have, while recognizing vulnerabilities and barriers. It focuses on understanding positive development within a context of adversity.

Although resilience research has focused largely on childhood and adolescence, how older adults cope with difficulties, yet experience positive outcomes, is important to deepen our understanding of development across the life course. Adult resilience has been studied within the contexts of daily stress, normative life events, and trauma such as the death of a loved one, chronic illness, caregiving, and natural disasters (Bonanno, 2004; Brewin, Andrews, & Valentine, 2000; Ong, Bergeman, & Boker, 2009; Phifer, 1990; Windle, Woods, & Markland, 2010; Zautra, Johnson, & Davis, 2005). Outcomes of resilience processes include recovery (Greene, Hantman, Sharabi, & Cohen, 2012; Mancini & Bonanno, 2010), the capacity to move forward and sustain positive meaning (Zautra, Hall, & Murray, 2010), and transformation growth as in gerotranscendence (Tornstam, 1994).

Developmental research in resilience spans four decades and continues to wrestle with descriptive and explanatory challenges inherent in a multidimensional and contextualized construct. These struggles are understandable, given the ever-broadening lens that attempts to model resilience from "cells to society" (Anderson, 1998) as well as "society to cells" (Szanton, Gill, & Thorpe, 2010). We briefly review the historical progression of research followed by several current definitions of resilience. We then turn to current tensions in understanding resilience in later life. Specifically, we consider the contributions of hedonic and eudaimonic well-being in the processes of resilience in later life and offer a new definition of resilience. Finally, we explore the importance of culturally sensitive approaches to research that emphasize essential elements to understand the heterogeneity and homogeneity of resilience processes and outcomes.

History of Resilience Research

Early research in resilience attempted to understand the development of children raised in adverse environments. Landmark longitudinal studies observed unanticipated cases of competence and an absence of psychopathology in children raised in situations perceived to be of high risk, such as parents with severe mental illness (Garmezy, 1991; Garmezy & Streitman, 1974), poverty, and family instability (Rutter, 1985; Werner, 1993,

1995). Details of this rich history exceed the limits of this chapter (see Ryff, Singer, Love, & Essex, 1998), but the results represent three waves of research that evolved from descriptive to prescriptive (Masten & Wright, 2010).

The first wave of studies was primarily descriptive and focused on attributes of resilience such as individual traits associated with positive outcomes (Garmezy, 1991; Rutter, 1979; Werner, 1993). Examples of individual capabilities that have continued to demonstrate protective value include a sense of agency or self-efficacy (Ryan & Deci, 2001), healthy brain development (Posner, Rothbart, Sheese, & Tang, 2007), and self-regulation (Masten & Coatsworth, 1998). Similarly, there has been an effort in the study of adult resilience to identify individual attributes associated with resilience as reflected in various measures of resilience (for a review, see Windle, Nennett, & Noyes, 2011). Although there is a consensus that resilience is not a trait of the individual, certain individual-level attributes such as a persons' capacity to regulate their emotions may be especially useful at any time in the life course in order to navigate the environment. In adults, emotion regulation is necessary for contemplation, planning, and control over emotions under stress (Urry & Gross, 2010).

A second wave of research moved from relatively static individual-level attributes to processes and pathways of influence associated with successful adaptation such as family cohesion (Garmezy, 1993) and support from peers or elders (Werner, 1995). Protective processes that have continued to demonstrate consistency in promoting positive development in the context of adversity include healthy attachments and relationships (see Masten & Obradovic, 2008), cultural traditions (Crawford, Wrights, & Masten, 2006), and a coherent sense of meaning (Janoff-Bulman, 1992; Park, 2010; Werner & Smith, 2001). Of these, relationships are a powerful protective factor. Luthar (2006) reviewed decades of child development research and concluded that "resilience rests, fundamentally, on relationships" (p. 780). Social relations are an important resilience resource in adults under stress as well (Fuller-Iglesias, Sellars, & Antonucci, 2008; Kahn & Antonucci, 1980; King, King, Fairbank, Keane, & Adams, 1998). A meta-analysis of trauma-exposed adults found the absence of social support was a leading risk factor in the development of posttraumatic stress disorder (Brewin et al., 2000).

The third wave in childhood resilience saw the development of interventions and this continues today with interventions targeted to improve protective factors such as effective parenting (e.g., Sandler, Schoenfelder, Wolchik, & MacKinnon, 2011) and executive control (e.g., Diamond & Lee, 2011). The ultimate goal in adult resilience research is also the development of culturally relevant interventions that foster resilience (Southwick, Bonanno, Masten, Panter-Brick, & Yehuda, 2014).

The fourth and current wave in child, youth, and adult resilience research is described as "integrative" (Masten & Wright, 2010, p. 214). At a 2013 plenary panel at the International Society for Traumatic Stress Studies, leading researchers agreed that the study of resilience included "genetic, epigenetic, developmental, demographic, cultural, economic, and social variables" (Southwick et al., 2014, p. 1). Ecological models of resilience attempt to consider multiple levels, bidirectional relationships, and the complex individual. However, our understanding of resilience in this manner is "nascent" (Ungar, 2011, p. 1)—and, without specifying structural relationships, may be overly broad.

Current Definitions of Resilience

Popular and academic uses of the term "resilience" have generated numerous definitions and applications (Allen, Haley, Harris, Fowler, & Pruthi, 2011), and this has contributed to the inconsistent usage of "resilience" as an individual trait, a process, and an outcome. Although the early child-development literature initially took more of a trait-based approach (Garmezy, 1991), currently, resilience is defined as a "dynamic process encompassing positive adaptation within the context of significant adversity" (Luthar, Cicchetti, & Becker, 2000, p. 543), suggesting that resilience is both process and outcome. That is, resilience is not a trait of the individual but "arises from many processes and interactions that extend beyond the boundaries of the individual organism, including close relationships and social support" (Masten & Wright, 2010, p. 215). From a life-span developmental perspective, Lerner et al. (2012) similarly stated that resilience is not a quality of a person but is "a dynamic attribute of the relationship between an individual and his or her multilevel and integrated (relational) developmental system" (p. 276) represented as individual ←→ context transaction.

Resilience in Later Life

Efforts to understand resilience in later life have been wide ranging, in part because the criteria for successful development in later life is unclear. Positive adult development can be conceptualized as well-being that is hedonic or eudaimonic in tone (Friedman & Ryff, 2012; Ryff & Singer, 2008). Hedonic well-being is commonly associated with happiness, subjective well-being, and characterized by seeking positive affective states (Staudinger & Bowen, 2010). The ability to maintain positive affect in the presence of serious difficulties, such as illness, has been studied as an attribute of resilience in later life (Zautra et al., 2005, 2010). Much of the literature supports the benefits of positive affect for recovery from challenges in life (for a review, see Pressman & Cohen, 2005) via improved problem solving, perseverance (Isen, 2003), and successful emotion regulation (Charles & Carstensen, 2014; Stawski, Sliwinski, Almeida, & Smyth, 2012).

In contrast, eudaimonic well-being is often described as having a sense of purpose, mastery, and accomplishment (Ryff & Singer, 2008). Following a major stressful event, how a person makes sense of life is central to prominent theories of posttraumatic growth (Janoff-Bulman, 1992, 2004; Linley & Joseph, 2004; Tedeschi & Calhoun, 2004) and stress-related growth (Aldwin & Levenson, 2004). Making sense of life involves a philosophy of life that is articulated in assumptions, beliefs, values, and worldviews (Schwartz & Boehnke, 2004; Wong, 2012). The importance of meaning in life to resilience is demonstrated in a qualitative study of 24 older women (age range 67–92 years) who had successfully adjusted to a major loss. Although not limited to later life, five themes emerged: equanimity, perseverance, self-reliance, meaningfulness of life, and "existential aloneness" (sense of freedom and uniqueness; Wagnild & Young, 1990, p. 254). Hedonic and eudaimonic well-being are not mutually exclusive, but how they work together in the resilience process is not well understood.

Resilience in later life has also been conceptualized as successful aging (Harris, 2008; Hochhalter, Smith, & Ory, 2011). The term "successful aging" was first used by Havighurst (1961) and defined in terms of maximal life satisfaction. Thus, a person's ability to experience positive outcomes in the face of challenges such as bereavement and changes in health can be considered a demonstration of successful aging (Depp, Vahia, & Jeste, 2010; Montross et al., 2006). Early theories of successful aging focused on life satisfaction (Havighurst, 1961) and were contrasted with Rowe and Kahn's (1997) greater attention to the contributions of good physical health. However, reviews of this extensive literature (Aldwin & Gilmer, 2013; Depp et al., 2010; Friedman & Ryff, 2012) suggest that understanding the process of responding to late life challenges may be more informative than criteria of physical, psychological, or emotional health (Aldwin & Igarashi, 2015). The World Health Organization defined successful aging as "the process of optimizing opportunities for health, participation and security in order to enhance quality of life as people age" (2002, p. 12).

New Definition of Resilience in Adulthood

A new definition of resilience in later life is necessary, one that is broad enough to permit multiple types of successful aging as well as equifinality, but specific enough to support the development of psychometrically adequate measures. This approach reflects the current paradigm shift in developmental science away from causal, reductionistic models and toward a relational developmental perspective (Aldwin, 2014; Antonucci & Webster, 2014; Lerner, Agans, DeSourza, & Hershberg, 2014).

We define resilience as *the ability to recognize, utilize, and develop or modify resources at the individual, community, and sociocultural levels in the service of three goal-related processes.* First, resilience includes effective coping efforts directed toward maintaining functional ability (e.g., physical, cognitive, and psychological health), given current strengths and limitations. Second, resilience in late life includes the development of a comfortable life structure (see Cruikshank, 2013) that affords not only basic human needs but also sufficient social interaction, as well as physical and cognitive stimulation, to support continued positive adaptation. Finally, resilience processes in late life often draw upon and are informed by a sense of purpose in life, which allows for the possibility of greater self-knowledge and integration, a meaningful existence, self-transcendence, and the development of wisdom.

Ecological Model of Resilience: Applications to Later Life

As indicated earlier, the newer models of resilience focus on the individual ←→ context transaction, with the implication that resilience in later life results from a dynamic transaction between individuals and their contexts, whether in the immediate community or in the larger sociocultural context (Lerner et al., 2012; Ungar, Ghazinour, & Richter, 2012). Aldwin and Igarashi (2012) developed a contextualized, transactional model of the resilience process. Rather than competing definitions as to whether resilience is a resource, a process, or an outcome, we attempted to develop a model that shows the structural relations between these different aspects of resilience. For this chapter, we have modified this figure to better represent the CARA model (see Figure 28.1). Note that the model follows a systems perspective. Although we have divided this into three panels or levels (resources, processes, and outcomes), from a systems perspective, these are somewhat arbitrary designations, because all levels of the system can transact both within and across levels to create change over time.

The panel on the left indicates the different types of *resilience resources,* which exist at the individual, community, and larger sociocultural levels. Individual resources include factors such as intelligence, emotional stability, a positive developmental history, and physical fitness. Community resources include family and social support, local religious and medical institutions, as well as public resources, including senior centers, information and referral services, age-friendly built environments, and the like. Sociocultural resources include aging-supportive institutions and policies.

The middle panel represents the *resilience outcomes.* Over the course of a lifetime of coping with stress, individuals can develop generalized resistance resources (GRRs;

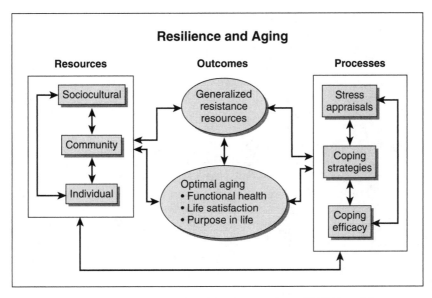

FIGURE 28.1 The Coping, Appraisal, and Resilience in Aging (CARA) model.

Antonovsky, 1987) that include both social capital (e.g., social support systems, finan-cial resources) and individual capital (e.g., mastery, values, purpose in life). The devel-opment of GRRs, however, does not result solely from stress and coping processes, but rather occurs within a larger context. It is influenced also by individual, commu-nity, and sociocultural resources. The ability to use these resources, GRRs, and to use appropriate appraisal and coping strategies, all feed into optimal aging and its three related goal processes: functional health, life satisfaction, and purpose in life. Thus, optimal aging in this model can be seen as the ultimate outcome of these processes, but it also feeds back into both the stress and coping process, as well as the development of resources for both one's self and for the community and perhaps culture as a whole.

Resilience processes are depicted in the panel on the right. As mentioned earlier, older adults may choose not to appraise situations as problems or as very stressful. For exam-ple, Aldwin et al. (1996) found that older men who were caregiving for their spouses did not perceive this to be a "problem" unless their usual management strategies did not work and/or there was a crisis of some sort such as a visit to the emergency room. When they do need to cope with problems, they may do so in a way that minimizes expendi-ture of resources but still maintains efficacy. Stress-related growth theory (e.g., Aldwin & Levenson, 2004; Park et al., 2008) holds that individuals can develop resources such as coping skills, mastery, social support, self-knowledge, and spirituality through coping with difficulties, which can then be used in future stressful episodes.

Age stereotypes are a sociocultural factor that can influence individual functional health. Children are presented with culturally constructed views of what it means to be old through books, movies, television, and the general cultural milieu that are internalized across the life span (Levy & Banaji, 2002). Although beliefs about older age include positive assumptions such as increased wisdom, the most pernicious ste-reotypes assume an inevitable and progressive deterioration of physical and cognitive health during adulthood (Masoro, 2006). These stereotypes can become self-perceptions (i.e., internalized), which can predict all-cause mortality when quantified as a person's satisfaction with aging (Levy, Slade, Kunkel, & Kasl, 2002). In a prospective study of participants 70 years and older, those with more negative age stereotypes at baseline (i.e., below median score) had a 50% greater likelihood of hospitalization than those with above median scores 10 years later (Levy, Slade, Chung, & Gill, 2015). However, individuals' own actions can defy negative age stereotypes, as when older adults continue to work, engage in community activities, run marathons, produce artwork, and so on. Potentially, perceptions of aging could be transformed into a resilience resource by engagement in transactional dialogues where our language and images of what it means to grow older are represented by a full spectrum.

The second resilience-related goal is the development of a comfortable life structure that supports basic needs and sufficient social interaction, as well as physical and cognitive stimulation. For example, Greene (2010) studied Holocaust survivors who benefited from U.S. immigration policies for displaced persons to illustrate how people navigate toward resources: "We were hopeful because the States offered so many possibilities we didn't have" (Greene, 2010, p. 418). Governmental policies can support individuals' efforts to meet basic needs and develop comfortable life structures. However, older individuals can and do influence government policy, and have been very successful in garnering supportive policies, such as Medicare and Meals on Wheels.

The community and the larger sociocultural milieu can provide opportunities for older adults to develop the third resilience-related goal, purpose in life. Although individuals often have their own individual or family-related goals, communities can provide opportunities for volunteer work, as many local hospitals and museums do, or through programs such as the Retired and Senior Volunteer Program (RSVP) or the Library of Congress's effort to collect oral histories from veterans and survivors of various conflicts in the past century. For example, some Holocaust survivors developed a purpose in life by using their stories in an attempt to promote peace: "I talked a lot about the past…maybe teach the world a lesson not to hate or kill but to be kind to each other" (Greene, 2010, p. 420). Sharing this message of kindness and hope is one way in which an individual can not only influence his or her social environment but also manifest self-transcendence in terms of having a broader goal than simply one's own well-being. The influence of beliefs, values, and meaning at the various levels of society, community, family, and individual is woven throughout CARA. Just as age stereotypes develop outside of our awareness, explicit understanding of implicit belief systems is the task of meaningful studies about how resilience may differ in diverse groups of people.

Ethnic and Cultural Diversity in Resilience

An important consideration is whether or not there are cultural and ethnic differences in conceptions and processes of resilience. There is surprisingly little work done on resilience in older ethnic groups, although more work has been done with adolescents (Ungar et al., 2007, 2008). We know that religiousness/spirituality (Chatters, Nguyen, & Taylor, 2014), social support/family embeddedness (Dilworth-Anderson & Hilliard, 2014), and optimism (Baldwin, Jackson, Okoh, & Cannon, 2010) are extremely important for minority elders in the United States. However, these constructs have also been shown to be important for optimal aging in most groups (Aldwin & Igarashi, 2015).

Becker and Newsom (2005) examined how racism and discrimination influenced the "philosophy of resilience" in 38 older African Americans (ages 65–91 years) who were living with chronic illness. All respondents shared a philosophy of resilience based on equality and personal autonomy, which was "root[ed] in their long struggle for freedom and equality" and from "situational contexts such as poverty to evolve over the life course into highly specific ways of viewing the world" (p. 221). Cultural values of religiosity, independence, and survival were linked to their current perseverance. Race and ethnicity provided some of the cultural meaning, but historical time and geographic location also define a dynamic context that shapes resilience.

A handful of studies have examined the importance of culturally specific constructs in conceptions of optimal aging. For example, "fictive kin" are particularly important in promoting resilience in African Americans at risk (Hall, 2013). Cross-nationally, two such constructs are *lojong* (the Buddhist practice of cultivating compassion through refining motivations and attitudes) in Tibetan culture and the notion of "harmonious aging" in broader Asian cultures. Lewis (2013) interviewed Tibetan refugees in India, one of whom described a resilient person as someone who is compassionate, humble, does not exaggerate negative emotions, and "has a flexible, vast, and spacious mind" (*lojong*; Lewis, p. 322). At first glance, these characteristics seem far afield from Western notions of resilience as competence, control, and self-esteem (Windle et al., 2010). But further understanding of *lojong* and its incorporation into daily life reveal engagement in a traditional practice to transform suffering (Lewis, 2013) that suggests a type of competence and control. An older female respondent stated, "These people are very skillful because they don't disturb others with their many problems" (Lewis, p. 322).

Among Asian cultures, the notion of harmonious aging has been raised as an alternative to Western ideals of successful aging (Liang & Luo, 2012). From Liang and Luo's perspective, the emphasis is on recognizing both the challenges and opportunities of the aging process, as well as the dialectic between activity and disengagement. It also emphasizes integrating the mind and the body, and the interconnectedness of all humans. Becvar (2013) published a book on family resilience that included research reviews on ethnic family systems, including Latinos (Bermudez & Mancini, 2013), African Americans (Hollingsworth, 2013), Koreans (Rigazio-DiGilio & Ki, 2013), and Native Americans (Robbins, Robbins, & Stennerson, 2013). Although Gallant, Spitze, and Grove (2010) argue that such deep cultural understanding is important in developing culturally appropriate interventions, McCubbin and McCubbin (2013) pointed out that studies that seek to understand ethnic differences in constructs such as resilience run the risk of promoting stereotypes among minorities and ignoring the considerable individual differences within ethnic groups.

The approach taken by Ungar et al. (2007) attempted to address this issue of deep cultural understanding. In a study of 11 countries, they identified seven dimensions, identified as tensions that work with each other to create processes associated with resilience (Ungar et al., 2007, 2012). Emergent tensions included: (a) access to material resources; (b) relationships; (c) identity (sense of self); (d) cohesion (balance between responsibility to self and others); (e) power/control (agency); (f) cultural adherence (adherence/opposition of global and local culture, values, beliefs); and (g) social justice (social equality, meaningful role in society; Ungar et al., see p. 295).

As an illustration, Ungar et al.'s (2007) tensions can be applied to Panter-Brick and Eggerman's (2012) study of Afghan youth and their families, in which resilience was defined as the ability to navigate and negotiate both local and global cultures within a context of chronic human-made and natural crises. For both youth and their unemployed fathers, cultural values such as obligations of service to the family and community (coherence, cultural adherence) and social respectability (identity, cultural adherence) were tensions to be resolved when economic realities (material resources) forced students to quit school and go to work to support their families (relationships; coherence, cultural adherence). Attaining an education (material resource, agency) is seen by some as "a gateway to success" for individuals and their families (p. 381), which instilled hope (social justice), in spite of an infrastructure that was not able to provide better jobs for those who graduate (material resource).

Ungar et al. (2012) argued that these dimensions were common across the cultures they studied, but that the cultures differed in their relative emphasis. We argue that the definition of resilience in late life presented in this chapter may provide the same framework to understanding cultural differences in resilient or optimal aging. So, for example, the Tibetan and Asian definitions of resilient aging cited earlier appear to focus more on the eudaimonic dimension of resilience in aging, while others may emphasize the more functional health or hedonic aspects of aging.

■ FUTURE DIRECTIONS

Resilience is an inherently developmental construct. Although most definitions include some notion of positive development under adversity, there is as yet no consensus as to what that positive development consists of, whether resilience in early life differs from what is considered to be resilience in later life, or how cultural and sociohistorical factors may influence the construct of resilience. Although this profusion of issues reflects the richness of the construct, it creates measurement difficulties. The identification of the three dimensions of resilient aging here—effective coping in the service of maintenance of functional health, development of a comfortable life structure, and a sense of meaning or purpose in life and wisdom—provides a framework that is specific enough to afford the development of measures, yet broad enough to be able to reflect cultural differences in their relative emphases.

However, the model is at best an initial framework, which needs to be further developed. First, in keeping with the transactional nature of this model, we need to extend our understanding of how individuals' stress and coping processes affect others in their community, as well as the larger sociocultural repercussions. Second, we need to develop a "tool box" of measures that can tap these three dimensions of optimal aging and thus promote future research into the predictors, consequences, and diversity of resilience in late life. Finally, wisdom, which involves self-knowledge (Levenson & Aldwin, 2013), is important for aging across cultures (Lee, Choun, Aldwin, & Levenson, 2015). Thus, it is important to include this construct in our understanding of optimal or resilient aging. Future research should investigate whether individual wisdom may have positive effects, not only for individuals and their families, but for the broader community. Some Taoists believe that the main purpose of longevity is to develop wisdom. Understanding the role of wisdom in resilience, and the role of wise elders in community well-being, is the next important theoretical step.

■ ACKNOWLEDGMENTS

Preparation of this chapter was supported by National Institute on Aging (NIA) grant R01 AG032037.

REFERENCES

Abele, A. E., & Wiese, B. S. (2008). The nomological network of self-management strategies and career success. *Journal of Occupational and Organizational Psychology, 81*(4), 733–749.

Aldag, L. D. P. (1997). *Is use of selective optimization with compensation associated with successful aging?* (Doctoral dissertation), University of California, Davis, CA.

Aldwin, C. M. (1991). Does age affect the stress and coping process? Implications of age differences in perceived control. *Journal of Gerontology: Psychological Sciences, 46*, 174–180.

Aldwin, C. M. (2007). *Stress, coping, and development: An integrative perspective* (2nd ed.). New York, NY: Guilford Press.

Aldwin, C. M. (2011). Stress and coping across the lifespan. In S. Folkman (Ed.), *The Oxford handbook of stress, health, and coping* (pp. 15–24). New York, NY: Oxford University Press.

Aldwin, C. M. (2014). Rethinking developmental science. *Research in Human Development, 11*, 247–254.

Aldwin, C. M., & Gilmer, D. F. (2013). *Health, illness, and optimal aging: Biological and psychosocial perspectives* (2nd ed.). New York, NY: Springer Publishing Company.

Aldwin, C. M., & Igarashi, H. (2012). An ecological model of resilience in late life. *Annual Review of Gerontology & Geriatrics, 32*, 115–130.

Aldwin, C. M., & Igarashi, H. (2015). Successful, optional, and resilient aging: A psychosocial perspective. In B. T. Mast, P. A. Lichtenberg, & B. D. Carpenter (Eds.), *APA handbook of clinical geropsychology* (pp. 331–359). Washington, DC: American Psychological Association.

Aldwin, C. M., & Levenson, M. R. (2004). Posttraumatic growth: A developmental perspective. *Psychological Inquiry, 15*, 19–22.

Aldwin, C. M., Park, C. L., & Spiro, A. III (Eds.). (2007). *Handbook of health psychology and aging*. New York, NY: Guilford Press.

Aldwin, C. M., Sutton, K. J., Chiara, G., & Spiro, A. (1996). Age differences in stress, coping, and appraisal: Findings from the normative aging study. *The Journals of Gerontology, Series B, 51*, 179–188.

Aldwin, C. M., & Yancura, L. (2011). Stress, coping, and adult development. In R. J. Contrada & A. Baum (Eds.), *The handbook of stress science: Biology, psychology, and health* (pp. 263–274). New York, NY: Springer Publishing Company.

Allen, R. S., Haley, P. P., Harris, G. M., Fowler, S. N., & Pruthi, R. (2011). Resilience: Definitions, ambiguities, and applications. In B. Resnick, L. P. Gwyther, & K. A. Roberto (Eds.), *Resilience in aging: Concepts, research, and outcomes* (pp. 1–13). New York, NY: Springer Publishing Company.

Anderson, N. B. (1998). Levels of analysis in health science. A framework for integrating sociobehavioral and biomedical research. *Annals of the New York Academy of Sciences, 840*, 563–576.

Antonovsky, A. (1987). *Unraveling the mystery of health: How people manage stress and stay well.* San Francisco, CA: Jossey-Bass.

Antonucci, T. C., & Webster, N. J. (2014). Rethinking cells to society. *Research in Human Development, 11,* 309–322.

Baldwin, D. R., Jackson, D., Okoh, I., & Cannon, R. L. (2010). Resiliency and optimism: An African American senior citizen's perspective. *Journal of Black Psychology, 37,* 24–41.

Baltes, P. B., Lindenberger, U., & Staudinger, U. M. (2006). Life span theory in developmental psychology. In W. Damon & R. M. Lerner (Eds.), *Handbook of child psychology: Volume one theoretical models of human development* (6th ed., pp. 569–664). New York, NY: John Wiley.

Baltes, P. B., & Smith, J. (1999). Multilevel and systemic analyses of old age: Theoretical and empirical evidence for a fourth age. In V. L. Bengtson & K. W. Schaie (Eds.), *Handbook of theories of aging* (pp. 153–173). New York, NY: Springer Publishing Company.

Baltes, P. B., & Staudinger, U. M. (2000). Wisdom: A metaheuristic (pragmatic) to orchestrate mind and virtue toward excellence. *The American Psychologist, 55*(1), 122–136.

Becker, G., & Newsom, E. (2005). Resilience in the face of serious illness among chronically ill African Americans in later life. *The Journals of Gerontology, Series B, 60,* S214–S223.

Becvar, D. S. (2013). *Handbook of family resilience.* New York, NY: Springer Science+Business Media.

Berg, C. A., & Upchurch, R. (2007). A developmental-contextual model of couples coping with chronic illness across the adult life span. *Psychological Bulletin, 133,* 920–954.

Bermudez, J. M., & Mancini, J. A. (2013). Familias fuertes: Family resilience among Latinos. In D. S. Becvar (Ed.), *Handbook of family resilience* (pp. 215–227). New York, NY: Springer Science+Business Media.

Blanchard-Fields, F., & Coats, A. H. (2008). The experience of anger and sadness in everyday problems impacts age differences in emotion regulation. *Developmental Psychology, 44,* 1547.

Boeninger, D. K., Shiraishi, R. W., Aldwin, C. M., & Spiro, A. III. (2009). Why do older men report low stress ratings? Findings from the Veterans Affairs Normative Aging Study. *International Journal of Aging and Human Development, 68,* 149–170.

Bonanno, G. A. (2004). Loss, trauma, and human resilience: Have we under-estimated the human capacity to thrive after extremely aversive events? *The American Psychologist, 59,* 20–28.

Brandtstädter, J., Rothermund, K., Kranz, D., & Kühn, W. (2010). Final decentrations: Personal goals, rationality perspectives, and the awareness of life's finitude. *European Psychologist, 15*(2), 152–163.

Brewin, C. R., Andrews, B., & Valentine, J. D. (2000). Meta-analysis of risk factors for posttraumatic stress disorder in trauma-exposed adults. *Journal of Consulting and Clinical Psychology, 68*(5), 748–766.

Byrne, D. (1964). Repression-sensitization as a dimension of personality. In B. A. Maher (Ed.), *Progress in experimental personality research* (Vol. 1, pp. 169–220). New York, NY: Academic Press.

Carver, C. S., & Connor-Smith, J. (2010). Personality and coping. *Annual Review of Psychology, 61,* 679–704.

Carver, C. S., Scheier, M. F., & Weintraub, J. K. (1989) Assessing coping strategies: A theoretically based approach. *Journal of Personality and Social Psychology, 56,* 267–283.

Charles, S. T. (2010). Strength and vulnerability integration: A model of emotional well-being across adulthood. *Psychological Bulletin, 136,* 1068–1091.

Charles, S. T., & Carstensen, L. L. (2014). Emotion regulation and aging. In J. Gross (Ed.), *Handbook of emotion regulation* (2nd ed., pp. 203–218). New York, NY: Guilford Press.

Chatters, L. M., Nguyen, A. M., & Taylor, R. J. (2014). Religion and spirituality among older African Americans, Asians, and Hispanics. In K. E. Whitfield & T. A Baker (Eds.), *Handbook of minority aging* (pp. 47–64). New York, NY: Springer Publishing Company.

Coats, A. H., & Blanchard-Fields, F. (2008). Emotion regulation in interpersonal problems: The role of cognitive-emotional complexity, emotion regulation goals, and expressivity. *Psychology and Aging, 23,* 39–51.

Cramer, P. (2000). Defense mechanisms in psychology today: Further processes for adaptation. *The American Psychologist, 55,* 637–646.

Cramer, P. (2015). Defense mechanisms: 40 Years of empirical research. *Journal of Personality Assessment, 97,* 114–122.

Crawford, E., Wright, M. O., & Masten, A. S. (2006). Resilience and spirituality in youth. In E. C. Roehlkepartain, P. E. King, L. Wagener, & P. L. Benson (Eds.), *The handbook of spiritual development in childhood and adolescence* (pp. 355–370). Thousand Oaks, CA: Sage.

Cruikshank, M. (2013). *Learning to be old: Gender, culture, and aging* (3rd ed.). New York, NY: Rowman & Littlefield.

Depp, C., Vahia, I. V., & Jeste, D. (2010). Successful aging: Focus on cognitive and emotional health. *Annual Review of Clinical Psychology, 6,* 527–550.

Diamond, A., & Lee, K. (2011). Interventions shown to aid executive function development in children 4 to 12 years old. *Science, 333*(6045), 959–964.

Diaz, A., & Eisenberg, N. (2015). The process of emotion regulation is different from individual differences in emotion regulation: Conceptual arguments and a focus on individual differences. *Psychological Inquiry, 26,* 37–47.

Diehl, M., Chui, H., Hay, E. L. Lumley, M. A., Grühn, D., & Labouvie-Vief, G. (2014). Change in coping and defense mechanisms across adulthood: Longitudinal findings in a European American sample. *Developmental Psychology, 50,* 634–648.

Diehl, M., Marsiske, M., Horgas, A. L., Rosenberg, A., Saczynski, J. S., & Willis, S. L. (2005). The revised Observed Tasks of Daily Living: A performance-based assessment of everyday problem solving in older adults. *Journal of Applied Gerontology, 24,* 211–230.

Dilworth-Anderson, P., & Hilliard, T. S. (2014). Social networks and minority elders. In K. E. Whitfield & T. A Baker (Eds.), *Handbook of minority aging* (pp. 405–426). New York, NY: Springer Publishing Company.

Dockendorff, D. C. T. (2014). Healthy ways of coping with losses related to the aging process. *Educational Gerontology, 40*, 363–384.

Folkman, S., & Lazarus, R. S. (1980). An analysis of coping in middle-aged community sample. *Journal of Health and Social Behavior, 21*, 219–239.

Folkman, S., Lazarus, R. S., Pimley, S., & Novacek, J. (1987). Age differences in stress and coping processes. *Psychology and Aging, 2*, 171–184.

Freud, A. (1966). *The ego and the mechanisms of defense* (Rev. ed.). New York, NY: International Universities Press.

Freund, A. M. (2008). Successful aging as management of resources: The role of selection, optimization, and compensation. *Research in Human Development, 5*, 94–106.

Freund, A. M., & Baltes, P. B. (1998). Selection, optimization, and compensation as strategies of life management: Correlations with subjective indicators of successful aging. *Psychology and Aging, 13*(4), 531–543.

Friedman, E. M., & Ryff, C. D. (2012). Living well with medical co-morbidities: A biopsychosocial perspective. *The Journals of Gerontology, Series B, 67*, 535–544.

Fuller-Iglesias, H., Sellars, B., & Antonucci, T. C. (2008). Resilience in old age: Social relations as a protective factor. *Research in Human Development, 5*, 181–193.

Gallant, M. P., Spitze, G., & Grove, J. G. (2010). Chronic illness self-care and the family lives of older adults: A synthesis review across four ethnic groups. *Journal of Cross Cultural Gerontology, 25*, 21–43.

Garmezy, N. (1991). Resiliency and vulnerability of adverse developmental outcomes associated with poverty. *American Behavioral Scientist, 34*, 416–430.

Garmezy, N. (1993). Vulnerability and resistance. In D. C. Funder, R. D. Parke, C. Tomlinson-Keasey, & K. Widaman (Eds.), *Studying lives through time: Personality and development* (pp. 377–398). Washington, DC: American Psychological Association.

Garmezy, N., & Streitman, S. (1974). Children at risk: The search for the antecedents of schizophrenia: I. Conceptual models and research methods. *Schizophrenia Bulletin, 1*, 14–90.

Greene, R. R. (2010). Holocaust survivors: Resilience revisted. *Journal of Human Behavior in the Social Environment, 20*, 411–422.

Greene, R. R., Hantman, S., Sharabi, A., & Cohen, H. (2012). Holocaust survivors: Three waves of resilience research. *Journal of Evidence-Based Social Work, 9*, 481–497.

Gutmann, D. L. (1974). Alternatives to disengagement: The old men of the Highland Druze. In R. A. LeVine (Ed.), *Culture and personality: Contemporary readings* (pp. 232–245). Chicago, IL: Aldine.

Hall, J. C. (2013). Resilience despite risk: Understanding African-American ACOAS' kin and fictive kin relationships. In D. S. Becvar (Ed.), *Handbook of family resilience* (pp. 481–494). New York, NY: Springer Science+Business Media.

Harris, P. B. (2008). Another wrinkle in the debate about successful aging: The undervalued concept of resilience and the lived experience of dementia. *International Journal of Aging and Human Development, 67*, 43–61.

Havighurst, R. J. (1961). Successful aging. *The Gerontologist, 1*, 8–13.

Hobfoll, S. E. (2004). *Stress, culture, and community: The psychology and philosophy of stress.* New York, NY: Springer Science+Business Media.

Hochhalter, A., Smith, M. L., & Ory, M. G. (2011). Successful aging and resilience: Applications for public healh and health care. In B. Resnick, L. P. Gwyther, & K. Roberto (Eds.), *Resilience in aging: Concepts, research, and outcomes* (pp. 15–29). New York, NY: Springer Publishing Company.

Hollingsworth, L. D. (2013). Resilience in Black families. In D. S. Becvar (Ed.), *Handbook of family resilience* (pp. 229–243). New York, NY: Springer Science+Business Media.

Isen, A. M. (2003). Positive affect as a source of human strength. In L. G. Aspinwall & U. M. Staudinger (Eds.), *A psychology of human strengths: Fundamental questions and future directions for a positive psychology* (pp. 179–195). Washington, DC: American Psychological Association.

Janoff-Bulman, R. (1992). *Shattered assumptions: Towards a new psychology of trauma.* New York, NY: Free Press.

Janoff-Bulman, R. (2004). Posttraumatic growth: Three explanatory models. *Psychological Inquiry, 15*(1), 30–34.

Johnson, C. I., & Barer, B. M. (1993). Coping and a sense of control among the oldest old. *Journal of Aging Studies, 7*, 67–80.

Kahn, R. L., & Antonucci, T. C. (1980). Convoys over the life course: Attachment, roles and social support. In P. B. Baltes & O. B. Brim (Eds.), *Life-span development and behavior* (Vol. 3, pp. 253–268). New York, NY: Academic Press.

King, L. A., King, D. W., Fairbank, J. A., Keane, T. M., & Adams, G. A. (1998). Resilience–recovery factors in post-traumatic stress disorder among female and male Vietnam veterans: Hardiness, postwar social support, and additional stressful life events. *Journal of Personality and Social Psychology, 74*, 420–434.

Kliewer, W., Sandler, I. N., & Wolchik, S. (1994). Family socialization of threat appraisal and coping: Coaching, modeling, and family context. In K. Hurrelmann & F. Festmann (Eds.), *Social networks and social support in childhood and adolescence* (pp. 271–291). Berlin, DE: Walter de Gruyter.

Lang, F. R., Rohr, M. K., & Williger, B. (2011). Modeling success in life-span psychology: The principles of selection, optimization, and compensation. In K. L. Fingerman, C. A. Berg, J. Smith, T. C. Antonucci, & C. Toni (Eds.), *Handbook of life-span development* (pp. 57–85). New York, NY: Springer Publishing Company.

Lazarus, R. S., & Folkman, S. (1984). *Stress, appraisal, and coping.* New York, NY: Springer Publishing Company.

Lee, S., Choun. S., Levenson, M. R., & Aldwin, C. M. (2015). Cross-cultural comparison of self-transcendent wisdom between the United States and Korea. *Journal of Cross-Cultural Gerontology 30*, 143–161. doi: 10.1007/s10823-015-9259-8

Lerner, R. M., Agans, J. P., DeSourza, L. M., & Hershberg, R. M. (2014). Developmental science in 2025: A predictive review. *Research in Human Development, 11,* 255–272.

Lerner, R. M., Weiner, M. B., Arbeit, M. R., Chase, P. A., Agans, J. P., Schmid, K. L., & Warren, A. E. A. (2012). Resilience across the lifespan. *Annual Review of Gerontology/Geriatrics, 32,* 275–299.

Levenson, M. R., & Aldwin, C. M. (2013). The transpersonal in personal wisdom. In M. Ferrari & N. M. Westrate (Eds.), *The scientific study of personal wisdom: From contemplative traditions to neuroscience* (pp. 213–228). New York, NY: Springer.

Levenson, M. R., Aldwin, C. M., & Cupertino, A. P. (2001). Transcending the self: Towards a liberative model of adult development. In A. I. Neri (Ed.), *Maturidade & Velhice: Um enforque multidisciplinar* (pp. 99–116). Sao Paulo, BR: Papirus.

Levy, B. R., & Banaji, M. B. (2002). Implicit ageism. In T. D. Nelson (Ed.), *Ageism: Stereotyping and prejudice against older persons* (pp. 49–75). Cambridge, MA: MIT Press.

Levy, B. R., Slade, M. D., Chung, P. H., & Gill, T. M. (2015). Resiliency over time of elders' age stereotypes after encountering stressful events. *The Journals of Gerontology, Series B, 70*(6), 886–890. doi:10.1093/geronb/gbu082

Levy, B., Slade, M. D., Kunkel, S. R., & Kasl, S. V. (2002). Longevity increased by positive self-perceptions of aging. *Journal of Personality and Social Psychology, 83,* 261–270.

Lewis, S. E. (2013). Trauma and the making of flexible minds in the Tibetan exile community. *ETHOS, 41,* 313–336.

Liang, J., & Luo, B. (2012). Toward a discourse shift in social gerontology: From successful aging to harmonious aging. *Journal of Aging Studies, 26,* 327–334.

Linley, P. A., & Joseph, S. (2004). Positive change following trauma and adversity: A review. *Journal of Traumatic Stress, 17,* 11–21.

Logan, S. M., Pelletier Hibbert, M., & Hodgins, M. (2006). Stressors and coping of in-hospital haemodialysis patients aged 65 years and over. *Journal of Advanced Nursing, 56,* 382–391.

Luthar, S. S. (2006). Resilience in development: A synthesis of research across five decades. In D. Cicchetti & D. J. Cohen (Eds.), *Developmental psychopathology: Risk, disorder, and adaptation* (Vol. 3, 2nd ed., pp. 739–795). Hoboken, NJ: John Wiley.

Luthar, S. S., Cicchetti, D., & Becker, B. (2000). The construct of resilience: A critical evaluation and guidelines for future work. *Child Development, 71,* 543–562.

Mancini, A. D., & Bonanno, G. A. (2010). Resilience to potential trauma: Toward a lifespan approach. In J. W. Reich, A. J. Zautra, & J. S. Hall (Eds.), *Handbook of adult resilience* (pp. 258–280). New York, NY: Guilford Press.

Masoro, E. J. (2006). Are age-associated diseases an integral part of aging? In E. J. Masoro & S. N. Austad (Eds.), *Handbook of the biology of aging* (6th ed., pp. 43–62). New York, NY: Academic Press.

Masten, A. S., & Coatsworth, J. (1998). The development of competence in favorable and unfavorable environments: Lessons from research on successful children. *The American Psychologist, 53,* 205–220.

Masten, A. S., & Obradovic, J. (2008). Disaster preparation and recovery: Lessons from research on resilience in human development. *Ecology and Society, 13*(9). Retrieved from http://www.ecologyandsociety.org/vol13/iss1/art9

Masten, A. S., & Wright, M. O. (2010). Resilience over the lifespan: Developmental perspectives on resistance, recovery, and transformation. In J. W. Reich, A. J. Zautra, & J. S. Hall (Eds.), *Handbook of adult resilience* (pp. 213–237). New York, NY: Guilford Press.

McCrae, R. R. (1989). Age difference and changes in the use of coping mechanisms. *Journal of Gerontology, 44*, 161–169.

McCubbin, L. D., & McCubbin, H. I. (2013). Resilience in ethnic family systems: A relational theory for research and practice. In D. S. Becvar (Ed.), *Handbook of family resilience* (pp. 175–195). New York, NY: Springer Science+Business Media.

Miller, S. (1980). When is a little information a dangerous thing? Coping with stressful events by monitoring vs. blunting. In S. Levine & H. Ursin (Eds.), *Coping and health* (pp. 145–170). New York, NY: Plenum Press.

Montross, L. P., Depp, C., Daly, J., Reichstadt, J., Golshan, S., Moore, D...Jeste, D. V. (2006). Correlates of self-rated successful aging among community-dwelling older adults. *American Journal of Geriatric Psychiatry, 14*(1), 43–51.

Newth, S., & DeLongis, A. (2004). Individual differences, mood, and coping with chronic pain in rheumatoid arthritis: A daily process analysis. *Psychology and Health, 19*(3), 283–305.

Nolen-Hoeksema, S. (2000). The role of rumination in depressive disorders and mixed anxiety/depressive symptoms. *Journal of Abnormal Psychology, 109*, 504–511.

Ong, A. D., Bergeman, C. S., & Boker, S. M. (2009). Resilience comes of age: Defining features in later adulthood. *Journal of Personality, 77*, 1777–1804.

Panter-Brick, C., & Eggerman, M. (2012). Understanding culture, resilience, and mental health: The production of hope. In M. Ungar (Ed.), *The social ecology of resilience: A handbook of theory and practice* (pp. 369–386). New York, NY: Springer Publishing Company.

Pargament, K. I., Koenig, H. G., Tarakeshwar, N., & Hahn, J. (2004). Religious coping methods as predictors of psychological, physical and spiritual outcomes among medically ill elderly patients: A two-year longitudinal study. *Journal of Health Psychology, 9*, 713–730.

Park, C. L. (2010). Making sense of the meaning literature: An integrative review of meaning making and its effects on adjustment to stressful life events. *Psychological Bulletin, 136*, 257–301.

Park, C. L., Aldwin, C. M., Fenster, J., & Snyder, L. (2008). Pathways to post-traumatic growth versus post-traumatic stress: Exposure, coping and emotional reactions following the September 11, 2001, terrorist attacks. *American Journal of Orthopsychiatry, 78*, 300–312.

Phifer, J. F. (1990). Psychological distress and somatic symptoms after natural disaster: Differential vulnerability among older adults. *Psychology and Aging, 5*, 412–420.

Posner, M. I., Rothbart, M. K., Sheese, B. E., & Tang, Y. (2007). The anterior cingulate gyrus and the mechanism of self-regulation. *Cognitive, Affective, and Behavioral Neuroscience, 7*, 391–395.

Pressman, S. D., & Cohen, S. (2005). Does positive affect influence health? *Psychological Bulletin, 131*, 925–971.

Ptacek, J. T., Pierce, G. R., & Thompson, E. L. (2006). Finding evidence of dispositional coping. *Journal of Research in Personality, 40*, 1137–1151.

Rigazio-DiGilio, S., & Ki, P. (2013). Resilience relative to Korean families. In D. S. Becvar (Ed.), *Handbook of family resilience* (pp. 245–266). New York, NY: Springer Science+Business Media.

Robbins, R., Robbins, S., & Stennerson, B. (2013). Native American family resilience. In D. S. Becvar (Ed.), *Handbook of family resilience* (pp. 197–213). New York, NY: Springer Science+Business Media.

Roth, S., & Cohen, L. J. (1986). Approach, avoidance, and coping with stress. *The American Psychologist, 41*, 813–819.

Rothermund, K., & Brandstädter, J. (2003). Coping with deficits and losses in later life: From compensatory action to accommodation. *Psychology and Aging, 18*, 492–505.

Rowe, J., & Kahn, R. (1997). Successful aging. *The Gerontologist, 37*, 433–440.

Rutter, M. (1979). Protective factors in children's responses to stress and disadvantage. *Annals of the Academy of Medicine, Singapore, 8*, 324.

Rutter, M. (1985). Resilience in the face of adversity: Protective factors and resistance to psychiatric disorder. *British Journal of Psychiatry, 147*, 598–611.

Ryan, R. M., & Deci, E. L. (2001). On happiness and human potentials: A review of research on hedonic and eudaimonic well-being. *Annual Review of Psychology, 52*, 141–166.

Ryff, C. D., & Singer, B. H. (2008). Know thyself and become what you are: A eudaimonic approach to psychological well-being. *Journal of Happiness Studies, 9*, 13–39.

Ryff, C. D., Singer, B. H., Love, G. D., & Essex, M. (1998). Resilience in adulthood and later life: Defining features and dynamic processes. In J. Lomranz (Ed.), *Handbook of aging and mental health* (pp. 69–96). New York, NY: Springer Science+Business Media.

Sandler, I., Schoenfelder, E., Wolchik, S., & MacKinnon, D. (2011). Long-term impact of prevention programs to promote effective parenting: Lasting effects but uncertain processes. *Annual Review of Psychology, 62*, 299–329.

Schulz, R., & Heckhausen, J. (1999). Aging, culture and control: Setting a new research agenda. *The Journals of Gerontology, Series B, 54*, 139–145.

Schwartz, S. H., & Boehnke, K. (2004). Evaluating the structure of human values with confirmatory factor analysis. *Journal of Research in Personality, 38*, 230–255.

Skaff, M. M. (2007). Sense of control and health: A dynamic duo in the aging process. In C. M. Aldwin, C. L. Park, & A. Spiro III (Eds.), *Handbook of health psychology and aging* (pp. 186–209). New York, NY: Guilford Press.

Skinner, E. A., Edge, K., Altman, J., & Sherwood, H. (2003). Searching for the structure of coping: A review and critique of category systems for classifying ways of coping. *Psychological Bulletin, 129*(2), 216.

Skinner, E., & Edge, K. (2002). Parenting, motivation, and the development of children's coping. *Nebraska Symposium on Motivation, 48*, 77–143.

Southwick, S. M., Bonanno, G. M., Masten, A. S., Panter-Brick, C., & Yehuda, R. (2014). Resilience definitions, theory, and challenges: Interdisciplinary perspectives. *European Journal of Psychotraumatology, 5*(10), 3402. Retrieved from http://www .ejpt.net/index.php/ejpt/article/view/25338

Staudinger, U., & Bowen, C. (2010). Life-span perspectives on positive personality development in adulthood and old age. In M. E. L. Lamb & A. M. Freund (Eds.), *The handbook of life-span development* (pp. 254–297). Hoboken, NJ: John Wiley.

Stawski, R. S., Sliwinski, M. J., Almeida, D. M., & Smyth, J. M. (2012). Reported exposure and emotional reactivity to daily stressors: The roles of adult-age and global perceived stress. *Psychology and Aging, 23*, 52–61.

Szanton, S. L., Gill J. M., & Thorpe, R. J. Jr. (2010). The society-to-cells model of resilience in older adults. *Annual Review of Gerontology and Geriatrics, 32*, 5–34.

Tedeschi, R. G., & Calhoun, L. G. (2004). Posttraumatic growth: Conceptual foundations and empirical evidence. *Psychological Inquiry, 15*(1), 1–18.

Tornstam, L. (1994). Gerotranscendence: A theoretical and empirical exploration. In L. E. Thomas & S. A. Eisenhandler (Eds.), *Aging and the religious dimension* (pp. 203–225). Westport, CT: Greenwood Publishing Group.

Ungar, M. (2011). The social ecology of resilience: Addressing contextual and cultural ambiguity of a nascent construct. *American Journal of Orthopsychiatry, 81*, 1–17.

Ungar, M., Brown, M., Liebenberg, L., Othman, R., Kwong, W. M., Armstrong, M., & Gilgun, J. (2007). Unique pathways to resilience across cultures. *Adolescence, 42*, 287–310.

Ungar, M., Ghazinour, M., & Richter, J. (2012). Annual research review: What is resilience within the social ecology of human development? *Journal of Child Psychology and Psychiatry, 54*, 348–366.

Ungar, M., Liebenberg, L., Boothroyd, R., Kwong, W. M., Lee, T. Y., Leblanc, J…Makhnach, A. (2008). The study of youth resilience across cultures: Lessons from a pilot study of measurement development. *Research in Human Development, 5*, 166–180.

Urry, H. L., & Gross, J. J. (2010). Emotion regulation in older age. *Current Directions in Psychological Science, 19*, 352–357.

Ursano, R. J., Wheatly, R., Sledge, W., Rahe, A., & Carlson, E. (1986). Coping and recovery styles in the Vietnam era prisoner of war. *Journal of Nervous and Mental Disease, 175*, 273–275.

Vaillant, G. E. (1977). *Adaptation to life: How the best and the brightest came of age*. Boston, MA: Little, Brown.

Vaillant, G. E. (1993). *The wisdom of the ego*. Cambridge, MA: Harvard University Press.

Vaillant, G. E., Bond, M., & Vaillant, C. O. (1986). An empirically-validated hierarchy of defense mechanisms. *Archives of General Psychiatry, 43*(8), 786–794.

Wagnild, G. M., & Young, H. M. (1990). Resilience among older women. *Journal of Nursing Scholarship, 22*, 252–255.

Werner, E. E. (1993). Risk, resilience, and recovery: Perspectives from the Kauai Longitudinal Study. *Development and Psychopathology, 5,* 503–515.

Werner, E. E. (1995). Resilience in development. *Current Directions in Psychological Science, 4,* 81–85.

Werner, E. E., & Smith, R. S. (2001). *Journeys from childhood to midlife: Risk, resilience, and recovery.* Ithaca, NY: Cornell University Press.

Windle, G., Nennett, K. M., & Noyes, J. (2011). A methodological review of resilience measurement scales. *Health and Quality of Life Outcomes, 9*(8). Retrieved from http://www/hqlo.com/content/9/1/8

Windle, G., Woods, R. T., & Markland, D. A. (2010). Living with ill-health in older age: The role of a resilient personality. *Journal of Happiness Studies, 11,* 763–777.

Wong, P. T. P. (2012). Toward a dual-systems model of what makes life worth living. In P. T. Wong (Ed.), *The human quest for meaning: Theories, research, and applications* (2nd ed., pp. 3–22). New York, NY: Routledge.

World Health Organization (WHO). (2002). *The World Health Report 2002; reducing risks, promoting healthy life.* Retrieved from http://www.who.int/whr/2002

Zautra, A. J., Hall, J. S., & Murray, K. E. (2010). Resilience: A new definition of health for people and communities. In J. W. Reich, A. J. Zautra, & J. S. Hall (Eds.), *Handbook of adult resilience* (pp. 3–34). New York, NY: Guilford Press.

Zautra, A. J., Johnson, L. M., & Davis, M. C. (2005). Positive affect as a source of resilience for women in chronic pain. *Journal of Consulting and Clinical Psychology, 73,* 212–220.

Zautra, A. J., & Wrabetz, A. B. (1991). Coping success and its relationship to psychological distress for older adults. *Journal of Personality and Social Psychology, 61,* 801–810.

CHAPTER 29

Religion, Spirituality, and Aging
Peter G. Coleman, Elisabeth Schröder-Butterfill, and John H. Spreadbury

The subject of religion and the related topic of spirituality have become of increasing interest to gerontologists in the 21st century. This has resulted in conceptual and theoretical developments alongside empirical data collection. In this chapter, we focus on three major areas of investigation into the role of religion and spirituality in older people's lives: age differences in the nature of religious and spiritual belief and practice; health benefits that accrue to older people who profess a religious faith and engage in spiritual activities; and influences on social and intergenerational relationships and support resulting from membership of a faith tradition.

The study of religion and spirituality with age would benefit from greater investment in comparative research. Excellent examples are provided by studies of Black and White older Americans (Krause, 2002; Taylor, Chatters, & Jackson, 2007), but there remains a huge untapped potential for detailed investigation of differences relating to ethnicity, gender, education, religious socialization and other demographic factors in addition to age. The vast majority of studies into older people's spiritual beliefs and practices over the past 50 years have been conducted in Western societies and with those socialized into Christian traditions (notable exceptions include Lamb, 2000; MacKinlay, 2010; Mehta, 1997; Traphagan, 2004). This has inevitably given a biased understanding of the relationships among religion, spirituality, and aging. We therefore conclude this chapter with a stress on the importance of conducting research on religion, spirituality, and aging in non-Western and non-Christian cultures, and also with the need for connecting theorizing more strongly to concepts of aging held by the various religious traditions themselves.

However, we must first acknowledge, if only briefly, changing relationships between the conceptions of religion and spirituality. Whereas these were previously closely intertwined concepts, developments in Western thought over the last century have led to a loss of alignment between them (Heelas & Woodhead, 2005; Hogan, 2014; Lynch, 2007). Certain understandings of the term "spirituality" no longer imply belief in a transcendent power such as is characteristic of most religious traditions. Moreover, factors other than initial religious socialization increasingly influence the development of individual spiritual beliefs. Religions indeed are often criticized for being closed and over-authoritarian systems of belief and practice, whereas "spiritualities" tend to be depicted positively as ways of experiencing meaning in being alive that reflect authentic personal choice rather than cultural or family habit (Pargament, 1999). New developmental concepts have been formulated, such as "spiritual seeking" (Dillon & Wink, 2007). At the same time nontheistic understandings of religion have also been proposed that are more consistent with some of the newer definitions of spirituality (Waschenfelder, 2012).

However, it is important to note that recent generations of older people in Western societies tend to have retained the closely connected understandings of religion and spirituality into which they were socialized when young (Bengtson, Putney, & Harris, 2013). Therefore, most of the relevant studies in this field have been conducted on older people's religious beliefs and practices rather than on possible new forms of spirituality. The consequences for later life of the current shift, which has taken place especially in Western Europe, from a predominance of traditional religious to new spiritual understandings of life will become evident only with the aging of the post–World War II (WWII) "baby boom" generation (Coleman, 2011). Most quantitative research on religion and aging has also been limited by its focus on a relatively restricted number of dimensions of affiliation, belief, and practice. The practice of religious fasting, for example, which plays an important part in many religions, has been relatively little studied in relation to aging (Coleman, Begum, & Jaleel, 2011). The role that the various types of religious ritual play in older people's lives has also been neglected (Coleman, Koleva, & Bornat, 2013; Traphagan, 2000, 2004).

■ EXPLANATIONS FOR AGE DIFFERENCES IN RELIGION AND SPIRITUALITY

The greater religiosity of older people compared with younger adults is evident from numerous surveys conducted in the United States and in several European societies since the 1970s (Moberg, 2001, 2005; Voas & Doebler, 2011). Older people attend religious services more and express firmer belief in a personal God to whom one can turn for assistance. However, the evidence points most strongly to cohort rather than developmental changes underpinning the observed age differences in religious participation in Western countries. The generational differences in turn result from the major societal shifts in attitudes to religion characteristic of Western societies since at least the 1960s. As a result, it seems very unlikely that current cohorts of young or middle-aged people, especially in Western Europe, will show the same levels of religious engagement when they grow old as current older people display. Nevertheless, there does appear to be potential for spiritual change in persons as they age. In the following pages, we first consider explanations for the existing evidence on age differences in religious attitudes followed by an examination of theories on spiritual development with age.

Distinguishing Cohort and Development Change in Religious and Spiritual Attitudes

Researchers have investigated age differences in religiosity by attempting to separate out age, period, and cohort effects in order to identify more clearly the social facts requiring explanation. Analyses of major British social surveys present a picture of continuous religious decline throughout the 20th century, with no evident differences in the rate of decline among measures of affiliation, attendance at worship, and expressed belief (Voas & Crockett, 2005). Altogether, the evidence suggests an explanation in terms of intergenerational decline with each successive generation being less successful in transmitting religious faith and practice to succeeding generations. As Crockett and Voas (2006) point out, the aging of the U.K. population does not seem to have significantly affected this downward trend. The greater religiosity of the increasing number of immigrants is a more likely mitigating factor. Many other Western European countries show similar trends, and secularization theory continues to provide the major explanatory framework for these changes (Brown & Snape, 2010; Bruce, 1996; see also Gorski, 2000, for a wider historical arch).

One line of theorizing argues that religious decline in Western Europe is only apparent, an artifact of a narrow focus on variables of religious *participation*. According to the "believing without belonging" thesis, more inclusive indicators of spirituality, morality, or belief in the supernatural point toward a persistent private importance of religiosity even among younger people (Davie, 2002, 2006; Luckmann, 1990). Davie (2007) also uses the term "vicarious religion" to refer to the phenomenon of approval for religious services by those not attending. Certainly, religious ceremonies continue to be seen as important responses at times of national, as well as personal, loss and celebration. Research on religion in Bulgaria and Romania, for example, attests to the continuing commitment to religious ritual in otherwise nonreligious older people, including the determination to "die Orthodox (Christian)" (B dic , 2013; Koleva, 2013). In a similar vein, anthropologists drawing on ethnographic data have tended to argue for changes in the *nature* of religious beliefs and practices, rather than wholesale abandonment of religion (Day, 2013a). But at least Western European studies using more inclusive measures of "belief," as opposed to just "belonging," fail to reverse the strong impression of generational decline in religiosity (Crockett &Voas, 2006; Gill, Hadaway, & Marler 1998).

U.S. data analysis also shows historical decline in religious affiliation and attendance at worship although, compared with the United Kingdom, to a much lesser degree and only beginning in the post-WWII years (Putnam & Campbell, 2010). Indeed the continuing large differences in religiosity between the United States and Europe already suggest that "Eurosecularity" is unlikely to be a model for the rest of the world (Berger, Davie, & Fokas, 2008). However, North American data do support the view that distinct birth cohorts can be identified according to the degree to which they associate spiritual practices with religious institutions, regard religion and spirituality as distinct, and have conceptions of God which tend toward the transcendent or immanent (Bengtson et al., 2013).

Only three substantial longitudinal studies on attitudes to religion involving older people have been conducted, all three in California (Bengtson, Silverstein, Putney, & Harris, 2015; Dillon & Wink, 2007; McCullough, Enders, Brion, & Jain, 2005). They reflect historical changes among birth cohorts in declining religious identification, but do not report significant and consistent changes in religious faith and practice within cohorts. Rather religious commitments appear to be established by early adulthood and to remain fairly stable thereafter. However, some U.S. post-WWI birth cohort groups have shown an increase in religious intensity in midlife and later (Bengtson et al., in press),whereas a longitudinal study of a British pre-WWI birth cohort showed a significant decline in the numbers of participants attributing importance to religious faith in their later years (Coleman, Ivani-Chalian, & Robinson, 2004).

Nevertheless, there are suggestions that development in religious and spiritual belief and practice with advanced age may become apparent with the use of more sensitive quantitative and qualitative indicators. Dillon and Wink reported a significant increase with age in "spiritual seeking" within their 1920s birth cohort, a process that they found to begin already in midlife. Their participants also came to express a more universalizing and more faith-based (and less social-based) meaning to their beliefs as they grew older (Dillon & Wink, 2007). The U.K. longitudinal study also found evidence for the more central role of religious self-descriptions in the one half of the sample that retained religious convictions as they grew older (Coleman, Ivani-Chalian, & Robinson, 2015). Studies on persons in the last years of their lives indicate a tendency to increased expressions of the value of religion to them (Idler, Kasl, & Hays, 2001). There is therefore reason to continue to explore changes in religion and spirituality in later life despite the strong evidence for stability of basic religious disposition across adulthood. What is needed is more theory-led and hypothesis-driven research.

Developmental Theories of Aging, Religion, and Spirituality

Religion and spirituality have constituted a significant element in general theorizing on life-span development. Particularly noteworthy are the mid-20th-century writings of the psychoanalyst Carl Jung, who emphasized a shift from exterior to interior purposes in objectives as people reached middle age and the importance of cultural and religious myths in this process (Jung, 1938, 1972). Among the next generation of theorists, Erik Erikson, in his influential psychosocial framework of life stages from birth to death, attributed a significant role to religious faith and belonging both as a unifying component across the life span and as a bridge between generations (Erikson, 1950). Of Erikson's many students, David Gutmann has been most explicit in pointing to the value of older people's role in religious transmission within traditional societies and linking this to intrinsic psychological changes in motivation, for example in the more passive stance men displayed as they aged (Gutmann, 1987, 1997). Less well known but indicative of changing attitudes to the concept of spirituality in the later 20th century is the addition Abraham Maslow made to his theory of hierarchy of needs (Maslow, 1943) later in his career. This originally peaked with "self-actualization" but Maslow subsequently added the pursuit of "intrinsic values," classifying them as "metaneeds," spiritual in character rather than biologically rooted as are the other needs (Maslow, 1971).

The latter part of the 20th century also saw the beginnings of explicit theorizing about stages of adult spiritual development (Fowler, 1981; Moody & Carroll, 1997). The most specifically related to the processes of aging is Lars Tornstam's concept of "gerotranscendence" (Tornstam, 1994, 2005) that strongly advocates the importance of spiritual development in later life. He defines gerotranscendence as a shift in perspective from a materialistic and rational view on life to a more cosmic and transcendent one. This brings with it increased feeling of affinity with nature and with past and future generations, and an increased wish for quiet and meditation. Robert Atchley (2003, 2009) has integrated much of this literature in proposing a model of later life spiritual "saging," connected to the stages of aging: development and growth of persons in their 60s, learning to be "rooted in their being"; becoming actualized sages in their 70s and early 80s, "fully in touch with their spiritual nature"; and transcendent sages "radiantly at peace" from their mid-80s onward. Among the many guidebooks produced on developing spirituality in old age, Edmund Sherman's (2010) *Contemplative Aging: A Way of Being in Later Life* stands out, also because of the author's long career in studying aging and adjustment. He was one of the first to stress the importance of developing a "psychophilosophy," a well-considered way of thinking and feeling about life that enables the person to face the existential challenges of later life (Sherman, 1981).

However, future empirical study on change in religious and spiritual attitudes with age will also need to link with general theorizing about the psychological and social functions of religion. For example, Sedikides and Gebauer (2013) provide a thorough analysis of evidence for the various potential benefits that religion provides to the self: enhancing not only self-esteem but also personal and compensatory control, reducing uncertainty, and providing secure attachment figures together with a sense of belonging and meaning. All of these various human needs are accentuated in the course of aging, and one might therefore on these grounds alone expect some degree of increased religious expression and practice in older people's lives. Research hypotheses in the field of religion and aging need to be similarly specific in conceptualization.

A good example is provided by Hayward and Krause's (2013b) study on age-related changes in sense of God-mediated control. Both maintenance of a sense of control and the ability when needed to change strategies of control are central aspects of contemporary theorizing about adjustments to aging (Baltes & Smith, 2003; Brandtstädter, 2006; Rowe & Kahn, 1998). But as Hayward and Krause point out, almost no attention has been given to the role of religion in maintaining sense of control with aging. They hypothesized that religious belief provides resources to cognitively reappraise the older person's situation so that loss of personal control is compensated by a stronger belief in God-mediated control. Their longitudinal survey over 7 years found results consistent with this hypothesis.

■ EXPLAINING THE HEALTH BENEFITS OF OLDER PEOPLE'S RELIGIOUS PRACTICE

There is now a significant body of empirical research with mainly Christian samples that demonstrates that different dimensions of religion and spirituality can have a positive influence on physical and mental health (Koenig, King, & Carson, 2012; Koenig, McCullough, & Larson, 2001). In the context of older adults, some of the most striking findings show religious service attendance (Hill, Angel, Ellison, & Angel, 2005; Lutgendorf, Russell, Ullrich, Harris, & Wallace, 2004), private religious practice (Helm, Hays, Flint, Koenig, & Blazer, 2000), and religious participation (Zhang, 2008) to be related to lower risk of mortality; religious service attendance (Norton et al., 2008) and intrinsic religiosity (Payman & Ryburn, 2010) to be associated with lower depression; religious service attendance (Benjamins, 2004; Park et al., 2008) to be associated with reduced physical functioning limitations; religious involvement (Idler, McLaughlin, & Kasl, 2009) to be associated with increased quality of life; participation in religious and spiritual activities, importance of and comfort from religion, and religious support (Fry, 2000) and spiritual belief (Kirby, Coleman, & Daley, 2004) to be associated with increased psychological well-being; and daily spiritual experience (Whitehead & Bergeman, 2012) to be associated with protection against stress and promotion of a positive mood.

There is a debate about the terms "religion" and "spirituality" and their relationship with one another; for example, whether they represent separate yet overlapping constructs, which is the broader or narrower construct, or whether they can be combined and perhaps used interchangeably (Moberg, 2005; Pargament, 1999). Indeed, a recent observed trend in the literature, perhaps for the sake of brevity or expedience, is of theorists simply referring to religion and spirituality as "RS." Both constructs are often considered as being a social or psychosocial resource that older adults can draw on in coping and in adjusting or adapting to age-related challenges or demands. Both are also frequently conceptualized as being multidimensional in terms of their constituent elements (e.g., affiliation, belief, practice). This multidimensional conceptualization can also be extended in terms of how the influence of religion and spirituality is experienced by the individual believer or community (e.g., cognitively, emotionally, and behaviorally).

How religion and spirituality are conceptualized has significance for researchers related to how these constructs are defined, understood by participants, and measured. Some conceptualizations may be difficult to operationalize and thus may not be drawn on in research despite being intellectually enlightening. In other circumstances, there may be a mismatch or disparity between conceptualizations and the lived experience of believers. Some believers may feel that theories, definitions, and questionnaire items do not represent adequately enough the breadth, depth, or richness of their thoughts, emotions, and behaviors. Conceptualizations of religion may lend themselves to being readily measured and quantified because of associations with traditional beliefs (e.g., belief in a God) and practices (e.g., attendance at church services) and named denominations or affiliations, and may therefore be considered relatively stable or consistent over time. In contrast, conceptualizations of spirituality, which can be related or unrelated to religion, are often associated with transcendent human experiences that can be difficult to measure. Spiritual conceptualizations can be sensitive to epoch and cultural influences and are therefore susceptible to change and development, making them less consistent over time or in producing cohort differences.

It can be discerned that the body of gerontological empirical research to focus on religion and spirituality is rarely characterized by explicit reference to theory, but instead identifies a number of explanatory mechanisms (Benjamins, 2004; George, Larson, Koenig, & McCullough, 2000) that can account for how religion and spirituality can have a beneficial influence on health and well-being. One of the main ways religion and spirituality are theorized to influence health is by encouraging healthy lifestyles and behaviors (Fitchett, Benjamins, Skarupski, & de Leon, 2013; George et al., 2000; George, Kinghorn, Koenig, Gammon, & Blazer, 2013). As several theorists have pointed out, most religious groups tend to discourage the use of substances (e.g., tobacco, alcohol, illegal drugs) and behaviors (e.g., unsafe sexual activity, violence) that might be detrimental to health (Fitchett et al., 2013; George et al., 2000, 2013), while encouraging activities related to diet, exercise, and social interaction that may promote optimal health. It is these healthy lifestyles and behaviors practiced throughout life that may contribute toward the avoidance or delay of disease and disability (Fitchett et al., 2013; Zhang, 2008).

Another main way religion and spirituality are theorized to influence health and well-being is through the social interaction and support accessible from one's religious congregation (George et al., 2000). Two main types of support theorized as important in later life are labelled as "instrumental" or "tangible" support, which refers to practical forms of support such as help with transportation or finances; and "emotional" support, which may take the form of care or empathy, with older adults being both the potential recipients and providers (Hayward & Krause, 2013a). Other important features derived from significant integration in one's religious congregation can include identity and belonging processes (e.g., providing a source of self-esteem, roles and routines, purpose in life, and secure attachment; see also section on social relationships, as follows); support in conforming with prescribed medical care (e.g., help getting to and from medical appointments, assistance in convalescing following illness or medical procedure); peer encouragement in engaging in health-promoting behaviors (overlapping with adhering to a healthy lifestyle); and in peer reinforcement of group-held beliefs.

The explanatory mechanism suggested by George et al. (2000) to have the most influence in accounting for the relationship between religion and health appears to be at the cognitive level and comes from the sense of meaning or meaning-making processes that can be derived from religion and spirituality. Park (2005) discusses, in the context of coping and stress models, how religious and spiritual beliefs may be used in a number of cognitive ways, such as in appraisals, reappraisals, reattributions, and reinterpretations, to understand or perceive stressful or distressing life events in more manageable or less threatening ways. These ways of thinking may then reduce the potentially harmful effects of stress, physiologically.

Religious and Spiritual Influences on Processes of Grief in Later Life

As useful as these explanatory mechanisms are, from a psychology of religion and spirituality perspective, they reveal little about the content of religious and spiritual belief, about what beliefs are being drawn on and how they are being used to exert positive influences. One area that has produced some interesting insight in this respect is in the religion and bereavement literature. Reviews of the empirical research suggest that religion and spirituality can have a potentially beneficial influence on people experiencing significant bereavement or grief (Becker et al., 2007; Wortmann & Park, 2008). In the context of older adults, Fry (2001), using a cross-sectional study of Canadian older adults bereaved from a spouse in the previous 24 months, found that importance of religion, spiritual beliefs and practices, and religious support contributed to psychological well-being. In a large prospective cohort study of American older adults, Brown, Nesse, House, and Utz (2004) identified that the experience of spousal bereavement could produce more frequent church attendance and an increase in importance of religious or spiritual belief, with the latter being related to reduced grief; this effect was seen as being particularly salient in those with an insecure attachment style.

Explanations for the beneficial influence of religion in circumstances of bereavement include that most religions contain beliefs related to issues of death and practices that can be used in the expression of grief and mourning. Research by Spreadbury and Coleman (2011) with religious British older adults who had experienced spousal bereavement found that religious cognition such as belief in a life after death, life after death reunion, and belief in a protective, omniscient and omnipresent God were used in ongoing coping and adjustment. Participants were able to make sense of their bereavement by interpreting it as part of a purpose or plan known to God and found benefit in beliefs that their spouses were in a life-after-death location free from suffering and had achieved their spiritual goal of reaching their desired afterlife.

Participants were also able to use religious rituals such as prayer and receiving Communion/Eucharist to facilitate continuing bonds processes (Klass, Silverman, & Nickman, 1996) with their deceased spouses. Through religious rituals participants felt that they were able to continue or maintain a cognitive and emotional relationship with the deceased and feel a sense of psychological and emotional closeness, as well as through rituals helping participants to regulate grief-related emotions. Participants were also able to draw on diverse Biblical content and use this in multiple ways to support sense-making processes and to bolster their coping.

Religion may also allow believers to find personal meaning in bereavement. Coleman, McKiernan, Mills, and Speck (2007) found in a longitudinal study of British older adults who had experienced recent spousal bereavement that those scoring high on religious belief tended to have higher personal meaning and lower depression compared with those of moderate and low religious belief during the second year of bereavement.

Another line of theorizing comes from the application of attachment theory to understanding both religious behavior (Kirkpatrick, 2005) and grief (Bowlby, 1980). With regard to religion, God, or any other religious deity or religious figure (e.g., Jesus), is in most circumstances comparable to a secure attachment figure, one who can provide feelings of everyday security (similar to a secure base) and protection in times of distress (similar to a haven of safety), and in which religious behaviors such as prayer or church attendance can be seen as attachment figure proximity seeking behaviors (Kirkpatrick, 2005). Within attachment theory, grief can be considered as a response to the permanent separation from an attachment figure, and significant bereavement such as the loss of a spouse, a type of attachment figure, is thought to elicit a decrease in felt security and trigger attachment responses (Kirkpatrick, 2005). Under these circumstances, these attachment responses may manifest themselves in an increase in the importance of God, or religious belief and behavior, in an attempt to find an alternative attachment figure and to emotionally compensate for the loss (Kirkpatrick, 2005). The study by Brown et al. (2004; see earlier discussion) provides some empirical support for this theorizing related to a reduction in grief.

Religious and Spiritual Influences on Cognitive Functioning and Dementia

Research has now begun to investigate whether the potential beneficial influence of religion and spirituality may apply to other areas important in later life such as cognitive functioning and dementia, with the latter now recognized as a worldwide public health problem (Prince et al., 2013). Indeed, we would predict that here is where there will be an increase in religious gerontological research over the next decade, as researchers, in the absence of more effective dementia medication, attempt to investigate whether psychosocial resources and interventions can delay the onset or slow down symptom progression related to cognitive impairment and dementia. A small number of high-quality studies including a focus on religious and spiritual variables have already begun to produce some thought-provoking findings in this area.

In the context of cognitive functioning, a study conducted by Hill, Burdette, Angel, and Angel (2006) has found that, in a sample of more than 3,000 American older adults of Mexican ethnicity, more frequent religious attendance was related to slower cognitive decline over an 8-year period as measured by the Mini Mental State Examination (MMSE—a neuropsychological instrument widely used in the assessment of different aspects of cognitive functioning). In the context of dementia, a study by Kaufman, Anaki, Binns, and Freedman (2007) found that, in a sample of Canadian patients diagnosed with probable Alzheimer's disease, more frequent engagement in private religious practices and greater self-rated spirituality, but not religious attendance, contributed to slower cognitive decline, again measured using the MMSE, over a 1-year period. More recently, a study by Coin et al. (2010) using a sample of Italian older adults with probable Alzheimer's disease has found that, compared with those categorized as high in religiosity (measured by increased frequency of participation in religious activities), those low in religiosity showed increased cognitive decline (measured by the MMSE) and increased behavioral disturbances (measured by the Neuropsychiatric Inventory) over a 1-year period. This study also showed that, over the same period, caregivers to patients low in religiosity showed increased caregiver burden and distress compared to caregivers of patients high in religiosity. Coin et al. (2010) concluded that, in circumstances of patients with an established religious belief, they should be encouraged in their religious practice with any potential advantages likely to be experienced by caregivers as well as patients.

There is also the earlier longitudinal research by Snowdon (2008), the "nun study," that has provided evidence for the argument that living a life of daily prayer and contemplation may contribute to the preventative effects relative to the development of Alzheimer's disease, and also improve the condition of those among the sisters who had already contracted the disease. Moreover, there is currently a developing literature indicating that meditation, which can form part of religious and spiritual practice as well as secular spirituality and activity, may have a beneficial influence on cognitive functioning in later life (Gard, Hölzel, & Lazar, 2014) and in neurodegenerative diseases (Newberg et al., 2014).

Despite this area of religion, spirituality, and health research being arguably one of the most exciting for theory development and potentially far reaching in its applied implications, there is still a lack of detailed theorizing about how religion and spirituality may influence cognitive functioning and dementia. However, some discourse does suggest that religion and spirituality may have a beneficial influence by encouraging regular cognitive stimulation, and thus stimulating and reinforcing underlying neural networks.

In comparison with secular activities, religious and spiritual involvement may be considered distinctive or unique in a number of ways, for example in the combination of both public and private activities, in the combination of evocative stimuli involved (e.g., use of music, vocalization, clothing, incense, iconography/imagery, symbolism, narrative), and involving different thought processes. Indeed, common religious and spiritual activities can include attending church services; interacting with one's congregation; remembering and commemorating religious holidays, saints' days, festivals, and anniversaries; reading or listening to religious scripture or stories; engaging in prayer; singing hymns; and performing and participating in religious rituals.

It is hypothesized that religious activities may be cognitively stimulating in several ways; for example: by encouraging cognitive activity such as concentration, introspection, meditation, perspective taking (McNamara, 2002), abstract thinking (Koenig et al., 2012), and contemplation (Hill et al., 2006); by encouraging activity in different cognitive modalities such as perception, comprehension, production, and emotion (Van Ness & Kasl, 2003); by engaging the use of different types of memory processes (Koenig et al., 2012); and by stimulating frontal lobe activity, in particular the activity of the prefrontal cortex associated with attentional processes and working memory (McNamara, 2002).

In general, Alzheimer's disease and vascular dementia are considered to be the two most common types of dementia affecting those older than 65 years. Koenig et al. (2012) have indicated that future research and theorizing needs to establish the mechanisms by which religion and spirituality may influence these dementias; for example, whether religion and spirituality can have an influence on the underlying pathology of neurodegeneration in Alzheimer's disease involving amyloid proteins and brain inflammation, or whether the healthy lifestyles and behaviors associated with religion and spirituality can reduce the risk of the development of vascular dementia.

■ THEORIES OF RELIGION, SOCIAL RELATIONSHIPS, AND AGING

Social gerontology's recent concern with religion and spirituality in later life has had a relatively limited impact on theorizing about aging and social relationships. This is particularly surprising, given that early "giants" of social theorizing (e.g., Max Weber, Emile Durkheim, and William James) were heavily concerned with religion as a key dimension of the social world and its influence on individual behavior (Idler, 2006). The richest theoretical seams can be found in two main areas of inquiry. These can be captured by the following theoretically motivated questions: First, how is religious identity and practice transmitted across generations, and how does religion shape intergenerational relationships? Second, why are religious communities sources of support in later life?

Religious Transmission and Identity in Intergenerational Relationships

Earlier we drew attention to the fact that religious identity remains relatively stable in adulthood, but that over recent decades successive cohorts in Western societies have appeared less religious. This suggests that religious identity is formed in childhood and adolescence, but that intergenerational transmission of religious identities and practices is becoming less complete over time. This raises important questions about how religious identities are formed and transmitted and the role of families and communities within this process.

An important but underexplored element in intergenerational transmission of religion concerns teaching about ritual practice, both of a religious and secular nature. Older people the world over have traditionally played an important part in transmitting religious rituals to future generations (Mehta, 1997; Traphagan, 2004), although this role has been diminished in modern societies. Comparative study can be particularly useful in understanding the different processes at work. Recent research conducted in both Western Europe (U.K.) and Eastern Europe (Bulgaria and Romania) has demonstrated the much greater involvement of older people in birth and death rituals within Eastern European countries, and reflected on the historical, educational, and cultural explanations for these differences (Coleman et al., 2013). Religious socialization varied greatly among the countries. "Sunday school," provided by churches, and Christian school assemblies had been major institutions in British society until the 1960s, and their past importance was strongly reflected in the interviews conducted with older British people. In Eastern Europe, by contrast, partly as a result of the discouragement or outright persecution of religious practice by the socialist state during the 20th century, faith and religious practice had been communicated solely within families, with especially grandmothers playing a key role (Koleva, 2013). In both Bulgaria and Romania, older people have remained active participants in the religious ritual practices around birth, marriage, and death (Bădică, 2013). Their physical enactment of faith traditions, for example through kissing icons and lighting candles, remains a model for younger generations that is at least as important as verbal teaching about religious doctrine.

Numerous studies have attested to the importance of early socialization in the development of religious identities and practices (Crockett & Voas, 2006; Day, 2013b; Wuthnow, 1999), although they differ in the relative role attributed to familial and wider networks. In her ethnography of older people's faith in Connecticut, Eisenhandler (2003) draws on terms like "folkways of faith" and "bedrock socialization" to convey the extent to which religious initiation among her locally rooted prewar generation was embedded in social relationships and community life. The result is a "reflexive" rather than "reflective" faith in later life. Without explicitly invoking the notion of culture, Eisenhandler's evidence supports an interpretation of religion as part of a cultural system of symbols, meanings, and practices that shape a person's ethos, social world, and way of life (Geertz, 1973/1993). Drawing on Geertz and on the theologian Paul Tillich's notion of religion as "ultimate concern," Traphagan applies such a cultural approach to religion and ritual in Japan. Older Japanese people play a vital role in enacting religious rituals on behalf of their families and communities, and in doing so they express individual and collective concern. As Traphagan (2004, pp. 180–181) argues,

> Ritual action reenacts in bodily form emotive meanings associated with the well-being of oneself and one's friends, family, and community.... The practice of ritual performance in Japan is the practice of concern. And it is the elderly who are the ones central in the *observation* of the rituals through which concern is reified.

A conceptualization of religion as part of a cultural system helps to make sense of both persistence and declines in religious identification over time. For example, Bengtson et al. (2013) found intergenerational familial transmission of faith to be particularly high among religious communities with pronounced social boundaries, internal solidarity, and social control. Such groups can be seen as not only sharing a religion but inhabiting a subculture in which familial and congregational institutions and practices reinforce each other and produce a distinct way of life. At the micro-level of individual families, shared (familial) cultures also appear to be important for successful religious transmission. For example, Voas and Crockett (2005) found for the United Kingdom that where *both* parents attend church or identify with a religious group, adult children are twice as likely to be religious than if just one parent attends or is religiously affiliated. Similarly, U.S. evidence suggests that grandparental influence on grandchildren's religiosity is greatest where it is consistent with parental religious socialization (Bengtson et al., 2013; Copen & Silverstein, 2007). By contrast, religious groups characterized by greater openness, heterodoxy, and tolerance, and families that are religiously heterogeneous appear to be less successful in religious transmission, possibly because their approach to religion lacks the coherence of a cultural system (Bengtson et al., 2013; Voas & Doebler, 2011).

Theories of parenting and intergenerational solidarity have further proven fruitful for shedding light on religious transmission within intergenerational families. For example, Bengtson et al. (2013) found parental role modeling in religious teaching and practice and warm and affirming parenting styles as central to explaining successful transmission, whereas distant or authoritarian parenting and inconsistency in moral behavior resulted in religious divergence or rejection of religion altogether (see also King, Burgess, Akinyela, Counts-Spriggs, & Parker, 2006, for the role of grandparenting styles). Given the value that many families attach to their religious identity (or to a lack thereof), it is surprising that not more studies have investigated religion as an important dimension of intergenerational solidarity or conflict (Bengtson, Giarrusso, Mabry, & Silverstein, 2002; Katz & Lowenstein, 2010; Merz, Özeke-Kocabas, Oort, & Schuengel, 2009). Bengtson et al.'s (2013) recent work provides a promising starting point for such theorizing by modeling relationship quality as an explanatory factor for religious transmission. Future work could in turn model religious "harmony" or "disharmony" as an aspect of consensual or affectual intergenerational solidarity and examine its impact on intergenerational support between elderly parents and adult children. Early work tentatively suggests not only that religious children are more supportive (Gans, Silverstein, & Lowenstein, 2009), but also that shared religious culture between parents and children accentuates intergenerational support provision (King, Ledwell, & Pearce-Morris, 2013).

Religious Communities as Sources of Support

A growing body of literature indicates that older people belonging to religious congregations are more likely to receive support than those who do not (George et al., 2000; Hayward & Krause, 2013a; Park, Roh, & Yeo, 2012). Within religious congregations, those who participate more actively and provide support are most likely to benefit from support from coreligionists (Krause & Hayward, 2014; Lee, 2014). As noted earlier, religious affiliation and participation appear to be sources of well-being for older people and to contribute health and longevity. These findings raise the question as to *why* religious communities should represent particular sources of support. The most promising theoretical avenues to explaining these social facts draw on social network theory and social identity theory.

Religious congregations are social networks connecting people on the basis of a shared religion (McIntosh, Sykes, & Kubena, 2002). Religious networks share many of the features of other social networks (e.g., their openness and fluidity), but additionally display specific characteristics that make them particularly significant as sources of support. Religious networks typically connect people over long periods of time (often over decades; Eisenhandler, 2003; Idler, 2006), and unlike many other networks are intergenerational and age integrated in nature (Idler, 2006). They are more heterogeneous than kinship or friendship networks in terms of socioeconomic status and ethnicity. Like family networks, they are locally rooted, but they also transcend local concerns and manifestations and develop important translocal and even transnational linkages (Kreager, 2009). Their foundation in shared values, particularly values centered on altruism, provide them with an explicit concern for human welfare beyond the confines of family networks (Gans et al., 2009; Krause, 2006, 2015; Kreager, 2009). For these reasons, religious networks are often seen as exemplars of civil society institutions (or "mediating structures," cf. Berger & Neuhaus, 1977) that operate in the social spaces between "formal" and "informal" or "public" and "private" welfare institutions (Benda-Beckmann et al., 1988; Thelen, Leutloff-Grandits, & Peleikis, 2009).

The long history of interactions among members of a congregation, combined with their shared values, nurture the development of strong trust or "social capital" within religious networks (Lewis, MacGregor, & Putnam, 2013; Merino, 2014). It is this social capital that is easily and readily translated into support to members in need and may account for the heightened availability of support to older members who have often contributed to religious congregations for many years and are thus considered "deserving" recipients of support (Schröder-Butterfill, 2015; Thelen et al., 2009).

Three further aspects of religious congregations as social networks deserve mention. First, their relative heterogeneity means that they are composed of both weak and strong ties, and thereby embody both bridging and bonding capital (Granovetter, 1973; Hayward & Krause, 2013a; Wellman & Wortley, 1989). The former may facilitate access to information or links to formal welfare structures, while the latter gives rise to emotional and practical support. Second, people who are part of religious congregations tend to have larger nonkin networks than those who are not, which in turn increases an older person's potential avenues to support (Ellison & George, 1994). Research on old-age support in rural Indonesia has shown, for example, that charitable support (especially *zakat*) from religious networks specifically targets elders with inadequate kinship networks and thus compensates for a lack of familial assistance (Benda-Beckmann, 1988; Kreager, 2009; Schröder-Butterfill & Kreager, 2005). Third, social networks are not only sources of support and integration, but also institutions of social control (Bott, 1957), with control seen as divinely sanctioned in the case of religious networks. This can, on the one hand, result in certain individuals or groups being excluded from support on account of reputation or nonadherence; on the other hand, it may serve to reinforce cooperative behavior among members (Crow, 2004).

Social identity theories are related to social network theories in that they consider (intense) interaction and participation as generative of social value from which support may then flow (Eisenhandler, 2003; Krause & Bastida, 2011). The greater the involvement of a person in a group, be that in terms of participation, interaction, or contribution, so the argument runs, the greater will be the sense of similarity with group members (Eisenhandler, 2003; Oyserman, 2007). This results in stronger social identification with the group and greater trust and willingness to cooperate within the group. For example, it has been argued that the particularly strong social support dimension within religious networks of African American older people is related to their common experience of discrimination, which has heightened social identification and a willingness to share support (Krause & Hayward, 2014).

■ FUTURE THEORY DEVELOPMENT

The vast majority of theories and research studies cited in this chapter have been based on Western samples and populations with a predominantly Christian socialization. This is an insufficient basis on which to develop the study of religion, spirituality, and aging. Despite the danger of invidious comparisons, there is much to be learned from systematic study of older persons with different and no religious views (MacKinlay 2010). This is especially so if the comparison enables theory testing, for example on the aspects of religious and spiritual beliefs and practices that produce beneficial effects (Hui & Coleman, 2012; Mehta, 1997; Wilkinson & Coleman, 2010).

A further limitation of recent theory formulation is the absence of close engagement with traditional religious teachings on the meaning and challenges of later life. Buddhist teaching appears to have had some influence on recent studies on coping with loss in later life, particularly in the application of mindful practice (Sherman, 2010). This is appropriate as confrontation with old age, disease, and death is represented in the very foundation story of Buddhism. Yet as Bodhi (2011) points out, there are dangers in extracting particular principles of religious teaching without paying attention to its original context. Hinduism is also widely regarded as an age-friendly religion, which ascribes a distinct more mature stage of being to the last stages of life, in preparation for the transition to a new life beyond death (Lamb, 2000; Ram-Prasad, 1995; Tilak, 1989). However, when one considers the preponderance of studies on Christian older people, it is surprising how little evident is specifically Christian teaching on aging within the social gerontological literature on religion (Hauerwas, Stoneking, Meador, & Cloutier, 2003). This may reflect the loss of the penitential emphasis characteristic of medieval and later attitudes to old age (Aers, 2003) and the failure to provide equally compelling perspectives to Christians living long lives nowadays.

Nevertheless, Christianity as well as most of the world's religious traditions share a common exhortation to a greater intensity of spiritual life, including contemplation, as persons grow older. It would therefore seem appropriate to consider what can be learned from the long traditions of religious and spiritual life. For example, various authors have referred to old age as a "natural monastery" (McFadden, 2008; Moody, 1995; Thibault, 1993). Foulcher (2014) has recently drawn attention to the relevance of monastic experience to the challenges of aging: being alone, dealing with loss and deprivation, increasing awareness of one's own limitations, long periods of waiting, and encounters with disturbing and destructive thoughts. Despite the many differences between a life of voluntary renunciation and involuntary loss, older persons increasingly face some of the same issues as the religious person who has chosen to leave the world to pursue a spiritual way of life. They may need to find similar answers.

REFERENCES

Aers, D. (2003). The Christian practice of growing old in the middle ages. In S. Hauerwas, C. B. Stoneking, K. G. Meador, & D. Cloutier (Eds.), *Growing old in Christ* (pp. 38–59). Grand Rapids, MI: William B. Eerdmans.

Atchley, R. (2003). Becoming a spiritual elder. In M. A. Kimble & S. H. McFadden (Eds.), *Aging, spirituality and religion: A handbook* (pp. 2, 33–46). Minneapolis, MN: Fortress Press.

Atchley, R. (2009). *Spirituality and aging*. Baltimore, MD: Johns Hopkins University Press.

Bădică, S. (2013). 'I will die Orthodox': Religion and belonging in life stories of the socialist era in Romania and Bulgaria. In P. G. Coleman, D. Koleva, & J. Bornat (Eds.), *Ageing, ritual and social change. Comparing the secular and religious in eastern and western Europe* (pp. 43–65). Farnham, UK: Ashgate.

Baltes, P. B., & Smith, J. (2003). New frontiers in the future of aging: From successful aging of the young old to the dilemmas of the fourth age. *Gerontology, 49*(2), 123–135.

Becker, G., Xander, C. J., Blum, H. E., Lutterbach, J., Momm, F., Gysels, M., & Higginson, I. J. (2007). Do religious or spiritual beliefs influence bereavement? A systematic review. *Palliative Medicine, 21*(3), 207–217.

Benda-Beckmann, F. V. (1988). Islamic law and social security in an Ambonese village. In F. V. Benda-Beckmann, K. V. Benda-Beckmann, B. O. Bryde, & F. Hirtz (Eds.), *Between kinship and the state: Social security and law in developing countries* (pp. 339–366). Dordrecht, The Netherlands: Foris.

Benda-Beckmann, F. V., Benda-Beckmann, K. V., Casino, E., Hirtz, F., Woodman, G. R., & Zacher, H. (1988). *Between kinship and the state: Social security and law in developing countries*. Dordrecht, The Netherlands: Foris.

Bengtson, V. L., Giarrusso, R., Mabry, J. B., & Silverstein, M. (2002). Solidarity, conflict, and ambivalence: Complementary or competing perspectives on intergenerational relationships? *Journal of Marriage and Family, 64*, 568–576.

Bengtson, V. L., Putney, N. P., & Harris, S. C. (2013). *Families and faith: How religion is passed down across generations*. New York, NY: Oxford University Press.

Bengtson, V. L., Silverstein, M., Putney, N. P., & Harris, S. C. (2015). Does religiousness increase with age? Age changes and generational differences over 35 years. *Journal of the Scientific Study of Religion, 52*(2), 363–379.

Benjamins, M. R. (2004). Religion and functional health among the elderly: Is there a relationship and is it constant? *Journal of Aging and Health, 16*(3), 355–374.

Berger, P. L., & Neuhaus, R. H. (1977). *To empower people: The role of mediating structures in public policy*. Washington, DC: American Enterprise Institute for Public Policy Research.

Berger, P., Davie, G., & Fokas, E. (2008). *Religious America, secular Europe? A theme and variations*. Farnham, UK: Ashgate.

Bodhi, B. (2011). What does mindfulness really mean? A canonical perspective. *Contemporary Buddhism, 12*, 19–39.

Bott, E. (1957). *Family and social network: Roles, norms and external relationships in ordinary urban families*. London, UK: Tavistock.

Bowlby, J. (1980). *Attachment and loss, volume 3: Loss; sadness and depression*. New York, NY: Basic Books.

Brandtstädter, J. (2006). Adaptive resources in later life: Tenacious goal pursuit and flexible goal adjustment. In M. Csikszentmihalyi & I. S. Csikszentmihalyi (Eds.), *A life worth living. Contributions to positive psychology* (pp. 143–164). New York, NY: Oxford University Press.

Brown, C. G., & Snape, M. (Eds.). (2010). *Secularisation in the Christian world*. Farnham, UK: Ashgate.

Brown, S. L., Nesse, R. M., House, J. S., & Utz, R. L. (2004). Religion and emotional compensation: Results from a prospective study of widowhood. *Personality and Social Psychology Bulletin, 30*(9), 1165–1174.

Bruce, S. (1996). *Religion in the modern world: From cathedrals to cults*. Cambridge, MA: Cambridge University Press.

Coin, A., Perissinotto, E., Najjar, M., Girardi, A., Inelmen, E. M., Enzi, G.,… Sergi, G. (2010). Does religiosity protect against cognitive and behavioral decline in Alzheimer's dementia? *Current Alzheimer Research, 7*(5), 445–452.

Coleman, P. G. (2011). The changing social context of belief in later life. In P. G. Coleman, *Belief and ageing: Spiritual pathways in later life* (pp. 11–33). Bristol, UK: Policy Press.

Coleman, P. G., Begum, A., & Jaleel, S. (2011). Religious difference and age: The growing presence of other faiths. In P. G. Coleman, *Belief and ageing: Spiritual pathways in later life* (pp. 139–55). Bristol, UK: Policy Press.

Coleman, P. G., Ivani-Chalian, C., & Robinson, M. (2004). Religious attitudes among British older people: Stability and change in a 20-year longitudinal study. *Ageing and Society, 24*, 167–88.

Coleman, P. G., Ivani-Chalian, C., & Robinson, M. (2015). *Self and meaning in the lives of older people. Case studies over 20 years*. Cambridge, UK: Cambridge University Press.

Coleman, P. G., Koleva, D., & Bornat, J. (Eds.). (2013). *Ageing, ritual and social change. Comparing the secular and religious in eastern and western Europe*. Farnham, UK: Ashgate.

Coleman, P. G., McKiernan, F., Mills, M., & Speck, P. (2007). In sure and uncertain faith: Belief and coping with loss of spouse in later life. *Ageing and society, 27*(06), 869–890.

Copen, C., & Silverstein, M. (2007). Transmission of religious beliefs across generations: Do grandparents matter? *Journal of Comparative Family Studies, 38*(4), 497–510.

Crockett, A., & Voas, D. (2006). Generations of decline: Religious change in 20th-century Britain. *Journal for the Scientific Study of Religion, 45*(4), 567–584.

Crow, G. (2004). Social networks and social exclusion: An overview of the debate. In C. Phillipson, G. Allan, & D. Morgan (Eds.), *Social networks and social exclusion* (pp. 7–19). Aldershot, UK: Ashgate.

Davie, G. (2002). *Europe the exceptional case: Parameters of faith in the modern world.* London, UK: Darton, Longman and Todd.

Davie, G. (2006). Religion in Europe in the 21st century: The factors to take into account. *Archives of European Sociology, 47*, 271–296.

Davie, G. (2007). Vicarious religion: A methodological challenge. In N. T. Ammerman (Ed.), *Everyday religion: Observing modern religious lives* (pp. 21–36). New York, NY: Oxford University Press.

Day, A. (2013a). Varieties of belief over time: Reflections from a longitudinal study of youth and belief. *Journal of Contemporary Religion, 28*(2), 277–293.

Day, A. (2013b). The problem of generalizing generation. *Religion and Society: Advances in Research, 4*(1), 109–124.

Dillon, M., & Wink, P. (2007). *In the course of a lifetime. Tracing religious belief, practice and change.* Berkeley: University of California Press.

Eisenhandler, S. (2003). *Keeping the faith in late life.* New York, NY: Springer Publishing Company.

Ellison, C., & George, L. K. (1994). Religious involvement, social ties, and social support in a southeastern community. *Journal for the Scientific Study of Religion, 33*(1), 46–61.

Erikson, E. H. (1950). *Childhood and society.* New York, NY: W. W. Norton.

Fitchett, G., Benjamins, M. R., Skarupski, K. A., & Mendes de Leon, C. F. (2013). Worship attendance and the disability process in community-dwelling older adults. *The Journals of Gerontology, Series B, 68*(2), 235–245.

Foulcher, L. (2014). Aging, humility, and the monastery. *Journal of Religion, Spirituality and Aging, 26*, 148–159.

Fowler, J. W. (1981). *Stages of faith.* San Francisco, CA: Harper and Row.

Fry, P. S. (2000). Religious involvement, spirituality and personal meaning for life: Existential predictors of psychological well being in community-residing and institutional care elders. *Aging and Mental Health, 4*(4), 375–387.

Fry, P. S. (2001). The unique contribution of key existential factors to the prediction of psychological well-being of older adults following spousal loss. *The Gerontologist, 41*(1), 69–81.

Gans, D., Silverstein, M., & Lowenstein, A. (2009). Do religious children care more and provide more care for older parents? A study of filial norms and behaviors across five nations. *Journal of Comparative Family Studies, 40*(2), 187–201.

Gard, T., Hölzel, B. K., & Lazar, S. W. (2014). The potential effects of meditation on age-related cognitive decline: A systematic review. *Annals of the New York Academy of Sciences, 1307*, 89–103.

Geertz, C. (1993). *The interpretation of cultures*. London, UK: Fontana Press. (Original work published 1973)

George, L. K., Kinghorn, W. A., Koenig, H. G., Gammon, P., & Blazer, D. G. (2013). Why gerontologists should care about empirical research on religion and health: Transdisciplinary perspectives. *The Gerontologist, 53*(6), 898–906.

George, L. K., Larson, D. B., Koenig, H. G., & McCullough, M. E. (2000). Spirituality and health: What we know, what we need to know. *Journal of Social and Clinical Psychology, 19*(1), 102–116.

Gill, R., Hadaway, C. K., & Marler, P. L. (1998). Is religious belief declining in Britain? *Journal for the Scientific Study of Religion, 37*(3), 507–516.

Gorski, P. S. (2000). Historicizing the secularization debate: Church, state, and society in late medieval and early modern Europe, ca. 1300 to 1700. *American Sociological Review, 65*(1), 138–167.

Granovetter, M. (1973). The strength of weak ties. *American Journal of Sociology, 78*(6), 1360–1380.

Gutmann, D. (1987). *Reclaimed powers: Towards a new psychology of men and women in later life*. New York, NY: Basic Books.

Gutmann, D. L. (1997). *The human elder in nature, culture and society*. Boulder, CO: Westview Press.

Hauerwas, S., Stoneking, C. B., Meador, K. G., & Cloutier, D. (Eds.). (2003). *Growing old in Christ*. Grand Rapids, MI: William B. Eerdmans.

Hayward, R. D., & Krause, N. M. (2013a). Changes in Church-based social support relationships during older adulthood. *The Journals of Gerontology, Series B, 68*(1), 85–96.

Hayward, R. D., & Krause, N. M. (2013b). Trajectories of late-life change in God-mediated control. *The Journals of Gerontology, Series B, 68*, 49–58.

Heelas, P., &Woodhead, L. (2005). *The spiritual revolution: Why religion is giving way to spirituality*. Oxford, MA: Blackwell.

Helm, H. M., Hays, J. C., Flint, E. P., Koenig, H. G., & Blazer, D. G. (2000). Does private religious activity prolong survival? A six-year follow-up study of 3,851 older adults. *The Journals of Gerontology, Series A, 55*(7), M400–M405.

Hill, T. D., Angel, J. L., Ellison, C. G., & Angel, R. J. (2005). Religious attendance and mortality: An 8-year follow-up of older Mexican Americans. *The Journals of Gerontology, Series B, 60*(2), S102–S109.

Hill, T. D., Burdette, A. M., Angel, J. L., & Angel, R. J. (2006). Religious attendance and cognitive functioning among older Mexican Americans. *The Journals of Gerontology, Series B, 61*(1), P3–P9.

Hogan, M. (2014). *The culture of our thinking in relation to spirituality*. New York, NY: Nova Science.

Hui, V. K., & Coleman, P. G. (2012). Do reincarnation beliefs protect older adult Chinese Buddhists against personal death anxiety. *Death Studies, 36,* 949–958.

Idler, E. (2006). Religion and aging. In R. Binstock, L. K. George, S. J. Cutler, J. Hendricks, & J. Schulz (Eds.), *Handbook of aging and the social sciences* (pp. 277–300). Burlington, MA: Academic Press.

Idler, E. L., Kasl, S. V., & Hays, J. C. (2001). Patterns of religious practice and belief in the last year of life. *The Journals of Gerontology, Series B, 56*(6), S326–S334.

Idler, E. L., McLaughlin, J., & Kasl, S. (2009). Religion and the quality of life in the last year of life. *The Journals of Gerontology, Series B, 64*(4), 528–537.

Jung, C. G. (1938). *Psychology and religion.* New Haven, CT: Yale University Press.

Jung, C. G. (1972). The transcendent function. In H. Read, M. Fordham, G. Adler, & W. McGuire (Eds.), *The structure and dynamics of the psyche: Volume 8. The collected works of C.G. Jung* (2nd ed., pp. 67–91). London, UK: Routledge and Kegan Paul.

Katz, R., & Lowenstein, A. (2010). Theoretical perspectives on intergenerational solidarity, conflict and ambivalence. In M. Izuhara (Ed.), *Ageing and intergenerational relations: Family reciprocity from a global perspective* (pp. 29–56). Bristol, UK: Policy Press.

Kaufman, Y., Anaki, D., Binns, M., & Freedman, M. (2007). Cognitive decline in Alzheimer disease: Impact of spirituality, religiosity, and QOL. *Neurology, 68*(18), 1509–1514.

King, S., Burgess, E., Akinyela, M., Counts-Spriggs, M., & Parker, N. (2006). The religious dimensions of the grandparent role in three-generation African American households. *Journal of Religion, Spirituality and Aging, 19*(1), 75–96.

King, V., Ledwell, M., & Pearce-Morris, J. (2013). Religion and ties between adult children and their parents. *The Journals of Gerontology, Series B, 68*(5), 825–836.

Kirby, S. E., Coleman, P. G., & Daley, D. (2004). Spirituality and well-being in frail and nonfrail older adults. *The Journals of Gerontology, Series B, 59*(3), P123–P129.

Kirkpatrick, L. A. (2005). *Attachment, evolution, and the psychology of religion.* New York, NY: Guilford Press.

Klass, D., Silverman, P., & Nickman, S. (1996). *Continuing bonds: New understandings of grief.* New York, NY: Taylor & Francis.

Koenig, H., King, D., & Carson, V. (2012). *Handbook of religion and health.* Oxford, UK: Oxford University Press.

Koenig, H., McCullough M., & Larson D. (2001). *Handbook of religion and health.* Oxford, UK: Oxford University Press.

Koleva, D. (2013). Performing social normativity: Religious rituals in secular lives. In P. G. Coleman, D. Koleva, & J. Bornat (Eds.), *Ageing, ritual and social change. Comparing the secular and religious in eastern and western Europe* (pp. 111–132). Farnham, UK: Ashgate.

Krause, N. (2002). Church-based social support and health in old age: Exploring variations by race. *The Journals of Gerontology, Series B, 57*(6), S332–S347.

Krause, N. (2015). Assessing the religious roots of volunteer work in middle and late life. *Research on Aging, 37*(5), 439–463.

Krause, N. M. (2006). Church-based social support and mortality. *The Journals of Gerontology, Series B, 61*(3), 140–46.

Krause, N. M., & Bastida, E. (2011). Church-based social relationships, belonging, and health among older Mexican Americans. *Journal for the Scientific Study of Religion, 50*(2), 397–409.

Krause, N. M., & Hayward, D. (2014). Work at church and church-based emotional support among older Whites, Blacks, and Mexican Americans. *Journal of Religion, Spirituality and Aging, 26*(1), 22–40.

Kreager, P. (2009). Ageing, finance and civil society: Notes for an agenda. In E. N. Arifin & A. Ananta (Eds.), *Older persons in Southeast Asia: An emerging asset* (pp. 361–391). Singapore: Institute of Southeast Asian Studies.

Lamb, S. (2000). *White saris and sweet mangoes: Aging, gender, and body in North India.* Berkeley, CA: University of California Press.

Lee, E. S. (2014). The impact of social and spiritual connectedness on the psychological well-being among older Americans. *Journal of Religion, Spirituality and Aging, 26*(4), 300–319.

Lewis, V. A., Macgregor, C. A., & Putnam, R. D. (2013). Religion, networks, and neighborliness: The impact of religious social networks on civic engagement. *Social Science Research, 42*(2), 331–346.

Luckmann, T. (1990). Shrinking transcendence, expanding religion? *Sociological Analysis, 50*(2), 127–138.

Lutgendorf, S. K., Russell, D., Ullrich, P., Harris, T. B., & Wallace, R. (2004). Religious participation, interleukin-6, and mortality in older adults. *Health Psychology: Official Journal of the Division of Health Psychology, American Psychological Association, 23*(5), 465–475.

Lynch, G. (2007). *The new spirituality. An introduction to progressive belief in the twenty-first century.* London, UK: Tauris.

MacKinlay, E. (Ed.). (2010). *Ageing and spirituality across faiths and cultures.* London, UK: Jessica Kingsley.

Maslow, A. H. (1943). A theory of human motivation. *Psychological Review, 50,* 370–396.

Maslow, A. H. (1971). *The farther reaches of human nature.* New York, NY: Viking Press.

McCullough, M. E., Enders, C. K., Brion, S. L., & Jain, A. R. (2005). The varieties of religious development in adulthood: A longitudinal investigation of religion and rational choice. *Journal of Personality and Social Psychology, 89*(1), 78–89.

McFadden, S. H. (2008). Mindfulness, vulnerability, and love: Spiritual lessons from frail elders, earnest young pilgrims, and middle-aged rockers. *Journal of Aging Studies, 22,* 132–9.

McIntosh, W. A., Sykes, D., & Kubena, K. S. (2002). Religion and community among the elderly: The relationship between the religious and secular characteristics of their social networks. *Review of Religious Research, 44*(2), 109–125.

McNamara, P. (2002). The motivational origins of religious practices. *Zygon, 37*(1), 143–160.

Mehta, K. (1997). The impact of religious beliefs and practices on aging: A cross-cultural comparison. *Journal of Aging Studies, 11*, 101–115.

Merino, S. M. (2014). Social support and the religious dimensions of close ties. *Journal for the Scientific Study of Religion, 53*(3), 595–612.

Merz, E. M., Ozeke-Kocabas, E., Oort, F. J., & Schuengel, C. (2009). Intergenerational family solidarity: Value differences between immigrant groups and generations. *Journal of Family Psychology: JFP: Journal of the Division of Family Psychology of the American Psychological Association (Division 43), 23*(3), 291–300.

Moberg, D. (2001). Research on spirituality. In D. Moberg (Ed.), *Aging and spirituality. Spiritual dimensions of aging theory, research, practice, and policy* (pp. 55–69). New York, NY: Haworth Press.

Moberg, D. (2005). Research in spirituality, religion, and aging. In H. R. Moody (Ed.), *Religion, spirituality, and aging: A social work perspective* (pp. 11–40). Birmingham, NY: Haworth Press.

Moody, H. R. (1995). Mysticism. In M. A. Kimble, S. H. McFadden, J. W. Ellor, & J. J. Seeber (Eds.). *Aging, spirituality, and religion: A handbook* (Vol. 1, pp. 87–101). Minneapolis, MN: Fortress Press.

Moody, H. R., & Carroll, D. (1997). *The five stages of the soul: Charting the spiritual passages that shape our lives.* New York, NY: Doubleday.

Newberg, A. B., Serruya, M., Wintering, N., Moss, A. S., Reibel, D., & Monti, D. A. (2014). Meditation and neurodegenerative diseases. *Annals of the New York Academy of Sciences, 1307*, 112–123.

Norton, M. C., Singh, A., Skoog, I., Corcoran, C., Tschanz, J. T., Zandi,…Steffens, D. C.; Cache County Investigators. (2008). Church attendance and new episodes of major depression in a community study of older adults: The Cache County study. *The Journals of Gerontology, Series B, 63*(3), P129–P137.

Oyserman, D. (2007). Social identity and self-regulation. In A. Kruglanski & T. Higgin (Eds.), *Handbook of social psychology* (pp. 432–453). New York, NY: Guilford Press.

Pargament, K. I. (1999). The psychology of religion *and* spirituality? Yes and no. *International Journal for the Psychology of Religion, 9*, 3–16.

Park, C. L. (2005). Religion and meaning. In R. F. Paloutzian & C. L. Park (Eds.), *Handbook of the psychology of religion and spirituality* (pp. 295–314). New York, NY: Guilford Press.

Park, J., Roh, S., & Yeo, Y. (2012). Religiosity, social support, and life satisfaction among elderly Korean immigrants. *The Gerontologist, 52*(5), 641–649.

Park, N. S., Klemmack, D. L., Roff, L. L., Parker, M. W., Koenig, H. G., Sawyer, P., & Allman, R. M. (2008). Religiousness and longitudinal trajectories in Elders' functional status. *Research on Aging, 30*(3), 279–298.

Payman, V., & Ryburn, B. (2010). Religiousness and recovery from inpatient geriatric depression: Findings from the PEJAMA Study. *Australian and New Zealand Journal of Psychiatry, 44*(6), 560–567.

Prince, M., Bryce, R., Albanese, E., Wimo, A., Ribeiro, W., & Ferri, C. P. (2013). The global prevalence of dementia: A systematic review and metaanalysis. *Alzheimer's & Dementia: The Journal of the Alzheimer's Association, 9*(1), 63–75.e2.

Putnam, R., & Campbell, D. (2010). *American grace: How religion divides and unites us.* New York, NY: Simon and Schuster.

Ram-Prasad, C. (1995). A classical Indian philosophical perspective on ageing and the meaning of life. *Ageing and Society, 15,* 1–36.

Rowe, J. W., & Kahn, R. L. (1998). *Successful aging.* New York, NY: Pantheon/Random House.

Schröder-Butterfill, E. (2015). Networks, strata and ageing: Towards a compositional demography of vulnerability. In P. Kreager, B. Winney, S. Ulijaszek, & C. Capelli (Eds.), *Population in the human sciences: Concepts, models, evidence* (pp. 257–291). Oxford, UK: Oxford University Press.

Schröder-Butterfill, E., & Kreager, P. (2005). Actual and de facto childlessness in old age: Evidence and implications from East Java, Indonesia. *Population and Development Review, 31*(1), 19–55.

Sedikides, C., & Gebauer, J. E. (2013). Religion and the self. In V. Saroglou (Ed.), *Religion, personality, and social behavior* (pp. 46–70). New York, NY: Psychology Press.

Sherman, E. (1981). *Counseling the aging: An integrative approach.* New York, NY: Free Press.

Sherman, E. (2010). *Contemplative aging: A way of being in later life.* New York, NY: Gordion Knot Books.

Snowdon, D. (2008). *Aging with grace: What the nun study teaches us about leading longer, healthier, and more meaningful lives.* New York, NY: Bantam Books.

Spreadbury, J. H., & Coleman, P. G. (2011). Religious responses in coping with spousal bereavement. In P. G. Coleman (Ed.), *Belief and ageing: Spiritual pathways in later life* (pp. 79–96). Bristol, UK: Policy Press.

Taylor, R. J., Chatters, L. M., & Jackson, J. S. (2007). Religious and spiritual involvement among older African Americans, Caribbean Blacks, and non-Hispanic Whites: Findings from the national survey of American life. *The Journals of Gerontology, Series B, 62*(4), S238–S250.

Thelen, T., Leutloff-Grandits, C., & Peleikis, A. (2009). Social security in religious networks: An introduction. In C. Leutloff-Grandits, A. Peleikis, & T. Thelen (Eds.), *Social security in religious networks.* New York, NY: Berghahn.

Thibault, J. M. (1993). *A deepening love affair: The gift of God in later years.* Nashville, TN: Upper Room Books.

Tilak, S. (1989). *Religion and aging in the Indian tradition.* Albany, NY: State University of New York Press.

Tornstam, L. (1994). Gerotranscendence: A theoretical and empirical exploration. In L. E. Thomas & S. A. Eisenhandler (Eds.), *Aging and the religious dimension* (pp. 203–225). Westport, CT: Greenwood.

Tornstam, L. (2005). *Gerotranscendence: A developmental theory of positive aging.* New York, NY: Springer Publishing Company.

Traphagan, J. W. (2000). Reproducing elder male power through ritual performance in Japan. *Journal of Cross-Cultural Gerontology, 15*(2), 81–97.

Traphagan, J. W. (2004). *The Practice of concern: Ritual, well-being and aging in rural Japan.* Durham, NC: Carolina Academic Press.

Van Ness, P. H., & Kasl, S. V. (2003). Religion and cognitive dysfunction in an elderly cohort. *The Journals of Gerontology, Series B, 58*(1), S21–S29.

Voas, D., & Crockett, A. (2005). Religion in Britain: Neither believing nor belonging. *Sociology, 39*(1), 11–28.

Voas, D., & Doebler, S. (2011). Secularization in Europe: Religious change between and within birth cohorts. *Religion and Society in Central and Eastern Europe, 4*(1), 39–62.

Waschenfelder, J. (2012). The world suffices: Spiritualities without the supernatural. *Journal for the Study of Spirituality, 1*, 171–186.

Wellman, B., & Wortley, S. (1989). Brothers' keepers: Situating kinship relations in broader networks of social support. *Sociological Perspectives, 32*(3), 273–306.

Whitehead, B. R., & Bergeman, C. S. (2012). Coping with daily stress: Differential role of spiritual experience on daily positive and negative affect. *The Journals of Gerontology, Series B, 67*(4), 456–459.

Wilkinson, P. J., & Coleman, P. G. (2010). Strong beliefs and coping in old age: A case-based comparison of atheism and religion. *Ageing and Society, 30*, 337–361.

Wortmann, J. H., & Park, C. L. (2008). Religion and spirituality in adjustment following bereavement: An integrative review. *Death Studies, 32*(8), 703–736.

Wuthnow, R. (1999). *Growing up religious: Christians and Jews and their journeys of faith.* Boston, MA: Beacon Press.

Zhang, W. (2008). Religious participation and mortality risk among the oldest old in China. *The Journals of Gerontology, Series B, 63*(5), S293–S297.

CHAPTER 30

Theories of Wisdom and Aging

Monika Ardelt and Hunhui Oh

What is wisdom and does it come with age as many people assume, or is it a relatively rare quality even among the older population? How do people develop wisdom throughout life and what might be its benefits in old age? Empirical evidence suggests that wisdom in old age is positively related to subjective well-being and less fear of death, even in the face of physical disability or the nearing of death (Ardelt, Landes, Gerlach, & Fox, 2013). In fact, it appears that wisdom is most beneficial for subjective well-being under conditions of adversity and stress, when external means to increase well-being are less available (Ardelt, 2005; Ardelt & Edwards, in press). Wisdom tends to provide a sense of mastery and meaning in life that sustains well-being even under adverse circumstances (Etezadi & Pushkar, 2013; Glück & Bluck, 2013).

In this chapter, we first provide a brief summary of explicit and implicit wisdom theories. After examining the relation between wisdom and age, we shed light on the contextual life-course approach to address the divergent trajectories of personal wisdom development, with focus on the importance of social support networks and role models. Last, we explore the associations among wisdom and culture, religion/spirituality, and well-being in old age.

■ THEORIES OF WISDOM

Numerous theories have been provided to define wisdom based either on the literature or personal narratives. For example, wisdom has been defined as

- Expert knowledge in the meaning and conduct of life (Baltes & Smith, 1990)
- Tacit knowledge to achieve a common good by balancing personal, interpersonal, and social interests (Sternberg, 1998)
- Understanding the deeper meaning of common knowledge (Kekes, 1983)
- Perceiving things as they really are by seeing through the illusion of wrong beliefs (McKee & Barber, 1999)
- The art of questioning (Arlin, 1990)
- The balance between knowing and doubting (Meacham, 1990)
- Expertise in dealing with the cognitive, emotional, and behavioral aspects of uncertainty (Brugman, 2000)
- The balance between emotion and detachment, action and inaction, and knowledge and doubt in dealing with life's vicissitudes (Birren & Fisher, 1990)
- The integration of cognitive reasoning with holistic, affective, and experiential knowing (Labouvie-Vief, 1990)
- The integration of cognitive, reflective, and affective/compassionate personality qualities (Ardelt, 1997; Clayton & Birren, 1980)

- The virtue that results from resolving the eighth psychosocial task of integrity versus despair in Erikson's (1982) stage model of psychosocial development
- Self-transcendence (Levenson, Jennings, Aldwin, & Shiraishi, 2005) or
- Daily decision making about, for instance, which school to apply to, which companies to work for, and which retirement fund to invest in (Hall, 2010)

Despite the various ways of defining wisdom, the central theme shared by the majority of wisdom literature is that wisdom is multidimensional and consists of cognitive, reflective, and benevolent components that are mutually interdependent and benefit the wise person, others, and society as a whole (Ferrari & Weststrate, 2013; Sternberg, 1990b; Sternberg & Jordan, 2005). In the following, we present evidence for these overarching themes and describe explicit or "expert" wisdom theories and implicit or "lay" wisdom theories in Western and Eastern cultures.

Explicit Wisdom Theories

Explicit wisdom theories have been developed by "experts" in the field with the goal of obtaining a gold standard for the utopian concept of wisdom (Baltes & Smith, 1990; Baltes & Staudinger, 2000). This orientation attempts to explicate the essential features of wisdom as an ideal endpoint of human development (Baltes & Kunzmann, 2004).

Among the Western approaches to wisdom, the Berlin Wisdom Paradigm, led by the late Paul Baltes since the early 90s, is probably the most prominent explicit wisdom model to date. Specifically, Baltes et al. define wisdom as an expert knowledge system in life planning, life management, and life review, related to the meaning and conduct of life (Baltes & Smith, 1990, 2008; Baltes & Staudinger, 2000; Baltes, Staudinger, Maercker, & Smith, 1995; Dittmann-Kohli & Baltes, 1990; Smith & Baltes, 1990; Smith, Staudinger, & Baltes, 1994). It is assessed as a performance measure by asking research participants to think aloud about ill-structured hypothetical life problems that have no easy solution (e.g., "A 15-year-old girl wants to go get married right away. What could one/she consider and do?"). Transcribed answers are rated on five criteria and then averaged: (a) rich factual knowledge about human nature and the life course; (b) rich procedural knowledge about ways of dealing with life problems; (c) life-span contextualism, that is, an awareness of the many contexts of life, including social relations; (d) value relativism and tolerance, that is, acknowledging individual, social, and cultural differences in values and life priorities, and (e) knowledge about handling uncertainty, including the limits of one's own knowledge and the knowledge of the world at large (Baltes & Staudinger, 2000).

The Berlin Wisdom Paradigm attempts to assess general wisdom-related knowledge that is independent of individuals rather than personal wisdom. Another measure of general wisdom-related knowledge is the reflective judgment interview (RJI). According to Kitchener and Brenner (1990, p. 226), high scoring responses to ill-structured problems related to the dilemmas of knowing in historical, scientific, religious, and everyday context "reflect a recognition of the limits of personal knowledge, an acknowledgment of the general uncertainty that characterizes human knowing, and a humility about one's own judgments in the face of such limitations."

Whereas general wisdom-related knowledge refers to life insight that is usually activated through advice giving and support of others, personal wisdom refers to self-insight and is activated in coping behavior and life management situations (Staudinger, 2013). To assess personal wisdom, Staudinger et al. (Mickler & Staudinger, 2008; Staudinger,

Dörner, & Mickler, 2005) developed a wisdom measure that asks participants about their behavior, strengths, and weaknesses as a friend and then rate the transcribed responses on five self-related criteria modeled after the Berlin Wisdom Paradigm: (a) rich self-knowledge; (b) rich procedural knowledge about personal growth and self-regulation, including emotions regulation and the development and maintenance of close social relationships; (c) knowledge about the causes of one's emotions and behavior and the nature of interdependence; (d) self-relativism, which requires reflection, self-reflection, and the acceptance of self and others, and (e) tolerance of ambiguity and uncertainty.

Sternberg's (1998) balance theory of wisdom is another prominent explicit wisdom theory. According to Sternberg (1990a, 1998), sagacity is the most distinguishing dimension between wisdom and intelligence. A person who possesses sagacity, developed through self-reflection and learning from others, displays concern for others, considers advice, and understands people by listening and observing. Sagacity helps people to know themselves and to grow further in wisdom by having the courage to admit making mistakes and the motivation to correct the mistakes. Sagacity, thus, forms the tacit knowledge that balances intrapersonal, interpersonal, and extrapersonal interests. As Sternberg (1998, p. 354) remarked, "Wisdom is involved when practical intelligence is applied to maximizing not just one's own or someone else's self-interest, but rather a balance of various self-interests (intrapersonal) with the interests of others (interpersonal) and of other aspects of the context in which one lives (extrapersonal), such as one's city or country or environment or even God." Although the balance theory of wisdom is theoretically promising, it lacks an approach to measure wisdom.

Most wisdom literature concurs that advanced cognitive development is necessary but not sufficient for wisdom to arise. For example, Pascual-Leone (1990) argued that wisdom requires a dialectical integration of cognition, reflection, affect, and personality, combining the authority of reason with a harmonious view of the world. A dialectical integration of personality weakens self-centered characteristics and strengthens other-centeredness and prosocial behavior. Kramer (1990) equally emphasized the importance of the integration of cognition, affect, and reflection as a highly developed form of functioning that is central to wisdom.

Ancient Eastern wisdom definitions have also stressed the integration of cognitive, reflective, affective, and prosocial characteristics as essential elements of wisdom. For example, in the Bhagavad Gita, a Hindu text that was written between 500 and 200 BCE (Zaehner, 1969), the domains of wisdom as identified by Jeste and Vahia (2008) include knowledge of life, emotional regulation, control over desires, decisiveness, love of God, duty and work, self-contentedness, yoga or integration of personality, compassion or sacrifice, and insight or humility. The teachings of the Buddha (born between 563 and 463 BCE) highlight that striving for equanimity, (self-)insight, and compassion are most important in the development of wisdom (Hart, 1987; Ñanamoli, 2001). In ancient China, Lao-Tzu (born between 600 and 300 BCE) taught that the development of intuition, self-knowledge and compassion led to wisdom, whereas Confucius (551–479 BCE) favored learning and reflecting on the learned material in combination with compassion and personal morality as the pathway to wisdom (Birren & Svensson, 2005; Riegel, 2006).

Although the most prominent Western approaches to wisdom tend to emphasize cognition and analytic abilities, the Eastern approaches view wisdom more holistically as comprising the whole person, including behavioral conduct in the form of morality and compassion toward others. Yet, some Western explicit theories, such as those by Pascual-Leone (1990) and Kramer (1990), also describe wisdom in more holistic terms as an integration of cognition, reflection, affect, and a less self-centered personality. Takahashi and Overton (2005) argued that wisdom definitions should transcend cultural egocentrism and incorporate wisdom descriptions that are culturally inclusive and broad. Hence, their explicit wisdom model consists of the integration of an analytical mode (consisting of knowledge and abstract reasoning abilities) and a synthetic mode (comprising reflective understanding, emotional empathy, and emotional regulation) to combine the dominant explicit wisdom theories in the West and East (Takahashi & Overton, 2002). After reviewing the world's philosophical, religious, and psychological wisdom traditions, Curnow (1999) came to the conclusion that the core features of wisdom consist of self-knowledge, detachment, self-integration, and self-transcendence. Levenson et al. (2005) viewed those core features as developmental stages that are recursive and reinforce each other in their theory of wisdom as self-transcendence. According to this theory, wisdom is a mode of being rather than knowing or doing (Levenson & Aldwin, 2013). It encompasses the whole person. As Moody (1986, p. 142) remarked, "One can *have* theoretical knowledge without any corresponding transformation of one's personal being. But one cannot 'have' wisdom without *being* wise" (emphasis in the original). This implies that it might be possible to have general wisdom-related knowledge, but personal wisdom requires a transformation of one's personality in the form of decreased self-centeredness and increased self-transcendence and other-centeredness. Personal wisdom entails a paradigm shift that enables people to not just know more about life but also to perceive the world differently as they grow wiser.

Overall, explicit wisdom theories have contributed to the research on adult human development by proposing ideal forms of human maturation and behaviors that few individuals can hope to attain in perfection. Yet, wisdom is not considered a binary quality but a continuum with people being closer or farther away from this ideal state (Ardelt, 2004b).

Implicit Wisdom Theories

Integrative features of wisdom have also been found in studies of how laypeople define the concept of wisdom. The rationale of implicit wisdom theories is that individuals know implicitly who and what is wise (Bluck & Glück, 2005).

For example, Clayton and Birren's (1980) seminal research presented participants of three age groups (31 young, 23 middle-aged, and 29 older adults) with the words "wise," "aged," and "myself" and a list of 12 wisdom-related adjectives, generated in an earlier study by a different set of research participants, and asked them to rate the similarity of all possible word pairs. A multidimensional scaling analysis of the similarities resulted in three wisdom dimensions, comprising cognition (knowledgeable, experienced, intelligent, pragmatic, and observant), reflection (introspective and intuitive), and affect/compassion (understanding, empathetic, peaceful, and gentle).

Similarly, Holliday and Chandler (1986) found that research participants' implicit wisdom theories included not only exceptional cognitive judgmental skills but also interpersonal skills and social unobtrusiveness. They first asked adults of three age groups (50 young, 50 middle-aged, and 50 old) to describe wisdom and then another group of 150 adults of the same age composition to rate the obtained wisdom characteristics on a scale from "almost never true of wise people" to "almost always true of wise people." The result of a principal component factor analysis indicated that wisdom was perceived as a mixture of (a) exceptional understanding of essences, contexts, and the self (e.g., learning from experience and seeing things in a larger context); (b) judgment and communication skills (e.g., the ability to understand and judge correctly in matters of daily living); (c) general competencies (e.g., intelligent and educated); (d) interpersonal skills (e.g., sensitive and sociable); and (e) social unobtrusiveness (discrete and nonjudgmental).

Sternberg's (1985) multidimensional scaling analysis based on descriptors of ideal intelligent, creative, and wise individuals collected from both college professors and laypersons showed that wise individuals were perceived to have analytical reasoning ability similar to intelligent individuals. Yet, wise persons were ascribed a certain sagacity that was not necessarily attributed to intelligent persons. In addition, wise individuals were characterized as having good judgment skills, perspicacity, and the ability to learn from ideas and the environment and to make expeditious use of information. This suggests that an open-minded attitude and reflective capacity run parallel with reasoning ability and sagacity for wise individuals to make clear, sensible, and fair judgments.

Although the approaches and measurements were different (and thus the list of wisdom characteristics that was generated and subsequently rated was not identical in the studies), cognitive, reflective, and prosocial benevolent wisdom characteristics were dominant descriptors endorsed by most research participants. Bluck and Glück's (2005) review of five studies on implicit wisdom theories, including the three studies mentioned earlier, concluded that cognitive ability, insight, reflective attitude, concern for others, and real-world skills are considered important elements in Western lay theories of wisdom. However, Glück & Bluck's (2011) subsequent study and cluster analysis with an age-diverse sample revealed that two different groups of people exist with conceptually distinct implicit wisdom theories. Similar to the Berlin Wisdom Paradigm, the *cognitive conception* group endorsed primarily cognitive characteristics (knowledge, life experience, and cognitive complexity) and reflective characteristics (self-reflection and acceptance of others' values) as central to wisdom, whereas the *integrative conception* group additionally endorsed affective/compassionate characteristics, such as benevolence, empathy, love for humanity, and concern for others.

The integrative definition of wisdom more closely resembles Eastern implicit wisdom theories, which tend to emphasize the affective/compassionate component of wisdom as much as or even more than its cognitive component (Takahashi & Overton, 2005). In addition, modesty and unobtrusiveness seem to be important elements of Eastern implicit wisdom theories that are not necessarily found in Western implicit wisdom theories. For example, Taiwanese Chinese adults from various age groups described wisdom as a combination of competencies, knowledge, benevolence, compassion, openness, profundity, modesty, and unobtrusiveness (Yang, 2001). Similarly, Takahashi and Bordia (2000) found that Indian and Japanese undergraduate students tended to rate the word "wise" as most similar to "discreet," whereas American and Australian students tended to rate "wise" closer to "experienced" and "knowledgeable."

Wisdom Theories That Combine Implicit and Explicit Approaches

Some researchers have used implicit wisdom theories as the basis for their explicit wisdom model. For example, Yang's (2008) theory of wisdom as a real-life process emerged from her research on contemporary Eastern implicit wisdom theories (Yang, 2001). In the theory of wisdom as a real-life process, wisdom is understood as a process requiring the cognitive integration of sometimes contradictory ideas, interests, and personality, whereas the embodiment of wisdom occurs in everyday life through action that ultimately results in positive outcomes for oneself and others.

In an attempt to create a culturally inclusive wisdom theory, Ardelt (1997, 2003, 2004b) developed the Three-Dimensional Wisdom Model based on Clayton and Birren's (1980) pioneering research on implicit wisdom theories. The model integrates the cognitive, reflective, and affective/compassionate dimensions of wisdom. The *cognitive wisdom dimension* entails a desire to know the truth and encompasses a deep and thorough understanding of life, particularly regarding issues that relate to one's own person and one's relationship with others, as well as knowledge and acceptance of the positive and negative aspects of human nature, of the inherent limits of knowledge, and of life's unpredictability and uncertainty. The *reflective wisdom dimension* refers to the ability to perceive phenomena and events from multiple perspectives, including one's own self, which requires self-examination, self-awareness, and self-insight and the ability to see through illusion (McKee & Barber, 1999) to overcome subjectivity and projections. Rather than blaming other people and circumstances for their own faults and failures (Bradley, 1978; Green & Gross, 1979; Riess, Rosenfeld, Melburg, & Tedeschi, 1981; Sherwood, 1981), wise people are able to accept reality as it is, which tends to reduce self-centeredness and contribute to a greater understanding of life and others. A more thorough understanding of life and the human condition combined with a reduction in self-centeredness tends to generate sympathetic and compassionate love for others and the motivation to foster others' well-being, which are characteristics of the *compassionate wisdom dimension* (Achenbaum & Orwoll, 1991; Clayton & Birren, 1980; Csikszentmihalyi & Rathunde, 1990; Holliday & Chandler, 1986; Kramer, 1990; Levitt, 1999; Orwoll & Achenbaum, 1993; Pascual-Leone, 1990). The Three-Dimensional Wisdom Model has the advantages of being relatively parsimonious and also able to encompass both implicit and explicit wisdom theories from the West and the East (Curnow, 1999; Sternberg, 1990b; Sternberg & Jordan, 2005; Takahashi & Bordia, 2000).

■ PSYCHOSOCIAL CORRELATES OF WISDOM IN OLD AGE AND ITS DEVELOPMENT

How is wisdom related to age, the social context, culture, religion or spirituality, and well-being? To some extent, the answers to this question depend on the definition and measurement of wisdom, which, as delineated earlier, vary widely. Still, some general trends are observable.

Wisdom and Age

Does wisdom increase with age? Theoretically, wisdom is considered a lifelong human developmental process, exemplified by Kekes' (1983, p. 286) statement that "one can be old and foolish, but a wise man is likely to be old, simply because such growth takes time." Erikson (1982) identified wisdom as the virtue that arises after the successful mastery of the eighth psychosocial development task of *ego integrity versus despair* in old age. Older adults who can accept the life they have lived, including missed opportunities and failures in the past, can achieve ego integrity that will help them to accept the physical, mental, and social challenges during the later years and the finitude of life. Hence, Erikson (1964, p. 133) defined wisdom as "informed and detached concern with life itself in the face of death itself," which requires a balance between active involvement in life and the acceptance of aging-related declines and the nearing of death without despairing over physical, mental, and social losses.

Although Erikson outlined a lifelong developmental path toward wisdom, Staudinger's (1999) earlier work and Sternberg's (2005) review of the literature on the relationship between age and wisdom describe various theoretical trajectories of wisdom development with age. It is possible that wisdom (a) continues to increase across the life span; (b) remains stable from early adulthood into old age; or (c) decreases with age after an initial increase in youth and young adulthood. In fact, it is likely that the development of wisdom varies for different people. Some people might grow in wisdom throughout life, while others remain stable after reaching a certain wisdom level or even decline with age (Sternberg, 2005). This suggests that multiple life-course factors, such as the promotion of wisdom in the family and the larger society, in combination with certain personality qualities might influence the trajectory of wisdom development.

Empirical evidence from cross-sectional data shows that mean levels of wisdom-related knowledge tend to increase with age throughout adolescence and young adulthood up to the age of about 24 years, then remain relatively stable, until they appear to decline after the age of 80 years (Baltes et al., 1995; Pasupathi, Staudinger, & Baltes, 2001; Staudinger, 1999). However, age was weakly and positively related to wisdom-related knowledge among individuals between the ages of 20 and 87 years who scored above the median level on moral reasoning (Pasupathi & Staudinger, 2001), which suggests that wisdom-related knowledge might increase with age if people are motivated to engage in positive personality development (Staudinger & Kunzmann, 2005).

A longitudinal study that used the RJI to assess wisdom as recognizing and understanding the limits and uncertainty of human knowledge found that RJI scores increased, on average, from age 16 to 20 years and from age 20 to 24 years. At age 28 years, many of the highly educated study participants already scored at or near the top of the RJI scale, but for those lower on the scale, RJI scores tended to increase further from age 28 to 32 years (Kitchener & Brenner, 1990; Kitchener, King, Wood, & Davison, 1989). Longitudinal research by Wink and Helson (1997) revealed that practical wisdom (measured by self-reported cognitive, reflective, and mature adjectives from the Adjective Check List) tended to increase between the ages of 27 and 52 years, particularly for clinical psychologists, indicating that wisdom might increase until at least middle age.

Wisdom, measured by the 39-item Three-Dimensional Wisdom Scale (3D-WS) as the integration of cognitive, reflective, and affective/compassionate personality qualities based on the Three-Dimensional Wisdom Model (Ardelt, 2003) or by Webster's (2003, 2007) 40-item noncognitive Self-Assessed Wisdom Scale (SAWS) as the combination of critical life experiences, reflectiveness/reminiscence, emotional regulation, openness to experience, and humor, has shown a curvilinear relationship with age in cross-sectional research, with the highest mean level scores at midlife rather than early adulthood (Bergsma & Ardelt, 2012; Webster, Westerhof, & Bohlmeijer, 2014). Yet, another study found that older college-educated adults had significantly higher mean-level scores on the 3D-WS than current undergraduate college students, whereas older adults without a college degree tended to score significantly lower on the 3D-WS than younger or older college-educated adults (Ardelt, 2010). Again, this suggests that wisdom might grow with age only among those individuals who have the opportunity, support, and motivation to pursue its development. Longitudinal studies have also documented that socioeconomic status, psychological mindedness, and openness to experience in early adulthood have a positive association with later life wisdom (Ardelt, 1998; Wink & Dillon, 2003; Wink & Helson, 1997), supporting the idea that favorable social conditions and certain personality dispositions can facilitate wisdom development.

It appears that the most important "building blocks" for wisdom emerge during adolescence and young adulthood (Richardson & Pasupathi, 2005). To better understand the relation between wisdom and age, it is critical to investigate how the seeds of wisdom were planted upfront, from whom individuals seek guidance, and to what extent older adults act as life consultants and wisdom mentors over the life course (Edmondson, 2012). Jordan (2005) argued that, although the factors that might lead to gains in wisdom with age in adolescence and young adulthood are well studied, such as the development of cognition, moral reasoning, and personality, there is a dearth of research on factors that might limit the growth of wisdom over the life span or even lead to a decline in wisdom during the later years.

Social Contexts and Wisdom Nominees

What are some of the factors that might promote or prevent growth in wisdom with age? Wisdom is a socially developed construct (Staudinger & Baltes, 1996), because a person cannot gain wisdom without the direct or indirect teachings of others (Jordan, 2005). The development of wisdom and wise decision making is fostered by the presence of and in consultation with other wise individuals (Edmondson, 2012, 2013). Close intergenerational relations and friendships, for instance, may provide wisdom-conducive experiences and a conversational context (Edmondson, 2013) that allows for the exploration of limits and doubts involved in knowing (Kramer, 1990; Meacham, 1990). Moreover, Erikson's (1963) psychosocial stage theory of human development professes that the successful mastery of childhood developmental tasks depends on how and to what extent family members—especially, parents or grandparents—provide quality care, trust, comfort, security, belongingness, and guidance. Therefore, family members can be wisdom role models for young children with long-lasting positive effects on the offspring's acquisition of wisdom. In contrast, the absence of kin support during the formative years might make the development of wisdom more challenging.

In addition, wisdom can be learned by growing up in a cultural setting where social interactions with older generations play central roles to generate and facilitate wisdom-related knowledge, experiences, and personality qualities over time. This implies that the development of wisdom is influenced not only by a certain personality makeup, such as openness to experiences and the motivation to gain deeper insight into the meaning and purpose of life and to engage in personality growth (Staudinger & Kunzmann, 2005), but also by having a wisdom role model from whom to seek advice in dealing with life's vicissitudes (Edmondson, 2012, 2013). Because wisdom is learned and expressed through social interactions, Edmondson (2012) argued that a person-centered research paradigm that focuses only on individuals' degree of wisdom cannot be considered optimal. Instead, given the social-interactive nature of wisdom, researchers need to study how wisdom is enacted in the social context through prosocial behaviors and compassionate concern for others, such as teaching, sharing, nurturing, encouraging, helping, and giving. This means that the acquisition of wisdom is likely to be facilitated by long-lasting personal relationships between apprentice and wisdom mentor (Staudinger & Baltes, 1996). One of the social deterrents to wisdom development of the young and wisdom maintenance of the old might be the isolation of older people.

Modern society's tendency to isolate their elders decreases the chances for social interactions and thus for passing on wisdom to younger generations.

In fact, research participants who were asked to nominate a person whom they perceived as wise were more likely to nominate someone who was older (50 years or above) and male, and the age of the wisdom nominee tended to increase with the age of the nominator (Ardelt, 2008a; Baltes et al., 1995; Denney, Dew, & Kroupa, 1995; Jason et al., 2001; Orwoll & Perlmutter, 1990). One study that examined people's general beliefs about characteristics of wisdom nominees revealed that 78% of the age-diverse respondents thought that wisdom was related to age, 16% to gender, and 68% to education (Perlmutter, Adams, Nyquist, & Kaplan, 1988). These findings indicate that people generally believe that wisdom is more prevalent in older and more educated people but not limited to one particular gender, although men tend to be nominated as wise more often than women. However, when asked to name the areas in which their wisdom nominees are particularly wise, female nominees dominate in interpersonal skill areas, whereas male nominees are prevalent in more cognitive skill areas, such as business or science (Denney et al., 1995). Indeed, a study that compared gender differences in 3D-WS scores among younger and older adults showed that women of both age groups tended to score higher on the compassionate wisdom dimension than men, but higher scores on the cognitive wisdom dimension for men compared to women were found only among the older age group, possibly reflecting changing and persistent cultural gender ideals and socialization practices (Ardelt, 2009). Whereas girls are still more likely than boys to be socialized to be nurturing and caring (Lytton & Romney, 1991), both genders are now encouraged to develop their cognitive capacities, as demonstrated by the more equal gender composition of university students, while in the past, intellectual endeavors were seen as more important for boys than for girls (Peter & Horn, 2005). However, the earlier study did not find significant gender differences in any of the three wisdom dimensions among the top 25% of 3D-WS scorers, indicating that relatively wise men and women tend to integrate the cognitive, reflective, and compassionate dimensions of wisdom (Ardelt, 2009).

Wisdom and Culture

Culture plays an important role in laypeople's understanding of wisdom and, therefore, might also affect the development of wisdom. In a culture where the self is expected to establish and control a clear identity and to actively engage in developmental tasks, a wise person is more likely to be characterized as upward (self-promoting) and inbound (self-controlling) and by cognitive, strategic, and analytic qualities. By contrast, in a culture where the self is considered wise when it examines itself and finds harmony in relations and sagacity in decisions and advice giving, wisdom tends to be characterized as downward (modest, self-critical) and outbound (communal, altruistic) and by affective, reflective, and synthetic qualities (Takahashi & Overton, 2005).

Unfortunately, contemporary studies of wisdom have not paid a lot of attention to the influence of culture or subculture on the development of wisdom (Edmondson, 2012, 2013). More specifically, if the local subculture, consisting of family, friends, and community, promotes a self-centered understanding of wisdom, individuals might be susceptible to comprehend wisdom as a purely cognitive dimension, which asks for excellence and mastery of knowledge about human life but is devoid of caring minds for others (Edmondson, 2012, 2013). Hence, if mastering wisdom-related knowledge about the fundamental pragmatics of life (e.g., life planning, life management, and life review) is regarded by one's culture as a more important wisdom dimension than the compassionate and self-reflective dimensions of wisdom, developing egocentric and self-empowering characteristics are likely more rewarded than fostering modest, pro-social behaviors and attitudes. In such a self-motivating culture, a lack of concern for others can be overlooked, while developing practical, self-oriented characteristics can appear to be wise (Csikszentmihalyi & Nakamura, 2005). In contrast, in a culture where the affective/compassionate domain is promoted for the sake of relational harmony and avoidance of social conflicts, growth in wisdom is more likely to be achieved through self-reflection and harmonious interpersonal relations (Takahashi & Overton, 2005; Tiberius, 2008). Yet, no matter in which culture a person grew up, a relatively wise individual comes to realize that there is no isolated self and that the self is mutually interdependent with others, which explains why wise decisions tend to be more harmonious than those that involve no concern for the welfare of others (Sternberg, 1998).

Wisdom, Religion, and Spirituality

One important (sub)culture that influences the development of wisdom is religion. Although many religious and spiritual traditions promote the development of wisdom (Walsh, 2014), certain forms of religion might repress aspirations for greater wisdom if beliefs are considered more important than the discovery of a deeper truth (Hall, 2010). For example, growing up in a religious culture that emphasizes love toward others might facilitate the development of the compassionate wisdom dimension, whereas being exposed to a religious culture that stresses unquestioning faith in the teachings of the Bible and the Church might impede growth in the cognitive and reflective wisdom dimensions. Baltes (2004, p. 56), for instance, argued that due to its commitment to a firm set of values, religion could be an "intellectual enemy" of wisdom, especially in the final stages of personal growth. He claimed that the development of wisdom is more likely to take place in diverse social contexts, in which generational and interpersonal values about the conduct and meaning of life are more freely interchanged than in religious disciplines.

Although both religion and spirituality involve a search for the sacred, religion is often practiced in an institutional setting with a group of likeminded people, whereas the experience and practice of spirituality might be more idiosyncratic and individualistic (Hill et al., 2000). In a longitudinal study by Wink and Dillon (2002, 2003), spirituality (defined in terms of noninstitutionalized religion or nontradition-centered beliefs and practices) but not religiousness (institutionalized or tradition-centered religious beliefs and practices) in late middle adulthood (50s to early 60s) and late adulthood (late 60s to late 70s) was significantly related to cognitive/reflective wisdom in late adulthood. Yet, individuals who were religious in early adulthood (in their 30s) tended to be rated higher on spirituality and cognitive/reflective wisdom in late adulthood than those who were less religious during their earlier years of life. This suggests that an earlier interest in religion might lead individuals on a spiritual quest that results in greater wisdom in old age.

Religion and spirituality are more likely to be associated with transcendent characteristics of wisdom than practical features. Practical wisdom, as exemplified by the Berlin Wisdom Paradigm, emphasizes wisdom-related knowledge in the pragmatics of daily living, advice, and action, whereas transcendent wisdom concerns mindfulness, intuitive insight, the transformation of consciousness, and detachment (Le, 2008; Levenson et al., 2005). A study with European American and Vietnamese American adults showed that the frequency of mystical experiences, such as a loss of sense of self and feelings of oneness, and belonging to a religious/spiritual community were associated with greater transcendent wisdom, assessed by ratings of self-knowledge, detachment, integration, and self-transcendence, but not more wisdom-related knowledge. However, religious and spiritual practices by themselves were unrelated to either form of wisdom (Le, 2008). In a study of older adults, wisdom, as measured by the 3D-WS, was also not associated with an intrinsic religious orientation (commitment to a religious/spiritual life) and even negatively related to an extrinsic religious orientation (using religion for self-enhancing purposes). Yet, those elders with the highest scores on the compassionate wisdom dimension and relatively high scores on the cognitive and reflective wisdom dimensions showed a strong intrinsic religious orientation, which they expressed through humility, gratitude, inner-centered guidance, and a commitment to love and help others (Ardelt, 2008b).

Overall, the findings suggest that religiosity might or might not lead to greater wisdom, although mystical experiences might foster the transformation of consciousness, insight, and detachment that characterizes self-transcendent wisdom. Although relatively wise older adults tend to be spiritual or exhibit an intrinsic religious orientation, deeply religious older adults are not necessarily wise. Moreover, relatively wise older adults are less likely than others to use their religion to achieve self-enhancing goals, such as improving one's standing in the community or to find friends and companionship. The religiosity of relatively wise persons appears to be committed to a higher purpose and intertwined with the wisdom path of specific religious traditions (Walsh, 2014).

Wisdom and Well-Being in Old Age

Wisdom is often described as an ideal endpoint of human development (Staudinger & Glück, 2011), both in secular as well as religious and spiritual terms, which implies that wisdom should lead to optimal living and aging well. Many researchers believe that wise people know "the art of living," which is a life that is good for self, others, and society as a whole (Baltes & Staudinger, 2000; Csikszentmihalyi & Nakamura, 2005; Hart, 1987; Kekes, 1995; Kramer, 2000; Kunzmann & Baltes, 2005; Kupperman, 2005; Sternberg, 1998). Moreover, the development of wisdom might also be intrinsically rewarding and joyful as it decreases the preoccupation with self-centered problems and leads to a greater connectedness with others and nature and a desire to help and avoid harm (Ardelt, 2008b; Csikszentmihalyi & Nakamura, 2005; Levenson & Aldwin, 2013). For example, Kunzmann and Baltes (2003) found that wisdom-related knowledge was positively related to "other-enhancing" values (i.e., values relating to the well-being of others, societal engagement, and ecological protection) and self-development values (i.e., orientation toward self-actualization and insight into life in general) but negatively associated with hedonistic values (e.g., materialistic and sensual). This finding corroborates the idea that "wisdom involves a joint orientation toward the personal and the common good and includes a spiritual orientation that extends beyond one's own physical states" (Kunzmann & Baltes, 2003, p. 1115).

Yet some researchers have argued that self-reflection and the ability to see reality clearly without a self-enhancing and positively biased life view might invoke negative emotions, because one recognizes how far away one is from the ideal state of wisdom, and, therefore, not necessarily enhance well-being (Mickler & Staudinger, 2008;

Staudinger et al., 2005; Staudinger & Glück, 2011). Indeed, the empirical evidence has been mixed, depending on the composition of the sample and the operationalization of wisdom and well-being.

In older adult samples of mixed educational and socioeconomic backgrounds, wisdom, assessed as analytic and synthetic wisdom modes (Takahashi & Overton, 2002) and an integration of cognitive, reflective, and compassionate wisdom dimensions (Ardelt, 2003; Bergsma & Ardelt, 2012; Le, 2011), was positively associated with subjective well-being, even after controlling for physical health, socioeconomic status, financial situation, physical environment, and social involvement (Ardelt, 1997). In addition, the 3D-WS was positively correlated with purpose in life, mastery, and less fear of death (Ardelt, 2003). In fact, it appears that a greater sense of mastery, control, and meaning in life is one possible pathway that at least partially explains the relation between wisdom and subjective well-being in old age (Ardelt & Edwards, in press; Etezadi & Pushkar, 2013).

Yet, in samples of highly educated White older adults, wisdom, measured as practical and transcendent wisdom (Wink & Helson, 1997), expertise in uncertainty (Brugman, 2000), and personal wisdom-related knowledge (Mickler & Staudinger, 2008), was unrelated to subjective well-being. It is possible that wisdom has a greater impact on subjective well-being in old age when life conditions are detrimental to a general sense of well-being. Most studies that did not find a positive association between wisdom and well-being included highly educated individuals of relatively privileged White adults who are more likely to be healthy (Martin, Schoeni, Freedman, & Andreski, 2007; Minkler, Fuller-Thomson, & Guralnik, 2006) and tend to have more options to enhance well-being than minorities and adults from lower socioeconomic backgrounds (Koster et al., 2006). Wisdom might be a psychosocial developmental resource that becomes most relevant during times of hardships and when extrinsic means to improve well-being, such as socializing, traveling, and consuming, are no longer possible. For example, the association between the 3D-WS and subjective well-being was significantly stronger in a sample of older nursing home residents and hospice patients than in a sample of relatively healthy older adults after controlling for subjective health, socioeconomic status, social involvement, age, gender, race, and marital status. Although nursing home residents and hospice patients tended to report lower well-being scores than relatively healthy older adults, the difference in average well-being scores disappeared among those participants with relatively high wisdom scores (Ardelt & Edwards, in press). Wise older adults seem to know how best to deal with hardship by using active rather than passive coping strategies and applying the life lessons they have learned in the past (Ardelt, 2005; Glück & Bluck, 2013). They also might engage in selection, optimization, and compensation (SOC) by selecting goals that are still possible, such as spending time in the company of dear family members and friends, to optimize well-being and compensate for health-related losses (Baltes & Freund, 2003).

In sum, knowing how to live a life that is good not only for oneself, but also for others and for the whole society helps wise individuals to feel in control of their lives, to perceive their lives as meaningful, and to feel satisfied and content even when faced with weakening physical, mental, and social capabilities (Ardelt, 2011).

■ CONCLUSION

Although a generally accepted theory of wisdom does not exist, explicit and implicit theories of wisdom might broadly be divided into two approaches. The first approach, exemplified by the explicit Berlin Wisdom Paradigm and the cognitive implicit wisdom theory, views wisdom in primarily cognitive and reflective terms, as expert knowledge about the conduct and meaning of life (Baltes & Staudinger, 2000). In this approach, wisdom is described as general knowledge that can be found in texts and is independent of individuals. In fact, individuals are considered only weak carriers of wisdom-related knowledge. The second approach, illustrated by the Three-Dimensional Wisdom Model and the integrative implicit wisdom theory, describes wisdom as a quality of persons who have integrated the cognitive, reflective, and benevolent characteristics of wisdom (Ardelt, 2004a, 2004b). Although most implicit and explicit wisdom theories of the East follow the integrative approach, the cognitive approach is favored by some of the Western explicit wisdom theories.

Although approaches to define and assess wisdom vary, empirical evidence supports the general agreement that wisdom does not automatically increase with age. The development of wisdom across the life course, however, is more likely for individuals who are open to new experiences, committed to psychosocial growth, and supported by wisdom role models and a secular and religious/spiritual culture that promotes wisdom-related qualities, such as the search for truth, a deeper understanding of life, the ability to engage in reflection, self-reflection, and self-examination, sympathetic and compassionate concern for others, and prosocial behaviors. Growing wiser is indeed a lifelong process insofar as planting the seeds of wisdom at an earlier stage of life can facilitate sagacity during the later years (Edmondson, 2013; Richardson & Pasupathi, 2005). For instance, the presence and absence of mentorship and guidance during the formative years can affect people's acquisition of wisdom decades later (Staudinger & Baltes, 1996). The rewards of wisdom in old age appear to be greater subjective well-being, particularly if life circumstances are less than optimal.

The social conditions for the development of wisdom have so far been largely ignored in research of human development (Jordan, 2005; Staudinger & Baltes, 1996; Sternberg, 2005). Jordan (2005, p. 181) claimed that what was missing in the psychology-dominant study of wisdom was an inquiry into "wisdom's trajectory...if certain environmental factors and challenges were absent or abated." Sternberg (2005) also noted a tendency to ignore the variations in individuals' paths toward wisdom across the life course, which might depend on culture, gender, and personality, resulting in interpersonal variances in manifestations of wisdom qualities.

Hence, a sociological approach to the study of wisdom is needed to comprehend the antecedents and consequences of wisdom more completely. Although individuals possess varying degrees of freedom to choose their paths, a phenomenon known as "human agency," these choices are not made in a social vacuum. As Elder (1994) and Dannefer (2003) noted, all life choices are contingent on the opportunities and constraints of social structures in which individuals are embedded over the life course. More specifically, Dannefer and Settersten (2010, p. 3) argued that human development and aging cannot be understood at either the individual or the societal level, "without paying attention to the cumulated life practices and experiences of aging individuals." The life-course perspective can help clarify generally applicable conditions and factors that contribute to the development of wisdom by investigating how wisdom is initially acquired, who helps in the development of wisdom over the life course, and how wisdom progresses toward successful aging. If we know the seeds and nutrients of wisdom, we can pinpoint resources necessary for the development of wisdom and thus develop ways to promote and teach wisdom in education (Ferrari & Potworowski, 2008), counseling (Ponterotto, 2010), and leadership (Pauleen & Küpers, 2013).

The theory of lifelong psychosocial growth in wisdom claims that people can still grow wiser with age even if they suffer disease, pain, and loss. Learning to value the lived wisdom of our elders might guide the younger generations to lead flourishing and meaningful lives while making wise decisions that improve the lives of the individual, others, and the whole society (Kupperman, 2005).

REFERENCES

Achenbaum, W. A., & Orwoll, L. (1991). Becoming wise: A psycho-gerontological interpretation of the Book of Job. *International Journal of Aging and Human Development*, 32(1), 21–39.

Ardelt, M. (1997). Wisdom and life satisfaction in old age. *The Journals of Gerontology, Series B*, 52(1), P15–P27.

Ardelt, M. (1998). Social crisis and individual growth: The long-term effects of the Great Depression. *Journal of Aging Studies*, 12(3), 291–314.

Ardelt, M. (2003). Empirical assessment of a three-dimensional wisdom scale. *Research on Aging*, 25(3), 275–324.

Ardelt, M. (2004a). Where can wisdom be found? A reply to the commentaries by Baltes and Kunzmann, Sternberg, and Achenbaum. *Human Development*, 47(5), 304–307.

Ardelt, M. (2004b). Wisdom as expert knowledge system: A critical review of a contemporary operationalization of an ancient concept. *Human Development*, 47(5), 257–285.

Ardelt, M. (2005). How wise people cope with crises and obstacles in life. *ReVision: A Journal of Consciousness and Transformation*, 28(1), 7–19.

Ardelt, M. (2008a). Being wise at any age. In S. J. Lopez (Ed.), *Positive psychology: Exploring the best in people* (Vol. 1: Discovering Human Strengths, pp. 81–108). Westport, CT: Praeger.

Ardelt, M. (2008b). Self-development through selflessness: The paradoxical process of growing wiser. In H. A. Wayment & J. J. Bauer (Eds.), *Transcending self-interest: Psychological explorations of the quiet ego* (pp. 221–233). Washington, DC: American Psychological Association.

Ardelt, M. (2009). How similar are wise men and women? A comparison across two age cohorts. *Research in Human Development*, 6(1), 9–26.

Ardelt, M. (2010). Are older adults wiser than college students? A comparison of two age cohorts. *Journal of Adult Development*, 17(4), 193–207.

Ardelt, M. (2011). Wisdom, age, and well-being. In K. W. Schaie & S. L. Willis (Eds.), *Handbook of the psychology of aging* (7th ed., pp. 279–291). Amsterdam, The Netherlands: Elsevier.

Ardelt, M., & Edwards, C. A. (in press). Wisdom at the end of life: An analysis of mediating and moderating relations between wisdom and subjective well-being. *The Journals of Gerontology, Series B*. Advance online publication. doi:10.1093/geronb/gbv051

Ardelt, M., Landes, S. D., Gerlach, K. R., & Fox, L. P. (2013). Rediscovering internal strengths of the aged: The beneficial impact of wisdom, mastery, purpose in life, and spirituality on aging well. In J. D. Sinnott (Ed.), *Positive psychology. Advances in understanding adult motivation* (pp. 97–119). New York, NY: Springer Publishing Company.

Arlin, P. K. (1990). Wisdom: The art of problem finding. In R. J. Sternberg (Ed.), *Wisdom: Its nature, origins, and development* (pp. 230–243). New York, NY: Cambridge University Press.

Baltes, P. B. (2004). *Wisdom as orchestration of mind and virtue.* Unpublished manuscript, Max Planck Institute for Human Development, Berlin, Germany. Retrieved from http://library.mpib-berlin.mpg.de/ft/pb/PB_Wisdom_2004.pdf

Baltes, P. B., & Freund, A. M. (2003). The intermarriage of wisdom and selective optimization with compensation: Two meta-heuristics guiding the conduct of life. In C. L. M. Keyes & J. Haidt (Eds.), *Flourishing: Positive psychology and the life well-lived* (pp. 249–273). Washington, DC: American Psychological Association.

Baltes, P. B., & Kunzmann, U. (2004). The two faces of wisdom: Wisdom as a general theory of knowledge and judgment about excellence in mind and virtue vs. wisdom as everyday realization in people and products. *Human Development, 47*(5), 290–299.

Baltes, P. B., & Smith, J. (1990). Towards a psychology of wisdom and its ontogenesis. In R. J. Sternberg (Ed.), *Wisdom: Its nature, origins, and development* (pp. 87–120). New York, NY: Cambridge University Press.

Baltes, P. B., & Smith, J. (2008). The fascination of wisdom: Its nature, ontogeny, and function. *Perspectives on Psychological Science: A Journal of the Association for Psychological Science, 3*(1), 56–64.

Baltes, P. B., & Staudinger, U. M. (2000). Wisdom. A metaheuristic (pragmatic) to orchestrate mind and virtue toward excellence. *The American Psychologist, 55*(1), 122–136.

Baltes, P. B., Staudinger, U. M., Maercker, A., & Smith, J. (1995). People nominated as wise: A comparative study of wisdom-related knowledge. *Psychology and Aging, 10*(2), 155–166.

Bergsma, A., & Ardelt, M. (2012). Self-reported wisdom and happiness: An empirical investigation. *Journal of Happiness Studies, 13*(3), 481–499.

Birren, J. E., & Fisher, L. M. (1990). The elements of wisdom: Overview and integration. In R. J. Sternberg (Ed.), *Wisdom: Its nature, origins, and development* (pp. 317–332). New York, NY: Cambridge University Press.

Birren, J. E., & Svensson, C. M. (2005). Wisdom in history. In R. J. Sternberg & J. Jordan (Eds.), *A handbook of wisdom. Psychological perspectives* (pp. 3–31). New York, NY: Cambridge University Press.

Bluck, S., & Glück, J. (2005). From the inside out: People's implicit theories of wisdom. In R. J. Sternberg & J. Jordan (Eds.), *A handbook of wisdom. Psychological perspectives* (pp. 84–109). New York, NY: Cambridge University Press.

Bradley, G. W. (1978). Self-serving biases in the attribution process: A reexamination of the fact or fiction question. *Journal of Personality and Social Psychology, 36*(1), 56–71.

Brugman, G. M. (2000). *Wisdom: Source of narrative coherence and eudaimonia.* Delft, The Netherlands: Eburon.

Clayton, V. P., & Birren, J. E. (1980). The development of wisdom across the life-span: A reexamination of an ancient topic. In P. B. Baltes & O. G. Brim, Jr. (Eds.), *Life-span development and behavior* (Vol. 3, pp. 103–135). New York, NY: Academic Press.

Csikszentmihalyi, M., & Nakamura, J. (2005). The role of emotions in the development of wisdom. In R. J. Sternberg & J. Jordan (Eds.), *A handbook of wisdom. Psychological perspectives* (pp. 220–242). New York, NY: Cambridge University Press.

Csikszentmihalyi, M., & Rathunde, K. (1990). The psychology of wisdom: An evolutionary interpretation. In R. J. Sternberg (Ed.), *Wisdom: Its nature, origins, and development* (pp. 25–51). New York, NY: Cambridge University Press.

Curnow, T. (1999). *Wisdom, intuition, and ethics.* Brookfield, VT: Ashgate.

Dannefer, D. (2003). Cumulative advantage/disadvantage and the life course: Cross-fertilizing age and social science theory. *The Journals of Gerontology, Series B, 58*(6), S327–S337.

Dannefer, D., & Settersten, R. A. (2010). The study of the life course: Implications for social gerontology. In D. Dannefer & C. Phillipson (Eds.), *Handbook of social gerontology* (pp. 3–19). Thousand Oaks, CA: Sage.

Denney, N. W., Dew, J. R., & Kroupa, S. L. (1995). Perceptions of wisdom: What is it and who has it? *Journal of Adult Development, 2*(1), 37–47.

Dittmann-Kohli, F., & Baltes, P. B. (1990). Toward a neofunctionalist conception of adult intellectual development: Wisdom as a prototypical case of intellectual growth. In C. N. Alexander & E. J. Langer (Eds.), *Higher stages of human development. Perspectives on adult growth* (pp. 54–78). New York, NY: Oxford University Press.

Edmondson, R. (2012). Intergenerational relations in the West of Ireland and sociocultural approaches to wisdom. *Journal of Family Issues, 33*(1), 76–98.

Edmondson, R. (2013). A social interpretation of personal wisdom. In M. Ferrari & N. M. Weststrate (Eds.), *The scientific study of personal wisdom: From contemplative traditions to neuroscience* (pp. 191–209). New York, NY: Springer Publishing Company.

Elder, G. H., Jr. (1994). Time, human agency, and social change: Perspectives on the life course. *Social Psychology Quarterly, 57*(1), 4–15.

Erikson, E. H. (1963). *Childhood and society.* New York, NY: W. W. Norton.

Erikson, E. H. (1964). *Insight and responsibility. Lectures on the ethical implications of psychoanalytic insight.* New York, NY: W. W. Norton.

Erikson, E. H. (1982). *The life cycle completed. A review.* New York, NY: W. W. Norton.

Etezadi, S., & Pushkar, D. (2013). Why are wise people happier? An explanatory model of wisdom and emotional well-being in older adults. *Journal of Happiness Studies, 14*(3), 929–950.

Ferrari, M., & Potworowski, G. (Eds.). (2008). *Teaching for wisdom: Cross-cultural perspectives on fostering wisdom.* New York, NY: Springer Publishing Company.

Ferrari, M., & Weststrate, N. M. (Eds.). (2013). *The scientific study of personal wisdom: From contemplative traditions to neuroscience.* New York, NY: Springer Publishing Company.

Glück, J., & Bluck, S. (2011). Laypeople's conceptions of wisdom and its development: Cognitive and integrative views. *The Journals of Gerontology, Series B, 66*(3), 321–324.

Glück, J., & Bluck, S. (2013). The MORE life experience model: A theory of the development of wisdom. In M. Ferrari & N. Weststrate (Eds.), *The scientific study of personal wisdom: From contemplative traditions to neuroscience* (pp. 75–97). New York, NY: Springer Publishing Company.

Green, S. K., & Gross, A. E. (1979). Self-serving biases in implicit evaluations. *Personality and Social Psychology Bulletin, 5*(2), 214–217.

Hall, S. S. (2010). *Wisdom: From philosophy to neuroscience*. New York, NY: Knopf.

Hart, W. (1987). *The art of living. Vipassana meditation as taught by S.N. Goenka*. San Francisco, CA: Harper.

Hill, P. C., Pargament, K. I., Hood, R. W., Jr., McCullough, M. E., Swyers, J. P., Larson, D. B., & Zinnbauer, B. J. (2000). Conceptualizing religion and spirituality: Points of commonality, points of departure. *Journal for the Theory of Social Behaviour, 30*(1), 51–77.

Holliday, S. G., & Chandler, M. J. (1986). *Wisdom: Explorations in adult competence*. Basel, Switzerland; New York, NY: Karger.

Jason, L. A., Reichler, A., King, C., Madsen, D., Camacho, J., & Marchese, W. (2001). The measurement of wisdom: A preliminary effort. *Journal of Community Psychology, 29*(5), 585–598.

Jeste, D. V., & Vahia, I. V. (2008). Comparison of the conceptualization of wisdom in ancient Indian literature with modern views: Focus on the Bhagavad Gita. *Psychiatry, 71*(3), 197–209.

Jordan, J. (2005). The quest for wisdom in adulthood: A psychological perspective. In R. J. Sternberg & J. Jordan (Eds.), *A handbook of wisdom. Psychological perspectives* (pp. 160–188). New York, NY: Cambridge University Press.

Kekes, J. (1983). Wisdom. *American Philosophical Quarterly, 20*(3), 277–286.

Kekes, J. (1995). *Moral wisdom and good lives*. Ithaca, NY: Cornell University Press.

Kitchener, K. S., & Brenner, H. G. (1990). Wisdom and reflective judgment: Knowing in the face of uncertainty. In R. J. Sternberg (Ed.), *Wisdom: Its nature, origins, and development* (pp. 212–229). New York, NY: Cambridge University Press.

Kitchener, K. S., King, P. M., Wood, P. K., & Davison, M. L. (1989). Sequentiality and consistency in the development of reflective judgment: A six-year longitudinal study. *Journal of Applied Developmental Psychology, 10*(1), 73–95.

Koster, A., Bosma, H., Kempen, G. I., Penninx, B. W., Beekman, A. T., Deeg, D. J., & van Eijk, J. T. (2006). Socioeconomic differences in incident depression in older adults: The role of psychosocial factors, physical health status, and behavioral factors. *Journal of Psychosomatic Research, 61*(5), 619–627.

Kramer, D. A. (1990). Conceptualizing wisdom: The primacy of affect-cognition relations. In R. J. Sternberg (Ed.), *Wisdom: Its nature, origins, and development* (pp. 279–313). New York, NY: Cambridge University Press.

Kramer, D. A. (2000). Wisdom as a classical source of human strength: Conceptualization and empirical inquiry. *Journal of Social and Clinical Psychology, 19*(1), 83–101.

Kunzmann, U., & Baltes, P. B. (2003). Wisdom-related knowledge: Affective, motivational, and interpersonal correlates. *Personality and Social Psychology Bulletin, 29*(9), 1104–1119.

Kunzmann, U., & Baltes, P. B. (2005). The psychology of wisdom: Theoretical and empirical challenges. In R. J. Sternberg & J. Jordan (Eds.), *A handbook of wisdom. Psychological perspectives* (pp. 110–135). New York, NY: Cambridge University Press.

Kupperman, J. J. (2005). Morality, ethics, and wisdom. In R. J. Sternberg & J. Jordan (Eds.), *A handbook of wisdom. Psychological perspectives* (pp. 245–271). New York, NY: Cambridge University Press.

Labouvie-Vief, G. (1990). Wisdom as integrated thought: Historical and developmental perspectives. In R. J. Sternberg (Ed.), *Wisdom: Its nature, origins, and development* (pp. 52–83). New York, NY: Cambridge University Press.

Le, T. N. (2008). Age differences in spirituality, mystical experiences and wisdom. *Ageing and Society, 28,* 383–411.

Le, T. N. (2011). Life satisfaction, openness value, self-transcendence, and wisdom. *Journal of Happiness Studies, 12*(2), 171–182.

Levenson, M. R., & Aldwin, C. (2013). The transpersonal in personal wisdom. In M. Ferrari & N. M. Weststrate (Eds.), *The scientific study of personal wisdom: From contemplative traditions to neuroscience* (pp. 213–228). New York, NY: Springer Publishing Company.

Levenson, M. R., Jennings, P. A., Aldwin, C. M., & Shiraishi, R. W. (2005). Self-transcendence: Conceptualization and measurement. *International Journal of Aging and Human Development, 60*(2), 127–143.

Levitt, H. M. (1999). The development of wisdom: An analysis of Tibetan Buddhist experience. *Journal of Humanistic Psychology, 39*(2), 86–105.

Lytton, H., & Romney, D. M. (1991). Parents' differential socialization of boys and girls: A meta-analysis. *Psychological Bulletin, 109*(2), 267–296.

Martin, L. G., Schoeni, R. F., Freedman, V. A., & Andreski, P. (2007). Feeling better? Trends in general health status. *The Journals of Gerontology, Series B, 62*(1), S11–S21.

McKee, P., & Barber, C. (1999). On defining wisdom. *International Journal of Aging and Human Development, 49*(2), 149–164.

Meacham, J. A. (1990). The loss of wisdom. In R. J. Sternberg (Ed.), *Wisdom: Its nature, origins, and development* (pp. 181–211). New York, NY: Cambridge University Press.

Mickler, C., & Staudinger, U. M. (2008). Personal wisdom: Validation and age-related differences of a performance measure. *Psychology and Aging, 23*(4), 787–799.

Minkler, M., Fuller-Thomson, E., & Guralnik, J. M. (2006). Gradient of disability across the socioeconomic spectrum in the United States. *The New England Journal of Medicine, 355*(7), 695–703.

Moody, H. R. (1986). Late life learning in the information society. In D. A. Peterson, J. E. Thornton & J. E. Birren (Eds.), *Education and aging* (pp. 122–148). Englewood Cliffs, NJ: Prentice-Hall.

Ñanamoli, B. (2001). *The life of the Buddha: According to the Pali Canon*. Seattle, WA: BPS Pariyatti Editions.

Orwoll, L., & Achenbaum, W. A. (1993). Gender and the development of wisdom. *Human Development, 36*, 274–296.

Orwoll, L., & Perlmutter, M. (1990). The study of wise persons: Integrating a personality perspective. In R. J. Sternberg (Ed.), *Wisdom: Its nature, origins, and development* (pp. 160–177). New York, NY: Cambridge University Press.

Pascual-Leone, J. (1990). An essay on wisdom: Toward organismic processes that make it possible. In R. J. Sternberg (Ed.), *Wisdom: Its nature, origins, and development* (pp. 244–278). New York, NY: Cambridge University Press.

Pasupathi, M., & Staudinger, U. M. (2001). Do advanced moral reasoners also show wisdom? Linking moral reasoning and wisdom-related knowledge and judgement. *International Journal of Behavioral Development, 25*(5), 401–415.

Pasupathi, M., Staudinger, U. M., & Baltes, P. B. (2001). Seeds of wisdom: Adolescents' knowledge and judgment about difficult life problems. *Developmental Psychology, 37*(3), 351–361.

Pauleen, D. J., & Küpers, W. (Eds.). (2013). *A handbook of practical wisdom: Leadership, organization and integral business practice*. Burlington, VT: Gower.

Perlmutter, M., Adams, C., Nyquist, L., & Kaplan, C. (1988). *Beliefs about wisdom*. Unpublished data. (Cited in Orwoll & Perlmutter, 1990)

Peter, K., & Horn, L. (2005). *Gender differences in participation and completion of undergraduate education and how they have changed over time (NCES 2005–169)*. U.S. Department of Education, National Center for Education Statistics. Washington, DC: U.S. Government Printing Office. Retrieved from http://nces.ed.gov/pubs2005/2005169.pdf

Ponterotto, J. G. (2010). *Handbook of multicultural counseling* (3rd ed.). Thousand Oaks, CA: Sage.

Richardson, M. J., & Pasupathi, M. (2005). Young and growing wiser: Wisdom during adolescence and young adulthood. In R. J. Sternberg & J. Jordan (Eds.), *A handbook of wisdom. Psychological perspectives* (pp. 139–159). New York, NY: Cambridge University Press.

Riegel, J. (2006). Confucius. In E. N. Zalta (Ed.), *The Stanford encyclopedia of philosophy*. Retrieved from http://plato.stanford.edu/archives/fall2006/entries/confucius

Riess, M., Rosenfeld, P., Melburg, V., & Tedeschi, J. T. (1981). Self-serving attributions: Biased private perceptions and distorted public descriptions. *Journal of Personality and Social Psychology, 41*(2), 224–231.

Sherwood, G. G. (1981). Self-serving biases in person perception: A reexamination of projection as a mechanism of defense. *Psychological Bulletin, 90*(3), 445–459.

Smith, J., & Baltes, P. B. (1990). Wisdom-related knowledge: Age/cohort differences in response to life-planning problems. *Developmental Psychology, 26*(3), 494–505.

Smith, J., Staudinger, U. M., & Baltes, P. B. (1994). Occupational settings facilitating wisdom-related knowledge: The sample case of clinical psychologists. *Journal of Consulting and Clinical Psychology, 62*(5), 989–999.

Staudinger, U. M. (1999). Older and wiser? Integrating results on the relationship between age and wisdom-related performance. *International Journal of Behavioral Development, 23*(3), 641–664.

Staudinger, U. M. (2013). The need to distinguish personal from general wisdom: A short history and empirical evidence. In M. Ferrari & N. M. Weststrate (Eds.), *The scientific study of personal wisdom: From contemplative traditions to neuroscience* (pp. 3–19). New York, NY: Springer Publishing Company.

Staudinger, U. M., & Baltes, P. B. (1996). Interactive minds: A facilitative setting for wisdom-related performance. *Journal of Personality and Social Psychology, 71*(4), 746–762.

Staudinger, U. M., Dörner, J., & Mickler, C. (2005). Wisdom and personality. In R. J. Sternberg & J. Jordan (Eds.), *A handbook of wisdom. Psychological perspectives* (pp. 191–219). New York, NY: Cambridge University Press.

Staudinger, U. M., & Glück, J. (2011). Psychological wisdom research: Commonalities and differences in a growing field. *Annual Review of Psychology, 62*, 215–241.

Staudinger, U. M., & Kunzmann, U. (2005). Positive adult personality development: Adjustment and/or growth? *European Psychologist, 10*(4), 320–329.

Sternberg, R. J. (1985). Implicit theories of intelligence, creativity, and wisdom. *Journal of Personality and Social Psychology, 49*(3), 607–627.

Sternberg, R. J. (1990a). Wisdom and its relations to intelligence and creativity. In R. J. Sternberg (Ed.), *Wisdom: Its nature, origins, and development* (pp. 142–159). New York, NY: Cambridge University Press.

Sternberg, R. J. (1998). A balance theory of wisdom. *Review of General Psychology, 2*(4), 347–365.

Sternberg, R. J. (2005). Older but not wiser? The relationship between age and wisdom. *Ageing International, 30*(1), 5–26.

Sternberg, R. J. (Ed.). (1990b). *Wisdom: Its nature, origins, and development.* New York, NY: Cambridge University Press.

Sternberg, R. J., & Jordan, J. (Eds.). (2005). *A handbook of wisdom: Psychological perspectives.* New York, NY: Cambridge University Press.

Takahashi, M., & Bordia, P. (2000). The concept of wisdom: A cross-cultural comparison. *International Journal of Psychology, 35*(1), 1–9.

Takahashi, M., & Overton, W. F. (2002). Wisdom: A culturally inclusive developmental perspective. *International Journal of Behavioral Development, 26*(3), 269–277.

Takahashi, M., & Overton, W. F. (2005). Cultural foundations of wisdom: An integrated developmental approach. In R. J. Sternberg & J. Jordan (Eds.), *A handbook of wisdom: Psychological perspectives* (pp. 32–60). New York, NY: Cambridge University Press.

Tiberius, V. (2008). *The reflective life: Living wisely with our limits.* New York, NY: Oxford University Press.

Walsh, R. (2014). *The world's great wisdom: Timeless teachings from religions and philosophies.* Albany, NY: University of New York Press.

Webster, J. D. (2003). An exploratory analysis of a self-assessed wisdom scale. *Journal of Adult Development, 10*(1), 13–22.

Webster, J. D. (2007). Measuring the character strength of wisdom. *International Journal of Aging & Human Development, 65*(2), 163–183.

Webster, J. D., Westerhof, G. J., & Bohlmeijer, E. T. (2014). Wisdom and mental health across the lifespan. *The Journals of Gerontology, Series B, 69*(2), 209–218.

Wink, P., & Dillon, M. (2002). Spiritual development across the adult life course: Findings from a longitudinal study. *Journal of Adult Development, 9*(1), 79–94.

Wink, P., & Dillon, M. (2003). Religiousness, spirituality, and psychosocial functioning in late adulthood: Findings from a longitudinal study. *Psychology and Aging, 18*(4), 916–924.

Wink, P., & Helson, R. (1997). Practical and transcendent wisdom: Their nature and some longitudinal findings. *Journal of Adult Development, 4*(1), 1–15.

Yang, S. Y. (2001). Conceptions of wisdom among Taiwanese Chinese. *Journal of Cross-Cultural Psychology, 32*(6), 662–680.

Yang, S. Y. (2008). A process view of wisdom. *Journal of Adult Development, 15*(2), 62–75.

Zaehner, R. C. (1969). *The Bhagavad-Gita, with a commentary based on the original sources.* Oxford, UK: Clarendon.

CHAPTER 31

Theories of Environmental Gerontology: Old and New Avenues for Person–Environmental Views of Aging
Hans-Werner Wahl and Frank Oswald

Development always happens in time and place. Although the time dimension has been extensively researched in developmental science, life-course research, and gerontology—conceptually, methodologically, and empirically (Baars, 2012; Baltes, Lindenberger, & Staudinger, 2006; Settersten, 2003)—the place aspect of development never became as central as the time dimension in social and behavioral aging research. However, it seems that the importance of space and place perspectives for aging is (re-)gaining prominence in gerontology (Rowles & Bernard, 2013; Wahl, Iwarsson, & Oswald, 2012). As we "move" (a spatial term) through our lives, we are also getting older, that is, getting more "distance" (another spatial term) from birth and less distance from death. We also start our lives in a broad variety of children playrooms, houses, apartments, gardens, and neighborhoods; then, we extend our life space to kindergarten and school environments; enjoy or suffer from job environments; buy or rent our own house or apartment in more self-selected physical–spatial areas (country of residence, urban, suburban, etc.) as compared to our early beginnings; execute our preferences for housing interiors, favorite objects, as well as for landscapes and leisure environments, for art and cultural environments, and for vibrant urban life or rural solitude.

Especially late in life, we probably meet unexpected spatial challenges (house too big, too many barriers, too distant from shopping area) and we may be forced to make a mostly undesirable transition to an assisted-living facility or a nursing home environment to spend another couple of years in what in the majority of cases is our "last refuge." It is also obvious that the place dimension of aging comes with cognitive–emotional ties, some of which resemble ties to intimate social partners (see also Wahl & Lang, 2004). We may "love" our home, garden, book, or music collection compiled over decades, or preferred landscape or region, and may connect strong feelings of familiarity and comfort with the places we belong to, which may have become even parts of our own identity.

As it seems, such cognitive–emotional ties to personal artifacts and places grow stronger as we age, and relocation late in life therefore frequently is a painful event that we try to avoid despite awareness of its imminence (Granbom et al., 2014). Hence, many people in advanced old age not only lose their spouses, but also the places and artifacts in and with which they have spent decades of their lives. Eventually, one may regard this late losing of one's long-standing environment as kind of a second "spatial widowhood."

On the other hand, aging in place is experienced by many older adults as a strong—if not the strongest indication and "spatial expression"—of preserving one's independence and autonomy. In a sense, one may even regard very old age to a large extent as a continuing struggle with the place in which one lives: How long can I as a frail and vulnerable person resist the hindrances of my place and when is the right point in time to leave this place-related "battle area"? Is housing adaptation a promising option? Or will I stay—whatever it takes—for me and possibly also my family? (Golant, 2015).

Places also shape our behaviors; they may, for example, stimulate or downgrade physical activity and provoke or hinder cognitive and emotional engagement at large. In old age, when functional competencies are on the decline, daily independence particularly depends on the quality of one's environment, for example, in terms of compensatory modalities, such as a low number of home hazards and easy-to-access public transport.

Going further, at the macro level, our "aging" lives are also embedded within mega trends, such as new technologies, environmental pollution, urbanization, and global warming, with important differentiations according to which region/country/continent aging takes its "place." For example, older adults belong to those subpopulations that are most vulnerable to global warming; this insight, together with demographical trends, may strongly impact how our urban environments—including sun shelter architectonic measures or cooling by water in cities—will look in the future.

Theoretical issues related to environmental gerontology have found substantial early treatment in gerontology (Lawton, 1982; Lawton & Nahemow, 1973) and the striving for conceptual models continued until recently (Golant, 2014; Scheidt & Windley, 2006; Wahl, 2001; Wahl et al., 2012; Wahl & Oswald, 2010; Wahl, Scheidt, & Windley, 2004). In this chapter, we hope to add and provide some integrative perspectives to some of the enduring conceptual challenges in the area, such as place dimension while we age; what available theories in the ecology of aging (early and more recent ones) are telling us; and what kind of new impulses (e.g., increasing use of technology environments in older adults) for theory refinement in this area are needed. Can gerontology and life-course research at large (e.g., for models of life-span developmental regulation) profit from theories on aging and environments?

We also make attempts at several locations of the chapter to link environmental gerontology thinking with developmental, life-span, and gerontology theorizing at large. Due to the nature of the chapter, we mostly refrain from the detailed consideration of empirical data speaking to person (P) and environment (E) relations as people age, although empirical verification is of course a major issue for environmental gerontology theorizing (see also Wahl et al., 2012; Wahl & Oswald, 2010).

We also need to confirm that some of our thoughts elaborated in this work have already been introduced in other places over the last decade, although from different perspectives and with various foci (Oswald & Wahl, 2004, 2013; Wahl et al., 2004; Wahl et al., 2012; Wahl & Gitlin, 2007; Wahl & Oswald, 2010; Wahl & Weisman, 2003). Finally, given that environmental gerontology emerged during the 1960s with now-classic work such as Lawton and Simon's (1968) early stating of the environmental docility hypothesis, we will refer to "classic" theoretical accounts still impacting current theory building and use, but also consider more recent ones, when it comes to conceptual contributions to environmental gerontology.

■ MULTIFACETED USE OF THE TERM "ENVIRONMENT" IN GERONTOLOGY: KEY EXAMPLES

"Environment" is a frequently used term in aging science across various disciplines and approaches, such as biogerontology, geropsychology, sociology of aging, geography of aging, or geriatric medicine. For example, environmental characteristics such as temperature, quantity of food, or environmental stress are of interest for biogerontology, because they may considerably shape the life span (Austad, 2009). Epigenetics, also a major branch of biogerontology, has come with a new and more differentiated understanding of gene–environment interactions, such as risk in family constellations or differences in economic setup that may or may not lead to gene expression (Campisi, 2005). Ryff and Singer (2009), in the last edition of the *Handbook of Theories of Aging*, have indeed made the intriguing argument that future behavioral research may be in a position to explain how people may select specific environments over their life course that may or may not elicit the expression of risk or protective genes.

Geropsychology argues that environment is primarily seen as an entity to be perceived and processed in order to come to adequate action as an aging individual. Environmental features are also researched mostly experimentally in geropsychology as "interference," as older adults may have more problems disregarding the "less important" components of the environmental input in information-processing tasks (and therefore have more difficulties in cognitive processing, becoming slower and more error-prone; Lindenberger, Marsiske, & Baltes, 2000). It is also frequently argued in the cognitive-aging literature (Hertzog, Kramer, Wilson, & Lindenberger, 2008) that environments such as the workplace influence cognitive trajectories via differential cognitive stimulation and challenges connected with such environments. From a life-span perspective, the quantity and quality of early-life educational context are seen as an important factor driving cognitive reserve that may make individuals late in life more resistant to cognitive loss (Richards & Sacker, 2003). Moreover, one might argue from a psychological perspective that the environment could be considered as a stimulus for the improvement of aging and the unfolding of latent reserves (Colcombe & Kramer, 2003). Here, also frequent use of the term "enriched environments" as important to unfold latent reserve capacities of older individuals is made. Furthermore, environmental stress also plays a major role in geropsychology and may influence, for instance, the experience of a negative affect (Diehl, Hay, & Chui, 2012).

Sociology of aging perspectives often focus on the role of class, cohort, or socioeconomic context for outcomes such as health, well-being, or death, and address issues of social inequality (Phillipson, 2007; Scharf, Phillipson, & Smith, 2005) or social capital (Nyqvist & Forsman, 2015) with respect to the environment. Furthermore, social sciences' perspectives mostly have social environments and social interactional patterns in mind. Environments have obviously always played a major role in *social gerontology* and *social relations* and aging research, but mostly as social environments (Antonucci, Birditt, & Akiyama, 2009). Considering interactions with one's spouse and examining its impact on cognitive functioning, for example, can also be observed as a new trend (Hoppmann & Gerstorf, 2009).

Geography of aging may be, in a fundamental sense, considered "the" discipline able to address the physical and spatial environment, because space and space use are among the major issues of geography at large. Notably, as we show subsequently, major conceptual and empirical input to environmental gerontology came from geographers (Golant, 2015; Peace, Holland, & Kellaher, 2006; Rowles &

Watkins, 2010). As part of what has been titled the "spatial and cultural turn in human geography," methods to explore person–environment relationships change, as well as interprofessional research interests (e.g., interlinks between geographical and educational research, with particular interest in aging research) have appeared on the scene (Butler & Hamnett, 2007). An emerging area also related to geography is research on climate warming and how it may affect older adults' health and behaviors (Wanka et al., 2014).

Geriatric medicine as well as related disciplines such as *academic occupational therapy* frequently predominantly use the concept of environment in relation to home hazards and gait and falls relevant to physical contexts. This understanding of the environment tends to be very concrete, for example, including the consideration/assessment of barriers at different loci in the house and light and floor conditions (Iwarsson, 2004). Geriatric medicine, geropsychology, and social gerontology also have invested interest in the role of long-term care institutions and special housing for older adults. Moreover, in the *health sciences* at large, evidence is increasing that active out-of-home behavior and healthy lifestyle (e.g., physical activity) may also depend on the nature of out-of-home environments that may foster or hinder such behavior (Tudor-Locke, Craig, Thyfault, & Spence, 2013).

With particular emphasis put on older adults with severe care needs, new understandings of the role and importance of environments have also been established recently; these understandings underscore the need to consider links among the individual, neighborhood, community, and society. The meaning of environment is enriched in these approaches by concepts such as mutual responsibility, concern, respect, belonging, trust, identity, and community participation, in order to create and maintain an independent and dignified living in the community until the end of life. In Germany, for example, the concept of "caring communities" has been established in this context (Klie, 2014).

The list of exemplary disciplines illustrates the diverse nature of using the term "environment" in gerontology. Building on the views of these overlapping disciplines, one can preliminarily conclude that the use of the concept of the environment in gerontology is a multilayered enterprise. For instance, environment is used very specifically (e.g., home hazards) or very abstractly (e.g., environment in person–gene interactions); in a social way (e.g., family as environmental context) or a physical–spatial way (e.g., navigating through the community); and as an entity not separable from the person (e.g., socioeconomic status) and as a separable entity (e.g., housing quality). Moving forward, we answer how environment is used in environmental gerontology, that is, in the subarea of gerontology that explicitly considers the aging person in his or her environment.

▪ PRINCIPLES AND EXPLANATORY AMBITION OF ENVIRONMENTAL GERONTOLOGY

Principles of Environmental Gerontology

As we see it, environmental gerontology rests on three main principles—two more related to the concept level and one more related to research strategy: (a) importance of P–E transaction and developmental co-construction; (b) importance of explicitly considering the environment, with a focus on the physical–spatial dimension; and (c) importance of optimizing ecological validity in research.

First, the classic formula—dating back to German psychologist Kurt Lewin, which states that behavior is a function of the person's characteristics, as well as those of the environment ($B = f[P, E]$)—remains to be a "conceptual given" in the social and behavioral sciences, and aging is no exception. Environmental gerontology theorizing may be characterized as the subdiscipline within gerontology which—in principal terms—has put equal emphasis on the consideration of P and E or may put more emphasis on E, presuming that other subdisciplines contributing to gerontology (e.g., geropsychology) are treating mostly the aging individual (P).

Environmental gerontology also had from the beginning close affinity with *environmental psychology*, in which the concept of "person–environment transaction" has gained much prominence (Altman & Rogoff, 1987; Wahl & Oswald, 2010). A key assumption inherent in this concept is that it is difficult to separate P from E and that the understanding of an ongoing complex and mutual shaping of P and E throughout the life span is adequate. Furthermore, it may be that this intimate intertwining of P and E increases across the life span and may indeed reach its climax in old age and very old age (often categorized as 65 and older or even 80 to 85 and older).

According to Bronfenbrenner's (1999) bio-ecological model of lifelong coping with environmental conditions, different layers of P–E interchange must be considered, that is, the microsystem (the interpersonal interactions within the immediate environment), the mesosystem (two or more microsystems directly impacting the developing individual), the exosystem (linkages among subsystems that indirectly influence the individual), and the macrosystem (values, norms, and legislation of a given society).

Furthermore, life-span development is seen as a never-ending sequence of ecological transitions, in which new P–E territories are continuously conquered, while other P–E territories are left behind. Prototypical examples include the transitions from school to the labor sphere, from the labor world to retirement, and from community-dwelling living to nursing home, assisted-living, or retirement community life. This reasoning closely coincides with developmental science's fundamental idea of developmental *co-construction*—that is, the assumption that developing individuals are constantly shaped by contexts and vice versa (Valsiner, 1994; Wahl & Lang, 2004).

Second, in his early landmark contributions to environmental gerontology, Powell M. Lawton (1977) has used a broad understanding of environment that included social others and social groups, as well as all its physical components (including both the natural or manmade ones). However, environmental gerontology "in action" has never treated both the physical and social components of the environment in similar intensity. Instead, the overall understanding of the environment in environmental gerontology as a subarea of gerontology has been the major emphasis on the physical and spatial environment (Wahl, 2001; Wahl et al., 2004, 2012).

It remains, however, quite clear that such emphasis does not ignore the social and cultural parts of environments of aging. Wahl and Gitlin (2007) have suggested the term *"physical–social* environment" to address this issue, that is, the physical component of the environment cannot be separated from its social component, and vice versa. For example, infrastructural characteristics in a nursing home may provoke or hinder social communication and objective spaces are not the least becoming meaningful places due to the social partners and processes being connected with them (e.g., family celebrations and rituals).

Third, environmental gerontology always argues for the importance of optimizing ecological validity in aging research (e.g., Wahl, 2001). Focusing on issues such as defining under which conditions older adults are "feeling at home" (Oswald & Wahl, 2005) or offering a detailed description of the role of environmental barriers in the home or immediate surrounding directly brings research to the daily ecology of old age. Older adults always operate in physical–social environments; therefore, making the environment the research target implies that reconstructing daily (or weekly) ecologies must have a high priority as a meta-idea of doing aging research (Kaspar, Oswald, Wahl, Voss, & Wettstein, 2015).

That said, it is an interesting development in gerontology (particularly in geropsychology) that ecological validity seems to have become more important over the past couple of decades. Major indicators include the emphasis now given to event-sampling in situ research strategies in geropsychology (Ram & Diehl, 2015) and the rapidly increasing trend to use ambulatory assessment as a way to assess aging individuals as closely as possible in their everyday world contexts (Hoppmann & Riediger, 2009; we refer to this point again in the following text).

Mission of Environmental Gerontology and Its Explanatory Ambition

In light of the principles described in the previous section, environmental gerontology strives for an in-depth understanding of the interrelations between aging persons and their physical–social environments and how these relationships shape aging outcomes (Wahl et al., 2012; Wahl & Gitlin, 2007; Wahl & Oswald, 2010). The overarching aim of environmental gerontology is thus to describe, explain, and modify/optimize the relationship between the aging person and his or her physical–social environment.

With regard to *description*, environmental gerontology puts, as already argued, strong emphasis on day-to-day contexts of aging individuals, reinforcing the notion that daily ecology settings deserve strong attention in gerontological research. First, older people—particularly those in advanced old age—spend most of their time (i.e., about three quarters of their daytime) at home and immediate home environment (Baltes, Maas, Wilms, Borchelt, & Little, 1999; Wahl & Oswald, 2010). As a consequence, housing characteristics as the predominant setting in which aging unfolds have been a major focus of research in environmental gerontology (Oswald & Wahl, 2004; Oswald & Wahl, 2013).

Second, older individuals tend to live in the same place for a long time; for example, in the German Aging Survey, nearly one third of those aged 65 years and older had already lived for more than 40 years in the same home (Motel, Künemund, & Bode, 2000). Such long-term living and aging at the same location seems to evoke rich cognitive and affective ties to the place one lives, coined in everyday language with the internationally known German term *Heimat* (homeland)—or, put in scholarly language, addressed as place identity and place attachment to the very specific idea of "my place." Other naturally occurring environmental changes over the course of the year—for example, lighting, temperature, weather conditions, smells, and noises—also contribute considerably to the environmental experience of the normal rhythm of life; the assumption is that such changes are of particular importance for older people, as they reflect the aging process and provide orientation in space and time.

Regarding *explanation*, the phenomena to be explained in environmental gerontology are, for one, classic outcomes in aging research and gero-epidemiology, such as well-being (Oswald, Jopp, Rott, & Wahl, 2011) and autonomy and identity (Oswald & Wahl, 2005; Wahl, Fänge, Oswald, Gitlin, & Iwarsson, 2009). In addition, the term "healthy aging" has been used in environmental gerontology work and includes outcomes, such as functional ability, falls, infections, cardiovascular disease, morbidity at large, and excess mortality (Oswald et al., 2007; Oswald & Wahl, 2004). The latter endpoints have been particularly linked with environmental conditions, such as heat waves, or risky living circumstances, such as moldiness in the house or noisy surroundings. Specific P–E constellations have also been linked with motor-behavior characteristics (e.g., extension of space in which one is acting) and activity patterns (e.g., frequency and quality of out-of-home activities, physical activity; Wettstein et al., 2015).

The focus on *optimization* reflects the ambition of environmental gerontology to provide a substantial and direct contribution to the improvement of quality of life in old age (Golant, 2015; Wahl et al., 2012) through means of intervention. The involvement of environmental gerontology in advancing evidence-driven home modifications is prototypical, adding to the development of new housing solutions for the diversity of aging individuals, or designing public spaces and "age-friendly" environments at large (e.g., Buffel et al., 2014).

■ EARLY THEORY BUILDING IN ENVIRONMENTAL GERONTOLOGY: OBJECTIVE AND EXPERIENTIAL P–E TRANSACTION SIDE BY SIDE

By "early theory building" in environmental gerontology, we mean predominantly classic work such as Lawton and Nahemow (1973) and Rowles (1978), which remains prominent in research and practice contexts (e.g., new housing solutions; community planning). As we see it, a major distinction can be made between those theories that focused on the "objective" environment "out there" versus those that emphasized the more experiential part of P–E relations for aging individuals.

Theoretical Focus on Objective Environments Supporting or Constraining Aging

A classic view that was influential until present is the Ecological Theory of Aging (ETA; Lawton, 1982; Lawton & Nahemow, 1973; Scheidt & Norris-Baker, 2004). The basic assumption of this theory has been that the capacity to adapt behaviorally to existing physical–social environmental pressure profoundly decreases as people age, due to an increasing number of functional limitations. According to the ETA, older individuals need to react to environmental pressure in order to remain independent and feel well (Lawton & Nahemow, 1973).

The original model describes behavior and well-being primarily as a function of the level of personal competence and environmental pressure (Lawton, 1982; Lawton & Nahemow, 1973). As has been argued by a number of scholars (e.g., Scheidt & Norris-Baker, 2004; Wahl & Gitlin, 2007), the ETA's assumptions and predictions still are of great heuristic value theoretically, as well as in applied perspective. First, the assumption that variability in autonomous behavior and well-being can increasingly be explained by physical environments (and not only by personal factors such as needs, personality traits, cognitive function, and goals) is an important addition to the understanding of development in old age.

Indeed, older adults may become "prisoners of space" (Rowles, 1978), with long-time life experiences dominated by the no-longer-fitting home environment and an unknown territory of new environments (e.g., a nursing home), which may be needed to enter in a not-too-far personal future. Thus, physical environments such as the home may play either the role of resource or risk to life satisfaction, depending on individual living circumstances and age (Oswald et al., 2011). A second interesting feature of the theory still worth considering is that environments slightly exceeding an older person's competence may indeed reveal latent reserves and new learning. It is somewhat disappointing however—in terms of the reception of the theory—that this optimization component of P–E relations in the ETA has found less attention as compared to the compensatory aspect, that is, environments that compensate for no-longer-available competencies.

Overall, considerable empirical support for the ETA and its variants is available in areas such as independence in activities of daily living, well-being, and depression (for review, see Iwarsson, 2004; Wahl & Oswald, 2010), although it remains difficult to make an estimation of the effect size of the role of the physical–social environment as compared to personal characteristics and the social environment.

Theoretical Focus on Perceived Environments Supporting or Constraining Aging

Major concepts in this area include place attachment, place identity, and the meaning of "home." Theories on place attachment and place identity—which have been long discussed (Altman & Low, 1992) and still inform environmental gerontology's conceptual and empirical platform (Rowles & Watkins, 2003; Wahl & Oswald, 2010)—point to a gamut of processes, operating when people form affective, cognitive, behavioral, and social bonds to the environment, thereby transforming "space" into "place." Often, these aspects of physical, social, and personal bonding are assessed by global attachment evaluations (e.g., on indoor versus outdoor place attachment; Oswald, Hieber, Wahl, & Mollenkopf, 2005), but there are also efforts to use qualitative methodology to approach place attachment and identity empirically (Peace, 2005).

Concepts on the meaning of "home" are directly related to place attachment, as they deal with the most frequent manifestation of attachment processes. For instance, since older adults often live in the same residence for long periods of time, cognitive and emotional aspects of the meaning of home are strongly linked to biography ("My home"; "My neighborhood"). Such social, cognitive, and emotional links may become manifest through processes of reflecting on the past, symbolically represented in certain places and cherished objects within the home. Meaning-of-home has been empirically targeted in earlier research via qualitative methodology (Rowles, 1983; Rubinstein, 1989), but recently there have also been successful efforts to quantify meaning-of-home aspects (Oswald et al. 2007; Oswald & Kaspar, 2012; Oswald et al., 2006).

Overall, this set of environmental gerontology theories has a strong descriptive notion, in that it provides conceptual dimensions to understand "place-making" processes as people age. In a sense, processes and outcomes are intertwined in these theories. For example, the goal is to describe and understand how an older person makes meaning out of his or her environment and feelings/evaluations, echoed in statements such as: "My home is the most important place in my life." There is also an empirical support for the assumption that meaning-of-home may depend on the older individual's health status; for example, functionally impaired older adults seem to value feelings of familiarization with their physical–social environment more strongly than unimpaired older adults (Oswald & Wahl, 2005, 2013).

■ RECENT THEORY BUILDING: SEARCHING FOR INTEGRATION OF OBJECTIVE AND SUBJECTIVE P–E TRANSACTIONAL ELEMENTS

The Model of Oswald and Wahl

Driven by the idea to integrate and extend both environmental concepts that focus on the objective and subjective physical–social environment, Wahl et al. (2012) suggest the framework depicted in Figure 31.1. At the core of this framework is the assumption that two fundamental processes, experience-driven P–E belonging and behavior-driven P–E agency, help increase the understanding and integration of existing P–E interchanges as people age. P–E belonging reflects a sense of mainly positive connection with the physical–social environment (e.g., Bakan, 1966; Baumeister & Leary, 1995), while P–E agency refers to the process of becoming a change agent in one's own life by means of intentional and proactive behaviors imposed on the physical–social environment (Bandura, 1991, 2006).

Going further, processes associated with P–E belonging account for the full range of subjective evaluations and interpretations of place and guide cognitive and emotional representations of P–E constellations related to places (Oswald & Wahl, 2005, 2013; Rowles & Watkins, 2003). Thus, belonging incorporates all non–goal-oriented cognitive and emotional aspects that make a space a place.

In contrast, processes of P–E agency include the full range of goal-directed behaviors related to making use of the objective physical–social environment, such as environment-related cognition and perceived control over the environment. They include reactive and proactive aspects of using, compensating, adapting, retrofitting, creating, and sustaining places, which is especially important in old age because of decreasing functional and cognitive capacity. The model also assumes that both P–E belonging *and* P–E

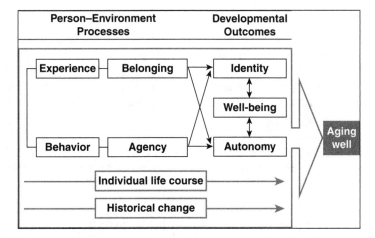

FIGURE 31.1 Model of Oswald and Wahl. The interplay between two fundamental processes, P–E belonging and P–E agency, is seen as a major driving force for identity, autonomy, and well-being in old age. This full P–E dynamic is embedded in individual life courses, as well as historical change.

Adapted from Wahl et al. (2012).

agency must be considered in any qualification of P–E relations in later life. Emerging empirical evidence for the model came from the "Enabling Autonomy, Participation and Well-Being in Old Age: The Home Environment as a Determinant for Healthy Ageing" (ENABLE-AGE) project, in which—for the first time—a maximum number of indicators regarding P–E belonging as well as P–E agency were assessed in parallel in advanced old age individuals in a range of European countries (Oswald et al., 2007).

As has been found to be empirically driven by this model, P–E fit processes and housing-related control processes that speak to objective constellations of remaining competence and respective objective physical–social home environments—as well as P–E belonging processes—contributed to the prediction of end points such as autonomy, well-being, and depression (Oswald et al., 2007). Furthermore, the model contributes to a better understanding of interactions among more person-based processes and environmentally based processes. For example, Wahl, Oswald, Schilling, and Iwarsson (2009) found that the link between lowered accessibility of the home environment and depression is higher in older adults aged older than 80 years, when they perceive their home situation overall as no longer under their control.

Other Recent Models

For one, Golant's model of Residential Normalcy has found much resonance in environmental gerontology and beyond, emphasizing residential decision-making processes in later life from an individual's perspective by highlighting subjective environmental experiences of residential comfort and mastery, as well as related adaptive coping strategies to maintain or achieve residential normalcy (Golant, 2011, 2015a, 2015b).

According to Golant's model, if older people feel comfortable and in control of their environment at home, they have already achieved residential normalcy and may no longer feel the need to change anything. However, if there is a perceived incongruence on the behavioral or experiential level, they perceive themselves as being out of their mastery and/or comfort zone. Consequently, they will try to achieve residential normalcy again by ways of assimilative or accommodative coping strategies (Brandtstädter & Greve, 1994) with respect to the immediate home environment. The model has also been adapted into real-life settings of relocation decision making—for instance, based on data from the European ENABLE-AGE study (Granbom et al., 2014).

Another intellectually and empirically promising approach is the yet unpublished model of "At-Oneness," which introduces a socio-spatial phenomenon in which the home evolves as both an individual and communal construct (Walsh, Rowles, & Scharf, 2014). The model of At-Oneness is based on qualitative narratives from rural Ireland; it is considered to be a multidimensional, interconnected construct, involving an evolving integration of the aging self and home across the life course. The model interweaves six dimensions of home in time and space as part of an evolving identity, that is, place of origin, inherited meaning, rhythm and routine, relational harmony, aesthetic functional landscape, and invested effort.

"New" Environments in Need of Consideration: Future Importance of Technology Environments

Technology developments that were not available to the cohorts of older adults considered in environmental gerontology's early theoretical work are now being developed, addressing an important new facet of the environment of older adults. Once again,

Lawton had taken strong action (see his keynote at the 1996 founding conference of the International Society for Gerontechnology in Helsinki) to support the critical role of technology for the quality of life in old age (Lawton, 1998).

The Internet, the "automation" of everyday technology (e.g., teller machines, ticket machines, computerized voice menus, car technology) and sensor- or GPS-based assistance are dramatically changing the way people organize and experience their everyday lives. Although the effect of technology was traditionally limited to a younger population, it is increasingly true for older adults as well (Schulz et al., 2014; Stokols, 1999). Robots accompany frail older adults while they stroll around the house or use the bathroom; personal computers provide cognitive or physical training programs; smart home environments support people with sensory, mobile, or cognitive decline; and robotic animals play a significant role in the social and emotional life of older people with dementia, although there is a lot of research to be done to provide better empirical evidence in this area (Kolling et al., 2013).

Future cohorts of older adults will benefit from a full range of technology products designed to support them as they "stay connected" and age well, despite accumulated loss experiences (Schulz et al., 2014). It is also possible that in the future, older adults (including those in advanced old age) will not only use robot care and other technological tools to support and compensate for lost competencies as an agency-relevant device (P–E agency), but may also feel emotionally attached to their robotic animal or enjoy virtual reality, which may become new means of experiencing environmental stimulation in the context of pronounced disability (P–E belonging).

Although this rapidly increasing role of technology as a means of P–E agency, as well as for P–E belonging purposes, is a challenge for theory building in gerontology at large (see Schulz et al., 2014), environmental gerontology is most directly affected by this challenge, with its direct emphasis on physical–social environments. For example, it may be heuristically fruitful to combine man-machine models in human factors research with ETA-inherent concepts such as environmental pressure and proactivity (Fozard & Wahl, 2012). It may also become an intellectually inspiring task to target linkages between P–E belonging and identity-building processes as highlighted in the Oswald–Wahl model (see again Figure 31.1) in relation to technology use by older adults. Will, for instance— as we currently see it in adolescents and even in older children—Internet use also serve important identity formation and social presentation purposes for aging individuals in the near future?

■ IMPLICATIONS OF ENVIRONMENTAL GERONTOLOGY THEORIZING FOR GERONTOLOGY'S THEORY BUILDING AT LARGE

Three major implications will be addressed in what follows: (a) implications for theories of life-span development and aging; (b) implications for the understanding of the cohort issue in aging research; and (c) implications for the understanding of the diversity and aging issue.

Environmental Gerontology Theorizing and Theories of Life-span Development and Aging

Despite the increasingly important role of the physical–social–technical environment for old and very old individuals, its role in the broader context of aging and life-span development is not well developed. For example, research connected with *social–emotional selectivity theory* (Carstensen, 2006) has confirmed that, with increasing age, people become increasingly selective, investing greater resources in goals and activities that maximize positive emotional experiences and minimize emotional risks.

Proactive use of environments, including use of technology, may indeed facilitate selection of desired people and contexts that support positive emotional interactions and help promote entertaining and engaging experiences. One may even argue that processes of socio-emotional selectivity can be seen not only at the level of social partners, but also in relation to the physical environment, expressed in increasingly stronger feelings of bonding to the home environment and familiar areas (e.g., location of one's vacation in old age; Wahl & Lang, 2004).

The *selective optimization with compensation model* (SOC; Baltes et al., 2006) focuses on how individuals allocate resources to promote growth and maintenance of functioning in the face of age-related declines/losses. According to the SOC model, successful aging involves selection of appropriate functional domains, optimizing developmental potential, and compensating for losses. It may be helpful to spell out in more detail how physical–social environments help or hinder SOC processes by using environmental gerontology theory. Regarding technology environments, Lindenberger et al. (2008) have used this general framework to discuss how intelligent assistive technology that continuously adjusts the balance between environmental support and individual capabilities can maximize the potential of an individual by "combining support with challenge, thereby enhancing motivation, social participation and a sense of autonomy" (p. 63).

The *motivational theory of lifespan development* (Heckhausen, Wrosch, & Schulz, 2010) proposes that the key criterion for adaptive development is the extent to which the individual realizes control of his or her environment (i.e., exerts primary control) across different domains of life. Striving for primary control is a constant and universal motivational drive throughout the life course. However, as individuals' capacity for primary control decreases in old age and some goals become unattainable, individuals need to have strategies that facilitate disengagement from unattainable goals in favor of pursuing other, more attainable ones.

A wide variety of cognitive strategies can be used to navigate these transitions, including adjusting expectations, values, and attributions so that losses in primary control do not undermine the individual's motivational resources for primary control striving in general. Environmental features, including technology, can compensate for declining primary control abilities through assistive and support devices; enhance control striving through task performance feedback that optimizes motivational engagement; and facilitate disengagement from unattainable goals by identifying appropriate alternative goals for a given level of functioning. Although such a role of the physical–social environment is frequently mentioned in the theory, the environmental part, as compared to the person part, is underaddressed and may profit from environmental gerontology theorizing.

Environmental Gerontology Theorizing and the Cohort Issue in Gerontology

Environmental gerontology's theory building and research may also be helpful when it comes to the understanding of cohort flow dynamics in gerontology. For example, new housing solutions for older adults—such as assisted living, retirement communities, or intergenerational arrangements, and new housing options for persons with dementia—have enhanced the fit between living preferences and needs (Wahl & Gitlin, 2003).

It is likely that future built environment solutions for older adults may not only, to take the model of Oswald and Wahl, better support P–E agency-related processes (e.g., enhancing daily autonomy even among older adults with disabilities), but also nurture or even "provoke" new forms of P–E belonging, including new relationships with the younger generation, friendships with persons with dementia, or even emotional attachment to robots. Similarly, new P–E interchange patterns are evident in out-of-home mobility and, at the more macro level, in the migration patterns of current and future cohorts of older people. Never before has there been an aging cohort with so much "world experience" and openness to new travel modes as there is today.

In the future, this lifestyle trend may become a more commonplace or take new directions, such as increasing "use" of virtual environmental realities. Migration or extensive traveling may become a major expression of older adults' agency-related behaviors, while also modifying the traditional view of "aging in place." Going further, it is also obvious that the technology environment issue as described earlier has considerable potential to deepen the discussion on ethical options and limits in aging, as well as to increase understanding of the needs, preferences, and "action modes" of future cohorts of older adults (Fozard & Wahl, 2012; Schulz et al., 2014).

Environmental Gerontology Theorizing and the Diversity of Aging

The understanding of age diversity remains a major conceptual issue in gerontology (Settersten & Trauten, 2009). Seen through the lenses of environmental gerontology, a major argument is that diversity may also mean diversity in terms of P–E constellations. However, the aging and diversity issue so far is treated mostly as interindividual differences at the person level. Such a context-free view of diversity has its limitations, because it ignores all the diversity on the side of the physical–social environment.

Aging people live in a range of housing characteristics, neighborhoods (again with a range of characteristics such as support potential, crime rate, cultural aspects, distances to public transport), green areas, and educational and cultural infrastructure. Some of these features are represented in classic SES notions, but definitely not all (see also the following discussion: issue of urbanization). It may thus be important to consider diversity in environments and thus in P–E constellations as people age because of two primary reasons.

First, diversity in key person variables, such as cognitive performance, may need to be qualified, depending on the environment. Indeed, strong differences in cognitive performance may level out at least to some extent because of compensatory and supportive environmental characteristics. An older person low in cognitive function may live in an ecology that is easy to handle at the home and out-of-home levels and his or her neighborhood may reveal all kinds of supporting activities, resulting in no significant differences in autonomy and independence (as compared to an older individual with high cognitive functioning).

Second, focusing P–E constellations as the unit of analysis may lead to a new understanding of diversity in aging at large. One implication of such a view could be that even quite homogeneous older individuals may be seen as quite diverse, when the environment is also taken into consideration.

■ SYNERGIES AMONG RECENT ADVANCEMENTS IN GERONTOLOGY AND ENVIRONMENTAL GERONTOLOGY THEORY BUILDING AND RESEARCH

In this final part of the chapter, we shortly highlight three key trends in gerontology at large in recent time, for which we see synergies with environmental gerontology perspectives: (a) event-sampling research designs and the trend toward ambulatory assessment; (b) bio-gerontology developments; and (c) aging and urbanization.

Environmental Gerontology and New Research Paradigms: The Case of Daily Experience-Sampling Methodology

We argue that the current trend toward intensive measurement designs in the daily ecology and the related increasing use of ambulatory assessment, taking into account short-term, interindividual variability in areas such as cognitive and emotional functioning, and daily stress experiences (Hoppmann & Riediger, 2009; Ram & Diehl, 2015), may benefit from environmental gerontology perspectives. This is so at a fundamental level, because it seems that measurement-burst designs reflect a more general trend—so far, mostly in the behavioral and medical sciences of aging—to consider the natural ecology of older adults as much as possible in their assessments (i.e., to increase what has been labeled "ecology validity").

As described earlier, such ecological validity is one of the basic premises of environmental gerontology; all the gathered research experience on the issue in this area may also become of profit for event-sampling research designs. At the same time, gathering data as closely as possible in naturally occurring ecologies means automatically that the data-assessment process happens in naturally occurring P–E constellations (Kaspar et al., 2015; Wettstein et al., 2015). Therefore, it may be also good in event-sampling designs to describe ("assess") the physical–social environment systematically; herein lies another layer where environmental gerontology research and assessment efforts may become important.

Environmental Gerontology and Bio-Gerontology: The Case of Neuro-Aging

The intersection of environmental gerontology and bio-gerontology and the neurosciences also demands more research attention. For example, a stronger liaison would enable better understanding of possible interactions between environmental input and cognitive and affective functioning at various levels, including brain processes as we age. Although research on the relationship between cognitive functioning and enriched environments indicates the importance of environments for normal aging and Alzheimer's disease (Arendash et al., 2004; Lores-Arnaiz et al., 2006), scant research regarding P–E transactions exists (Hertzog et al., 2008).

In particular, we are not aware of any rigorous research that brings together the physical–social environment (e.g., various housing solutions in the assisted-living sector) and its impact on frontal lobe processes or brain areas that play a role in affective functioning (e.g., amygdala). A particularly interesting topic would be the better understanding of *novelty* in environments, as much novelty may influence brain development in later life. It seems that the fundamental argument of the neurosciences—that brain functions unfold in close correspondence with the environment—is mostly unexplored territory in human-aging research, which is in stark contrast to respective animal models designed to understand the aging process.

Environmental Gerontology and Globalization: The Case of Urbanization

Gerontology that includes environmental gerontology research has been predominantly urban research, though the implications are seldom made explicit (Phillipson, 2004). Urban environments as major living settings of aging people all over the world increasingly reveal similarities—particularly in terms of increasing ambivalences—which seem to become even sharper in the future.

One such ambivalence manifests in the trend toward "hypermobility" on the one hand (particularly for the young, well-educated, elite population) and the search for feelings of *Heimat* on the other hand (possibly more for those in advanced old age). Furthermore, there is reason to assume that urban settings, under the influence of globalization, economic pressure, and mega-diversity of their populations, launch social exclusion and inequalities in day-to-day quality of life, which may ultimately affect senior citizens. Environmental gerontology approaches may be helpful to understand better why older adults have a high likelihood of becoming the targets of such social exclusion processes (Scharf, Philipson, & Smith, 2007).

Similarly, current P–E-fit approaches predominantly applied to the housing domain (Iwarsson, 2004) deserve extension to livable communities or even countries; they may add to the better understanding of the role of ambiguities of aging in the city and to combine political requirements (e.g., age friendliness) with the need for conceptual strength and empirical evidence (Buffel et al., 2014). In other words, environmental gerontology theorizing and the theoretical approaches of a "re-vitalized" (Phillipson, 2004, p. 963) urban sociology and political science concerned with aging should merge their conceptual strengths.

■ CONCLUSION

As we argued throughout this chapter, environmental gerontology is an "old" and established area within gerontology theorizing and practice. Still—and this has much to do with changing environments due to scientific and societal developments, as well as demographical trends, the urbanization movement, globalization, climate change, and the discourse on social inequality—environmental gerontology needs fresh input and is currently undergoing major conceptual and empirical challenges in a changing world.

We also made a number of arguments to support the view that developmental science, life-span theorizing, and gerontology theory building at large may profit from environmental gerontology thinking and evidence and that there is an underused potential for cross-fertilization.

Going further, we strongly believe that new alliances among disciplines and scientific programs will further infuse environmental gerontology theory as well as respective empirical research, for example, liaisons with the neurosciences, the health sciences, and the technology and aging area. Consequently, it would be promising for future research if the importance of explicitly considering aging in the environment and the environment in aging—particularly in ongoing longitudinal studies of aging—would find better resonance; this would avoid the decontextualization of the aging individual, which is tempting, especially for geropsychology. On the other hand—from a methodological perspective—the trend toward event-sampling research designs and ambulatory assessment may bring unexpected new environmental gerontology infusing for geropsychology as well.

REFERENCES

Altman, I., & Low, S. M. (Eds.). (1992). *Human behavior and environment (Vol. 12): Place attachment*. New York, NY: Plenum.

Altman, I., & Rogoff, B. (1987). World views in psychology: Trait, interactionist, organismic, and transactional perspectives. In D. Stokels & I. Altman (Eds.), *Handbook of environmental psychology* (Vol. 1, pp. 1–40). New York, NY: Wiley.

Antonucci, T. C., Birditt, K. S., & Akiyama, H. (2009). Convoys of social relations: An interdisciplinary approach. In V. Bengtson, D. Gans, N. M. Putney, & M. Silverstein (Eds.), *Handbook of theories of aging* (pp. 247–260). New York, NY: Springer Publishing Company.

Arendash, G. W., Garcia, M. F., Costa, D. A., Cracchiolo, J. R., Wefes, I. M., & Potter, H. (2004). Environmental enrichment improves cognition in aged Alzheimer's transgenic mice despite stable beta-amyloid deposition. *Neuroreport, 15*(11), 1751–1754.

Austad, S. N. (2009). Making sense of biology theories of aging. In V. Bengtson, D. Gans, N. M. Putney, & M. Silverstein (Eds.), *Handbook of theories of aging* (pp. 147–162). New York, NY: Springer Publishing Company.

Baars, J. (2012). *Aging and the art of living*. Baltimore, MD: Johns Hopkins Press.

Bakan, D. (1966). *The duality of human existence*. Chicago, IL: Rand McNally.

Baltes, M. M., Maas, I., Wilms, H. U., Borchelt, M. F., & Little, T. (1999). Everyday competence in old and very old age: Theoretical considerations and empirical findings. In P. B. Baltes & K. U. Mayer (Eds.), *The Berlin aging study* (pp. 384–402). Cambridge, UK: Cambridge University Press.

Baltes, P. B., Lindenberger, U., & Staudinger, U. M. (2006). Life-span theory in developmental psychology. In W. Damon & R. M. Lerner (Eds.), *Handbook of child psychology* (6th ed., Vol. 1: Theoretical models of human development, pp. 569–664). New York, NY: Wiley.

Bandura, A. (1991). Human agency: The rhetoric and the reality. *The American Psychologist, 46*, 157–162.

Bandura, A. (2006). Toward a psychology of human agency. *Perspectives on Psychological Science, 1*, 164–180. doi:10.1111/j.1745-6916.2006.00011.x

Baumeister, R. F., & Leary, M. R. (1995). The need to belong: Desire for interpersonal attachments as a fundamental human motivation. *Psychological Bulletin, 117*(3), 497–529.

Brandtstädter, J., & Greve, W. (1994). The aging self: Stabilizing and protective processes. *Developmental Review, 14*, 42–80.

Bronfenbrenner, U. (1999). Environments in developmental perspective: Theoretical and operational models. In S. L. Friedman & T. D. Wachs (Eds.), *Measuring environment across the life span* (pp. 3–28). Washington, DC: American Psychological Association.

Buffel, T., McGarry, P., Phillipson, C., De Donder, L., Dury, S., De Witte,... Verté, D. (2014). Developing age-friendly cities: Case studies from Brussels and Manchester and implications for policy and practice. *Journal of Aging and Social Policy, 26*(1–2), 52–72.

Butler, T., & Hamnett, C. (2007). The geography of education: Introduction. *Urban Studies, 4*, 1161–1174.

Campisi, J. (2005). Senescent cells, tumor suppression, and organismal aging: Good citizens, bad neighbors. *Cell, 120*(4), 513–522.

Carstensen, L. L. (2006). The influence of a sense of time on human development. *Science, 312*(5782), 1913–1915.

Colcombe, S., & Kramer, A. F. (2003). Fitness effects on the cognitive function of older adults: A meta-analytic study. *Psychological Science, 14*(2), 125–130.

Diehl, M., Hay, E. L., & Chui, H. (2012). Personal risk and resilience factors in the context of daily stress. *Annual Review of Gerontology and Geriatrics, 32*(1), 251–274.

Fozard, J. L., & Wahl, H. W. (2012). Age and cohort effects in gerontechnology: A reconsideration. *Gerontechnology, 11*, 10–21.

Golant, S. M. (2011). The quest for residential normalcy by older adults: Relocation but one pathway. *Journal of Aging Studies, 25*, 193–205.

Golant, S. M. (2015a). Residential normalcy and the enriched coping repertoires of successfully aging older adults. *The Gerontologist, 55*(1), 70–82.

Golant, S. M. (2015b) *Aging in the right place*. Baltimore, MD: Health Professions Press.

Granbom, M., Himmelsbach, I., Haak, M., Löfqvist, C., Oswald, F., & Iwarsson, S. (2014). Residential normalcy and environmental experiences of very old people: Changes in residential reasoning over time. *Journal of Aging Studies, 29*, 9–19.

Heckhausen, J. H., Wrosch, C., & Schulz, R. (2010). A motivational theory of lifespan development. *Psychological Review, 117*, 32–60.

Hertzog, C., Kramer, A. F., Wilson, R. S., & Lindenberger, U. (2008). Enrichment effects on adult cognitive development: Can the functional capacity of older adults be preserved and enhanced? *Psychological Science in the Public Interest: A Journal of the American Psychological Society, 9*(1), 1–65.

Hoppmann, C., & Gerstorf, D. (2009). Spousal interrelations in old age: A mini-review. *Gerontology, 55*(4), 449–459.

Hoppmann, C., & Riediger, M. (2009). Ambulatory assessment in lifespan psychology: An overview of current status and new trends. *European Psychologist, 14*, 98–108.

Iwarsson, S. (2004). Assessing the fit between older people and their home environments: An occupational therapy research perspective. In H. W. Wahl, R. Scheidt, & P. Windley (Eds.), *Annual Review of Gerontology and Geriatrics, 23* (pp. 85–109). New York, NY: Springer Publishing Company.

Kaspar, R., Oswald, F., Wahl, H. W., Voss, E., & Wettstein, M. (2015). Daily mood and out-of-home mobility in older adults: Does cognitive impairment matter? *Journal of*

Applied Gerontology: The Official Journal of the Southern Gerontological Society, 34(1), 26–47.

Klie, T. (2014). *Wen kümmern die Alten? Auf dem Weg in eine sorgende Gesellschaft. [Who cares about the aged? On the way to a concerning society.]* Munich, Germany: Pattloch.

Kolling, T., Haberstroh, J., Kaspar, R., Pantel, J., Oswald, F., & Knopf, M. (2013). Methodological considerations for research in social and emotional robots: Input, outcome, and evaluation. *GeroPsych—The Journal of Gerontopsychlogy and Geriatric Psychiatry, 26*, 83–88.

Lawton, M. P. (1977). The impact of the environment on aging and behavior. In J. E. Birren & K. W. Schaie (Eds.), *Handbook of the psychology of aging* (pp. 276–301). New York, NY: Van Nostrand Reinhold.

Lawton, M. P. (1982). Competence, environmental press, and the adaptation of older people. In M. P. Lawton, P. G. Windley, & T. O. Byerts (Eds.), *Aging and the environment* (pp. 33–59). New York, NY: Springer Publishing Company.

Lawton, M. P. (1998). Future society and aging. In J. A. M. Graafmans, V. Taipale, & N. Charness (Eds.), *Gerontechnology: A sustainable investment in the future* (pp. 12–22). Amsterdam, The Netherlands: IOS Press.

Lawton, M. P., & Nahemow, L. (1973). Ecology and the aging process. In C. Eisdorfer & M. P. Lawton, (Eds.), *Psychology of adult development and aging* (pp. 619–674). Washington, DC: American Psychological Association.

Lindenberger, U., Lövdén, M., Schellenbach, M., Li, S. C., & Krüger, A. (2008). Psychological principles of successful aging technologies: A mini-review. *Gerontology, 54*(1), 59–68.

Lindenberger, U., Marsiske, M., & Baltes, P. B. (2000). Memorizing while walking: Increase in dual-task costs from young adulthood to old age. *Psychology and Aging, 15*(3), 417–436.

Lores-Arnaiz, S., Bustamante, J., Arismendi, M., Vilas, S., Paglia, N., Basso, N.,...Arnaiz, M. R. (2006). Extensive enriched environments protect old rats from the aging dependent impairment of spatial cognition, synaptic plasticity and nitric oxide production. *Behavioural Brain Research, 169*(2), 294–302.

Motel, A., Künemund, H., & Bode, C. (2000). Wohnen und Wohnumfeld älterer Menschen [Housing and neighborhood of older adults]. In M. Kohli & H. Künemund (Eds.), *Die zweite Lebenshälfte - Gesellschaftliche Lage und Partizipation im Spiegel des Alters-Survey* [The second part of life - Societal situation and participation in the mirror of the Aging-Survey data.] (pp. 124–175). Opladen: Leske & Budrich.

Nyqvist, F., & Forsman, A. K. (Eds.).(2015). *Social capital and health resource in later life: The relevance of context* (Vol. 11). New York, NY: Springer Publishing Company.

Oswald, F., Hieber, A., Wahl, H. W., & Mollenkopf, H. (2005). Ageing and person-environment fit in different urban neighbourhoods. *European Journal of Ageing, 2*, 88–97.

Oswald, F., Jopp, D., Rott, C., & Wahl, H. W. (2011). Is aging in place a resource for or risk to life satisfaction? *The Gerontologist, 51*(2), 238–250.

Oswald, F., & Kaspar, R. (2012). On the quantitative assessment of perceived housing in later life. *Journal of Housing for the Elderly, 26,* 72–93.

Oswald, F., Schilling, O., Wahl, H. W., Fänge, A., Sixsmith, J. & Iwarsson, S. (2006). Homeward bound: Introducing a four domain model of perceived housing in very old age. *Journal of Environmental Psychology, 26,* 187–201.

Oswald, F., & Wahl, H. W. (2004). Housing and health in later life. *Reviews on Environmental Health, 19*(3–4), 223–252.

Oswald, F., & Wahl, H. W. (2005). Dimensions of the meaning of home in later life. In G. D. Rowles & H. Chaudhury (Eds.), *Home and identity in later life. International perspectives* (pp. 21–46). New York, NY: Springer Publishing Company.

Oswald, F., & Wahl, H.-W. (2013). Creating and sustaining homelike places in own home environments. In G. D. Rowles & M. Bernard (Eds.), *Environmental Gerontology* (pp. 53–77). New York, NY: Springer Publishing Company.

Oswald, F., Wahl, H. W., Schilling, O., Nygren, C., Fänge, A., Sixsmith, A.,…Iwarsson, S. (2007). Relationships between housing and healthy aging in very old age. *The Gerontologist, 47*(1), 96–107.

Peace, S. M. (2005). *Environment and identity in later life.* Berkshire, UK: Open University Press.

Peace, S., Holland, C., & Kellaher, L. (2006). *Environment and identity in later life.* Maidenhead, UK: Open University Press.

Phillipson, C. (2004). Urbanisation and ageing: Towards a new environmental gerontology. *Ageing and Society, 24,* 963–972.

Phillipson, C. (2007). The "elected" and the "excluded": Sociological perspectives on the experience of place and community in old age. *Ageing and Society, 27,* 321–342.

Ram, N., & Diehl, M. (2015). Multiple-time-scale design and analysis: Pushing towards real-time modeling of complex developmental processes. In M. Diehl, K. Hooker, & M. J. Sliwinski (Eds.), *Handbook of intraindividual variability across the life span* (pp. 308–323). New York, NY: Routledge/Taylor & Francis.

Richards, M., & Sacker, A. (2003). Lifetime antecedents of cognitive reserve. *Journal of Clinical and Experimental Neuropsychology, 25*(5), 614–624.

Rowles, G. D. (1978). *Prisoners of space? Exploring the geographical experience of older people.* Boulder, CO: Westview Press.

Rowles, G. D. (1983). Geographical dimensions of social support in rural Appalachia. In G. D. Rowles & R. J. Ohta (Eds.), *Aging and milieu: Environmental perspectives on growing old* (pp. 111–130). New York, NY: Academic Press.

Rowles, G. D., & Bernard, M. (2013). *Environmental gerontology.* New York, NY: Springer Publishing Company.

Rowles, G. D., & Watkins, J. F. (2003). History, habit, heart and hearth: On making spaces into places. In K. W. Schaie, H. W. Wahl, H. Mollenkopf, & F. Oswald (Eds.), *Aging independently: Living arrangements and mobility* (pp. 77–96). New York, NY: Springer Publishing Company.

Rowles, G. D., & Watkins, J. F. (2010). The geography of aging and the aged. In B. F. Warf (Ed.), *Encyclopedia of geography* (Vol. 2, pp. 877–878). Thousand Oaks, CA: Sage.

Rubinstein, R. L. (1989). The home environments of older people: A description of the psychosocial processes linking person to place. *Journal of Gerontology, 44*(2), S45–S53.

Ryff, C. R., & Singer, B. (2009). Understanding healthy aging: Key components and their integration. In V. Bengtson, D. Gans, N. M. Putney, & M. Silverstein (Eds.), *Handbook of theories of aging* (pp. 117–144). New York, NY: Springer Publishing Company.

Scharf, T., Philippson, C., & Smith, A. (2007). Aging in a difficult place: Assessing the impact of urban deprivation on older people. In H. W. Wahl, C. Tesch-Römer & A. Hoff (Eds.), *New dynamics in old age: Individual, environmental and societal perspectives* (pp. 153–174). Amityville, NY: Baywood Publishing.

Scharf, T., Phillipson, C., & Smith, A. E. (2005). Social exclusion of older people in deprived urban communities of England. *European Journal of Ageing, 2,* 76–87.

Scheidt, R. J., & Norris-Baker, C. (2004). The general ecological model revisited: Evolution, current status, and continuing challenges. In H. W. Wahl, R. J. Scheidt, & P. G. Windley (Eds.), *Annual review of gerontology and geriatrics, 23* (pp. 35–48). New York, NY: Springer Publishing Company.

Scheidt, R. J., & Windley, P. G. (2006). Environmental gerontology: Progress in the post-Lawton era. In J. E. Birren & K. W. Schaie (Eds.), *Handbook of the psychology of aging* (6th ed., pp. 105–125). Amsterdam: Elsevier.

Schulz, R., Wahl, H. W., Matthews, J. T., De Vito Dabbs, A., Beach, S. R., & Czaja, S. J. (2015). Advancing the aging and technology agenda in gerontology. *The Gerontologist, 55*(5), 724–734.

Settersten, R. A. (2003). Propositions and controversies in life-course scholarship. In R. A. Settersten (Ed.), *Invitation to the life course: Toward new understandings of later life* (pp. 15–45). Amityville, NY: Baywood.

Settersten, R. A., & Trauten, M. E. (2009). The new terrain of old age: Hallmarks, freedoms, and risks. In V. Bengtson, D. Gans, N. M. Putney, & M. Silverstein (Eds.), *Handbook of theories of aging* (pp. 455–470). New York, NY: Springer Publishing Company.

Stokols, D. (1999). Human development in the age of the internet: Conceptual and methodological horizons. In S. L. Friedman, & T. D. Wachs (Eds.), *Measuring environment across the life span* (pp. 327–356). Washington, DC: American Psychological Associaton.

Tudor-Locke, C., Craig, C. L., Thyfault, J. P., & Spence, J. C. (2013). A step-defined sedentary lifestyle index: <5000 steps/day. *Applied Physiology, Nutrition, and Metabolism = Physiologie applique´e, nutrition et me´tabolisme, 38*(2), 100–114.

Valsiner, J. (1994). Irreversibility of time and the construction of historical developmental psychology. *Mind, Culture, and Activity, 1,* 25–42.

Wahl, H. W. (2001). Environmental influences on aging and behavior. In J. E. Birren & K. W. Schaie (Eds.), *Handbook of the psychology of aging* (5th ed., pp. 215–237). San Diego, CA: Academic Press.

Wahl, H. W., Fänge, A., Oswald, F., Gitlin, L. N., & Iwarsson, S. (2009). The home environment and disability-related outcomes in aging individuals: What is the empirical evidence? *The Gerontologist, 49*(3), 355–367.

Wahl, H. W., & Gitlin, L. (2003). Future developments in living environments for older people in the United States and Germany. In K. W. Schaie, H. W. Wahl, H. Mollenkopf, & F. Oswald (Eds.), *Aging independently: Living arrangements and mobility* (pp. 281–301). New York, NY: Springer Publishing Company.

Wahl, H. W., & Gitlin, L. N. (2007). Environmental gerontology. In J. E. Birren (Ed.), *Encyclopedia of gerontology* (2nd ed., pp. 494–502). Oxford, UK: Elsevier.

Wahl, H. W., Iwarsson, S., & Oswald, F. (2012). Aging well and the environment: Toward an integrative model and research agenda for the future. *The Gerontologist, 52*(3), 306–316.

Wahl, H. W., & Lang, F. (2004). Aging in context across the adult life course: Integrating physical and social environmental research perspectives. In H. W. Wahl, R. Scheidt, & P. Windley (Eds.), *Annual review of gerontology and geriatrics* (Vol. 23, pp. 1–33). New York, NY: Springer Publishing Company.

Wahl, H. W., & Oswald, F. (2010). Environmental perspectives on aging. In D. Dannefer & C. Phillipson (Eds.), *The SAGE handbook of social gerontology* (pp. 111–124). London, UK: Sage.

Wahl, H. W., Oswald, F., Schilling, O., & Iwarsson, S. (2009). The home environment and quality of life related outcomes in advanced old age: Findings of the ENABLE-AGE project. *European Journal of Ageing, 6*(2), 101–111.

Wahl, H. W., Scheidt, R., & Windley, P. (Eds.). (2004). *Annual review of gerontology and geriatrics* (Vol. 23). New York, NY: Springer Publishing Company.

Walsh, K., Rowles, G. D., & Scharf, T. (2014, November). *Constructing home over the life course: Toward a model of at-oneness.* Paper presented in the symposium "International perspectives on home, belonging and aging in the community" at the 67th Annual Scientific Meeting of the Gerontological Society of America, Washington, DC.

Wanka, A., Arnberger, A., Allex, B., Eder, R., Hutter, H. P., & Wallner, P. (2014). The challenges posed by climate change to successful ageing. *Zeitschrift für Gerontologie und Geriatrie, 47*(6), 468–474.

Wettstein, M., Wahl, H. W., Shoval, N., Oswald, F., Voss, E., Seidl, U.,…Landau, R. (2015). Out-of-home behavior and cognitive impairment in older adults: Findings of the SenTra Project. *Journal of Applied Gerontology: The Official Journal of the Southern Gerontological Society, 34*(1), 3–25.

CHAPTER 32

Theoretical Perspectives on Biodemography of Aging and Longevity

Leonid A. Gavrilov and Natalia S. Gavrilova

Biodemography of aging represents an area of research that integrates demographic and biological theory and methods and provides innovative tools for studies of aging and longevity. Biodemography of aging conducts comparative studies of aging and mortality in different species and addresses some key questions about aging, life course, and health. Biodemography of aging is the science of the mechanisms that determine the life span of organisms. Among its most interesting problems is the problem of the heritability and variability of lifetimes, the problem of sex differentials in lifetimes, and the problem of the changing life span of organisms in the process of evolution. Thus one of the objectives of the biodemography of aging is to explain the causes of individual differences in lifetimes, as well as the causes of interspecies differences. The practical interest of these studies is to open up the possibility of predicting and controlling the aging and longevity of organisms, and most importantly, to discover ways of extending the lives of human beings.

■ BIODEMOGRAPHY OF AGING AND LONGEVITY: A HISTORICAL REVIEW

Biodemography of aging and longevity was developed as an independent scientific discipline at the beginning of the 20th century, thanks to the classic investigations of the American scientist Raymond Pearl (Pearl, 1922; Pearl & Pearl, 1934). At this time, researchers used the term "biology of life span," which was suggested by one of Raymond Pearl's students, Professor Vladimir Alpatov (Alpatov, 1930). Because the study of the mechanisms that determine the length of life is closely linked with investigations into the processes of aging, biodemography of aging owed its subsequent development to the biology of aging and gerontology. It is worth noting that such famous gerontologists as Alex Comfort, Bernard L. Strehler, and George Sacher also made an invaluable contribution to the study of life span and biodemography of aging (Comfort, 1979; Sacher, 1977; Strehler, 1978). The ideas and methods of the biodemography of aging are so widely used in gerontology that some gerontologists regard it as one of the branches of their own discipline. However, the biodemography of aging and longevity, in distinction to gerontology, is just as much interested in the mechanisms that determine mortality and aging in wild animal populations (which are of great importance for ecology and the theory of evolution), and effects of external factors on mortality (which are of special interest also for toxicology and radiobiology). Thus, although the biodemography of aging and longevity is close to biogerontology, it nevertheless has its own specific goals and cannot be reduced to this latter science.

Moreover, the biodemography of aging has its own historical roots, which connect it with demography and population biology. The result is that the biodemography of aging and longevity has developed its own characteristic style of research: the use of precise quantitative methods, a probabilistic approach to natural phenomena, and a desire to explain the mechanisms of particular processes by their external manifestations in the population under investigation.

The beginnings of the field are straddled by such great scientists as Christian Huygens (1629–1695), Gottfried Wilhelm Leibniz (1646–1716), Edmund Halley (1656–1742), Leonard Euler (1707–1783), and Pierre Simon Laplace (1749–1827). The contribution of these men was basically related to the collection of statistical information concerning human mortality in the form of life tables. The well-known Belgian scientist, Adolphe Quetelet (1796–1874), became one of the founders of the modern method of constructing life tables. This initial historical stage in the development of the subject can be described as the "period of descriptive human mortality statistics."

The biodemography of aging and longevity was further developed in the works of a well-known English expert on mathematical statistics, one of the founders of biometry, Karl Pearson (1857–1936). In 1901, Pearson founded the journal *Biometrika*, remaining its editor until he died. In the first issue of this journal, Pearson published his article "On the Inheritance of the Duration of Life and on the Intensity of Natural Selection in Man" (Beeton & Pearson, 1901). This work signifies the beginning of truly biological research into life span. Nevertheless, the remarkable American scientist Raimond Pearl must be considered the real founder of the biodemography of aging. In our opinion, the biodemography of aging was born as an independent discipline in 1922 with the appearance of Pearl's book *The Biology of Death* (Pearl, 1922). This book is in fact not concerned at all with problems of death (the dying process), but is totally dedicated to problems of the biology of life span. Pearl published a total of several dozen works on this problem, including a large series of articles entitled "Experimental Studies on the Duration of Life." In his studies, Pearl dealt with practically all the problems in the biology of life span, including the genetic, ecological, physiological, and comparative-evolutionary aspects. Many of these works have preserved their importance and relevance to the present day, and methodologically almost all of Pearl's works can serve as a model for contemporary researchers. One of his famous studies is represented by the book *The Ancestry of Long-Lived* where he showed for the first time that longevity runs in families (Pearl & Pearl, 1934).

Because the biodemography of aging and longevity was founded by scholars having a strong background in mathematics (mathematicians, physicists, astronomers, statisticians), it is a discipline that, from the start, unlike most of the other areas of biology, began to take the shape of an exact science. In this regard it is related to such areas of biology as biometry, quantitative genetics, and biokinetics. Whereas in many areas of biology exceptional attention is paid to experimental techniques in the search for clear qualitative effects, in biodemography of aging primary importance is attached to the method of quantitative observation with subsequent mathematical analysis of the results. This approach, which is less "aggressive" toward the natural environment, may seem at first glance to be too indirect, formal, and unconvincing. However, its value has been demonstrated many times in the history of the natural sciences. For example, all the basic notions of genetics (the concept of genes and their mutations, the concept of allelic forms of genes and their pair-wise association [the diploid concept], the conclusion that genes are linearly ordered and organized into cohesive groups, chromosomes) were the result of this "formal" method, a statistical analysis of the transmission of the traits of an organism in subsequent generations. The desire to discover scientific truths "by pen and paper" was a characteristic feature of the founders of the biodemography of aging, and this tradition has been maintained to the present day. The historical development of the biodemography of aging is closely interwoven with the historical development of statistics, demography, and even the technical aspects of life insurance. This led to the discipline being formed as a statistical, population-based area of biology, which easily borrows the methods and ideas of other sciences. The biology of aging, like most of the other divisions of modern biology, is characterized by a "bottom-up" approach, while the biodemography of aging finds a "top-down" approach more natural, an explanation of mechanisms as they are revealed at the level of populations of organisms. Of course, these two approaches are not mutually exclusive. They complement each other, as the historical experience of the science development shows.

In the 1960s–1980s, the biodemography of aging studies seems to be scattered among a multitude of disciplines: gerontology and the biology of aging (Comfort, 1979; Strehler, 1978), demography (Bourgeois-Pichat, 1979; Manton, Stallard, & Vaupel, 1981; Olshansky & Carnes, 1997), ecology (Caughley, 1966; Hutchinson, 1978), radiobiology (Lindop, 1961; Sacher, 1956, 1966), and other disciplines. We need to acknowledge significant contributions by Bernard Strehler and George Sacher into the field. They not only established and analyzed existing mortality regularities, but also suggested mathematical theories of aging explaining these regularities (Sacher, 1977; Strehler & Mildvan, 1960). At that time, the biodemography of aging and longevity had suffered above all from the disconnectedness of biological and demographic studies. The clearest manifestation of this is the fact that the colossal archive of data on the human life span (hundreds of demographic life tables from a wide variety of the world's population groups) has been almost unused in human biology, despite the acute deficiency of factual information in the field. For a long time many biologists had no idea of the scale of this archive of accumulated demographic data, and of how it might be used to investigate the biology of life span.

The temporary loss of contact with demography has had the consequence that many researchers—biologists working on life span—lacked the necessary minimum demographic and statistical knowledge for the task. As a result, some biologists strongly believed in the concept of the species-specific life-span limit beyond which survival is impossible even for a second. It was also maintained that the species-specific human life-span limit "has remained unchanged across time, races and civilizations" (Economos, 1985). The theoretical unsoundness of this dogma has been frequently pointed out by demographers (Sauvy, 1961), by experts in probability theory (Feller, 1968), and by biologists who are qualified in statistical methods (Caughley, 1977). The failure of this concept to agree with the observed mortality data in humans was demonstrated in the book *The Biology of Life Span* (Gavrilov & Gavrilova, 1991). Publication of this book was considered as "the birth of modern biodemography" by renowned American demographer, S. J. Olshansky, in his thoughtful review essay on the history of biodemography (Olshansky, 1998). In this book the authors overviewed existing mortality laws; tested the validity of the Gompertz law of mortality using data on more than 100 life tables for humans, fruit flies, and other species; compared mortality across different species and historical periods; analyzed sex differentials in mortality among various species; suggested reliability theory of aging; and provided references for hundreds of published life tables. S. J. Olshansky himself (together with Bruce Carnes) was among the founders of contemporary biodemography of aging and made a significant contribution to the field (Carnes & Olshansky, 1997; Carnes, Olshansky, & Grahn, 1996; Olshansky & Carnes, 1997). In particular, the researchers tested the Gompertz law of mortality using data on humans and mice (Carnes et al., 1996). They also conducted a biologically motivated partitioning of mortality into endogenous and exogenous parts using cause-of-death data on humans and rodents (Carnes & Olshansky, 1997). Methodological studies of demographic indicators, which take into account health status of population (healthy life expectancy and active life expectancy), were another direction of research initiated during the 1980s and 1990s (Crimmins, Hayward, & Saito, 1996; Laditka & Laditka, 2009).

Publication of the monograph "Between Zeus and Salmon" in 1997 was a significant event in the history of biodemography of aging (Wachter & Finch, 1997). Besides topics already described earlier in *The Biology of Life Span* book (mortality laws, limit to individual life span, reliability theory of aging) this monograph established new research directions for biodemography of aging: evolutionary and ecological models of aging (Tuljapurkar, Partridge, Rose); intergenerational relations (Lee); evolution of the human life course (Kaplan); comparative biodemography (Austad, Finch, Carey); and biomarkers in population-based surveys (Wallace). The latter topic was further developed in other editions: *Biosocial Surveys* published in 2007 (Weinstein, Vaupel, & Wachter, 2007) and *Conducting Biosocial Surveys: Collecting, Storing, Accessing, and Protecting Biospecimens and Biodata* published in 2010 (Hauser, Weinstein, Pool, & Cohen, 2010). Study of biomarkers in population-based surveys is now one of the most rapidly developing areas of biodemographic research (Crimmins & Seeman, 2000; Crimmins & Vasunilashorn, 2011).

The scope of biodemography research is exceptionally broad and continues to expand. In recent years, especially intensive work has been carried out in genetics (Boardman, Barnes, Wilson, Evans, & Mendes de Leon, 2012; Gögele et al., 2011; Yashin et al., 2015), and comparative biodemography (Austad, 2009; Weinstein & Lane, 2014). Significant attention is paid to the effects of early-life conditions on late-life mortality, and to the problem of the evolution of life span (Hayward, Rickard, & Lummaa, 2013). Another promising area of research in biodemography of aging is related to biomarkers as predictors of health and longevity (Crimmins et al., 2014; Crimmins & Seeman, 2000; Karlamangla, Merkin, Crimmins, & Seeman, 2010).

■ BIODEMOGRAPHIC THEORIES ANSWERING THE "WHY DO WE AGE?" QUESTION

It is generally believed that evolutionary theory of aging is able to answer the question: Why do we age? (Le Bourg, 2014). Traditional evolutionary theory of aging explains aging as a result of declining force of natural selection (Robins & Conneely, 2014). According to this theory, death rates are increasing with age because a selection against deleterious mutations is weaker for later-acting mutations, thus shifting the mutation-selection balance to a higher equilibrium frequency of later-acting deleterious mutations. Evolutionary explanations of aging and limited longevity of biological species are based on two major evolutionary theories: the mutation accumulation theory (Medawar, 1958) and the antagonistic pleiotropy theory (Williams, 1957). These two theories can be briefly summarized as follows:

1. According to the mutation accumulation theory, aging is an inevitable result of the declining force of natural selection with age. For example, a mutant gene

that kills young children will be strongly selected against (will not be passed to the next generation) while a lethal mutation that affects only old people will experience no selection because people with this mutation will have already passed it to their offspring by that age. Over successive generations, late-acting deleterious mutations will accumulate, leading to an increase in mortality rates later in life.

2. According to the antagonistic pleiotropy theory, late-acting deleterious genes may even be favored by selection and be actively accumulated in populations if they have any beneficial effects early in life.

Note that these two theories of aging are not mutually exclusive, and both evolutionary mechanisms may operate at the same time. The main difference between the two theories is that, in the mutation accumulation theory, genes with negative effects at old age accumulate passively from one generation to the next, while in the antagonistic pleiotropy theory these genes are actively kept in the gene pool by selection (Le Bourg, 2014).

The evolutionary "disposable soma theory" (Kirkwood & Holliday, 1979) postulated a special class of gene mutations with the following antagonistic pleiotropic effects: These hypothetical mutations save energy for reproduction (positive effect) by partially disabling molecular proofreading and other accuracy-promoting devices in somatic cells (negative effect). The authors of the disposable soma theory argued that "it may be selectively advantageous for higher organisms to adopt an energy saving strategy of reduced accuracy in somatic cells to accelerate development and reproduction, but the consequence will be eventual deterioration and death" (Kirkwood & Holliday, 1979). Most researchers (including the authors themselves) agree that the disposable soma theory is a special, more narrowly defined variant of the antagonistic pleiotropy theory of aging.

Currently, some researchers started to challenge traditional evolutionary theories of aging pointing to the diversity of age-specific trajectories of mortality and fertility and suggesting the development of broader perspectives on the evolution of aging (Jones et al., 2014).

It should be noted that one of the first explanations of aging with evolutionary arguments was proposed by August Weismann (1834–1914), the great German theorist and experimental biologist of the 19th century. His initial idea was that there exists a specific death mechanism designed by a natural selection to eliminate the old, and therefore worn-out, members of a population (Gavrilov & Gavrilova, 2002). The purpose of this programmed death of the old is to clean up the living space and to free up resources for younger generations. Later the idea of programmed aging was abandoned by Weismann himself and criticized by gerontologists (Gavrilov & Gavrilova, 1991; Kirkwood, 1998; Kirkwood & Melov, 2011). One of the principal arguments against the theory of programmed death is a paucity of old individuals in the wild, so that the aging program could not evolve during evolution (Kirkwood & Melov, 2011). However, recent studies demonstrated that the process of senescence is nearly ubiquitous in the living world (Lemaître et al., 2015). Senescence patterns are highly variable among species and current evolutionary theories of aging propose that such variation can be accounted for by differences in allocation to growth and reproduction during early life rather than by programmed aging (Lemaitre et al., 2015). Nevertheless, the question of whether aging is programmed was debated by gerontologists (Austad, 2004; Bredesen, 2004) and some of them recognized the possibility of both programmatic and nonprogrammatic components of aging (Bredesen, 2004). Recently, more researchers have begun to consider aging as a programmed process (Mitteldorf & Martins, 2014; Skulachev, 2011), although the majority of gerontologists does not support this view.

The problem of the biological evolution of aging was initially studied in a purely theoretical, nonexperimental way by August Weismann, Ronald Fisher, Peter Medawar, George Williams, William Hamilton, Brian Charlesworth, and other researchers. The resulting evolutionary theories of aging were then partially tested by direct evolutionary experiments on laboratory fruit flies (Rose, 1991; Stearns, Ackermann, Doebeli, & Kaiser, 2000). Specifically, the researchers found that aging and life span do evolve in subsequent generations of biological species in a theoretically predicted direction, depending on particular living conditions. For example, a selection for later reproduction (artificial selection of late-born progeny for further breeding) produced, as expected, longer-lived fruit flies (Rose, 1991), while placing animals in a more dangerous environment with high extrinsic mortality redirected evolution, as predicted, to a shorter life span in subsequent generations (Stearns et al., 2000). Therefore, the early criticism of the evolutionary theory of aging, as merely theoretical speculation with limited and indirect supporting evidence obtained from retrospective and descriptive studies, has been overturned. On the contrary, the evolutionary plasticity of aging and longevity is now an established experimental fact.

■ TESTING EVOLUTIONARY THEORIES OF AGING WITH HUMAN DATA

Many biodemographic studies use human data to test predictions of evolutionary theories of aging. We consider here some of the most promising directions of research. Both antagonistic pleiotropy theory (Williams, 1957) and the disposable soma theory of aging (Westendorp & Kirkwood, 1998) argue that genetic investments in somatic maintenance increase longevity at the cost of reproductive success. According to these theories, one may expect that long-lived individuals should have less children on average compared to their shorter-lived peers. Some studies found support for these theories (Doblhammer & Oeppen, 2003; Lycett, Dunbar, & Voland, 2000; Westendorp & Kirkwood, 1998), while others found no relation between longevity and reproduction (Gavrilova, Gavrilov, Semyonova, & Evdokushkina, 2004), or even higher fertility among long-lived individuals (Goegele et al., 2011). This issue still remains to be resolved. For example, a recent study of Ashkenazi Jews found that centenarians have less children on average than controls (Tabatabaie et al., 2011) and the analysis of Framingham Heart Study data found negative phenotypic correlation between number of children ever born and life span (Wang, Byars, & Stearns, 2013). On the other hand, study of Swedish twins found no support for the disposable soma theory (Chereji, Gatz, Pedersen, & Prescott, 2013). Thus, more research is needed to resolve the existing controversies as suggested by the experts in this area (Gagnon, 2015).

Disposable soma theory of aging (Kirkwood, 1998) predicts a trade-off between investment in reproduction and a woman's own survival. An alternative approach, also supported by empirical findings from human populations, speculates that selection for increased reproductive success simultaneously may drive the selection of longevity (Müller, Chiou, Carey, & Wang, 2002; Perls, Alpert, & Fretts, 1997; Smith, Gagnon et al., 2009; Smith, Mineau, & Bean, 2002). It was postulated that postreproductive life extension is triggered by late births (reproductive potential hypothesis; Muller et al., 2002). Existing studies support the reproduction potential hypothesis: Women bearing children at advanced ages have been shown to have better postmenopausal survival (Grundy & Kravdal, 2008; Helle, Lummaa, & Jokela, 2005; Müller et al., 2002; Sun et al., 2015). In testing this hypothesis, it is important to consider the direction of causality between longevity and late reproduction: it could be a genuine causation effect (late childbirth extends maternal life) or a selection effect (longer-lived mothers lose their fertility later). Some insights into these issues can be gained by studying late reproduction in relatives (mothers or sisters) of long-lived women (Smith, Mineau, Garibotti, & Kerber, 2009).

Another interesting approach is to study sex composition of offspring and parental mortality and longevity. The trade-off between longevity and reproduction is often investigated by relating the total number of children to the total life span (Doblhammer & Oeppen, 2003). However, delivering sons compared with daughters is likely to be energetically more costly for the mothers (Helle, Lummaa, & Jokela, 2002). Indeed, maternal longevity was negatively related to having sons (Harrell, Smith, & Mineau, 2008; Helle & Lummaa, 2013; Helle et al., 2002; Jasienska, Nenko, & Jasienski, 2006; Van de Putte, Matthijs, & Vlietinck, 2004) and positively related to having daughters (Beise & Voland, 2002; Helle et al., 2002). Some studies found that having daughters increased paternal life span (Jasienska et al., 2006). This gender effect may be due to the lower direct physiological costs of daughters and to the fact that daughters more often become caregivers for older parents. These results demonstrate that both the direct effects of reproductive investment and the social effects of gender-biased family structure appear to be important in determining female life span.

■ BIODEMOGRAPHY OF AGING AND LIFE HISTORY THEORY

The evolutionary theory of aging may be considered as part of a more general life history theory (Stearns, 1992), which tries to explain how evolution designs organisms to achieve reproductive success (i.e., avoid extinction). Life history theory is based on mathematical methods of optimization models with specific biological constraints. Among the questions posed and answered by life history theory are (Stearns, 1992): Why are organisms small or large? Why do they mature early or late? Why do they have few or many offspring? Why do they have a short or a long life? Why must they grow old and die? The latter two questions represent the entire scientific agenda of the evolutionary theory of aging. Therefore, it could be said that the evolutionary theory of aging is a subset of the life history theory (Le Bourg, 2001). On the other hand, the evolutionary theory of aging is considered to be the intellectual core of the biodemography of aging and longevity (Carnes & Olshansky, 1993).

The "grandmother hypothesis" is one of the most widely known concepts among the life history topics. It suggests that the evolution of human life history proposes that grandmother effects promoted increase in life span without changes in the age of female fertility decline (Hawkes & Smith, 2010). Similar conclusions were made by using computer simulations of intergenerational transfers from postreproductive humans to their descendants. As a result, the growth and survival of descendants is enhanced, which in turn promotes selection for postreproductive survival (Lee, 2014). Effects of stressful environments characterized by high extrinsic mortality on life history evolution are another direction of research. It was shown that the speed of life histories is associated with family-level effects rather than with individual-level mortality experiences and that exposure to higher levels of mortality in the family leads to earlier marriage and reproduction (Störmer & Lummaa, 2014).

■ THEORIES ANSWERING THE "HOW DO WE AGE?" QUESTION

Theories of aging providing specific explanations of age-related changes attempt to answer the "How do we age?" question. Among these theories are the free radical theory, cell membranes theory, oxidative stress and mitochondria theory, cell communication theory, immunological theory, and others (Robert & Fulop, 2014). Many of these theories are focused on specific chemical processes that are damaging to the organism's organs and tissues, such as free radical damage or protein cross-linkage. In view of the existing numerous types of damage, Gladyshev suggested a model explaining aging through an imperfectness-driven nonrandom damage process pointing out that physicochemical properties preclude ideal biomolecules and perfect biological functions (Gladyshev, 2013). It should be noted that some aging theories are very general (e.g., free radical theory), while others may explain aging in a limited number of species (e.g., immunological theory). Discussing all existing specific explanations of aging is beyond the scope of this chapter, so we focus our review on some theories that are more specific for humans.

Neuroendocrine Theory of Aging

One theory, which has support from experiments on lower organisms, is the neuroendocrine theory of aging (Weinert & Timiras, 2003). This theory proposes that aging occurs due to changes in neural and endocrine functions. A particular emphasis in this theory is given to the hypothalamo–pituitary–adrenal (HPA) axis as the master regulator that signals the onset and termination of each life stage (Weinert & Timiras, 2003). One of the first versions of the neuroendocrine theory of aging was proposed by Vladimir Dilman who suggested that the key process in development and aging is a gradual elevation of the threshold of sensitivity of the hypothalamus to feedback suppression (Dilman, 1971; Dilman & Dean, 1992). More recent studies emphasize the role of lifelong exposure to stress, which can weaken the ability to adapt and lead to so-called diseases of adaptation. According to these studies, aging should be considered as a result of declining ability to resist stress (Weinert & Timiras, 2003).

Most studies now are focused on insulin/insulin-like growth factor I (IGF-I) signal response pathway as an evolutionarily conserved mechanism of longevity from yeast to humans. Animal experiments demonstrated that insulin/IGF-like signaling pathway controls aging in worms, insects, and mammals and that genetic down regulation or interruption of this signaling pathway can lead to significant life extension (Anisimov & Bartke, 2013). Biologists believe that rapid growth may be harmful, while delayed maturation would be beneficial for longevity and health (Rollo, 2002). Animal studies of different strains and breeds within biological species of dogs, rats, and mice showed that smaller animals live on average longer within a given species (Michell, 1999; Miller, Chrisp, & Atchley, 2000; Samaras, Elrick, & Storms, 2003). It is also well known that caloric restriction is a powerful way of life extension in animals (Finch, 2007). These biological findings agree with the recent studies of adverse effects of obesity on human mortality (Flegal, Kit, Orpana, & Graubard, 2013), particularly at younger ages (Wang, 2015). However, these biological data do not agree with the results obtained by historical demographers. Studies of demographers showed that an individual's height at a young adult age seems to be a good indicator of a person's nutritional and infectious disease history in the past (Alter, 2004; Alter, Neven, & Oris, 2004; Elo & Preston, 1992). Most studies, starting with Waaler's pioneer work, found a negative relationship between body height and mortality later in life (Elo & Preston, 1992; Waaler, 1984). A study of the Union Army veterans found that the relationship between height and subsequent mortality was negative, findings similar to a study of modern Norwegian males (Costa & Lahey, 2005; Fogel & Costa, 1997). Infectious diseases (and diarrhoeal diseases in particular) can result in growth retardation leading to shorter adult height. For example, conscripts from high-mortality districts of antebellum New York were shorter than those from healthier districts (Haines, Craig, & Weiss, 2003). Based on existing historical information, Crimmins and Finch hypothesized that both the decline in old-age mortality and the increase in height were promoted by a declining burden of infections and inflammatory causes rooted in the external environment (Crimmins & Finch, 2006). However, recent data on contemporary Japanese men demonstrated that height in midlife is positively associated with mortality and it was also associated with fasting insulin level pointing to the involvement of insulin/IGF signaling pathway in both aging and growth regulation (He et al., 2014). Similarly, higher longevity was found for shorter Sardinian men compared to their taller peers (Salaris, Poulain, & Samaras, 2012). It appears that environmental factors are able to modulate the existing biological link between height and life span.

■ LIFE-COURSE PERSPECTIVE IN AGING THEORIES

Early-life programming theory and cumulative risk theory apply life-course perspective for explaining old age diseases and mortality. A growing body of evidence documents that adverse early-life conditions negatively affect survival and health in later life (Ben-Shlomo & Kuh, 2002; Bengtsson & Mineau, 2009; Blackwell, Hayward, & Crimmins, 2001; Hamil-Luker & O'Rand, 2007; Hayward & Gorman, 2004). Two major explanations of these effects now exist in the scientific literature. The first explanation is related to direct effects of adverse childhood conditions on the human organism resulting in "scarring" (Elo & Preston, 1992; Preston, Hill, & Drevenstedt, 1998) or biological imprint in a way that makes it more susceptible to late-life diseases (Hamil-Luker & O'Rand, 2007). This theory, also known as the "latency model," suggests that early-life exposures can program permanent changes in an organism's physiology. A variant of this theory is the fetal origin hypothesis suggested by Barker (Barker, 1998) that the fetus may adapt to malnutrition or metabolic changes of maternal organism, but these changes may be accompanied with permanent damage of physiological systems resulting in premature chronic diseases (Hamil-Luker & O'Rand, 2007). Another variant of this theory is the idea of early-life inflammatory exposure (Finch, 2007; Finch & Crimmins, 2004).

The second theory explaining early-life effects on later-life mortality is the cumulative risk theory (Galobardes, Lynch, & Davy Smith, 2004), or pathway model (Hamil-Luker & O'Rand, 2007; Kuh & Ben-Shlomo, 1997), also called a theory of "cumulative disadvantage" in sociology (Ferraro & Kelley-Moore, 2003). For example, early-life social disadvantage may result in poor education and unhealthy behaviors and eventually limited job opportunities and low socioeconomic status in adulthood, which are known risk factors for poor health and mortality (Hamil-Luker & O'Rand, 2007). This theory considers an indirect mechanism among death risks across the life cycle that is attributable to their joint association with other variables (Preston et al., 1998). Both theories are not mutually exclusive.

Childhood exposure to infections (as a factor of elevated mortality later in life) deserves special attention. Finch and Crimmins (Finch & Crimmins, 2004) proposed a hypothesis that historical decline in chronic inflammation (due to decreasing exposure to early-life infections) has led to a decrease in morbidity and mortality resulting from chronic conditions in old age. Studies of rural 18th-century Sweden (Bengtsson & Lindstrom, 2000, 2003), U.S. Civil War veterans (Costa, 2000, 2002), and Americans in their 50s (Blackwell et al., 2001) demonstrated that exposure to infections early in life is associated with elevated mortality from chronic diseases at older ages. Existing historical evidence suggests that disease load in the early-20th-century United States was high (Preston & Haines, 1991). Many factors related to child mortality in 1900 (Preston & Haines, 1991) were found to be significant predictors of survival to advanced ages (Ferrie & Rolf, 2011; Preston et al., 1998; Stone, 2003). It was demonstrated that early-life mortality that is linked to exposure to infection and poor nutrition predicts both the estimated cohort mortality level at age 40 years and the subsequent Gompertz rate of mortality acceleration during aging (Beltrán-Sáncheza, Crimmins, & Finch, 2012). This suggests that early childhood infections in the late 19th and early 20th centuries represented a significant health hazard with potential harmful effects later in life.

Currently, studies of early-life predictors of longevity have become an important direction of research in biodemography of aging. It was demonstrated that such biodemographic factors as maternal age at person's birth (Gavrilov & Gavrilova, 2012; Gillespie, Russell, & Lummaa, 2013; Jarry, Gagnon, & Bourbeau, 2013); season of birth and ambient temperature (Bruckner, van den Berg, Smith, & Catalano, 2014; Gavrilov & Gavrilova, 2014); longevity of relatives (Gavrilov & Gavrilova, 2014; Sebastiani et al., 2013); and transgenerational responses to early-life experience (Pembrey, Saffery, & Bygren, 2014) are important predictors of longevity and health. In addition to that, research in the area of developmental psychology shed light on the relationships between personality, well-being, and health. Specifically, it was found that the basic five-factor personality dimensions (particularly conscientiousness, neuroticism, and extraversion, but also often agreeableness and openness) do predict multiple diseases and longevity (Friedman & Kern, 2014; Shanahan, Hill, Roberts, Eccles, & Friedman, 2014). Study of early-life factors of aging and longevity is an important area of biodemographic research, which continues to grow.

■ NEW DEVELOPMENTS IN BIODEMOGRAPHY OF AGING: STUDIES OF OLD-AGE MORTALITY

Attempts to develop a fundamental quantitative theory of aging, mortality, and life span have deep historical roots. In 1825, the English actuary (life insurance specialist), Benjamin Gompertz (1779–1865), published a work (Gompertz, 1825), which became the keystone of the biodemography of aging (see reviews in Gavrilov & Gavrilova, 1991; Kirkwood, 2015). Gompertz provided a theoretical foundation for the idea (and used concrete examples to demonstrate it) that the hazard rate (the relative rate at which a population dies out) increases with age according to the geometric progression law. Moreover, he noted that, alongside this mortality, there must also exist a chance mortality that does not depend on age. Gompertz's observation was taken into account in 1860 by another English actuary, William Makeham (1823–1891), who presented the age-related change in mortality as the sum of a constant (the Makeham term) and an exponential (the Gompertz function). This was the birth of the well-known Gompertz-Makeham equation, which has great importance for biodemography of aging to this day (Makeham, 1860). Currently, the Makeham term of the equation is called the "background mortality" (Gavrilov, Gavrilova, 1991) and the Gompertz term is called the "senescent mortality" (Bongaarts, 2009). An exponential (Gompertzian) increase in death rates with age is observed for many biological species including fruit flies *Drosophila melanogaster*, nematodes, mosquitoes, human lice *Pediculus humanus*, flour beetles *Tribolium confusum*, mice, rats, dogs, horses, mountain sheep, and baboons (see reviews in Gavrilov & Gavrilova, 1991, 2006).

It was also believed that exponential growth of mortality with age (Gompertz law) is followed by a period of deceleration, with slower rates of mortality increase at extreme old ages (Gavrilov & Gavrilova, 1991; Greenwood & Irwin, 1939). This mortality deceleration eventually produces the "late-life mortality leveling-off" and "late-life mortality plateaus" at extreme old ages. Greenwood and Irwin (Greenwood & Irwin, 1939) provided a detailed description of this phenomenon in humans and even made the first estimates for the asymptotic value of the upper limit to human mortality. The same phenomenon of "almost nonaging" survival dynamics at extreme old ages was described for other biological species, and in some species, like medfly and housefly, the mortality plateau can occupy a sizable part of their lives (Carey, Liedo, Orozco, & Vaupel, 1992; Gavrilov & Gavrilova, 2006).

According to some researchers, the late-life mortality plateau represents a distinct phase of life when the aging slows down or stops. They called the discovery of late-life mortality deceleration "a revolution for aging research" (Rose, Rauser, Mueller, & Benford, 2006). Evolutionary biologists suggest that aging is a result of declining forces of natural selection with age. When these forces eventually bottom up at extreme old ages, then the cessation of aging is expected according to this paradigm (Mueller, Rauser, & Rose, 2011). The lifelong heterogeneity theory is another, even more popular, explanation of mortality deceleration, which was first proposed by the British actuary Eric Beard in 1959 (Beard, 1959). As George Sacher explained, "sub-populations with the higher injury levels die out more rapidly, resulting in progressive selection for vigour in the surviving populations" (Sacher, 1966). Another explanation of this phenomenon comes from the reliability theory of aging that explains mortality leveling-off by an exhaustion of organism's redundancy (reserves) at extremely old ages, so that every additional random hit of damage results in death (Gavrilov & Gavrilova, 1991). There is also an opinion that lower (than predicted) risks of death for older people may be due to their less risky behavior (Greenwood & Irwin, 1939).

The existence of mortality plateaus is well described for a number of lower organisms, including medfly, house fly *Musca domestica*, fruit flies *Anastrepha ludens*, *Anastrepha obliqua*, *Anastrepha serpentine*, parasitoid wasp *Diachasmimorpha longiacaudtis*, and bruchid beetle *Callosobruchus maculates* (see review in Gavrilov & Gavrilova, 2006). In the case of mammals, however, data are much more controversial. Some researchers reported short-term periods of mortality deceleration in mice at advanced ages (Sacher, 1966). However, Austad later argued that rodents do not demonstrate mortality deceleration even in the case of very large samples with many animals surviving to old ages (Austad, 2001). Study of baboons found no mortality deceleration at older ages (Bronikowski et al., 2002). Longitudinal study of mortality among seven wild primate species failed to find mortality deceleration at older ages (Bronikowski et al., 2011). Thus, we may suggest that mortality deceleration is observed for many invertebrate species, but the evidence for mammals is controversial.

Due to painstaking efforts of Kannisto, Thatcher et al., it became possible to pool together and analyze data on mortality after age 80 years for Japan and 13 Western European countries. These data formed the basis of the Kannisto-Thatcher Database on Old Age Mortality. Analysis of these data demonstrated that mortality decelerates after age 80 years, reaching a maximum or ceiling around age 110 years (Horiuchi & Wilmoth, 1998; Thatcher, Kannisto, & Vaupel, 1998).

Recently, new developments happened in this research area thanks to the use of more detailed and more accurate data. In particular, the U.S. Social Security Administration Death Master File (DMF) was used to estimate hazard rates at extremely old ages using a more accurate method of extinct generations. Availability of month-of-birth and month-of-death information in this data source provides a unique opportunity to obtain more accurate hazard-rate estimates for every month of age. The study of 20 single-year extinct birth cohorts with good data quality found that mortality deceleration at advanced ages is negligible up to the advanced age of 106 years (Gavrilov & Gavrilova, 2011). This finding was further supported by additional studies of mortality in 22 single-year U.S. birth cohorts based on data from the Human Mortality Database (Gavrilova & Gavrilov, 2015). The same conclusion was made after analysis of mortality trajectories in 8 cohorts of laboratory mice, and 10 cohorts of laboratory rats (Gavrilova & Gavrilov, 2015). Thus, it turned out that for all three mammalian species, the Gompertz model fits mortality data significantly better than the "mortality deceleration" Kannisto model. Another recent study confirmed that mortality in the U.S. birth cohorts is compatible with the Gompertz-like mortality. The same results were obtained for Canada and Australia, although old-age mortality in European countries were more compatible with models predicting mortality deceleration with the onset of mortality deceleration occurring later in more recent birth cohorts (Bebbington, Green, Lai, & Zitikis, 2014).

It is not surprising why earlier studies (Gavrilov & Gavrilova, 1991; Horiuchi & Wilmoth, 1998; Thatcher et al., 1998) reported mortality deceleration and mortality leveling-off at advanced ages as early as at age 80 years. Most empirical studies of mortality trajectories were conducted in the 1990s when age reporting among aging cohorts was not as accurate as it is now. It was demonstrated that the age misreporting at older ages leads to mortality underestimation, which contributes to mortality deceleration (Preston, Elo, & Stewart, 1999). Also, it was found that mortality deceleration is more expressed in the case of data with poor quality compared to data with better quality (Gavrilov & Gavrilova, 2011). During the last decade, age reporting has significantly improved due to better registration and education in developed countries including large countries such as the United States and Canada.

These results suggest that mortality deceleration at advanced ages is not a universal phenomenon, and survival of many mammalian species follows the Gompertz law up to very old ages. This new finding represents a challenge to many aging theories, including the evolutionary theory that explains senescence by declining force of natural selection with age. New ideas are needed to explain why exactly the same exponential pattern of mortality growth is observed not only at reproductive ages, but also at very old post-reproductive ages (up to 106 years), long after the force of natural selection becomes negligible (when there is no room for its further decline). A new finding on wide applicability of the Gompertz law to adult ages leads to another burning research question: How is it possible for different diseases and causes of death to "negotiate" with each other in order to produce a simple exponential function for all-cause mortality (given that contribution of different causes of death in all-cause mortality changes dramatically with age)? Further biodemographic studies should provide an answer to this question.

■ IN SEARCH OF GENERAL BIODEMOGRAPHIC THEORY OF AGING

There is a growing interest in scientific explanations of aging and in the search for a general theory that can explain what aging is and *why* and *how* it happens. There is also a need for a general theoretical framework that would allow researchers to handle an enormous amount of diverse observations related to aging phenomena. To transform these numerous and diverse observations into a comprehensive body of knowledge, a general theory of species aging and longevity is required.

The quest for a general explanation of aging (age-related increase in failure rates), applicable both to technical devices and to biological systems, invites us to consider the general theory of systems failure known as "reliability theory" (Barlow & Proschan, 1975). Reliability theory was historically developed to describe failure and aging of complex electronic (military) equipment, but the theory itself is a very general theory based on mathematics (probability theory) and systems approach (Barlow & Proschan, 1975). It may therefore be useful to describe and understand the aging and failure of biological systems too. Reliability theory may be useful in several ways: first, by providing a kind of scientific language (definitions and cross-cutting principles) that helps to create a logical framework for organizing numerous and diverse observations on aging into a coherent picture. Second, it helps researchers to develop an intuition and an understanding of the main principles of the aging process through consideration of simple mathematical models, having some features of a real world. Third, reliability theory is useful for generating and testing specific predictions, as well as deeper analyses of already collected data. In this chapter, we review some applications of reliability theory to the problem of biological aging.

The reliability theory was first applied in the 1970s to explain aging of biological species (Abernethy, 1979; Gavrilov, 1978). Since that time, the reliability theory of aging has been developed further (Gavrilov & Gavrilova, 1991, 2001, 2006) leading to the following conclusions: (a) Redundancy is a key notion for understanding aging and the systemic nature of aging in particular. Systems, which are redundant in numbers of irreplaceable elements, do deteriorate (i.e., age) over time, even if they are built of nonaging elements. (b) An apparent aging rate or expression of aging (measured as age differences in failure rates, including death rates) is higher for systems with higher redundancy levels. (c) Redundancy exhaustion over the course of life explains the observed compensation law of mortality (mortality convergence at later life) as well as the observed late-life mortality deceleration, leveling-off, and mortality plateaus. (d) Living organisms seem to be formed with a high load of initial damage, and therefore their life spans and aging patterns may be sensitive to early-life conditions that determine this initial damage load during early development. The idea of early-life programming of aging and longevity may have important practical implications for developing early-life interventions promoting health and longevity.

There may be several different research strategies in attempts to understand the nature of the aging process. The prevailing research strategy now is to focus on the molecular level in the hope of understanding the proverbial nuts and bolts of the aging process. In accordance with this approach, many aging theories explain aging of organisms through aging of organisms' components. However, this circular reasoning of assuming aging in order to "explain" aging eventually leads to a logical dead end, because moving in succession from the aging of organisms to the aging of organs, tissues, and cells, we eventually come to atoms, which are known not to age. A good example of a broad vision of the aging problem is provided by the evolutionary theories of aging (Kirkwood & Holliday, 1979; Rose, 1991). Evolutionary perspective helps us to stay focused on a bigger picture, and to avoid being overwhelmed by billions of tiny details. Evolutionary theories demonstrate that taking a step back from too close consideration of the details over "the nuts and bolts" of the aging process helps to gain a broader vision of the aging problem. The remaining question is whether the evolutionary perspective represents the ultimate general theoretical framework for explanations of aging. Or perhaps there may be even more general theories of aging, one step further removed from the particular details. The main limitation of evolutionary theories of aging is that they are applicable to reproducing organisms only, because these theories are based on the idea of natural selection and on the declining force of natural selection with age. However, aging is a very general phenomenon—it is also observed in technical devices (such as cars), which do not reproduce and that are, therefore, not subject to evolution through natural selection. Thus, there may exist a more general explanation of aging, beyond the evolutionary theories.

The quest for a general explanation of aging (age-related increase in failure rates) applicable both to technical devices and biological systems invites us to consider the general theory of systems failure known as "reliability theory" (Gavrilov & Gavrilova, 2001, 2006). Interestingly, the reliability theory suggests that we need to reevaluate the old belief that aging is somehow related to limited economic or evolutionary investments in systems' longevity. The theory provides a completely opposite perspective on this issue: Aging is a direct consequence of investments into systems' reliability and durability through enhanced redundancy. This is an important statement, because it helps to explain why the expression of aging (age-associated differences in failure rates) might be more profound in more complicated redundant systems, designed for higher durability (Gavrilov & Gavrilova, 2006). For example, reliability approach may help to explain general mechanisms underlying lower mortality of women and their poorer health compared to men, which some researchers consider "elusive" (Austad & Bartke, 2015). Mortality patterns of men and women suggest that a female organism is more reliable because it has higher redundancy. However, organisms with higher redundancy are able to accumulate more damage and still stay alive. Hence women on average are able to survive with more diseases, which is a payment for higher redundancy of female organism. The theory also suggests that research on aging should not be limited to the studies of qualitative changes (e.g., age-related changes in gene expression), because changes in quantity (numbers of cells and other functional elements) could be an important driving force of the aging process. In other words, aging may be driven largely by a process of redundancy loss (de Grey, 2003; Gavrilov & Gavrilova, 2006).

Reliability theory of aging provides theoretical arguments explaining the importance of early-life conditions in later-life health outcomes (Gavrilov & Gavrilova, 2006). According to this theory, biological species (including humans) start their lives with extremely high initial damage load (HIDL hypothesis) and therefore should be sensitive to early-life conditions affecting the level of this damage. In this regard, reliability theory of aging is compatible with life-course theories (discussed earlier), which emphasize the role of childhood adversity on late-life health and mortality.

Reliability theory of aging is perfectly compatible with the idea of biological evolution, and it helps to identify key components that may be important for evolution of species reliability and durability (longevity): initial redundancy levels; initial damage load; rate of redundancy loss; and repair potential (Gavrilov & Gavrilova, 2006). Moreover, reliability theory helps evolutionary theories explain how the age of onset of diseases caused by deleterious mutations could be postponed to later ages during the evolution (as suggested by the mutation accumulation theory of aging)—this could be easily achieved by simple increase in the initial redundancy levels (e.g., initial cell numbers). From the reliability perspective, the increase in initial redundancy levels is the simplest way to improve survival at particularly early reproductive ages (with gains fading at older ages). This exactly matches with the higher fitness priority of early reproductive ages emphasized by evolutionary theories. Evolutionary and reliability ideas also help to understand why organisms seem to "choose" a simple but short-term solution of the survival problem through enhancing the system's redundancy, rather than more permanent but complicated solution based on rigorous repair (with a potential for negligible senescence).

Laird and Sherratt attempted to reconcile reliability and evolutionary models (Laird & Sherratt, 2009, 2010). They showed how a degree of redundancy (and more broadly an ability to deal with damage to system components) can evolve by natural selection, and that the resulting population equilibrium is sufficiently diverse to generate mortality trajectories with attributes that are observed in natural populations, but are not as readily understood by the late-acting deleterious effects of functioning genes (Laird & Sherratt, 2009). Another study applied a top-down approach to aging research and illustrated the potential of reliability-based models to investigate aging using an insect model (Boonekamp, Briga, & Verhulst, 2015). Researchers found that these models were able to fit data on flies subjected to food or temperature manipulations and provided new insights in the experimental results.

Aging is a complex phenomenon, and a holistic approach using reliability theory may help to analyze, understand, and perhaps control it. We suggest therefore that reliability theory should be added to the arsenal of methodological approaches applied in biodemographic research on aging.

■ CONCLUSION

Finding mechanisms of aging and longevity of organisms is an important task that will help to reduce morbidity and mortality and diminish the burden of care of the elderly in society. Biodemography that emerged at the intersection of biology and demography is a priority area of science and provides researchers with innovative methods for understanding the mechanisms of aging, mortality, and life span. During the last decade, biodemography of aging has broadened its scope and incorporated studies of longevity predictors (including biomarker studies), psychological measures, and research on morbidity and the disablement process. In addition to classic studies of mortality laws and regularities, a new research in genetic markers has been developed. Once emerged as a science analyzing mortality patterns at population level, biodemography of aging now incorporates studies at individual level with risk factor analysis.

In this chapter we reviewed biodemographic theories of aging that attempt to answer the proverbial "why" and "how" questions in gerontology. Evolutionary theories provide an answer to the "Why do we age?" question through the mechanisms of natural selection. They are able to make testable predictions regarding human longevity, mortality, and reproduction, which were discussed in this chapter. More specific theories attempt to answer the "How do we age?" question. Neuroendocrine theory of aging is particularly promising for explaining mechanisms of aging in view of recent findings that insulin/IGF-like signaling pathway controls aging in worms, insects, and mammals (Anisimov & Bartke, 2013). Life-course perspective offers another approach to unraveling the causes and mechanisms of aging that is more specific to humans. Reliability theory of aging provides a more general explanation of the aging process and suggests answers to both the "why" and the "how" questions about aging. It explains why aging occurs by identifying the key determinant of aging behavior: system redundancy in numbers of irreplaceable elements. Reliability theory also explains how aging occurs, by focusing on the process of redundancy loss over time as the major mechanism of aging.

Biodemographic theories advance our understanding of biological, social, and environmental factors that favor healthy aging and longevity, including early-life childhood conditions, which has implications for public health policy, population forecasting, and health planning. The growing number of persons living beyond age 80 years underscores the need for accurate studies of mortality at advanced ages and understanding the biosocial mechanisms of aging and longevity. These are important issues not only for demographic forecasts of mortality and population aging, policy implications on health care and pension expenditures, but also for improving our understanding of the fundamental mechanisms of human aging and longevity.

■ ACKNOWLEDGMENTS

This study was supported in part by the U.S. National Institutes of Health (NIH).

REFERENCES

Abernethy, J. D. (1979). The exponential increase in mortality rate with age attributed to wearing-out of biological components. *Journal of Theoretical Biology, 80*(3), 333–354.

Alpatov, W. W. (1930). Experimental studies on the duration of life. XIII. The influence of different feeding during the larval and imaginal stages on the duration of life of the imago of Drosophila melanogaster. *American Naturalist, 64*, 37–55.

Alter, G. (2004). Height, frailty, and the standard of living: Modelling the effects of diet and disease on declining mortality and increasing height. *Population Studies, 58*(3), 265–279.

Alter, G., Neven, M., & Oris, M. (2004). Stature in transition: A micro-level study from nineteenth-century Belgium. *Social Science History, 28*(2), 231–247.

Anisimov, V. N., & Bartke, A. (2013). The key role of growth hormone-insulin-IGF-1 signaling in aging and cancer. *Critical Reviews in Oncology/Hematology, 87*(3), 201–223.

Austad, S. N. (2001). Concepts and theories of aging. In E. J. Masoro & S. N. Austad (Eds.), *Handbook of the biology of aging* (5th ed., pp. 3–22). San Diego, CA: Academic Press.

Austad, S. N. (2004). Is aging programed? *Aging Cell, 3*(5), 249–251.

Austad, S. N. (2009). Is there a role for new invertebrate models for aging research? *The Journals of Gerontology, Series A, 64*(2), 192–194.

Austad, S. N., & Bartke, A. (2015). Sex differences in longevity and in responses to anti-aging interventions: A mini-review. *Gerontology, 62*(1), 40–46.

Barker, D. J. P. (1998). *Mothers, babies, and health later in life* (2nd ed.). London, UK: Churchill Livingstone.

Barlow, R. E., & Proschan, F. (1975). *Statistical theory of reliability and life testing: Probability models.* New York, NY: Holt, Rinehart & Winston.

Beard, R. E. (1959). Note on some mathematical mortality models. In E. W. Wolstenholme & M. O. O'Connor (Eds.), *The lifespan of animals* (pp. 302–311). Boston, MA: Little, Brown.

Bebbington, M., Green, R., Lai, C. D., & Zitikis, R. (2014). Beyond the Gompertz law: Exploring the late-life mortality deceleration phenomenon. *Scandinavian Actuarial Journal, 3*, 189–207.

Beeton, M., & Pearson, K. (1901). On the inheritance of the duration of life, and on the intensity of natural selection in man. *Biometrika, 1*, 50–89.

Beise, J., & Voland, E. (2002). Effect of producing sons on maternal longevity in premodern populations. *Science, 298*(5592), 317; author reply 317.

Beltrán-Sáncheza, H., Crimmins, E., & Finch, C. (2012). Early cohort mortality predicts the rate of aging in the cohort: A historical analysis. *Journal of Developmental Origins of Health and Disease, 3*(5), 380–386.

Ben-Shlomo, Y., & Kuh, D. (2002). A life course approach to chronic disease epidemiology: Conceptual models, empirical challenges and interdisciplinary perspectives. *International Journal of Epidemiology, 31*(2), 285–293.

Bengtsson, T., & Lindstrom, M. (2000). Childhood misery and disease in later life: The effects on mortality in old age of hazards experienced in early life, southern Sweden, 1760–1894. *Population Studies, 54*(3), 263–277.

Bengtsson, T., & Lindström, M. (2003). Airborne infectious diseases during infancy and mortality in later life in southern Sweden, 1766–1894. *International Journal of Epidemiology, 32*(2), 286–294.

Bengtsson, T., & Mineau, G. P. (2009). Early-life effects on socio-economic performance and mortality in later life: A full life-course approach using contemporary and historical sources. *Social Science and Medicine, 68*(9), 1561–1564.

Blackwell, D. L., Hayward, M. D., & Crimmins, E. M. (2001). Does childhood health affect chronic morbidity in later life? *Social Science and Medicine, 52*(8), 1269–1284.

Boardman, J. D., Barnes, L. L., Wilson, R. S., Evans, D. A., & Mendes de Leon, C. F. (2012). Social disorder, APOE-E4 genotype, and change in cognitive function among older adults living in Chicago. *Social Science and Medicine, 74*(10), 1584–1590.

Bongaarts, J. (2009). Trends in senescent life expectancy. *Population Studies, 63*(3), 203–213.

Boonekamp, J. J., Briga, M., & Verhulst, S. (2015). The heuristic value of redundancy models of aging. *Experimental Gerontology, 71*, 95–102.

Bourgeois-Pichat, J. (1979). Future outlook for mortality decline in the world. In *Prospects of population: Methodology and assumption* (pp. 227–266). *Population Studies, Series A, No. 67*, New York, NY: United Nations.

Bredesen, D. E. (2004). Rebuttal to Austad: "Is aging programmed?" *Aging Cell, 3*(5), 261–262.

Bronikowski, A. M., Alberts, S. C., Altmann, J., Packer, C., Carey, K. D., & Tatar, M. (2002). The aging baboon: Comparative demography in a non-human primate. *Proceedings of the National Academy of Sciences of the United States of America, 99*(14), 9591–9595.

Bronikowski, A. M., Altmann, J., Brockman, D. K., Cords, M., Fedigan, L. M., Pusey, A., . . . Alberts, S. C. (2011). Aging in the natural world: Comparative data reveal similar mortality patterns across primates. *Science, 331*(6022), 1325–1328.

Bruckner, T. A., van den Berg, G. J., Smith, K. R., & Catalano, R. A. (2014). Ambient temperature during gestation and cold-related adult mortality in a Swedish cohort, 1915–2002. *Social Science and Medicine, 119,* 191–197.

Carey, J. R., Liedo, P., Orozco, D., & Vaupel, J. W. (1992). Slowing of mortality rates at older ages in large medfly cohorts. *Science, 258*(5081), 457–461.

Carnes, B. A., & Olshansky, S. J. (1993). Evolutionary perspectives on human senescence. *Population and Development Review, 19*(4), 793–806.

Carnes, B. A., & Olshansky, S. J. (1997). A biologically motivated partitioning of mortality. *Experimental Gerontology, 32*(6), 615–631.

Carnes, B. A., Olshansky, S. J., & Grahn, D. (1996). Continuing the search for a law of mortality. *Population and Development Review, 22*(2), 231–264.

Caughley, G. (1966). Mortality patterns in mammals. *Ecology, 47*(6), 906–918.

Caughley, G. (1977). *Analysis of vertebrate populations.* London, UK: Wiley and Sons.

Chereji, E., Gatz, M., Pedersen, N. L., & Prescott, C. A. (2013). Reexamining the association between fertility and longevity: Testing the disposable soma theory in a modern human sample of twins. *The Journals of Gerontology, Series A, 68*(5), 499–509.

Comfort, A. (1979). *The biology of senescence* (3rd ed.). New York, NY: Elsevier.

Costa, D. L. (2000). Understanding the twentieth-century decline in chronic conditions among older men. *Demography, 37*(1), 53–72.

Costa, D. L. (2002). Changing chronic disease rates and long-term declines in functional limitation among older men. *Demography, 39*(1), 119–137.

Costa, D. L., & Lahey, J. (2005). Becoming oldest old: Evidence from historical U.S. data. *Genus, 61*(1), 125–161.

Crimmins, E. M., & Finch, C. E. (2006). Infection, inflammation, height, and longevity. *Proceedings of the National Academy of Sciences of the United States of America, 103*(2), 498–503.

Crimmins, E. M., Hayward, M. D., & Saito, Y. (1996). Differentials in active life expectancy in the older population of the United States. *The Journals of Gerontology, Series B, 51*(3), S111–S120.

Crimmins, E., Kim, J. K., McCreath, H., Faul, J., Weir, D., & Seeman, T. (2014). Validation of blood-based assays using dried blood spots for use in large population studies. *Biodemography and Social Biology, 60*(1), 38–48.

Crimmins, E. M., & Seeman, T. (2000). Integrating biology into demographic research on health and aging (with a focus on the MacArthur Study of Successful Aging). In

C. E. Finch, J. Vaupel, & K. Kinsella (Eds.), *Cells and surveys* (pp. 9–41). Washington, DC: National Academies Press.

Crimmins, E. M., & Vasunilashorn, S. (2011). Links between biomarkers and mortality. In R. G. Rogers & E. M. Crimmins (Eds.), *International handbook of adult mortality* (Vol. 2, pp. 381–398). New York, NY: Springer Publishing Company.

de Grey, A. D. N. J. (2003). An engineer's approach to the development of real anti-aging medicine. *Science of Aging Knowledge Environment: SAGE KE, 2003*(1), VP1.

Dilman, V. M. (1971). Age-associated elevation of hypothalamic, threshold to feedback control, and its role in development, ageing, and disease. *The Lancet, 1*(7711), 1211–1219.

Dilman, V. M., & Dean, W. (1992). *Neuroendocrine theory of aging*. Pensacola, FL: Center for Bio-Gerontology.

Doblhammer, G., & Oeppen, J. (2003). Reproduction and longevity among the British peerage: The effect of frailty and health selection. *Proceedings. Biological Sciences/The Royal Society, 270*(1524), 1541–1547.

Economos, A. C. (1985). Rate of aging, rate of dying and non-Gompertzian mortality—Encore. *Gerontology, 31*(2), 106–111.

Elo, I. T., & Preston, S. H. (1992). Effects of early-life conditions on adult mortality: A review. *Population Index, 58*(2), 186–212.

Feller, W. (1968). *An introduction to probability theory and its applications* (Vol. 1). New York, NY: Wiley and Sons.

Ferraro, K. F., & Kelley-Moore, J. A. (2003). Cumulative disadvantage and health: Long-term consequences of obesity? *American Sociological Review, 68*(5), 707–729.

Ferrie, J., & Rolf, K. (2011). Socioeconomic status in childhood and health after age 70: A new longitudinal analysis for the US, 1895–2005. *Explorations in Economic History, 48*(4), 445–460.

Finch, C. E. (2007). *The biology of human longevity: Inflammation, nutrition, and aging in the evolution of lifespans*. Amsterdam, The Netherlands: Elsevier.

Finch, C. E., & Crimmins, E. M. (2004). Inflammatory exposure and historical changes in human life-spans. *Science, 305*(5691), 1736–1739.

Flegal, K. M., Kit, B. K., Orpana, H., & Graubard, B. I. (2013). Association of all-cause mortality with overweight and obesity using standard body mass index categories: A systematic review and meta-analysis. *Journal of the American Medical Association, 309*(1), 71–82.

Fogel, R. W., & Costa, D. L. (1997). A theory of technophysio evolution, with some implications for forecasting population, health care costs, and pension costs. *Demography, 34*(1), 49–66.

Friedman, H. S., & Kern, M. L. (2014). Personality, well-being, and health. *Annual Review of Psychology, 65*, 719–742.

Gagnon, A. (2015). Natural fertility and longevity. *Fertility and Sterility, 103*(5), 1109–1116.

Galobardes, B., Lynch, J. W., & Davey Smith, G. (2004). Childhood socioeconomic circumstances and cause-specific mortality in adulthood: Systematic review and interpretation. *Epidemiologic Reviews, 26*, 7–21.

Gavrilov, L. A. (1978). [Mathematical model of aging]. *Doklady Akademii nauk SSSR, 238*(2), 490–492.

Gavrilov, L. A., & Gavrilova, N. S. (1991). *The biology of life span: A quantitative approach.* New York, NY: Harwood Academic Publisher.

Gavrilov, L. A., & Gavrilova, N. S. (2001). The reliability theory of aging and longevity. *Journal of Theoretical Biology, 213*(4), 527–545.

Gavrilov, L. A., & Gavrilova, N. S. (2002). Evolutionary theories of aging and longevity. *The Scientific World Journal, 2,* 339–356.

Gavrilov, L. A., & Gavrilova, N. S. (2006). Reliability theory of aging and longevity. In E. J. Masoro & S. N. Austad (Eds.), *Handbook of the biology of aging* (6th ed., pp. 3–42). San Diego, CA: Academic Press.

Gavrilov, L. A., & Gavrilova, N. S. (2011). Mortality measurement at advanced ages: A study of the Social Security Administration Death Master File. *North American Actuarial Journal, 15*(3), 432–447.

Gavrilov, L. A., & Gavrilova, N. S. (2012). Biodemography of exceptional longevity: Early-life and mid-life predictors of human longevity. *Biodemography and Social Biology, 58*(1), 14–39.

Gavrilov, L. A., & Gavrilova, N. S. (2015). New developments in biodemography of aging and longevity. *Gerontology, 61*(4), 364–371.

Gavrilova, N. S., & Gavrilov, L. A. (2015). Biodemography of old-age mortality in humans and rodents. *The Journals of Gerontology, Series A, 70*(1), 1–9.

Gavrilova, N. S., Gavrilov, L. A., Semyonova, V. G., & Evdokushkina, G. N. (2004). Does exceptional human longevity come with a high cost of infertility? Testing the evolutionary theories of aging. *Annals of the New York Academy of Sciences, 1019,* 513–517.

Gillespie, D. O., Russell, A. F., & Lummaa, V. (2013). The effect of maternal age and reproductive history on offspring survival and lifetime reproduction in preindustrial humans. *Evolution; International Journal of Organic Evolution, 67*(7), 1964–1974.

Gladyshev, V. N. (2013). The origin of aging: Imperfectness-driven non-random damage defines the aging process and control of lifespan. *Trends in Genetics: TIG, 29*(9), 506–512.

Gögele, M., Pattaro, C., Fuchsberger, C., Minelli, C., Pramstaller, P. P., & Wjst, M. (2011). Heritability analysis of life span in a semi-isolated population followed across four centuries reveals the presence of pleiotropy between life span and reproduction. *The Journals of Gerontology, Series A, 66*(1), 26–37.

Gompertz, B. (1825). On the nature of the function expressive of the law of human mortality and on a new mode of determining life contingencies. *Philosophical Transactions of the Royal Society of London, 115,* 513–585.

Greenwood, M., & Irwin, J. O. (1939). The biostatistics of senility. *Human Biology, 11,* 1–23.

Grundy, E., & Kravdal, Ø. (2008). Reproductive history and mortality in late middle age among Norwegian men and women. *American Journal of Epidemiology, 167*(3), 271–279.

Haines, M. R., Craig, L. A., & Weiss, T. (2003). The short and the dead: Nutrition, mortality, and the "antebellum puzzle" in the United States. *Journal of Economic History, 63*(2), 382–413.

Hamil-Luker, J., & O'Rand, A. M. (2007). Gender differences in the link between childhood socioeconomic conditions and heart attack risk in adulthood. *Demography, 44*(1), 137–158.

Harrell, C. J., Smith, K. R., & Mineau, G. P. (2008). Are girls good and boys bad for parental longevity?: The effects of sex composition of offspring on parental mortality past age 50. *Human Nature, 19*(1), 56–69.

Hauser, R. M., Weinstein, M., Pool, R., & Cohen, B. (2010). *Conducting biosocial surveys: Collecting, storing, accessing, and protecting biospecimens and biodata.* Washington, DC: National Academies Press.

Hawkes, K., & Smith, K. R. (2010). Do women stop early? Similarities in fertility decline in humans and chimpanzees. *Annals of the New York Academy of Sciences, 1204*, 43–53.

Hayward, A. D., Rickard, I. J., & Lummaa, V. (2013). Influence of early-life nutrition on mortality and reproductive success during a subsequent famine in a preindustrial population. *Proceedings of the National Academy of Sciences of the United States of America, 110*(34), 13886–13891.

Hayward, M. D., & Gorman, B. K. (2004). The long arm of childhood: The influence of early-life social conditions on men's mortality. *Demography, 41*(1), 87–107.

He, Q., Morris, B. J., Grove, J. S., Petrovitch, H., Ross, W., Masaki, K. H.,... Willcox, B. J. (2014). Shorter men live longer: Association of height with longevity and FOXO3 genotype in American men of Japanese ancestry. *PloS One, 9*(5), e94385.

Helle, S., & Lummaa, V. (2013). A trade-off between having many sons and shorter maternal post-reproductive survival in pre-industrial Finland. *Biology Letters, 9*(2), 20130034.

Helle, S., Lummaa, V., & Jokela, J. (2002). Sons reduced maternal longevity in preindustrial humans. *Science, 296*(5570), 1085.

Helle, S., Lummaa, V., & Jokela, J. (2005). Are reproductive and somatic senescence coupled in humans? Late, but not early, reproduction correlated with longevity in historical Sami women. *Proceedings. Biological Sciences/The Royal Society, 272*(1558), 29–37.

Horiuchi, S., & Wilmoth, J. R. (1998). Deceleration in the age pattern of mortality at older ages. *Demography, 35*(4), 391–412.

Hutchinson, G. E. (1978). *An introduction to population ecology.* New Haven, CT: Yale University Press.

Jarry, V., Gagnon, A., & Bourbeau, R. (2013). Maternal age, birth order and other early-life factors: A family-level approach to exploring exceptional survival. *Vienna Yearbook of Population Research, 11*, 263–284.

Jasienska, G., Nenko, I., & Jasienski, M. (2006). Daughters increase longevity of fathers, but daughters and sons equally reduce longevity of mothers. *American Journal of Human Biology: The Official Journal of the Human Biology Council, 18*(3), 422–425.

Jones, O. R., Scheuerlein, A., Salguero-Gómez, R., Camarda, C. G., Schaible, R., Casper, B. B., . . . Vaupel, J. W. (2014). Diversity of ageing across the tree of life. *Nature, 505*(7482), 169–173.

Karlamangla, A. S., Merkin, S. S., Crimmins, E. M., & Seeman, T. E. (2010). Socioeconomic and ethnic disparities in cardiovascular risk in the United States, 2001–2006. *Annals of Epidemiology, 20*(8), 617–628.

Kirkwood, T. B. (1998). Biological theories of aging: An overview. *Aging, 10*(2), 144–146.

Kirkwood, T. B. L. (2015). Deciphering death: A commentary on Gompertz (1825) "On the nature of the function expressive of the law of human mortality, and on a new mode of determining the value of life contingencies." *Philosophical Transactions of the Royal Society B-Biological Sciences, 370*(1666), 8.

Kirkwood, T. B., & Holliday, R. (1979). The evolution of ageing and longevity. *Proceedings of the Royal Society of London: Series B, Biological Sciences, 205*(1161), 531–546.

Kirkwood, T. B., & Melov, S. (2011). On the programmed/non-programmed nature of ageing within the life history. *Current Biology: CB, 21*(18), R701–R707.

Kuh, D., & Ben-Shlomo, B. (1997). *A life course approach to chronic disease epidemiology.* Oxford: Oxford University Press.

Laditka, S. B., & Laditka, J. N. (2009). Active life expectancy: A central measure of population health. In P. Uhlenberg (Ed.), *International handbook of the demography of aging* (pp. 543–565). New York, NY: Springer Publishing Company

Laird, R. A., & Sherratt, T. N. (2009). The evolution of senescence through decelerating selection for system reliability. *Journal of Evolutionary Biology, 22*(5), 974–982.

Laird, R. A., & Sherratt, T. N. (2010). The evolution of senescence in multi-component systems. *Bio Systems, 99*(2), 130–139.

Le Bourg, E. (2001). A mini-review of the evolutionary theories of aging. *Demographic Research, 4*(1), 1–28.

Le Bourg, E. (2014). Evolutionary theories of aging can explain why we age. *Interdisciplinary Topics in Gerontology, 39*, 8–23.

Lee, R. (2014). Intergenerational transfers, social arrangements, life histories, and the elderly. In M. Weinstein & M. A. Lane (Eds.), *Sociality, hierarchy, health: Comparative biodemography* (pp. 223–246). Washington, DC: National Academies Press.

Lemaître, J. F., Berger, V., Bonenfant, C., Douhard, M., Gamelon, M., Plard, F., & Gaillard, J. M. (2015). Early-late life trade-offs and the evolution of ageing in the wild. *Proceedings of the Royal Society of London: Series B, Biological Sciences, 282*(1806), 20150209.

Lindop, P. J. (1961). Growth rate, lifespan and causes of death in SAS/4 mice. *Gerontologia, 5*, 193–208.

Lycett, J. E., Dunbar, R. I., & Voland, E. (2000). Longevity and the costs of reproduction in a historical human population. *Proceedings of the Royal Society of London: Series B, Biological Sciences, 267*(1438), 31–35.

Manton, K. G., Stallard, E., & Vaupel, J. W. (1981). Methods for comparing the mortality experience of heterogeneous populations. *Demography, 18*(3), 389–410.

Medawar, P. B. (1958). Old age and natural death. In *The uniqueness of the individual* (pp. 17–43). New York, NY: Basic Books.

Michell, A. R. (1999). Longevity of British breeds of dog and its relationships with sex, size, cardiovascular variables and disease. *The Veterinary Record, 145*(22), 625–629.

Miller, R. A., Chrisp, C., & Atchley, W. (2000). Differential longevity in mouse stocks selected for early life growth trajectory. *The Journals of Gerontology, Series A, 55*(9), B455–B461.

Mitteldorf, J., & Martins, A. C. (2014). Programmed life span in the context of evolvability. *The American Naturalist, 184*(3), 289–302.

Mueller, L. D., Rauser, C. L., & Rose, M. R. (2011). *Does aging stop?* Oxford, UK: Oxford University Press.

Müller, H. G., Chiou, J. M., Carey, J. R., & Wang, J. L. (2002). Fertility and life span: Late children enhance female longevity. *The Journals of Gerontology, Series A, 57*(5), B202–B206.

Olshansky, S. J. (1998). On the biodemography of aging: A review essay. *Population and Development Review, 24*, 381–393.

Olshansky, S. J., & Carnes, B. A. (1997). Ever since Gompertz. *Demography, 34*(1), 1–15.

Pearl, R. (1922). *The biology of death.* Philadelphia, PA: Lippincott Williams & Wilkins.

Pearl, R., & Pearl, R. D. W. (1934). *The ancestry of the long-lived.* Baltimore, MD: The John Hopkins Press.

Pembrey, M., Saffery, R., Bygren, L. O., & Network in Epigenetic Epidemiology. (2014). Human transgenerational responses to early-life experience: Potential impact on development, health and biomedical research. *Journal of Medical Genetics, 51*(9), 563–572.

Perls, T. T., Alpert, L., & Fretts, R. C. (1997). Middle-aged mothers live longer. *Nature, 389*(6647), 133.

Preston, S. H., Elo, I. T., & Stewart, Q. (1999). Effects of age misreporting on mortality estimates at older ages. *Population Studies: A Journal of Demography, 53*(2), 165–177.

Preston, S. H., & Haines, M. R. (1991). *Fatal years. Child mortality in late nineteenth-century America.* Princeton, NJ: Princeton University Press.

Preston, S. H., Hill, M. E., & Drevenstedt, G. L. (1998). Childhood conditions that predict survival to advanced ages among African-Americans. *Social Science and Medicine, 47*(9), 1231–1246.

Robert, L., & Fulop, T. (2014). *Aging: Facts and theories* (Vol. 39). Basel, Switzerland: Karger.

Robins, C., & Conneely, K. N. (2014). Testing evolutionary models of senescence: Traditional approaches and future directions. *Human Genetics, 133*(12), 1451–1465.

Rollo, C. D. (2002). Growth negatively impacts the life span of mammals. *Evolution and Development, 4*(1), 55–61.

Rose, M. R. (1991). *Evolutionary biology of aging.* New York, NY: Oxford University Press.

Rose, M. R., Rauser, C. L., Mueller, L. D., & Benford, G. (2006). A revolution for aging research. *Biogerontology, 7*(4), 269–277.

Sacher, G. A. (1956). On the statistical nature of mortality, with especial reference to chronic radiation mortality. *Radiology, 67*(2), 250–258.

Sacher, G. A. (1966). The Gompertz transformation in the study of the injury-mortality relationship: Application to late radiation effects and ageing. In P. J. Lindop & G. A. Sacher (Eds.), *Radiation and aging* (pp. 411–441). London, UK: Taylor & Francis.

Sacher, G. A. (1977). Life table modification and life prolongation. In C. E. Finch & L. Hayflick (Eds.), *Handbook of the biology of aging* (1st ed., pp. 582–638). New York, NY: Van Nostrand Reinhold.

Salaris, L., Poulain, M., & Samaras, T. T. (2012). Height and survival at older ages among men born in an inland village in Sardinia (Italy), 1866–2006. *Biodemography and Social Biology, 58*(1), 1–13.

Samaras, T. T., Elrick, H., & Storms, L. H. (2003). Is height related to longevity? *Life Sciences, 72*(16), 1781–1802.

Sauvy, A. (1961). *Les Limites de la Vie Humaine.* Paris, FR: Hachette.

Sebastiani, P., Sun, F. X., Andersen, S. L., Lee, J. H., Wojczynski, M. K., Sanders, J. L., …Perls, T. T. (2013). Families enriched for exceptional longevity also have increased health-span: Findings from the long life family study. *Frontiers in Public Health, 1,* 38.

Shanahan, M. J., Hill, P. L., Roberts, B. W., Eccles, J., & Friedman, H. S. (2014). Conscientiousness, health, and aging: The life course of personality model. *Developmental Psychology, 50*(5), 1407–1425.

Skulachev, V. P. (2011). Aging as a particular case of phenoptosis, the programmed death of an organism (a response to Kirkwood and Melov "On the programmed/non-programmed nature of ageing within the life history"). *Aging, 3*(11), 1120–1123.

Smith, K. R., Gagnon, A., Cawthon, R. M., Mineau, G. P., Mazan, R., & Desjardins, B. (2009). Familial aggregation of survival and late female reproduction. *The Journals of Gerontology, Series A, 64*(7), 740–744.

Smith, K. R., Mineau, G. P., & Bean, L. L. (2002). Fertility and post-reproductive longevity. *Social Biology, 49*(3–4), 185–205.

Smith, K. R., Mineau, G. P., Garibotti, G., & Kerber, R. (2009). Effects of childhood and middle-adulthood family conditions on later-life mortality: Evidence from the Utah Population Database, 1850–2002. *Social Science and Medicine, 68*(9), 1649–1658.

Stearns, S. C. (1992). *The evolution of life histories.* Oxford: Oxford University Press.

Stearns, S. C., Ackermann, M., Doebeli, M., & Kaiser, M. (2000). Experimental evolution of aging, growth, and reproduction in fruitflies. *Proceedings of the National Academy of Sciences of the United States of America, 97*(7), 3309–3313.

Stone, L. (2003). *Early-life conditions and survival to age 110 in the U.S.* Paper presented at the workshop "Early Life Conditions and Longevity. Reconstructive Lives from Cradle to Grave," Geneva.

Störmer, C., & Lummaa, V. (2014). Increased mortality exposure within the family rather than individual mortality experiences triggers faster life-history strategies in historic human populations. *PloS One, 9*(1), e83633.

Strehler, B. L. (1978). *Time, cells, and ageing* (2nd ed.). New York, NY: Academic Press.

Strehler, B. L., & Mildvan, A. S. (1960). General theory of mortality and aging. *Science, 132*(3418), 14–21.

Sun, F., Sebastiani, P., Schupf, N., Bae, H., Andersen, S. L., McIntosh, A.,…Perls, T. T. (2015). Extended maternal age at birth of last child and women's longevity in the Long Life Family Study. *Menopause, 22*(1), 26–31.

Tabatabaie, V., Atzmon, G., Rajpathak, S. N., Freeman, R., Barzilai, N., & Crandall, J. (2011). Exceptional longevity is associated with decreased reproduction. *Aging, 3*(12), 1202–1205.

Thatcher, A. R., Kannisto, V., & Vaupel, J. W. (1998). *The force of mortality at ages 80 to 120* (Vol. 5). Odense, Denmark: Odense University Press.

Van de Putte, B., Matthijs, K., & Vlietinck, R. (2004). A social component in the negative effect of sons on maternal longevity in pre-industrial humans. *Journal of Biosocial Science, 36*(3), 289–297.

Waaler, H. T. (1984). Height, weight and mortality. *Acta Medica Scandinavica,* Suppl. No. 679.

Wachter, K. W., & Finch, C. E. (1997). *Between Zeus and the salmon. The biodemography of longevity.* Washington, DC: National Academies Press.

Wang, X., Byars, S. G., & Stearns, S. C. (2013). Genetic links between post-reproductive lifespan and family size in Framingham. *Evolution, Medicine, and Public Health, 2013*(1), 241–253.

Wang, Z. Q. (2015). Age-dependent decline of association between obesity and mortality: A systematic review and meta-analysis. *Obesity Research and Clinical Practice, 9*(1), 1–11.

Weinert, B. T., & Timiras, P. S. (2003). Theories of aging. *Journal of Applied Physiology, 95*(4), 1706–1716.

Weinstein, M., & Lane, M. A. (2014). *Sociality, hierarchy, health: Comparative biodemography: Papers from a workshop.* Washington, DC: National Academies Press.

Weinstein, M., Vaupel, J. W., & Wachter, K. W. (2007). *Biosocial surveys.* Washington, DC: National Research Council.

Westendorp, R. G. J., & Kirkwood, T. B. L. (1998). Human longevity at the cost of reproductive success. *Nature, 396*(6713), 743–746.

Williams, G. C. (1957). Pleiotropy, natural selection and the evolution of senescence. *Evolution, 11,* 398–411.

Yashin, A. I., Wu, D., Arbeeva, L. S., Arbeev, K. G., Kulminski, A. M., Akushevich, I.,…Ukraintseva, S. V. (2015). Genetics of aging, health, and survival: Dynamic regulation of human longevity related traits. *Frontiers in Genetics, 6,* 122.

CHAPTER 33

The Multiplicity of Aging: Lessons for Theory and Conceptual Development From Longitudinal Studies

Dario Spini, Daniela S. Jopp, Stéphanie Pin, and Silvia Stringhini

This chapter offers a new perspective on the development of theories of aging by proposing that the complexity of the aging process requires accounting for its multiplicity, specifically, its multiple time frames, multidirectionality, multidimensionality and interplay of factors, and multilevel influences. Complementing earlier proposals from life-span developmental psychology (Baltes, Staudinger, & Lindenberger, 1999) and life-course research (Elder, Johnson, & Crosnoe, 2003; Settersten Jr., 2003), we propose some key theoretical principles that should be considered in future research to advance our understanding of aging within the context of the social sciences.

Given the complexity of the phenomenon of aging, the breadth of research in this field, and the rapid development of this field, we cannot present a comprehensive model of development and aging in this chapter. After decades of relying on cross-sectional studies in which insights into age-related changes were derived from age-group comparisons, a great number of longitudinal studies that enable a better understanding of development have been recently conducted. More than ever, there is a need to discuss how the empirical findings of longitudinal studies can be integrated and incorporated into aging theories. One of the major strengths of longitudinal studies is that they allow an analysis of intraindividual changes, interindividual differences in intraindividual changes, and their determinants (Baltes & Nesselroade, 1979). We build the current chapter on this strength.

During recent decades, an increasing number of longitudinal studies that examine variable durations, different trajectories (e.g., health, cognition, well-being, personality) and different life periods have emerged (Schaie & Hofer, 2001). This development in the field is related to the understanding of or interest in empirically testing whether aging is aligned with prior development or is a consequence of occurrences during earlier life phases. Some of these studies were initiated and continued because of the foresight of visionary researchers who followed their study participants for their entire scientific career. Such researchers include Schaie (1993), who conducted the Seattle Longitudinal Study, and George Vaillant (2012), who conducted the Harvard Grant Study.

Other longitudinal data sets exist because researchers retrieved long-lost (or ignored) data that were assessed during adult patients' childhoods, understood the importance and uniqueness of these data, and then linked them to existing adult databases that included the same participants or initiated follow-up assessments with the remainder of the now elderly sample. Examples include Elder's (1974) and Clausen's (1995) classic sociological life-course studies on the children of the Great Depression, which were based on the Berkeley Guidance Study and the Oakland Growth Study. More recent examples include the Nun Study by Snowdon et al. (1996) and the Lothian Birth Cohort Studies by Deary, Whalley, and Starr (2009), which follow up the Scottish Mental Surveys of 1932 and 1947. Finally, longitudinal studies and national panels are now regularly financed by national or international funding agencies. Importantly, many of these studies have also been conducted by multidisciplinary teams with the aim of capturing the multidimensionality of the aging process and the interdependence of the domains of function (Levy & Pavie Team, 2007).

The development of theories that capture aging processes is an interdisciplinary endeavor that should include diverse disciplines, such as biology, medical sciences, psychology, epidemiology, and sociology and such interdisciplinary fields as gerontology and life-course studies. Here, we will rely primarily on the contributions that these interdisciplinary fields, in addition to social sciences and life span psychology, have made to the understanding of intraindividual processes. Four main theoretical key principles will be covered: (a) multiple time frames; (b) multidirectionality and heterogeneity; (c) multidimensionality and the interplay of factors; and (d) multilevel influences.

■ MULTIPLE TIME FRAMES

One central feature of development and aging is the time frame in which aging occurs. Most aging researchers currently agree that aging does not occur only once an individual has reached retirement age. Rather, "aging" can be considered equal to "development," which begins even before a person's birth. We will use here the concepts "aging" and "development" interchangeably, as they are highly interrelated; the only difference between them is that development refers to the more general concept of individual change, whereas aging more strongly implies a connection between individual changes and chronological age. These developmental/aging processes happen on different time scales: some can be observed over the course of a long time, while others present as lagged effects with a very short duration.

Unfortunately, there is no established language for describing these processes; thus, communication about them is somewhat difficult. For example, long-term effects, such as the long-lasting effect of childhood and socioeconomic circumstances on health (Galobardes, Lynch, & Smith, 2004; Kuh, Hardy, Langenberg, Richards, & Wadsworth, 2002), can span several decades and several developmental phases, while short-term effects may span a shorter period of time, such as a few years. For example, critical life events, such as marriage, may raise life satisfaction for approximately a year, whereas widowhood appears to lower life satisfaction for half a decade on an average. Other events, such as unemployment, apparently result in a long-term reduction in life satisfaction (Diener, Lucas, & Scollon, 2006). Finally, micro-longitudinal studies, such as daily diaries and experience-sampling studies, offer detailed insights into short-term variability of functioning (Dautovich, Dzierzewski, & Gum, 2014; Gerstorf, Hoppmann, & Ram, 2014). Importantly, these micro-changes are often embedded within midterm developments, which are in turn embedded within more long-term developments. However, for most domains of functioning, we have little knowledge about the time frames of developmental processes, which complicates the selection of the optimal assessment periods for studying those aging processes.

Regarding the long-lasting influence of early-life conditions on health and aging, three interconnected processes have been proposed: (a) a lifelong biological impact of adverse conditions experienced during critical or sensitive periods in early life; (b) the accumulation of adverse exposures across the life course; and (c) the impact of early-life conditions on an individual's trajectories across his or her life course (Ben-Shlomo & Kuh, 2002).

The first model, also called the "critical" or "sensitive" period model, assumes that exposure to adverse events/circumstances during particularly developmentally sensitive (or critical) periods early in life may influence certain biological parameters that have a long-lasting influence on health. A classic example (and the one from which the "fetal origins hypothesis" originated) is low birth weight, which is considered a consequence of in utero exposure to a range of factors (including socioeconomic ones) and is associated with a higher lifetime risk of cardiometabolic disorders (Barker, 2004; Eriksson, Forsen, Tuomilehto, Osmond, & Barker, 2001). In addition to low birth weight, accumulating evidence has found that exposure to a plethora of events during early life (in utero in particular) impacts physical and cognitive functions and shapes the majority of aging-related diseases (Barker, 2004) through mechanisms of biological adaptation to the individual's anticipated environment during maturity (Huang, Li, Wang, & Martorell, 2010). Recently reported evidence suggests that epigenetic modifications that occur as a consequence of early life exposures may be among the mechanisms through which early-life conditions are remembered and stored; thus, such modifications affect the aging process throughout life (McGuinness et al., 2012; Stringhini et al., 2015). A second example of the idea of sensitive periods related to critical life events in childhood is child abuse or maltreatment, which have been found to be related to mental health issues, poor cognitive functioning, and poor health (Dube et al., 2001; Irving & Ferraro, 2006; Shaw & Krause, 2002). The mechanisms of such outcomes include long-lasting changes in the stress-related hormonal system, that is, the hypothalamus–pituitary–adrenal (HPA) axis (Bremner & Narayan, 1998), which may result in structural changes to the brain (Cohen et al., 2006); both the hormonal changes and the resulting structural changes are likely to have lifelong effects. For example, maltreatment and abuse during childhood have been linked to decreases in the volume of multiple areas of the hippocampus, including the dentate gyrus, which plays a key role in neurogenesis (Teicher, Anderson, & Polcari, 2012). As a consequence, childhood abuse has been found to result in poorer childhood cognition and impairments in learning and memory capacity that persist through old age (Kim & Diamond, 2002).

The second model, also called the "accumulation model," states that events that are experienced across the life course may accumulate and impact aging in a dose-response manner (Dannefer, 2003; Ferraro & Shippee, 2009; Kuh & Ben-Shlomo, 1997). For example, exposure to adverse socioeconomic circumstances may accumulate across the life course: A person who is born into a household with low socioeconomic status and who grows up in an area of town with little access to healthy food and quality schools may develop poor health habits, receive a poor education, and have poor employment opportunities. A second example is the cumulative exposure to smoke or other environmental insults that individuals with low socioeconomic status experience from childhood to old age. These cumulative conditions are assumed to have an impact on diseases of aging, such as type 2 diabetes and cardiovascular disease (Stringhini et al., 2013).

The third model, also called the "pathway model," asserts that a number of circumstances to which individuals are exposed during early life may influence their adult life conditions (e.g., by impacting their social mobility), which in turn negatively affects their health and aging. In contrast to the sensitive period models, this model does not necessarily consider changes in the biological system caused by childhood conditions or events; rather, it considers the impact of early life events and experiences in shaping individuals' socioeconomic and behavioral trajectories into adult life. For example, individuals who attend poor-quality schools in early life may be less likely to have a successful educational path and, in turn, more likely to be employed in unskilled occupations. In this case, the negative consequences on health would result from adverse occupational exposures in adulthood (among other factors). Although this model does not consider early-life conditions as direct determinants of one's health and aging, one's occupational position in adult life is determined by early-life conditions; thus, the pathway model reflects an indirect link between early-life circumstances and adult health. Most importantly, the pathway model is centered on social pathways from early to adult life rather than on biological pathways, as in the critical period model. If the critical period model implies a certain degree of determinism, in the sense that early-life conditions may directly and permanently affect biological systems, the pathway model is more probabilistic and remains open to positive pathways that would redeem individuals from the poor conditions to which they were exposed as children.

In practice, the three life-course models are not competing hypotheses. Rather, these models are strongly interrelated; thus, it is often difficult to empirically delineate them (Baltes et al., 1999). A potential method for integrating the three models into a general theory of aging considers the pathway model as representing the general social process that drives life-course trajectories and the critical period and accumulation models as representing the biological processes of disease causation (Blane, Netuveli, & Stone, 2007).

Another important timing aspect that should be considered is the impact of life transitions (i.e., the precise point in an individual's life when he or she experiences transitions) on health and aging. An effective example is the impact of work transitions on health. Acute work events, such as job loss or retirement, may permanently affect an individual's health and aging (Gallo, Bradley, Siegel, & Kasl, 2000). On the one hand, the variety of positive latent functions associated with everyday work (i.e., the work-related structuring of the day, one's identity, and one's interpersonal contacts) is terminated when an individual's job ends. On the other hand, for some individuals, job loss or retirement may represent a termination of exposures that have an adverse impact on health. Regarding unemployment, it is important to consider that this experience may affect groups of individuals differently depending on their age and stage of life. A large body of evidence, particularly from longitudinal studies, has documented the long-lasting detrimental effects of unemployment on physical and mental health (Gallo et al., 2000; Mathers & Schofield, 1998). Regarding retirement, longitudinal studies, such as the French GAZEL Cohort Study and the Finnish Public Sector Study have documented improvements in self-rated health, mental health, and physical fatigue among individuals after they leave work (Oksanen et al., 2011; Westerlund et al., 2009). Not surprisingly, these health improvements have been reported mostly for individuals who lost jobs with poor working conditions (Westerlund et al., 2009).

■ MULTIDIRECTIONALITY AND HETEROGENEITY

One of the central tenets of life-span developmental theory is multidirectionality (Baltes et al., 1999): that is, the view that development is characterized by positive (gain-related) and negative (loss-related) trajectories as well as stability/continuity. We can observe multidirectionality within and across domains; changes can be successively positive, negative, or nonexistent, resulting in a trajectory of successive states. The second key concept is heterogeneity, or interindividual differences in the resulting intraindividual changes (Kelley-Moore & Lin, 2011), which indicates the degree to which there are variations in the direction of development across individuals or groups. As we will now review, multidirectionality and heterogeneity are key theoretical issues when examining the complexity of aging processes.

When the entire life course is considered, many theoretical models describe the shape of development of various dimensions but do not take into account the fact that individuals at all ages can show different trajectories of change. Typically, these theories propose a developmental curve that represents the average trajectory of human development. For example, Strachan and Sheikh (2004) proposed a two-state model to describe life-course influences on aging that resulted in an inverse-U-shaped curve for health. During the first phase, health (e.g., strength, immune function) is accumulated, and during the second phase, health is progressively lost (i.e., through aging). Aging trajectories are then influenced both by the state of health that is achieved during the first phase (the starting level) and by the rate at which health is lost during the second phase (Blane, Kelly-Irving, d'Errico, Bartley, & Montgomery, 2013). The first stage is defined as "build-up" and spans the time from conception and the early intrauterine environment to late adolescence or early adult life (i.e., up to the age of 30 years); it is characterized by rapid successions of developmentally and socially sensitive periods (Bartley, Blane, & Montgomery, 1997). The second stage, "decline," starts during early adulthood and is defined as a period of decline from the maximum attained capacity to a loss of function, disease, and death. Exposures to health risks and life events during the second stage can influence the rate at which proper function is lost. This interesting model, which was originally developed for respiratory and allergic diseases, can be applied as a prototypical example of general models of aging.

Similar examples of general curves based on longitudinal studies can be found in psychology for such domains as self-esteem (Trzesniewski, Brent Donnellan, & Robins, 2003), the "big five" personality dimensions (Roberts & Mroczek, 2008; Roberts, Walton, & Viechtbauer, 2006), and well-being (Blanchflower & Oswald, 2008). During recent years, changes in well-being have been discussed in the context of "one shape fits all" approaches (notably by economists) and can be taken as an example of the general shape of development that we aim to discuss in more detail. Specifically, well-being is described by some as a linear (stable or increasing) or curvilinear trajectory (with more evidence of a U-shape curve with relatively lower levels between 30 and 50 years of age and at sometimes near the end of life; see Ulloa, Møller, & Sousa-Poza, 2013). Despite extensive analyses, there is currently no consensus regarding the shape of the development of well-being. In addition to cohort effects and measurement issues (e.g., subjective/objective, general or domain-specific assessment), a major debate concerns the way that aging should be conceived, that is, is well-being a "pure" age effect controlled by other variables (e.g., socioeconomic status, health, and gender), or does it lack independence from other trajectories? For example, should we consider that well-being may depend on health, which changes considerably in older age? Even if general trajectories across the life course appear useful for gaining a preliminary description of the general shape and commonality of the aging process, there are serious limitations in this line of research because the idea of a single average general model of development cannot account for the heterogeneity of aging processes.

As a result of the development of longitudinal studies and statistical methods designed to examine trajectories, aging theories can increasingly take multidirectionality and heterogeneity into account in their formulations. One of the central findings of aging and longitudinal research is that although some developments such as loss of a cognitive function or declining health in old age can be observed for *most* individuals, there is substantial interindividual variability. In fact, because of the heterogeneity in aging, the differences in function among individuals of the same age can be greater than those observed between individuals of very different ages; plasticity (within-person modifiability) plays an important role in function (Baltes, 1987). The assumption that all individuals of a particular socioeconomic environment, gender, age, social class, and personality would share the same aging processes is less heuristic than a theoretical perspective that takes multidirectionality and heterogeneity into consideration. The questions of when, where, and for whom changes related to age occur are of utmost importance in theory building. Theories about aging should question the generalizability and validity of the explanations of events across different social groups and time points in the life course and in relation to relevant transitions.

Another interesting aspect derived from developmental theories is that many developmental trajectories can occur at any age. Even centenarians have been found to not only lose cognitive functioning over time but also improve their performance (Kliegel, Moor, & Rott, 2004). Moreover, models must consider developmental phases that are characterized by little individual change. For example, the largest groups of centenarians demonstrated stability in cognitive functioning, either at a high or very low level (Kliegel et al., 2004). With a few exceptions, theories underestimate the stability and continuity that occur in wide phases of the life span and, for many people, persist until the very last stages of life. This is illustrated in the Swiss Interdisciplinary Longitudinal Study on the Oldest Old (SWILSOO) in terms of such dimensions as self-reported health trajectories and religious beliefs (Lalive d'Epinay & Spini, 2008; Lalive d'Epinay, Guilley, Guillet, & Spini, 2008).

Thus, as mentioned, an important issue that must be taken into consideration when formulating theories of aging is the heterogeneity of individual trajectories. We will elaborate on an example to show how considering multidirectionality and heterogeneity in our theories and analyses of well-being trajectories can change our view of a well-known phenomenon: the well-being paradox (Kunzmann, Little, & Smith, 2000). The basic idea of this theory is that, despite an accumulation of losses during older age, individuals maintain a relatively stable and positive level of well-being. This paradox has been observed in numerous studies and is typically considered a robust finding (Fiske, Gatz, & Pedersen, 2003; Idler, 1993; Leinonen, Heikkinen, & Jylhä, 1998; Rodin & McAvay, 1992; Rothermund & Brandtstädter, 2003b).

There is a large amount of evidence that older adults successfully use strategies, including the adjustment of self-appraisals, and influence their environment to maintain a relatively high and stable level of well-being despite losses in functional health; however, different studies describe the limits of the extent to which the paradox of well-being applies.

First, Swift et al.'s (2014) study of the 2008 to 2009 wave of the European Social Survey showed that gross domestic product (GDP) measured at the country level had a much stronger effect on the subjective well-being of older people than on younger individuals and that the paradox of well-being was observed only in the wealthiest countries. This suggests that the paradox of well-being may not be a universal phenomenon and that theories should specify the level of universality and generalizability that they address, an issue that is often overlooked (Norenzayan & Heine, 2005).

Moreover, it appears that, while the paradox of well-being may be true at a general level (e.g., a representative sample), a different profile emerges when health transitions or groups are considered. In an investigation of SWILSOO participants who were 80 years old and older, Girardin Keciour and Spini (2006) considered the specific health transitions that individuals experience and how these transitions were related to well-being (Lalive d'Epinay et al., 2008). At the mean level, the paradox of well-being again emerged; while the number of incapacities increased across waves and with advancing age, the level of well-being was relatively stable and did not vary with age or time at the intraindividual level. However, when individual transitions from different states of health (independent, frail, and dependent) were considered, a different result emerged. Those who experienced a trajectory that included independence (stable independence, independence to frailty, or frailty to independence, 54% of trajectories) showed relatively high levels of well-being. Those who were frail at two successive waves (33% of trajectories) showed moderate levels of well-being. Interestingly, those who experienced a period of dependence (stable dependence or frailty to dependence, 13% of trajectories) showed low levels of well-being. Notably, 72% of the observed health trajectories remained in the same state across two waves (stable independence, frailty, or dependence). It appears that, when the paradox accounts for the heterogeneity of trajectories, it is no longer paradoxical. Stability and high levels of well-being occur because a majority of aging individuals experience a relatively stable and positive health trajectory, even in old-old age (Guilley, Ghisletta, Armi, Berchtold, & Lalive d'Epinay, 2008); however, when health is deteriorated, levels of well-being are relatively lower.

More generally, we argue that theories of aging should systematically consider multidirectionality and heterogeneity. Furthermore, theories should always specify to whom a given model applies and, perhaps even more importantly, to whom it may not apply. Fortunately, method development has aided in a more systematic analysis that includes multidirectionality and heterogeneity by offering techniques for modeling individual trajectories or groups of trajectories, such as latent growth curve models and latent class analyses (George, 2009), sequence analyses (Blanchard, Bühlmann, & Gauthier, 2014) and emerging methods for longitudinal data mining (McArdle & Ritschard, 2013). Re-analyses of existing longitudinal data have led to the confirmation that not all individuals follow the same health trajectories and that various factors, including birth cohort, socioeconomic status, gender, and migration trajectories, help to differentiate the trajectories (Ayyagari et al., 2012; Hybels, Blazer, Landerman, & Steffens, 2011; Jivraj, Nazroo, Vanhoutte, & Chandola, 2014; Taylor & Lynch, 2011; Wickrama, Mancini, Kwag, & Kwon, 2013).

Multidimensionality and Interplay of Factors

When considering the factors that shape individual development over the life course, scholars often focus on aspects that hinder normal or positive development, such as critical life events or deprived environments (see as follows). Theories about dependence (Wood, 1975), frailty (Spini, Ghisletta, Guilley, & Lalive d'Epinay, 2007), and vulnerability (Schröder-Butterfill & Marianti, 2006) primarily focus on loss of function. Although this may seem appropriate given that aging is characterized by many losses, it nevertheless retains the risk of ignoring potential positive developments that may arise from different factors. Consider, for example, the experience of positive and negative effect, which have been shown to be unrelated, that is, the experience of positive emotions is not related to the absence of negative emotions, and vice versa (Kunzmann et al., 2000; Zautra, Potter, & Riech, 1997). These two types of affect exhibit differential reactivity to events (Röcke, Li, & Smith, 2009) and have been shown to have different trajectories over the life course (Charles, Reynolds, & Gatz, 2001). Relative independence and differential developmental trajectories could be attributed to two different brain systems that are responsible for the two types of emotions. As a consequence, different aspects may contribute to positive versus negative effect, as different channels may lead to one outcome or the other (Lawton, 1983). Empirical studies indeed support this latter point (Isaacowitz & Smith, 2003).

Another example of the utility of considering the multidimensionality of specific constructs is the difference between subjective and objective aspects of health. Objective health aspects, such as the number of illnesses, increase steadily with chronological age. In contrast, the perception of health, namely, the individual's subjective self-evaluation of his or her health status, is much more stable and does not necessarily represent objective health conditions (Galenkamp, Deeg, Braam, & Huisman, 2013; Idler, 1993). Furthermore, health is a good example of a topic that demonstrates the importance of interdisciplinary collaboration to investigate aging. In addition to the importance of objective health conditions, it is essential to track how individuals experience these conditions. Currently, the following question remains: Why is subjective health a better predictor of mortality in advanced age than objective health (Benyamini, 2011)? Examinations of the multidimensionality of development in terms of both developmental predictors and outcomes are useful for gaining a comprehensive understanding of the phenomenon.

Objective conditions, such as exposure to critical life events, can lead to various outcomes depending on other factors, such as the individual's evaluation of the situation and the available resources. These conditions represent the key assumption of stress theory (Lazarus & Folkman, 1984) and cast a particular light on the effects of life events. Events that are either negative or positive have been considered as disruptors of development and triggers for adaptation, as previously discussed. Therefore, assuming that childhood adversity and traumatic events or an accumulation of stress across the life span lead to vulnerability (Turner, Wheaton, & Lloyd, 1995), the correlation between life events and well-being is rather weak (typically ranging between 0.10 and 0.30). This has led to the conclusion that "differential exposure to stressful events is substantially less important than differential vulnerability to stress in determining the relationships between mental health and social class, gender, and marital status" (Turner et al., 1995, pp. 105–106). In this context, the concept of resilience was developed to identify (individual) factors related to reactivity and recovery after exposure to a potentially disruptive event (Rutter, 2000).

Complementing this view of risk factors, theoretical approaches that have considered both factors related to dealing with loss and those that promote positive development appear in the context of psychological life-span developmental theories and successful aging theories. Such factors are mostly individual ones, including basic resources such as health, cognitive capacity, and social engagement, as proposed in Rowe and Kahn's (1997) popular model of successful aging; psychological aspects, such as the preference for specific goal-setting and life-management strategies (Baltes & Baltes, 1990) or coping tendencies (Rothermund & Brandstädter, 2003a), as proposed by the more recent life-span developmental theories (for an overview, see Boerner & Jopp, 2007), are also frequently considered. There is substantial evidence that these factors are related to positive development and aging. Health and cognitive functioning represent important features that are related to aging well. For example, super centenarians were found to have had good health for most of their lives (Andersen, Sebastiani, Dworkis, Feldman, & Perls, 2012). There is also a strong evidence base indicating that social partners are essential resources over the life course; they have concrete and cumulative effects on well-being and health (Antonucci, Ajrouch, & Birditt, 2014) and function as a buffer against various stressors (Berkman & Glass, 2000; Moren-Cross & Lin, 2006; Wrzus, Hänel, Wagner, & Neyer, 2013). Similarly, studies have demonstrated that the use of adaptive strategies is associated with higher functioning and higher well-being (Jopp & Smith, 2006; Li, Lindenberger, Freund, & Baltes, 2001); thus, strategic behavior and cognitions represent important mechanisms of successful development.

In addition to these general positive effects, studies on successful aging have developed more complex models that consider moderation and mediation effects. For example, there is evidence that the role of specific resources changes according to age. Using subjective well-being as an indicator of successful aging, health appears to be less important for centenarians than for younger individuals (Jopp & Rott, 2006), and social resources, such as regular phone calls, became more important in very old individuals relative to their young-old counterparts (Jopp, Rott, & Oswald, 2008). Similar age-differential predictions were found for life-management strategy selection, optimization, and compensation (SOC; Baltes & Baltes, 1990); in terms of well-being, very old individuals with poor resources experienced the greatest benefit from using SOC (Jopp & Rott, 2006). One of the few longitudinal studies on life-management strategies also showed that not only a person's age but also his or her available resources determines the effectiveness of the strategies; for example, older individuals with poorer resources who used life-management strategies were as satisfied with their aging 1 year later as individuals who had previously reported having many resources (Jopp & Rott, 2006). A study of younger adults also provided evidence that disengagement, a strategy that would typically be considered more adaptive in older age, can be very beneficial under particular circumstances. Specifically, when individuals felt under considerable pressure with respect to career choices or when they lived in disadvantaged regions, letting go of career goals was linked to increases in their well-being (Tomasik & Silbereisen, 2012). In another study, the number of rooms in an individual's house (used as a proxy for housing resources) changed from being positively linked to life satisfaction in young–old age to having a negative effect in old–old age (Oswald, Jopp, Rott, & Wahl, 2011). This effect may imply that the reduced mobility of the very old made a large apartment not only less enjoyable but also a hassle. Thus, whether a specific resource or strategy is beneficial or detrimental may depend on a third variable beyond age or health status.

To understand the mechanisms underlying development, it is important to identify how specific determinants of successful development may relate to each other, or how they may influence each other over time. In a longitudinal study that sought to disentangle the influence of specifically linked determinants on different developmental outcomes, Taylor (2010) investigated the role of sociodemographic resources, including education and income, in the onset versus trajectories of a specific age-related aspect of development, namely, disability in late life. He found that education had a preventive effect on disability onset but not on its progression once income was controlled, whereas income was related to both onset and progression. In addition, he found that men and White individuals were able to delay the onset of disability for a longer period of time than women and non-White study participants; however, men did not experience a slower decline after onset. Furthermore, to gain a better understanding of developmental dynamics, a consideration of how the determinants of development influence one another over time is very useful. Measurement-burst studies aiming to link stress experience and cognition found that individuals showed reduced performance on demanding cognitive tasks on days with daily stressors (Sliwinski, Smyth, Hofer, & Stawski, 2006) and that these effects were more pronounced in older adults. Finally, investigations of lagged effects also help to disentangle causal relations. Using data from the Berlin Aging Study, Lövdén, Gishletta, and Lindenberger (2005) showed that social activities predicted perceptual speed over time, suggesting that social activities have a positive effect on cognitive functioning, whereas cognitive functioning was not related to future participation in social activities.

Inspired by successful aging models, a few longitudinal studies have also developed more complex models that consider various groups of predictors (resources, strategies, and beliefs) and their concurrent interplay, leading to a more specific understanding of the conditions under which specific mechanisms may work. One longitudinal study of middle-aged individuals examined the role of resources, coping strategies, and control beliefs in the context of critical life events (Jopp & Rott, 2006). Resources were negatively related to prospective critical life events and positively related to use of coping strategies 4 years later. Individuals who experienced more critical life events were also more likely to use assimilative strategies to directly address their problems and were even more likely to use accommodative strategies, including more passive strategies, such as the adjustment of goals and standards. Notably, when comparing individuals with a high perception of control and those with a low perception of control, the direct effect of life events was stronger for those who did not feel in control, which might indicate that those individuals were not protected by control beliefs. At the same time, the positive effect of assimilative coping was significant only for those who felt in control, indicating that only those who believed that they were in control benefited from their active coping efforts. These psychological models could, however, be further refined by sociological approaches because they typically do not take into account variables such as gender. A study conducted in Taiwan found what appear to be substantial sex differences in the trajectories of depression after life events; these differences were related to gender-specific disadvantages in terms of social position and employment and in the selected living arrangement (Glei, Goldman, Liu, & Weinstein, 2013).

In summary, given the key characteristic of multidirectionality of development, it is not sufficient to focus on resilience and the prevention of negative development. Rather, studies should be more strongly inspired by models of successful aging. However, more longitudinal studies are needed to examine the development of life-management and coping strategies and other determinants of successful aging, as their changes over the life span are poorly understood and require further investigation. Additionally, given the complexity and dynamics of the underlying mechanisms of development and aging, models of simple main effects are less likely to represent the reality. Initial studies show that combining variables that have been found to be individually meaningful into models that specify the interplay among individual variables, such as resources, strategies, and beliefs, is likely to increase the amount of explained variance in successful aging outcomes and to foster our understanding of the underlying mechanisms of development and aging.

Multilevel Influences

In our opinion, the multilevel processes that craft developmental trajectories represent an additional perspective that must be considered more systematically in theories of aging, a position that was first stated in the 1970s (Gubrium, 1973; Lawton & Nahemow, 1973; Lawton, 1980). The first generation of socioecological research was based primarily on cross-sectional studies, and it produced different representations of the cross-level influences on aging and development (Bronfenbrenner, 1986; Dahlgren & Whitehead, 2006): Namely, older people appear to be embedded in various contexts, which can be pictured as concentric circles around the person at the intrapersonal level, the interpersonal level (e.g., social networks, social capital), the community level (e.g., characteristics of the living and physical environments, neighborhood), and the societal level (e.g., institutions, social policies, social norms and social representations, cultural specificities). During the past 10 years, scholars who have employed the ecological perspective have moved toward longitudinal studies and have used prospective designs to systematically explore the influence of these different contextual levels on individual trajectories.

Social capital is an important proximal resource during aging that has been investigated in this line of research. Following a sociological perspective, social capital combines cognitive and structural dimensions (Islam, Merlo, Kawachi, Lindström, & Gerdtham, 2006). Longitudinal research examining the dynamics between social capital and individual outcomes found inconsistent results regarding the direction of relationships (De Silva, McKenzie, Harpham, & Huttly, 2005; Murayama, Fujiwara, & Kawachi, 2012; Sirven & Debrand, 2012). On the one hand, highly educated older people who engaged in informal or structured social activities were found to have a lower risk of developing chronic diseases or disabilities and had higher levels of well-being than socially disadvantaged older people (Belley et al., 2013; Murayama et al., 2012; Sirven & Debrand, 2012). On the other hand, diseases, functional limitations, and disabilities were found to hinder the social participation of older people and to contribute to the diminution of social capital during aging (Sirven & Debrand, 2012).

At a larger level, a set of structures (e.g., the characteristics of living and physical environments, the social stratification system, institutional fields, social norms, and social policy arrangements) can affect virtually all aspects of aging. Recent developments contribute to a better understanding of the interplay between more distant levels and individual outcomes. Some studies, such as the Canadian VoisiNuAge study (Gauvin et al., 2008; Payette & Shatenstein, 2005) and English Longitudinal Study of Ageing (ELSA) (Bell et al., 2014), establish that the stability of physical activity levels or changes in nutritional habits depend on the main physical or material characteristics of the neighborhood, such as the presence and good condition of pavement, bright lighting, and the availability of sports facilities; even the aesthetic appearance of urban facilities or the countryside were of importance. In these studies, country specificities present a higher order environmental level that is increasingly examined in aging research. This trend can be partially explained by the appearance of multicountry surveys or paired surveys that use similar methods and questionnaires (e.g., Health and Retirement Study [HRS], ELSA, and Survey of Health, Ageing and Retirement in Europe [SHARE]). Using parallel surveys, these studies primarily examine the influence of socioeconomic (e.g., gross national product, poverty rates) and institutional (e.g., public policies, public pension amounts) factors on health or well-being trajectories (Angelini & Laferrère, 2012; Dragano, Siegrist, & Wahrendorf, 2010).

Earlier ecological models were criticized mainly for their lack of comprehensiveness and their lack of emphasis on contextual changes. Recent developments attempt to enhance the integration of ecological principles by adding behavioral, cultural, or sociohistorical dimensions (Glass & Vander Plaats, 2013). Moreover, taking an ecological perspective into account has enabled some innovative methodological developments;

for example, life calendars that consider trajectories and that are informed by social or geographical information (Elcheroth et al., 2013). Contemporary definitions of ecological models have reinforced their relevance to the field of public health. In particular, the resurgence of interest in social inequalities in health has underlined the central role of larger contextual determinants of health, such as socioeconomic factors, gender, and other environmental influences (Richard, Gauvin, & Raine, 2011). Recent position statements by leading scientific bodies, including the National Institutes of Health, the National Academy of Sciences, and the Institute of Medicine, are based on ecological models as frameworks that characterize and encourage multidisciplinary work in the health sciences. In addition to providing enhanced understanding via innovative results, such recommendations underscore the importance of the ecological perspective for health prevention efforts and aging policies.

■ DISCUSSION AND CONCLUSION

This chapter takes advantage of the increasing number of longitudinal studies in the aging and developmental field to outline some lessons about the way theories on aging may be developed in the future to gain a more comprehensive picture of development and aging. The challenges of generating a more realistic view of aging are substantial, as the factors that explain development originate from different domains (biological, psychological, and social) and are interrelated both causally and systemically. The complexity of aging processes across the life course will likely not be fully theorized, but we need to find ways to better understand these processes. This need suggests that we should reflect on how to frame theories and studies to formulate questions that advance the understanding of aging processes. This chapter is written with the intent of sharing some reflections on how dynamic theories about aging can be heuristically framed. We retained four key central features that seem to us central to deriving lessons for future theory development: (a) multiple time frames; (b) multidirectionality and heterogeneity; (c) multidimensionality and the interplay among determinants; and (d) multilevel analyses. In our view, the lessons derived from these aspects are essential to promoting a life-course understanding of aging processes, understanding the diversity of aging, fostering multi- or interdisciplinarity, and contextualizing trajectories within contexts, respectively.

Taking the dynamics of development into serious consideration must become a guiding principle for aging research both within (Spini, Elcheroth, & Figini, 2008) and across disciplines. Consequently, research questions and hypotheses should be crafted to specify the time frame of the phenomenon under investigation. Specifically, this process could include identifying the exact point in time at which factors are expected to have effects, determining the duration of exposure that is required for the effects to be evident, and establishing the duration of these effects. Most theories do not take into account these questions or do not have the precision to tackle such questions. We have derived some proposals regarding how longitudinal studies can inform our theories. Serious consideration of time matters should both encourage researchers to reflect on how temporal issues impact the phenomena of interest and structure how they decide to frame their study, particularly the length of the study (e.g., number of waves, age of participants) and the time among waves of observation (e.g., years, months, regular or irregular intervals; Taris & Kompier, 2014).

The question of multidirectionality and heterogeneity prompts our second central lesson; the discussion of these two principles lead us to assumptions about the universality that underlies many theories of aging. We do not argue that describing a general average shape of development is useless; indeed, it is useful to have a baseline model against which to compare the trajectory of different individuals or groups. However, this type of general model should be only one component of our research efforts. Much effort must be devoted to describing the different shapes that developmental trajectories take at different times (considering age, time to death, and long- or short-term trajectories, among other parameters). Moreover, the question of heterogeneity (i.e., interindividual differences in intraindividual changes) should enrich theories of aging by exploring and systematically analyzing the diversity of trajectories in relation to differences in temporal factors, including age, cohort, or period effects and biological, psychological, or social factors.

Furthermore, we propose the principle of multidimensionality and interplay of factors as a third way of developing heuristic theories. We need to have a critical perspective on the outcomes that we consider in our research and to consider multidimensionality in our measures (e.g., subjective/objective, positive/negative framing, mixed methods in approaching the outcome). As discussed, multidimensionality is important but often overlooked, as the factors that have an effect on one dimension of an outcome may not be the same factors that impact a different measure of the outcome. Moreover, the multiplicity of aging also relates to the interplay of factors. Aging is a complex and systemic phenomenon that cannot be fully understood by considering only disciplinary perspectives. Disciplinary research is essential for selecting and measuring the factors with the greatest influence on a given trajectory. However, we have reviewed several longitudinal studies that show that an interplay between biological, psychological, and social factors affects important outcomes, such as subjective health or well-being. A more systematic evaluation of mediating and moderating effects across different types of determining factors of aging should enable theories to enlarge their assumptions and better capture the actual complexity of aging.

Developmental trajectories do not take place in a vacuum. This assumption leads us to propose a fourth key perspective, which focuses on the need to develop multilevel analyses of aging trajectories. Aging trajectories are related to social relationships and networks and to the physical and societal environments in which these relationships and networks are embedded. For example, it is well established that life expectancy and well-being are related to socioeconomic environments, yet many theories of aging focus on personal characteristics and individually based explanations rather than considering them in the context of or in relation to environmental factors. This consideration leads us to encourage researchers to complement aging explanations that are based on changes in individual characteristics with changes in environmental characteristics at a shared and more collective level (and vice versa). Importantly, we propose that there are levels of explanations that are not reducible to the individual and that need to be articulated. The study of multiple interactions among individual aging and ecological factors from a dynamic perspective is an emerging field in longitudinal research that should provide innovative and useful information about the multiplicity of aging processes, and this information will influence both theories of aging and the transfer of knowledge to policy makers.

Overall, the multiplicity of aging processes calls for collaborations and articulations at different levels: (a) theory; (b) disciplines and interdisciplinarity; and (c) organization of research. At the theoretical level, the multiplicity of aging processes calls for an articulation of different levels of explanation. Development is influenced by micro- to macro-factors (from cells to society) and by temporal (age/period/cohort), biological, psychological, and social dynamics. Clearly, theories and models cannot integrate all of these aspects easily.

Researchers from different disciplines and with different epistemological backgrounds are needed to address these theoretical challenges. However, to integrate these different perspectives that capture developmental diversity, there must be some consensus regarding the focus of attention among the involved fields of study to produce interdisciplinary outputs that advance the field. This is the function of theoretical syntheses: to look for key developments and possibly provide some consensus about the directions of research projects and programs. However, the bottom-up process of collecting and synthesizing empirical findings from different disciplines into shared theoretical advances should be developed further. We have tried to do so in this chapter, which was written by a life-span psychologist, a social psychologist, a sociologist, and an epidemiologist. The inverse top–down movement, the management of interdisciplinary research, is even less organized; it follows informal rules and individual or team efforts that do not always appear rational. Reflecting on the two other mentioned levels—disciplines and interdisciplinarity and the organization of research—may help to more efficiently structure the development of key perspectives from the past, such as the ones we developed here.

In addition to increasing awareness of the issues that we find essential for the future advancement of theories of aging, we believe that we could also encourage the development of more comprehensive models of aging by considering a few practical issues, such as enhancing the education of young scientists and creating interdisciplinary research networks. The training of researchers and the creation of academic research positions is a primary issue. It is certain that disciplinary training and doctoral education form the foundations of our scientific knowledge. Nonetheless, exposure to other disciplines and training in multi- or interdisciplinary research must gain increased importance in the education of future generations of scientists if we mean to advance the field of aging research. However, this raises the question of when should we introduce knowledge from other disciplines and interdisciplinary syntheses into the curricula: Should this occur at the bachelor's, master's, or doctoral education levels or later, when finding a tenured academic position is no longer a concern? Claims that interdisciplinarity is important often remain empty. Many view interdisciplinary work as a waste of time and may even consider it detrimental to an academic career, which is often defined as a specialization process within a discipline. Moreover, disciplinary journals tend to have higher impact factors than interdisciplinary ones, and the gap between the average impact factors of the top social sciences journals compared with that of medical journals, for example, is very substantial (Rafols et al., 2012). Unfortunately, such realities and perceptions are important structural barriers to interdisciplinarity.

Additional opportunities that favor advances in research on aging and development include the creation of interdisciplinary research networks. For example, there is a clear push from funding agencies to heavily finance projects on aging that come from interdisciplinary and international networks. For example, we at the Swiss National Centre of Competence in Research LIVES (www.lives-nccr.ch) have been financed for several years to analyze vulnerability across the life course; our center includes approximately 150 researchers in psychology, social psychology, sociology, demography, social economy, medicine, social policies, and statistics organized in interdisciplinary subgroups. Ongoing meetings and activities among researchers from different fields and our project structure and goals (including shared theoretical concepts, goals, publications, data, and research agendas) promote continual exchanges and interdisciplinary developments.

There are examples of similar network programs, such as National Education Panel Study (NEPS; www.neps-data.de/en-us/home.aspx) in Germany and Midlife in the United States (MIDUS; www.midus.wisc.edu/). The integration of efforts from different fields or disciplines, when it happens, must first occur and be evaluated at the theoretical level. It is not yet clear whether these types of heavily financed programs really make a difference in the integration of knowledge about the complex issues of explaining development and aging. We are still learning by doing, and the future will tell what we have learned and transmitted to future generations of researchers in the process.

■ ACKNOWLEDGMENTS

This publication benefited from the support of the Swiss National Centre of Competence in Research LIVES—Overcoming Vulnerability: Life Course Perspectives. Silvia Stringhini is supported by an Ambizione Grant (number PZ00P3_147998). The authors are grateful to the Swiss National Science Foundation for its financial support.

REFERENCES

Andersen, S. L., Sebastiani, P., Dworkis, D. A., Feldman, L., & Perls, T. T. (2012). Health span approximates life span among many supercentenarians: Compression of morbidity at the approximate limit of life span. *The Journals of Gerontology, Series A, 67*(4), 395–405.

Angelini, V., & Laferrère, A. (2012). Residential mobility of the European elderly. *CESifo Economic Studies, 58*(3), 544–569.

Antonucci, T. C., Ajrouch, K. J., & Birditt, K. S. (2014). The convoy model: Explaining social relations from a multidisciplinary perspective. *The Gerontologist, 54*(1), 82–92.

Ayyagari, P., Ullrich, F., Malmstrom, T. K., Andresen, E. M., Schootman, M., Miller, J. P.,...Wolinsky, F. D. (2012). Self-rated health trajectories in the African American health cohort. *PloS One, 7*(12), e53278.

Baltes, P. B. (1987). Theoretical propositions of life-span developmental psychology: On the dynamics between growth and decline. *Developmental Psychology, 23*(5), 611–626.

Baltes, P. B., & Baltes, M. M. (1990). Psychological perspectives on successful aging: The model of selective optimization with compensation. In P. B. Baltes & M. M. Baltes (Eds.), *Successful aging: Perspectives from the behavioral sciences* (Vol. 1, pp. 1–34). Cambridge, MA: Cambridge University Press.

Baltes, P. B., & Nesselroade, J. R. (1979). History and rationale of longitudinal research. In J. R. Nesselroade & P. B. Baltes (Eds.), *Longitudinal research in the study of behavior and development* (pp. 1–39). New York, NY: Academic Press.

Baltes, P. B., Staudinger, U. M., & Lindenberger, U. (1999). Lifespan psychology: Theory and application to intellectual functioning. *Annual Review of Psychology, 50*, 471–507.

Barker, D. J. (2004). The developmental origins of adult disease. *Journal of the American College of Nutrition, 23*(6, Suppl.), 588S–595S.

Bartley, M., Blane, D., & Montgomery, S. (1997). Health and the life course: Why safety nets matter. *British Medical Journal, 314*(7088), 1194–1196.

Bell, C. L., Chen, R., Masaki, K., Yee, P., He, Q., Grove, J., ... Willcox, B. J. (2014). Late-life factors associated with healthy aging in older men. *Journal of the American Geriatrics Society, 62*(5), 880–888.

Belley, A. M., Parisien, M., Nour, K., Bier, N., Ferland, G., Guay, D., ... Laforest, S. (2013). An ecological perspective on the determinants of the cognitive vitality of seniors. *Canadian Journal on Aging, 32*(3), 240–249.

Ben-Shlomo, Y., & Kuh, D. (2002). A life course approach to chronic disease epidemiology: Conceptual models, empirical challenges and interdisciplinary perspectives. *International Journal of Epidemiology, 31*(2), 285–293.

Benyamini, Y. (2011). Why does self-rated health predict mortality? An update on current knowledge and a research agenda for psychologists. *Psychology and Health, 26*(11), 1407–1413.

Berkman, L. F., & Glass, T. (2000). Social integration, social networks, social support, and health. In L. F. Berkman & I. Kawachi (Eds.), *Social epidemiology* (Vol. 1, pp. 137–173). Oxford, UK: Oxford University Press.

Blanchard, P., Bühlmann, F., & Gauthier, J. A. (2014). *Advances in sequence analysis: Theory, method, applications* (Vol. 2). New York, NY: Springer Publishing Company.

Blanchflower, D. G., & Oswald, A. J. (2008). Is well-being U-shaped over the life cycle? *Social Science and Medicine, 66*(8), 1733–1749.

Blane, D., Kelly-Irving, M., d'Errico, A., Bartley, M., & Montgomery, S. (2013). Social-biological transitions: How does the social become biological? *Longitudinal and Life Course Studies, 4*(2), 136–146.

Blane, D., Netuveli, G., & Stone, J. (2007). The development of life course epidemiology. *Revue d'Epidémiologie et de Santé Publique, 55*(1), 31–38.

Boerner, K., & Jopp, D. (2007). Improvement/maintenance and reorientation as central features of coping with major life change and loss: Contributions of three life-span theories. *Human Development, 50*(4), 171–195.

Bremner, J. D., & Narayan, M. (1998). The effects of stress on memory and the hippocampus throughout the life cycle: Implications for childhood development and aging. *Development and Psychopathology, 10*(4), 871–885.

Bronfenbrenner, U. (1986). Ecology of the family as a context for human development: Research perspectives. *Developmental Psychology, 22*(6), 723–742.

Charles, S. T., Reynolds, C. A., & Gatz, M. (2001). Age-related differences and change in positive and negative affect over 23 years. *Journal of Personality and Social Psychology, 80*(1), 136–151.

Clausen, J. A. (1995). *American lives: Looking back at the children of the great depression.* Oakland: University of California Press.

Cohen, R. A., Grieve, S., Hoth, K. F., Paul, R. H., Sweet, L., ... Williams, L. M. (2006). Early life stress and morphometry of the adult anterior cingulate cortex and caudate nuclei. *Biological Psychiatry, 59*(10), 975–982.

Dahlgren, G., & Whitehead, M. (2006). *European strategies for tackling social inequities in health: Levelling up part 2* (p. 149). Copenhagen, Denmark: World Health Organization.

Dannefer, D. (2003). Cumulative advantage/disadvantage and the life course: Cross-fertilizing age and social science theory. *The Journals of Gerontology, Series B, 58*(6), 327–337.

Dautovich, N. D., Dzierzewski, J. M., & Gum, A. M. (2014). Older adults display concurrent but not delayed associations between life stressors and depressive symptoms: A microlongitudinal study. *The American Journal of Geriatric Psychiatry, 22*(11), 1131–1139.

De Silva, M. J., McKenzie, K., Harpham, T., & Huttly, S. R. (2005). Social capital and mental illness: A systematic review. *Journal of Epidemiology and Community Health, 59*(8), 619–627.

Deary, I. J., Whalley, L. J., & Starr, J. M. (2009). *The Scottish mental surveys of 1932 and 1947.* Washington, DC: American Psychological Association.

Diener, E., Lucas, R. E., & Scollon, C. N. (2006). Beyond the hedonic treadmill: Revising the adaptation theory of well-being. *The American Psychologist, 61*(4), 305–314.

Dragano, N., Siegrist, J., & Wahrendorf, M. (2011). Welfare regimes, labour policies and unhealthy psychosocial working conditions: A comparative study with 9917 older employees from 12 European countries. *Journal of Epidemiology and Community Health, 65*(9), 793–799.

Dube, S. R., Anda, R. F., Felitti, V. J., Chapman, D. P., Williamson, D. F., & Giles, W. H. (2001). Childhood abuse, household dysfunction, and the risk of attempted suicide throughout the life span: Findings from the Adverse Childhood Experiences Study. *Journal of the American Medical Association, 286*(24), 3089–3096.

Elcheroth, G., Penic, S., Fasel, R., Giudici, F., Glaeser, S., Joye, D.,…Spini, D. (2013). Spatially weighted context data and their application to collective war experiences. *Sociological Methodology, 43*(1), 364–411.

Elder, G. H. (1974). *Children of the great depression: Social change in life experience.* Boulder, CO: Westview Press.

Elder, G. H., Jr., Johnson, M. K., & Crosnoe, R. (2003). The emergence and development of life course theory. In J. T. Mortimer & M. J. Shanahan (Eds.), *Handbook of the life course* (pp. 3–19). New York, NY: Springer Publishing Company.

Eriksson, J. G., Forsén, T., Tuomilehto, J., Osmond, C., & Barker, D. J. (2001). Early growth and coronary heart disease in later life: Longitudinal study. *British Medical Journal, 322*(7292), 949–953.

Ferraro, K. F., & Shippee, T. P. (2009). Aging and cumulative inequality: How does inequality get under the skin? *The Gerontologist, 49*(3), 333–343.

Fiske, A., Gatz, M., & Pedersen, N. L. (2003). Depressive symptoms and aging: The effects of illness and non-health-related events. *The Journals of Gerontology, Series B, 58*(6), 320–328.

Galenkamp, H., Deeg, D. J., Braam, A. W., & Huisman, M. (2013). "How was your health 3 years ago?" Predicting mortality in older adults using a retrospective change measure of self-rated health. *Geriatrics and Gerontology International, 13*(3), 678–686.

Gallo, W. T., Bradley, E. H., Siegel, M., & Kasl, S. V. (2000). Health effects of involuntary job loss among older workers: Findings from the health and retirement survey. *The Journals of Gerontology, Series B, 55*(3), 131–140.

Galobardes, B., Lynch, J. W., & Davey Smith, G. (2004). Childhood socioeconomic circumstances and cause-specific mortality in adulthood: Systematic review and interpretation. *Epidemiologic Reviews, 26*(1), 7–21.

Gauvin, L., Riva, M., Barnett, T., Richard, L., Craig, C. L., Spivock, M.,...Gagné, S. (2008). Association between neighborhood active living potential and walking. *American Journal of Epidemiology, 167*(8), 944–953.

George, L. K. (2009). Conceptualizing and measuring trajectories. In G. H. Elder, Jr. & J. Z. Giele (Eds.), *The craft of life course research* (pp. 163–186). New York, NY: Guilford Press.

Gerstorf, D., Hoppmann, C. A., & Ram, N. (2014). The promise and challenges of integrating multiple time-scales in adult developmental inquiry. *Research in Human Development, 11*(2), 75–90.

Girardin Keciour, M., & Spini, D. (2006). Well-being and frailty process in later life: An evaluation of the effectiveness of downward social comparison. *Schweizerische Zeitschrift für Soziologie, 32*(3), 389–406.

Glass, A. P., & Vander Plaats, R. S. (2013). A conceptual model for aging better together intentionally. *Journal of Aging Studies, 27*(4), 428–442.

Glei, D. A., Goldman, N., Liu, I. W., & Weinstein, M. (2013). Sex differences in trajectories of depressive symptoms among older Taiwanese: The contribution of selected stressors and social factors. *Aging and Mental Health, 17*(6), 773–783.

Gubrium, J. F. (1973). *The myth of the golden years: A socio-environmental theory of aging.* Springfield, IL: Thomas.

Guilley, E., Ghisletta, P., Armi, F., Berchtold, A., & Lalive d'Epinay, C. J. (2008). Individual health transitions between robustness ADL-independent frailty and ADL-dependence in late life. In E. Guilley & C. J. Lalive d'Epinay (Eds.), *The closing chapters of long lives* (pp. 29–36). New York, NY: Nova Science Publishers.

Huang, C., Li, Z., Wang, M., & Martorell, R. (2010). Early life exposure to the 1959–1961 Chinese famine has long-term health consequences. *The Journal of Nutrition, 140*(10), 1874–1878.

Hybels, C. F., Blazer, D. G., Landerman, L. R., & Steffens, D. C. (2011). Heterogeneity in symptom profiles among older adults diagnosed with major depression. *International Psychogeriatrics, 23*(6), 906–922.

Idler, E. L. (1993). Age differences in self-assessments of health: Age changes, cohort differences, or survivorship? *Journal of Gerontology, 48*(6), 289–300.

Irving, S. M., & Ferraro, K. F. (2006). Reports of abusive experiences during childhood and adult health ratings: Personal control as a pathway? *Journal of Aging and Health, 18*(3), 458–485.

Isaacowitz, D. M., & Smith, J. (2003). Positive and negative affect in very old age. *The Journals of Gerontology, Series B, 58*(3), P143–P152.

Islam, M. K., Merlo, J., Kawachi, I., Lindström, M., & Gerdtham, U. G. (2006). Social capital and health: Does egalitarianism matter? A literature review. *International Journal for Equity in Health, 5*, 3.

Jivraj, S., Nazroo, J., Vanhoutte, B., & Chandola, T. (2014). Aging and subjective well-being in later life. *The Journals of Gerontology, Series B, 69*(6), 930–941.

Jopp, D., & Rott, C. (2006). Adaptation in very old age: Exploring the role of resources, beliefs, and attitudes for centenarians' happiness. *Psychology and Aging, 21*(2), 266–280.

Jopp, D., Rott, C., & Oswald, F. (2008). Valuation of life in old and very old age: The role of sociodemographic, social, and health resources for positive adaptation. *The Gerontologist, 48*(5), 646–658.

Jopp, D., & Smith, J. (2006). Resources and life-management strategies as determinants of successful aging: On the protective effect of selection, optimization, and compensation. *Psychology and Aging, 21*(2), 253–265.

Kelley-Moore, J. A., & Lin, J. (2011). Widening the view: Capturing "unobserved" heterogeneity in studies of age and the life course. In R. A. Settersten & J. L. Angel (Eds.), *Handbook of sociology of aging* (pp. 51–68). New York, NY: Springer Publishing Company.

Kim, J. J., & Diamond, D. M. (2002). The stressed hippocampus, synaptic plasticity and lost memories. *Nature Reviews: Neuroscience, 3*(6), 453–462.

Kliegel, M., Moor, C., & Rott, C. (2004). Cognitive status and development in the oldest old: A longitudinal analysis from the Heidelberg Centenarian Study. *Archives of Gerontology and Geriatrics, 39*(2), 143–156.

Kuh, D., & Ben-Shlomo, Y. (1997). A lifecourse approach to the etiology of chronic diseases. In D. Kuh & Y. Ben-Shlomo (Eds.), *A lifecourse approach to chronic disease epidemiology* (pp. 3–14). Oxford, UK: Oxford University Press.

Kuh, D., Hardy, R., Langenberg, C., Richards, M., & Wadsworth, M. E. (2002). Mortality in adults aged 26–54 years related to socioeconomic conditions in childhood and adulthood: post war birth cohort study. *British Medical Journal, 325*(7372), 1076–1080.

Kunzmann, U., Little, T. D., & Smith, J. (2000). Is age-related stability of subjective well-being a paradox? Cross-sectional and longitudinal evidence from the Berlin Aging Study. *Psychology and Aging, 15*(3), 511–526.

Lalive d'Epinay, C., & Spini, D. (2008). *Les années fragiles: La vie au-delà de quatre-vingt ans* [The frailty years: Life beyond 80 years old]. Québec, Canada: Presses Universitaires de Laval.

Lalive d'Epinay, C. J., Guilley, E., Guillet, L., & Spini, D. (2008). The Swiss interdisciplinary longitudinal study on the oldest-old: Design and population. In E. Guilley & C. J. Lalive d'Epinay (Eds.), *The closing chapters of long lives* (pp. 9–26). New York, NY: Nova Science Publishers.

Lawton, M. P. (1980). *Environment and aging*. Monterey, CA: Brooks/Cole Publishing Company.

Lawton, M. P. (1983). Environment and other determinants of well-being in older people. *The Gerontologist, 23*(4), 349–357.

Lawton, M. P., & Nahemow, L. (1973). Ecology and the aging process. In C. Eisdorfer & M. P. Lawton (Eds.), *Psychology of adult development and aging* (pp. 619–674). Washington, DC: American Psychology Association.

Lazarus, R. S., & Folkman, S. (1984). *Stress, coping and adaptation*. New York, NY: Springer Publishing Company.

Leinonen, R., Heikkinen, E., & Jylhä, M. (1998). Self-rated health and self-assessed change in health in elderly men and women: A five-year longitudinal study. *Social Science and Medicine, 46*(4–5), 591–597.

Levy, R., & Pavie Team. (2007). Why look at life courses in an interdisciplinary perspective? In R. Levy, P. Ghisletta, J. M. Le Goff, D. Spini, & E. Widmer (Eds.), *Towards an interdisciplinary perspective on the life course* (Vol. 10, pp. 3–32). Amsterdam, The Netherlands: Elsevier.

Li, K. Z., Lindenberger, U., Freund, A. M., & Baltes, P. B. (2001). Walking while memorizing: Age-related differences in compensatory behavior. *Psychological Science, 12*(3), 230–237.

Lövdén, M., Ghisletta, P., & Lindenberger, U. (2005). Social participation attenuates decline in perceptual speed in old and very old age. *Psychology and Aging, 20*(3), 423–434.

Mathers, C. D., & Schofield, D. J. (1998). The health consequences of unemployment: The evidence. *Medical Journal of Australia, 168*(4), 178–182.

McArdle, J. J., & Ritschard, G. (2013). *Contemporary issues in exploratory data mining in the behavioral sciences*. Oxford, UK: Routledge.

McGuinness, D., McGlynn, L. M., Johnson, P. C., MacIntyre, A., Batty, G. D., Burns, H.,…Shiels, P. G. (2012). Socio-economic status is associated with epigenetic differences in the pSoBid cohort. *International Journal of Epidemiology, 41*(1), 151–160.

Moren-Cross, J. L., & Lin, N. (2006). Social networks and health. In R. H. Binstock, L. K. George, S. J. Cutler, J. Hendricks, & J. H. Schulz (Eds.), *Handbook of aging and the social sciences* (Vol. 6, pp. 111–126). Salt Lake City, UT: Academic Press.

Murayama, H., Fujiwara, Y., & Kawachi, I. (2012). Social capital and health: A review of prospective multilevel studies. *Journal of Epidemiology, 22*(3), 179–187.

Norenzayan, A., & Heine, S. J. (2005). Psychological universals: What are they and how can we know? *Psychological Bulletin, 131*(5), 763–784.

Oksanen, T., Vahtera, J., Westerlund, H., Pentti, J., Sjösten, N., Virtanen, M.,…Kivimäki, M. (2011). Is retirement beneficial for mental health?: Antidepressant use before and after retirement. *Epidemiology, 22*(4), 553–559.

Oswald, F., Jopp, D., Rott, C., & Wahl, H. W. (2011). Is aging in place a resource for or risk to life satisfaction? *The Gerontologist, 51*(2), 238–250.

Payette, H., & Shatenstein, B. (2005). Determinants of healthy eating in community-dwelling elderly people. *Canadian Journal of Public Health, 96*(Suppl. 3), 27–31.

Rafols, I., Leydesdorff, L., O'Hare, A., Nightingale, P., & Stirling, A. (2012). How journal rankings can suppress interdisciplinary research: A comparison between innovation studies and business & management. *Research Policy, 41*(7), 1262–1282.

Richard, L., Gauvin, L., & Raine, K. (2011). Ecological models revisited: Their uses and evolution in health promotion over two decades. *Annual Review of Public Health, 32*, 307–326.

Roberts, B. W., & Mroczek, D. (2008). Personality trait change in adulthood. *Current Directions in Psychological Science, 17*(1), 31–35.

Roberts, B. W., Walton, K. E., & Viechtbauer, W. (2006). Patterns of mean-level change in personality traits across the life course: A meta-analysis of longitudinal studies. *Psychological Bulletin, 132*(1), 1–25.

Röcke, C., Li, S.-C., & Smith, J. (2009). Intraindividual variability in positive and negative affect over 45 days: Do older adults fluctuate less than young adults? *Psychology and Aging, 24*(4), 863–878.

Rodin, J., & McAvay, G. (1992). Determinants of change in perceived health in a longitudinal study of older adults. *Journal of Gerontology, 47*(6), 373–384.

Rothermund, K., & Brandtstädter, J. (2003a). Coping with deficits and losses in later life: From compensatory action to accommodation. *Psychology and Aging, 18*(4), 896–905.

Rothermund, K., & Brandtstädter, J. (2003b). Depression in later life: Cross-sequential patterns and possible determinants. *Psychology and Aging, 18*(1), 80–90.

Rowe, J. W., & Kahn, R. L. (1997). Successful aging. *The Gerontologist, 37*(4), 433–440.

Rutter, M. (2000). Resilience reconsidered: Conceptual considerations, empirical findings, and policy implications. In J. P. Shonkoff & S. J. Meisels (Eds.), *Handbook of early childhood intervention* (2nd ed., Vol. 21, pp. 651–682). New York, NY: Cambridge University Press.

Schaie, K. W. (1993). The Seattle longitudinal studies of adult intelligence. *Current Directions in Psychological Science, 2*(6), 171–175.

Schaie, K. W., & Hofer, S. M. (2001). Longitudinal studies in aging research. In J. E. Birren & K. W. Schaie (Eds.), *Handbook of the psychology of aging* (5th ed., pp. 53–77). San Diego, CA: Academic Press.

Schröder-Butterfill, E., & Marianti, R. (2006). A framework for understanding old-age vulnerabilities. *Ageing and Society, 26*(1), 9–35.

Settersten, R. A., Jr. (2003). Invitation to the life course: The promise. In R. A. Settersten, Jr. (Ed.), *Invitation to the life course* (pp. 1–12). Amityville, NY: Baywood Publishing Company.

Shaw, B. A., & Krause, N. (2002). Exposure to physical violence during childhood, aging, and health. *Journal of Aging and Health, 14*(4), 467–494.

Sirven, N., & Debrand, T. (2012). Social capital and health of older Europeans: Causal pathways and health inequalities. *Social Science and Medicine, 75*(7), 1288–1295.

Sliwinski, M. J., Smyth, J. M., Hofer, S. M., & Stawski, R. S. (2006). Intraindividual coupling of daily stress and cognition. *Psychology and Aging, 21*(3), 545–557.

Snowdon, D. A., Kemper, S. J., Mortimer, J. A., Greiner, L. H., Wekstein, D. R., & Markesbery, W. R. (1996). Linguistic ability in early life and cognitive function and Alzheimer's disease in late life: Findings from the Nun Study. *Journal of the American Medical Association, 275*(7), 528–532.

Spini, D., Elcheroth, G., & Figini, D. (2008). Is there space for time in social psychology publications? A content analysis across five journals. *Journal of Community and Applied Social Psychology, 19*, 165–181.

Spini, D., Ghisletta, P., Guilley, E., & Lalive d'Epinay, C. (2007). Frail elderly. In J. E. Birren (Ed.), *Handbook of aging* (2nd ed., pp. 572–579). Oxford, UK: Elsevier.

Strachan, D. P., & Sheikh, A. (2004). A life course approach to respiratory and allergic diseases. In D. Kuh & Y. Ben-Shlomo (Eds.), *A life course approach to chronic disease epidemiology* (2nd ed., pp. 240–259). Oxford, UK: Oxford University Press.

Stringhini, S., Batty, G. D., Bovet, P., Shipley, M. J., Marmot, M. G., Kumari, M.,…Kivimäki, M. (2013). Association of lifecourse socioeconomic status with chronic inflammation and type 2 diabetes risk: The Whitehall II prospective cohort study. *PLoS Medicine, 10*(7), e1001479.

Stringhini, S., Polidoro, S., Sacerdote, C., Kelly, R. S., van Veldhoven, K., Agnoli, C., . . . Vineis, P. (2015). Life-course socioeconomic status and DNA methylation of genes regulating inflammation. *International Journal of Epidemiology, 44*(4), 1320–1330.

Swift, H. J., Vauclair, C. M., Abrams, D., Bratt, C., Marques, S., & Lima, M. L. (2014). Revisiting the paradox of well-being: The importance of national context. *The Journals of Gerontology, Series B, 69*(6), 920–929.

Taris, T. W., & Kompier, M. A. (2014). Cause and effect: Optimizing the designs of longitudinal studies in occupational health psychology. *Work & Stress, 28*(1), 1–8.

Taylor, M. G. (2010). Capturing transitions and trajectories: The role of socioeconomic status in later life disability. *The Journals of Gerontology, Series B, 65*(6), 733–743.

Taylor, M. G., & Lynch, S. M. (2011). Cohort differences and chronic disease profiles of differential disability trajectories. *The Journals of Gerontology, Series B, 66*(6), 729–738.

Teicher, M. H., Anderson, C. M., & Polcari, A. (2012). Childhood maltreatment is associated with reduced volume in the hippocampal subfields CA3, dentate gyrus, and subiculum. *Proceedings of the National Academy of Sciences of the United States of America, 109*(9), 563–572.

Tomasik, M. J., & Silbereisen, R. K. (2012). Beneficial effects of disengagement from futile struggles with occupational planning: A contextualist-motivational approach. *Developmental Psychology, 48*(6), 1785–1796.

Trzesniewski, K. H., Donnellan, M. B., & Robins, R. W. (2003). Stability of self-esteem across the life span. *Journal of Personality and Social Psychology, 84*(1), 205–220.

Turner, R. J., Wheaton, B., & Lloyd, D. A. (1995). The epidemiology of social stress. *American Sociological Review, 60*(1), 104–125.

Ulloa, B. F. L., Møller, V., & Sousa-Poza, A. (2013). How does subjective well-being evolve with age? A literature review. *Journal of Population Ageing, 6*(3), 227–246.

Vaillant, G. E. (2012). *Triumphs of experience.* Cambridge, MA: Harvard University Press.

Westerlund, H., Kivimäki, M., Singh-Manoux, A., Melchior, M., Ferrie, J. E., Pentti, J., . . . Vahtera, J. (2009). Self-rated health before and after retirement in France (GAZEL): A cohort study. *The Lancet, 374*(9705), 1889–1896.

Wickrama, K. K., Mancini, J. A., Kwag, K., & Kwon, J. (2013). Heterogeneity in multidimensional health trajectories of late old years and socioeconomic stratification: A latent trajectory class analysis. *The Journals of Gerontology, Series B, 68*(2), 290–297.

Wood, P. H. N. (1975). *International classification of impairments, disabilities, and handicaps.* Geneva, Switzerland: World Health Organization.

Wrzus, C., Hänel, M., Wagner, J., & Neyer, F. J. (2013). Social network changes and life events across the life span: A meta-analysis. *Psychological Bulletin, 139*(1), 53–80.

Zautra, A. J., Potter, P. T., & Riech, J. W. (1997). The independence of affect is context-dependent: An integrative model of the relationship between positive and negative affect. *Annual Review of Gerontology and Geriatrics, 17*(1), 75–103.

PART VII

Conclusion

CHAPTER 34

The Past as Prognosis: A Prismatic History of Theories of Aging

W. Andrew Achenbaum

The principle of Unripe Time is that people should not do at the present moment what they think right at that moment, because the moment which they think it is right has not yet arrived.

Cornford (1908, p. 64)

C. M. Cornford's observation is an apt epigraph for us. Several of gerontology's founders promulgated or borrowed theories to guide research on aging. Their approaches to theory building never proved quite timely, however. Those who applied grand theories rarely sustained explanations with acceptable data. Even now, most gerontological theories illuminate disciplinary-based perspectives more effectively than do interdisciplinary constructs.

Is Cornford's contention still relevant today? We do not need to inventory every theory to answer the question. Nor is another meta-theoretical analysis required (Achenbaum, 2009). What follows is a *prismatic* history (Weber & Orsborn, 2015)—a selective, select account of theory building in the field, which ideally stirs gerontological imaginations about future theoretical work.

■ LAYING THE FOUNDATIONS FOR THEORY BUILDING IN GERONTOLOGY

Cornford wrote *Microcosmographic academia* (1908) 5 years after Elie Metchnikoff first published *The Nature of Man* (1903). Philosophers and alchemists predated Metchnikoff by more than a millennium (Cole, 1992; Gruman, 1966), but it took that Nobel Laureate to coin the term "gerontology." Metchnikoff contended that "we must first understand the most intimate details of its mechanism" before "an optimistic philosophy of senescence" alleviated the ravages of age. Based on work in pathology, cytology, and immunology, Metchnikoff formulated "phagocytosis," an interdisciplinary theory of aging hypothesizing that large intestinal white blood cells destroyed microbes that hastened premature senility in humans, apes, dogs, and plants (Metchnikoff, 1908); the construct anticipated various degenerative and wear-and-tear theories. Peers discounted both Metchnikoff's attempt at grand theory making and his remedy (eating yoghurt, Metchnikoff believed, could kill pathological macrophages) all the while supporting his commitment to scientific method.

Acknowledging that Metchnikoff's theory was "the most prominent theory of age-ing today" (1914, p. 41), I. L. Nascher nevertheless proceeded differently in *Geriatrics*. Nascher, a physician who cared for aging patients in clinics and almshouses, challenged Metchnikoff's premise—one grounded in conventional wisdom—that old age was a chronic disease. Instead, Nascher identified later years as an age-specific, physiological stage of life. He weighed causes of aging in terms of averages.

Nascher distinguished normal processes of aging from diseases. "Many theories have been advanced to account for this ageing," Nascher declared (1914, p. 39). "A scientific theory of life must have a comprehensible basis though we may not be able to prove the theory or the existence of the basis, with our present methods of investigation." The observation underlined the paucity of efficacious theory building during gerontology's formative decades. (In 1926, Nascher admitted to being the only geriatrician in the United States.) Nascher proved more adept at debunking late-19th century theories about gland degeneration as a pathological cause of aging (as set forth by Sir Victor Horsley and by Arnold Lorand) than advancing his theory of tissue–cell evolution "based upon some facts and some assumptions" (Nascher, 1914, pp. 42–43; see also, Nascher, 1926). There were grounds for sharp disagreement about whether aging is a disease or whether senescence is a natural process.

■ EARLY CROSS-DISCIPLINARY AND DISCIPLINARY-BASED AGE-SPECIFIC APPROACHES TO THEORY BUILDING

Retired psychologist G. Stanley Hall melded his interests in old age and death in *Senescence* (1922), a bookend to his definitive two-volume exposition of *Adolescence* (1904). "There are few specialists in gerontology even among physicians," Hall realized (1922, p. 8). "I was alone, indeed in a new kind of solitude, and must pursue the rest of my life in a way in life by a more or less individual research as to how to keep well and at the top of my condition" (Hall, 1922, p. 15). A student of William James, Hall sought to smash "cheap and chipper paradoxes" (1922, p. 133) through inductive reasoning.

Chapters 2 and 3 of *Senescence* showcased cross-disciplinary research in gerontology, gleaning insights from historical and literary perspectives. Besides presenting cross-national statistics on old age, its care as well as medical interventions, Hall (1922, p. 257) critiqued efforts at theory building by Metchnikoff and other biomedical researchers. Hall then offered results from a survey in which he "selected a few score of names of mostly eminent and some very distinguished old people, both acquaintances and strangers" (Hall, 1922, p. 321). Responses revealed surprisingly diverse feelings about growing older, and practicalities about diet and hygiene, and intergenerational ties.

In lieu of grand theory, Hall delivered a "thesis" of aging that undercut prevailing notions of decline and obsolescence:

> Intelligent and well-conserved senectitude has very important social and anthropological functions in the modern world not hitherto utilized or even recognized. The chief of these is most comprehensively designated by the general term synthesis (Hall, 1922, p. 405).

Rather than equate senectitude with senility, *Senescence* looked forward to latter-day models of "successful aging." Furthermore, half a century before the Riley's analysis of aging and society (1969–1972), Hall demonstrated how structural and cultural lags impede meaningful aging. *Senescence* did not conclude on an uplifting note; the last

80 pages treat the psychology of death, bolstered with references from Scripture, science, and philosophy. Like Metchnikoff, Hall believed that gerontology must take account of finitude.

G. Stanley Hall tried to incorporate cross-disciplinary insights into a multifaceted model of aging; his contemporaries in the biomedical sciences held that any quest for a unified science of gerontology was futile (Achenbaum, 1995, pp. 54–84). To advance gerontological knowledge between the World Wars meant giving the best minds resources to solve complex puzzles, with results disseminated to the scientific community. A few learned societies and foundations promoted gerontology. "Here was virgin territory with broad implications for many of the biological, medical, and social sciences," recalled an officer of the Josiah Macy, Jr. Foundation (1950, p. 32). "Here was an opportunity for a foundation to assist in the development of a new field of science which, by its nature, demanded the integration of data, methods, and concepts from many special branches—a coordinate, multi-professional approach."

The Josiah Macy, Jr. Foundation invited Edmund V. Cowdry, an anatomist and cytologist who had compiled a handbook on arteriosclerosis, to assemble a team to probe *Problems of Ageing* (1939). Cowdry recruited 25 stars, men who knew each other's research from conferences at Woods Hole or through the Union of American Biologists. In 758 pages, the collaborators reported how their particular disciplines illuminated specific mechanisms or processes of aging—in plants, insects, invertebrates, and vertebrates. Others dealt with human cells, tissues, organs, functions, or systems. Cowdry commissioned one chapter on longevity, one each on anthropology and psychology, and a final contribution from a clinician. Significantly, no author proposed a cross- or inter-disciplinary theory of aging in *Problems of Ageing*, though investigators subsequently adapted for their own purposes the "ageing of homeostatic mechanisms" (Cannon, 1939, p. 624), which rested on theories of a 19th-century physiologist.

Reflexivity in Foundational Gerontological Theory Building

Two contributors to Cowdry's *Problems of Ageing* entertained issues of cause and effect in aging. Columbia University philosopher John Dewey insisted more work be done before surveying common ground across disciplines. "The present volume of studies is itself evidence of the new recognition of the importance of the problem of ageing," observed Dewey (1939, p. 22). "They provide the needed base line, for they disclose basic conditions which in any case must be taken into account." Investigators had to describe basic conditions as they determined methods and means that bridged the cellular and organic, biological processes, and cultural norms. "Biological processes are at the root of the problems and of the methods of solving them, but the biological processes take place in economic, political, and cultural contexts" (Dewey, 1939, p. 26). Dewey privileged biology because "biology as a science brings to the foreground of attention the significance of growth in a way in which underlying physical sciences do not" (Dewey, 1939).

Lawrence K. Frank, a Macy Foundation's program officer, emphasized interdisciplinary syntheses more than Dewey. Frank (like Metchnikoff and Nascher) wished to disentangle "cumulative but physiological involutions that inevitably take place in all individuals as they grow older, and pathological changes that occur in ageing individuals as the result of adverse environmental conditions" (Frank, 1939, p. 13). In three ways, Frank endeavored to reframe recent work in gerontology. First Frank, a social psychologist who studied child development, urged a life-course approach. He wanted to determine whether "changes represent the process of ageing or rather pathological deviations which conceivably might have been avoided or minimized in early years" (Frank, 1939, p. 16). Second, Frank (1946, p. 3) probed the relationship between time and aging: He shared Alexis Carrel's opinion that chronological time failed to differentiate rates of aging within and across organisms. Third, lacking a general theory of aging, Frank nonetheless urged gerontologists to consider the "fruitfulness of the 'field' concept in embryology" (Frank, 1939, p. 16) in measuring structural changes in organisms.

"The lack of theoretical clarity," declared Frank (1946, p. 7), hampered gerontology, "an enterprise calling for many and diversified studies." He added that "for an adequate formulation of the larger problem of aging, field theory may offer a much needed conceptual tool for grasping the totality of organic structures and functioning" through basic and applied research. Invoking Dr. George Morris Piersol's vision of "not more years to life, but more life to years," Frank recommended "creating new designs for living in and through which the aging individual can find what will be appropriate to his needs, capacities and interests" (Frank, 1946, p. 10). Multidisciplinary perspectives, he stressed, "command the interest and devotion of a variety of scientists, scholars, and professional workers, all of whom are needed to study such problems as human growth, development and aging, ecology and regional planning, mental hygiene, human conservation, or cultural change" (Frank, 1946, p. 1).

Postwar Pioneers Do Not Resolve Theoretical Debates in Gerontology

By the time that the third, expanded edition of *Cowdry's Problems of Ageing* appeared (Lansing, 1952), two scientific organizations—the American Geriatrics Society (1942) and the Gerontological Society of America (GSA, 1945)—had been organized. Among the newly emergent gerontologists, three individuals epitomize divergent engagements in theory building.

Physiologist Nathan W. Shock (1906–1989) did postdoctoral training with Lawrence K. Frank. Like Hall, he sought insights in gerontology from any reliable sources. Shock published more than 350 research articles on biochemical, behavioral, and physiological aspects of aging. He built the Gerontology Research Center and launched the Baltimore Longitudinal Studies in Aging.

Shock, however, did not emphasize theory building. "Research is a technical operation," Shock noted in *Trends in Gerontology* (1952, p. 114). "This formulation of questions and the design of adequately controlled procedure of adequately controlled procedures and observations are the essence of research." Measurements, he insisted, decomposed big issues into manageable questions. Shock encouraged trainees (including three future GSA presidents) to generate well-documented "facts" in measuring differences between aging and disease. "Give me a testable hypothesis," Shock stated. "It is worth a thousand theories" (Achenbaum & Albert, 1995, p. 324).

James E. Birren (1918–2016) collaborated on aging projects with Nathan Shock at the National Institutes of Health, and then spent most of his career based in Los Angeles, promoting research and training in gerontology, and "investigating how biological and environmental factors modulated behavioral expressions of physiological mechanisms" (Achenbaum & Albert, 1995, p. 35). In the scientific tradition of Cowdry's *Problems of Ageing*, Birren compiled multiple editions of aging handbooks and several encyclopedia of gerontology.

Like Cowdry, Birren favored expansively disciplinary inquiries that ultimately would advance an integrative science. "There is an opportunity for many kinds of significant research," declared Birren (1961, p. 40), "and in the diversity of our studies we should be increasingly explicit about our (sic) *problems, theories, designs, controls, methods,* and *analyses of results.*" Birren often repeated these keywords in terms of "counterpart theory," a pluralistic paradigm amenable to analyses of concepts and methods. He used metaphors such as "senescing," "eldering," and "geronting" to refer to biological, social, and psychological processes. Although advocating for unity in the gerontological sciences, Birren bemoaned the field's fragmentation. "Current theories in gerontology are actually microtheories," he declared (1988, p. 9), "they do not, in general embrace larger perspectives or information from different domains of the behavioral, social, and biological sciences or from the humanities."

Early in a career spent mainly in medical facilities, Robert Kastenbaum (1933–2013) emerged as an important theory builder in aging. Like Frank and Birren, he pursued the relationship of time to human development, as well as to habituation and death. "In Theories of Aging: The Search for a Conceptual Framework" (1965), Kastenbaum underscored the divergence between biomedical and psychosocial processes. "Aging is a multilevel phenomenon, either in a systematic or random sense" (1965, p.17).

Kastenbaum saw possibilities for convergence: "Although not all theories move with equal ease in all directions, there is also the shared conviction that one must somehow come to terms with phenomena at all levels of human behavior and experience" (1965, p. 35). Later Kastenbaum echoed Birren's concern about what his colleagues fragmentized: "I do not know which is more peculiar: disciplined biological research veering off into uncontrolled, speculative morality, or psychosocial theory concerned with the quality of inner experience and the entire network of human relationships" (1978, p. 62). Experts surely need to specialize, Kastenbaum affirmed, but they should also enrich understandings of aging's totality.

At least two consistent themes emerge from this prismatic perspective on the formative period of gerontological theory building. On the one hand, most writers grappled with distinguishing between aging and disease. "Everyone aspires to a long life, but no one wants to be old" (Shock, 1961, p. 14). On the other hand, gerontology's founders valued cross-disciplinary investigations as well as disciplinary-specific research. However aspects of aging were categorized—macro/micro, by genus or species, or in terms of biomedical/psychosocial—gerontologists wished to incorporate the most appropriate tools and techniques to address the particular problem of aging under investigation.

The field's founding fathers did not leave a clear, consistent set of opinions concerning the role of theory in explaining processes and mechanisms of senescence. Disparate approaches to problem solving presage conceptual disputes in gerontology today. To Shock and many contributors to Cowdry's *Problems of Ageing*, theories detracted attention from the pressing task of studying phenomena using appropriate measurements. To others, like Nascher and Cowdry, distinguishing between pathological and physiological dimensions sufficed. Metchnikoff, on the other hand, based investigations on theory. Frank thought the science of gerontology would flourish once investigators adopted a construct (like field theory) pliable in different scientific settings. Birren saw value in mini theories, though (like Cannon) he found models and metaphors adequate in the absence of formal theory. How ironic, then, that a grand theory of aging polarized gerontologists in the 1960s.

Theories of Successful Aging, Disengagement, and Adjustment/Activity

"The science of gerontology has its practical purpose," began Robert J. Havighurst in *The Gerontologist*'s premier issue. "In order to give good advice, it is essential that gerontology have a theory of successful aging" (Havighurst, 1961, p. 8). Havighurst's hortatory comment signaled a new phase in gerontological theory building. Theories were to be taken seriously as explanatory vehicles. Havighurst took steps to ensure that the behavioral and social sciences shaped ideas.

Long before Rowe and Kahn's *Successful Aging* (1998), Havighurst noted that two theories of successful aging prevailed in the field. Activity Theory, "favored by most of the practical workers in the field of gerontology" (Havighurst, 1961, p. 8), posited that maintaining attitudes and activities associated with middle age as long and as far as possible promoted successful aging. In contrast, proponents of Disengagement Theory hypothesized that successfully aging individuals accepted and acquiesced to the process of withdrawing from active life. Before privileging either competing model, recommended Havighurst, researchers had to settle on "an operational definition of successful aging and a method of measuring the degree to which people fit this definition" (Havighurst, 1961, p. 9).

Havighurst realized that his peers would resist, but until investigators could describe successful aging, they "should not assume that either activity or disengagement is desirable" (Havighurst, 1961). Theory testing would be difficult: "There are a number of procedures for the measurement of successful aging, and all of them have been criticized" (Havighurst, 1961). Havighurst nonetheless thought it "possible to develop an instrument [such as he constructed with Albrecht (Havighurst & Albrecht, 1953)] to measure the social acceptability of a person's behavior and consequently the degree of his success in aging" (Havighurst, 1961). "As long as there is disagreement as to what constitutes successful aging, caution must be used in selecting measures of successful aging" (Havighurst, 1961, p. 12).

Although gerontologists in 1961 had neither an overarching paradigm nor agreed-on measurements, Havighurst believed that merging elements of activity and disengagement theories could explain processes of aging:

> Undoubtedly there is a disengaging force operating on and within people as they pass 70 and 80. But they will still retain the personality-lifestyle characteristics of their middle years; those who were happy and satisfied by being active and productive then will continue to be happy and satisfied if they can maintain a considerable part of their activity and productiveness; and those who were happy and satisfied by being relatively passive and dependent in their middle years will be happy and satisfied if they can become even more disengaged in their later years (Havighurst, 1961)

Havighurst deployed integrative theory building in gerontology. "Successful aging," he believed, required a life-course perspective to explain diverse patterns of senescing. Attitudes and activities in later years vary; perspectives and values change over time. Nevertheless, advocates of the Disengagement Theory, Havighurst predicted, would reject measurement scales for Activity Theory, and vice versa.

At 61 years, Robert J. Havighurst was a respected idea-broker (Achenbaum & Albert, 1995, pp. 158–161). He chaired the University of Chicago's Committee on Human Development (CHD), after teaching physics and chemistry. In the 1930s, he was at the Rockefeller Foundation and then moved to the Macy Foundation to work with

Lawrence Frank. At Chicago, with colleagues in psychology, anthropology, sociology, and education, he made CHD a premier center for research and training in gerontology. Havighurst's own policy-relevant studies dealt with the personality development of Native American children. After World War II, Havighurst studied seniors' activities and resilience; he published *Personal Adjustment in Old Age* with Ruth Shonle Cavan (1949), *Older People* with Ruth Albrecht (1953), and *The Meaning of Work and Retirement* with E. A. Friedmann & R. J. Havighurst (1954). A grant from the Carnegie Corporation supported CHD faculty and students in the field, a decade-long inquiry in Kansas City into middle age and aging. Disengagement and Activity theorists gathered data that they interpreted radically differently.

Theoretical disagreements between the Disengagement and Activity teams have been ably analyzed (Achenbaum & Bengtson, 1994; Hochschild, 1975; Lynott & Lynott, 1996; Thornstam, 1989). Elaine Cumming and William Henry in *Growing Old: The Process of Disengagement* said that (a) they had developed "an inductive theory of aging to fit [their] data" and (b) postulated that "aging is an inevitable, mutual withdrawal or disengagement, resulting in decreased interaction between the aging person and others in the social system he belongs to" (Cumming & Henry, 1961, p. 14, 227). Disengagement Theory had merits. *Many* people did withdraw from everyday activities. Cumming and Henry (1961, p. 227) shared Shock's opinion that "there is nothing so practical as a good theory." *Growing Old*'s modus operandi resembled homeostatic maneuvers, moving from concept to data and then back again. "This [is] an important book," Talcott Parsons proclaimed in his Foreword, "probably the most serious attempt to put forward a general theoretical interpretation of the social and psychological nature of the aging process in American society."

Yet criticisms immediately surfaced about Disengagement Theory. At CHD debaters clashed over the operational definitions and measurements grounding gerontological theory. Intellectual jousting usually sharpens critical thinking, but protagonists held fast to their positions in Unripe Time. Havighurst thought the Kansas City data undercut the inexorability of disengagement; his investigators portrayed the old as active, adjusting sights to fit their stamina. Bernice Neugarten cautioned against falsely assuming that senescence was homogeneous; variations in gender, race, and class created disparate pathways to aging. To presume that biology is destiny (to her) was unfounded.

No theorist won the Disengagement–Activity debate. Cumming and Henry disengaged from gerontology. Havighurst pursued topics in aging while studying children and youth. Neugarten evenhandedly criticized Disengagement Theory in *Middle Age and Aging* (1968), while designing paradigms of age she would apply in federal policy circles. Disengagement Theory was shelved.

The controversy over *Growing Old* represents an important moment in the history of theories of age and aging. The debate underscored the necessity to unveil sound, empirically grounded ideas. However, most researchers sought promotions and raises in home departments over pursuing gerontological reputations. In the vagaries of Unripe Time, gerontologists could postpone theory building.

Disengagement Theory's fate, of course, was not the only disincentive to theory building in gerontology from (roughly) the mid-1960s to the 1980s. Bench scientists proposed scores of explanatory theories about cells, rarely useful to psychologists or social workers. In their rhetoric gerontologists lauded integrative puzzle solving, knowing that their efforts were vetted by peers in one of the Gerontological Society's divisions. Basic and applied researchers rarely collaborated.

The gerontology community prioritized microtheories, not grand syntheses, as building blocks. "The major new concern then came to be the dialectical relationship between fact and explanation," contended Lynott and Lynott (1996, p. 754); "our understanding of the facts of aging not only grows with their accumulation, but with the transformations in our understanding as well." Gerontologists honed existing modes of scientific measurement. "One's confidence in truth telling and knowledge building is contingent upon the reliability of evidence under scrutiny," observed Bookstein and Achenbaum (1993, p. 21). "Researchers must believe that the observations that they and their colleagues generate bear close correspondence to the reality they purport to describe."

Critiquing a Proliferation of Microtheories and Metatheories in Aging

Emergent Theories of Aging, edited by James Birren and Vern Bengtson, represents a major step to promote interest in gerontological theory building: "The present volume is an attempt by researchers to begin to address the data-rich but theory-poor state of the current research on aging, and to encourage cross-disciplinary interchange that focuses on theory development in aging" (1988, p. 9). Birren and Gary Kenyon (1986), unpublished prepared a catalog of roughly 225 works dealing with theories of aging in biology, psychology, sociology, and the humanities. "The wide scope of the field and, more recently, the high level of its activity and research productivity have resulted in the creation of islands of knowledge with little communication between them," stated Birren and Bengtson (1988, p. 9). "Current theories in gerontology are actually microtheories; they do not, in general, embrace larger perspectives or information from the different domains." Were the pair right that the time had come to stop treating theory building in gerontology as a secondary issue?

For more than 25 years, interest has grown in gerontological theory making. Increasing specialization and the advent of new (hybrid) fields of inquiry, however, entice researchers in aging to explain more and more about less and less. Practitioners still tend to use theories from their own or adjoining disciplines, although the aging community increasingly welcomes its own cross-disciplinary theories and interdisciplinary models.

Metatheories of aging have become important, because they embody "consilience": interlocking strands of principles and rules that describe and direct scientific exploration: "A balanced perspective cannot be acquired by studying disciplines in pieces; the consilience gives purpose to intellect. It promises that order not chaos lies beyond the horizon" (Wilson, 1988). Biologist Vincent Cristofalo (1996), endorsing no unified biological theory of aging, reduced models into groupings of stochastic and developmental-genetic theories. Joannes J. F. Schroots (1996, p. 743), who presented a dozen theories of aging, cited Birren's contention that "there is no major theory or underlying metaphor that links the various areas of psychology." Social scientists created normative models, linkages, and interpretations (Marshall, 1999, p. 438). Glenn Elder (1998) and Peter Uhlenberg (2004) trumpeted life-course theories, which prompted "Cumulative Advantage/Disadvantage" theory (Dannefer, 2000) and an "Aging and Cumulative Inequality" model (Ferraro & Shippee, 2009), respectively.

New voices joined the conversation, "identifying *themes of meaning* that emerge from their research" (Bengtson, Parrott, & Burgess, 1996, p. 769). First, experts in the humanities occasionally played Cassandra. *The Need for Theory: Critical Approaches to Social Gerontology* castigated both *Emergent Theories of Aging* and its successor (Bengtson & Schaie, 1999): "What emerged was a surprisingly atheoretical handbook on theory. Perhaps it is reflective of the historic nature of the field rather than the state of the art" (Biggs, Lowenstein, & Hendricks, 2003, p. 3; see also Krause & Bastida, 2009, p. 112). Second, as feminist theorists (Holstein,1999; Ray, 2006) listened to inner voices of aging, Carroll Estes (2001) dissected gendered dysfunctions in policy and practice. Third, macrotheorists bridged the gap among theory, observations, and practice: "A well-grounded theory and a well-theorized applied model hold great promise by generating further research by giving direction, articulating, and specifying more stringent conditions for the development of knowledge" (Hendricks, Applebaum, & Kunkel, 2010, p. 293).

"We feel that there is a need to reestablish the importance of theory in the discourse about problems of aging," announced Vern Bengtson and Warner Schaie in the first edition of the *Handbook of Theories of Aging*. "We feel it is valuable to emphasize the primacy of explanations in the vastly expanding scientific literature reporting empirical findings about aging" (Bengtson & Schaie, 1999, p. 9). Bengtson and his associate editors (2009, p. 22) showcased "attempts to explain" in the second edition of the *Handbook of the Theories of Aging*. Contributors were encouraged to cross disciplinary boundaries in explicating processes of aging. "Perhaps nowhere is this more visible than in the growth of cross-disciplinary studies concerning the mechanisms of aging" (Bengtson & Schaie, 2009, p. 21).

Despite much progress, cultural lags and structural barriers remained. Achenbaum and Levin (1989) recounted historical disputes over definitions of gerontology (see also, Bass, 2013, p. 7). Settersten and Dobransky (2000, p. 369) underscored different disconnects: "As biological phenomena are theorized, they are more isolated from the psychological and social; as psychological phenomena are theorized, they more often incorporate the biological; and as social phenomena are theorized, they are more often considered in the conjunction with the biological and psychological" (see also Bengtson et al., 1999, pp. 22–23). Kenneth Ferraro (2008, p. 4), reviewing the "greatest hits" cited in the *The Journals of Gerontology*, substantiated Shock's observation that "measurement is the basis of all science." From this perspective, methods trump ideas.

Theory's place in major texts on aging remains mixed. In the lead chapter of the *Cambridge Handbook of Age and Aging* (Johnson et al., 2005) addresses "the problem of theory in gerontology today" and devotes 20 lines to the topic in the index. Theorists Dale Dannefer and Chris Phillipson, in contrast, included neither a chapter nor references to "theory" in the index of their *The Sage Handbook of Social Gerontology* (Dannefer & Phillipson, 2010). In *Successful Aging*, John Rowe and Robert Kahn (1998, p. 12) were "committed to an interdisciplinary research program . . . which was actually a coherent set of dozens of individual research projects," not bound by any overarching theory of aging.

Connections deepen between theory and research—"When there is not a body of relevant theory, researchers often do not know where to turn" (Longino, 2005, p. 172)—yet impediments deter progress. "Part of gerontology's strength—its explicit drawing upon a range of disciplines to understand the aging individual within a societal context—has also been part of its difficulty in building fundamental theoretical constructs" (Bass, 2006, p. 139). Historical interpretations, which might inform theory building, appear more taxonomic than heuristic. Jon Hendricks (1992), weary of disembodied ideas, reconstructed the succession of scholarly attempts to study aging. Alluding to Hendricks's generational history, Vern Bengtson and associates argued (1997, p. 76) that "previous successes (and failures) at explanation provide crucial viewpoints from which to assess the adequacy of our own empirical efforts" (see also Marshall, 1999, p. 436).

■ IS IT WORTH RECONSTRUCTING A USEABLE PAST IN GERONTOLOGICAL THEORY BUILDING?

Gerontologists demolished Disengagement Theory in Unripe Time. Not even a giant like Robert Havighurst could salvage parts of Activity Theory in order to sustain his pioneering theory of successful aging. Ironically, in this highly competitive era for diminishing resources, it finally might prove timely to recover theories from our collective past. For instance, there are underappreciated corollaries in Cumming and Henry's *Growing old*, which could trigger investigations, such as the authors' explications of gender disparities (1961) and generational tensions (1961). Two other motifs merit elaboration:

First is the study of the "fourth age." "Very old people often have a surprisingly high level of social competence and seem able to maintain high spirits," Cumming and Henry declared (1961, pp. 201–202). "There may be a group of people who, more than being merely survivors, have a special biological invulnerability." Americans usually focus on the young and the old whereas many British scholars are fascinated with the dimensions of advanced years. Although "'old age' proper becomes tautologically synonymous with decline," notes Susan Pickard (2014, pp. 1279–1280),

> positive experiences of embodiment in the 'fourth age' point the way to extending the space of self-actualisation to the whole life span where currently the fear of ageing casts its long shadow far into youth, as well as encouraging increasing recognition of, and research focus upon, ambiguous categories such as the good life in old age. (Pickard, 2014, p. 1289)

The second issue deals with aging and death. "As a matter of fact, death is excluded from most of the literature on aging, and it emerges only occasionally as if by accident," Cumming and Henry (1961, p. 18) noted. "This is probably a direct consequence of the belief in the desirability of an ever-expanding life." (Pickard, 2014) Few theories yet conjoin gerontology and thanatology. "Whatever the reasons, there is a marked aversion to addressing end-of-life issues among researchers and writers on aging," opines Malcolm Johnson's Handbook (2009, p. 659).

> While we may describe our field of study as 'the study of aging and the life span,' comparatively little attention is given in the literature to the far end of life span— death—or psychosocial aspects of the endings of lives. (Johnson, 2009, p. 659)

Having arrived at Ripe Time, what should gerontologists do? Should they echo Henry Ford's claim that "history is bunk?" Or, should theoreticians reconstruct a useable past? At the least, it makes sense to revisit Metchnikoff and Hall who theorized about the old–old and death, incorporating dependency, debility, and demise into a web of positivist paradigms. The exercise might induce the current generation of gerontologists to think out of the box, to integrate gerontological insights with ideas advanced by disability experts or Queer theorists, whose theoretical literature is richer than ours. We might look inward to theories of global aging or legal/financial gerontology. There are bound to be pay-offs: "Time can and should play a more important role because it can change the ontological description and meaning of a theoretical construct and of the relationships between constructs" (George & Jones, 2000, p. 657). To the extent that past masters serve as prognosticators, empirically tested, historical nuggets might prompt a paradigm shift in how we perceive and experience aging. Rather than shelve what we deem to be obsolescent theories, emerging scholars' critical thinking about our roots just might advance gerontological theory building in fruitful and timely ways.

REFERENCES

Achenbaum, W. A. (1995). *Crossing frontiers: Gerontology emerges as a science*. New York, NY: Cambridge University Press.

Achenbaum, W. A. (2009). A metahistorical perspective on theories of aging. In V. L. Bengtson, N. Putney, D. Gans, & M. Silverstein (Eds.), *Handbook of theories of aging* (2nd ed., pp. 25–38). New York, NY: Springer Publishing Company.

Achenbaum, W. A., & Albert, D. M. (1995). *Profiles in gerontology*. Westport, CT: Greenwood.

Achenbaum, W. A., & Bengtson, V. L. (1994). Re-engaging the disengagement theory of aging. *The Gerontologist, 34*, 756–763.

Achenbaum, W. A., & Levin, J. S. (1989). What does gerontology mean? *The Gerontologist, 29*, 393–400.

Bass, S. A. (2006). Gerontological theory. *The Gerontologist, 46*, 139–144.

Bass, S. A. (2013). The state of gerontology. *The Gerontologist, 53*, 1–9.

Bengtson, V. L., Burgess, E. O., & Parrott, T. M. (1997). Theoretic experience and a third generation of theoretical development in social gerontology. *The Journals of Gerontology, Series B, 52*, S372–S388.

Bengtson, V. L., Parrott, T. M., & Burgess, E. O. (1996). Progress and pitfalls in gerontological theorizing. *The Gerontologist, 36*, 768–772.

Bengtson, V. L., & Schaie, K. W. (Eds.). (1999). *Handbook of theories of aging*. New York, NY: Springer Publishing Company.

Biggs, S., Lowenstein, A., & Hendricks, J. (Eds.). (2003). *The need for theory: Critical approaches to social gerontology*. Amityville, NY: Baywood Publishing.

Birren, J. E. (1961). Principles of research on aging. In J. E. Birren (Ed.), *Handbook of aging and the individual* (pp. 3–42). Chicago, IL: University of Chicago Press.

Birren, J. E., & Bengtson, V. L. (Eds.). (1988). *Emergent theories of aging*. New York, NY: Springer Publishing Company.

Bookstein, F. L., & Achenbaum, W. A. (1993). Aging as explanation. In T. R. Cole et al. (Eds.), *Voices and visions*. New York, NY: Springer Publishing Company.

Cannon, W. (1939). Ageing of homeostatic mechanisms. In E. V. Cowdry (Ed.), *Problems of ageing* (pp. 623–642). Baltimore, MD: Lippincott Williams & Wilkins.

Cavan, R. (1949). *Personal adjustment in old age*. New York, NY: Longmans, Green.

Cole, T. R. (1992). *The journey of life*. New York, NY: Cambridge University Press.

Cornford, C. M. (1908). *Microcosmographia academica: Being a guide to young academic politicians*. Cambridge, UK: Bowes and Bowes.

Cowdry, E. V. (1939). *Problems of ageing*. Baltimore, MD: Lippincott Williams & Wilkins.

Cristofalo, V. J. (1996). Ten years later. *The Gerontologist, 36*, 737–741.

Cumming, E., & Henry, W. E. (1961). *Growing old: The process of disengagement*. New York, NY: Basic Books.

Dannefer, D. (2000). Cumulative advantage/disadvantage and the life course. *The Journals of Gerontology, Series B, 58*, S327–S337.

Dannefer, D., & Phillipson, C. (Eds.). (2010). *The Sage handbook of social gerontology.* Thousand Oaks, CA: Sage.

Dewey, J. (1939). Introduction. In E. V. Cowdry (Ed.), *Problems of ageing* (pp. 19–27). Baltimore, MD: Lippincott Williams & Wilkins.

Elder, G. (1998). *The children of the great depression.* Chicago, IL: University of Chicago Press.

Estes, C. (2001). *Social policy & aging.* Thousand Oaks, CA: Sage.

Ferraro, K. E., & Schaefer, M. (2008). Gerontology's greatest hits. *The Journals of Gerontology, Series B, 63,* S83–S86.

Ferraro, K., & Shippee, T. P. (2009). Aging and cumulative inequality. *The Gerontologist, 49,* 333–343.

Frank, L. K. (1939). Foreword. In E. V. Cowdry (Ed.), *Problems of ageing* (pp. 13–18). Baltimore, MD: Lippincott Williams & Wilkins.

Frank, L. K. (1946). Gerontology. *Journal of Gerontology, 1,* 1–11.

Friedman, E. A., & Havighurst, R. J. (1954). *Meaning of work and retirement.* Chicago, IL: University of Chicago Press.

George, J. M., & Jones, G. R. (2000). The role of time in theory and theory building. *Journal of Management, 26,* 657–684.

Gruman, G. J. (1966). *A history of ideas about the prolongation of life.* New York, NY: The American Philosophical Society.

Gruman, G. J. (2003). *A history of ideas about the prolongation of life.* New York, NY: Springer Publishing Company (Reprint).

Hall, G. S. (1904). *Adolescence* (2nd Vol.). New York, NY: D. Appleton and Company.

Hall, G. S. (1922). *Senescence: The last half of life.* New York, NY: D. Appleton and Company.

Havighurst, R. J. (1961). Successful aging. *The Gerontologist, 1,* 8–13.

Havighurst, R. J., & Albrecht, R. (1953). *Older people.* New York, NY: Longmans, Green.

Hendricks, J. (1992). Generations and the generation of theory in social gerontology. *International Journal of Aging and Human Development, 35,* 31–47.

Hendricks, J., Applebaum, R., & Kunkel, S. (2010). A world apart? Bridging the gap between theory and applied social gerontology. *The Gerontologist, 50,* 284–293.

Holstein, M. (1999).Women and productive aging. In M. Minkler & C. L. Estes (Eds.), *Critical gerontology.* Amityville, NY: Baywood

Hochschild, A. R. (1975). Disengagement theory. *American Sociological Review, 40,* 553–569.

Johnson, M. L., Bengtson, V. L., Coleman, P. G., & Kirkwood, B. L. (Eds.). (2005). *The Cambridge handbook of age and ageing.* Cambridge, UK: Cambridge University Press.

Kastenbaum, R. (1965). Theories of human aging: The search for a conceptual framework. *Journal of Social Issues, 21,* 13–36.

Kastenbaum, R. (1978). Essay: Gerontology's search for understanding. *The Gerontologist, 18,* 59–63.

Krause, N. E. (1999). Deriving a sense of meaning in late life. In V. L. Bengtson, N. Putney, D. Gans, & M. Silverstein (Eds.), *Handbook of theories of aging* (2nd ed., pp. 101–116). New York, NY: Springer Publishing Company.

Krause, N. R., & Bastida, E. (2009). Religion, suffering, and health among older Mexican Americans. *Journal of Aging Studies, 23*(2), 114–123.

Lansing, A. I. (Ed.). (1952). *Cowdry's problems of ageing* (3rd ed.). Baltimore: Williams & Wilkins.

Longino, C. (2005). Exploring the connections. *The Journals of Gerontology, Series B, 60,* 172.

Lynott, R. J., & Lynott, P. P. (1996). Tracing the course of theoretical development in the sociology of aging. *The Gerontologist, 36,* 749–760.

Marshall, V. W. (1999). Theory informing public policy. In V. L. Bengtson, N. Putney, D. Gans, & M. Silverstein (Eds.), *Handbook of theories of aging* (2nd ed., pp. 573–594). New York, NY: Springer Publishing Company.

Metchnikoff, E. (1903). *The nature of man.* New York, NY: G. P. Putnam's Sons.

Metchnikoff, E. (1908). *The prolongation of life.* New York, NY: G. P. Putnam's Sons.

Nascher, I. L. (1914). *Geriatrics.* Philadelphia, PA: P. Blakiston's Son.

Nascher, I. L. (1926). A history of geriatrics. *Medical Review of Reviews, 32,* 281–284.

Neugarten, B. L. (1968). *Middle age and aging.* Chicago, IL: University of Chicago Press.

Pickard, S. (2014). Biology as destiny? *Ageing and Society, 34,* 1279–1291.

Ray, R. E. (2006). The personal as political. In T. M. Calasanti & K. F. Slevin (Eds.), *Age matters* (pp. 21–25). New York, NY: Routledge.

Riley, M. W., Johnson, M., & Foner, A. (1969–1972). *Aging and society* (Vol. 3). New York, NY: Russell Sage Foundation.

Rowe, J. W., & Kahn, R. L. (1998). *Successful aging.* New York, NY: Pantheon.

Schroots, J. J. F. (1996). Theoretical developments in the psychology of aging. *The Gerontologist, 36,* 742–746.

Settersten R. A., & Dobransky, L. M. (2000). On the unbearable lightness of theory in gerontology. *The Gerontologist, 40,* 367–373.

Shock, N. W. (1952). *Trends in gerontology* (2nd ed.). Stanford, CA: Stanford University Press.

Shock, N. W. (1961). The role of research in solving the problems of the aged. *Journal of Gerontology, 15,* 14–16.

Thornstam, L. (1989). Gero-transcendence. *Aging, 1,* 55–63.

Uhlenberg, P., & Gierveld, J. (2004). Age segregation in later life. *Ageing and Society, 24,* 5–28.

Weber, R. L., & Orsborn, C. (2015). *The power of age.* Rochester, VT: Inner Traditions.

Wilson, E. O. (1998). *Consilience.* New York, NY: Random House.

CHAPTER 35

Prospects for Future Theory Development in Aging

Richard A. Settersten, Jr., and Vern L. Bengtson

The rigor and maturity of a scholarly or scientific field can be judged by the strength of its theories. As described in Chapter 1, we have seen a progressive increase in theory development in aging since the first volume of theories of aging was published in 1988 (Birren & Bengtson, 1988). Particularly impressive has been the recent expansion in transdisciplinary scholarship, as traditional scientific boundaries and research paradigms have been bridged by investigators increasingly conversant with those working in adjacent fields. As the chapters of this handbook reveal, notable theory development has taken place both within and across disciplines during the past decade of research on a wide variety of topics in aging.

The process of theory development hinges on cumulative, coordinated, and integrated knowledge about aging. This is necessary to counter the threat of what James Birren (1963, p. 11) called "barefoot empiricism" in aging research—the proliferation of basically descriptive reports of studies about age-related contrasts that lack theoretical framing and interpretation. In the long run, these add relatively little to the cumulative knowledge development of a field, beyond factual information that is likely to be quickly outdated.

In this chapter, we look toward the future of theory development in research on aging, offering some perspectives that we hope will be helpful to graduate students, postdocs, and junior investigators. Although these projections are based on insights provided by the many authors who have contributed to this volume, it is not intended to be a summary or synthesis of the *Handbook*. Rather, we want to highlight some directions for theory development and theory-driven research and application that are likely to be the most fruitful arenas for explanatory inquiry in the decade to come. These include:

- Successful and positive aging
- Longevity, health, and well-being in aging
- Environments, and transactions among aging individuals and their environments
- The life course and its effects on aging
- Variations in trajectories of aging

These and other areas of theory development will become more transdisciplinary because a comprehensive science of aging requires it. The increased permeability of disciplinary boundaries should, in turn, give way to deeper theory-based understanding of aging as a multifaceted puzzle and, we hope, the identification of theory-based solutions to improving the health and well-being of aging individuals, aging families, and aging societies.

There is widespread agreement across chapters that aging phenomena are greatly interrelated. Outside of biology, where there is still much effort to unlock cellular mechanisms of aging, much research on aging does not attempt to isolate highly specific aspects of the aging process without at least some treatment of other interconnected dimensions of functioning or levels of analysis. As inquiry moves outward from cells to whole people, and to whole people living in extraordinarily complex social worlds, it becomes impossible to study aging without acknowledging these interdependencies.

■ THEORIZING SUCCESSFUL AND POSITIVE AGING

The last century saw marked increases of the human life span that were met with increased research interests in uncovering factors for a higher quality of life in old age. These interests were also actively promoted by gerontologists to offer a counterpoint to earlier views of aging as an "inevitably bleak and unrelieved landscape characterized by irretrievable loss," to use George Maddox's (1994, p. 767) words. Negative views of aging and associations with "unproductivity, inflexibility, and senility," said pioneering gerontologist Robert Butler (1974, p. 529), "must be changed if the elderly are to have more opportunities for successful aging."

The notion that the human aging process can to some degree be modified or controlled underlies one of the oldest and still active traditions in gerontology—that of successful aging. The term "successful aging" first appeared as the title of Robert Havighurst's (1961) article in the inaugural issue of *The Gerontologist*, which he defined as "the conditions of individual and social life under which the individual person gets a maximum of satisfaction and happiness" (p. 8). What constitutes and contributes to successful aging has been sharply debated in the decades since, but the idea that one can "succeed" at aging, and that some strategies and interventions might increase the chances of that success, has become almost an article of faith within gerontology today.

At any rate, "successful aging" has become one of the most widely used phrases in the history of gerontology in both popular and professional usage, prompted especially by the publication of Jack Rowe and Robert Kahn's (1987, 1997, 1998) prominent publications. Their biomedically based formulation of the successful aging concept has generated considerable attention in the scientific and applied communities—as well as vehement debate and criticism, most recently in a collection of papers from 2015 in *The Gerontologist*. Since the 1990s, the study of successful aging has been refined or expanded, often in response to the criticism of Rowe and Kahn's focus.

One major point of criticism of Rowe and Kahn's formulation relates to the limited three-part conceptualization of "success" as avoiding disease, maintaining physical and mental function, and staying socially engaged. In addition, it has been criticized for overemphasizing the role of individual choice in negotiating aging, neglecting social and environmental constraints and opportunities, not considering individuals' subjective interpretations of "success," and being elitist in promoting a model that is exhibited by and open to people who are more advantaged socially and economically, thereby discounting the hardships of those who are disabled, poor, or of minority status.

In response to these criticisms, Rowe (with Theodore Cosco, Chapter 27) acknowledges the need to reconceptualize successful aging in ways that address these concerns.

Their new efforts are also aimed at envisioning societal reforms that will allow and encourage more individuals to age successfully, and at probing the implications of successful aging for society's capacities and institutions and for the organization of the life course. These, too, are not new but harken back to the important issues first raised in Alan Pifer and Lydia Bronte's (1986) classic edited book, *Our Aging Society: Paradox and Promise*.

The challenge for researchers is to make inquiry in this tradition more theoretically and conceptually rich by expanding treatment of a wider spectrum of success and its measurement. Most important, however, is the theoretical task of explaining *why* some individuals and groups age more successfully than others and *how* successful aging can be nurtured in a wider population of individuals. Despite the growing variability in measures of successful aging, most approaches have nonetheless continued to have at their core variants of the first two components proposed by Rowe and Kahn: low probability of disease and disease-related disability and high cognitive and physical functional capacity. Much of the literature on successful aging also suggests that these outcomes can be influenced by individual effort and specific actions.

A parallel area that is ripe for theoretical development concerns what has come to be called "antiaging" science and medicine. As "successful aging" models were advanced and broadened within gerontology, the "antiaging" movement was gaining traction as a scientific, commercial, and public interest. Their co-occurrence is not a coincidence. The images and proscriptions for "successful aging" from gerontology challenged ageist beliefs and stereotypes by claiming that there were positivist methods that could be employed to create a "new" kind of aging, whereby the fruits of middle age could be enjoyed well into old age (Moody, 2005). Antiaging medicine targets the aging process via biomedical interventions in order to delay aging, which is also the focal point of much effort in biological science today (see Chapters 7 through 10). Indeed, recent advances in biology (see as follows) are all ultimately aimed at creating interventions to "delay aging" and "enhance longevity." The lesson, Brian Kennedy says in his introduction to Part II, is that "aging *is* modifiable." So, while mainstream gerontology and antiaging medicine have a long history of alienation and antagonism, antiaging medicine may be seen as offering a route to achieving successful aging, and in many ways successful aging and antiaging medicine are "two sides of the same coin" (Flatt, Settersten, Ponsaran, & Fishman, 2013).

We predict that the next few years will see important theoretical advances in more generally conceptualized "positive aging" dimensions as well. Although successful aging has recently dominated the literature, there are many other positive aspects of aging that have increasingly become topics of research and theorizing—and, importantly, that may be less value laden or politically volatile, more precise, easier to operationalize, and theoretically fecund. These include theories of "optimal" aging, coping, and resilience (Aldwin and Igarashi, Chapter 28), religion and spirituality (Coleman, Schröder-Butterfill, and Spreadbury, Chapter 29), and wisdom (Ardelt and Oh, Chapter 30). The linkages between religion and the course of later life, because of their well-documented connections to health and well-being, are particularly ripe for theoretical development (Bengtson, Silverstein, Putney, & Harris, 2015).

There can be a challenge, however, that must be faced by theories focusing on positive outcomes in aging. They may overemphasize the individual's role in making his or her aging experience, whereby it becomes the responsibility and even moral imperative of individuals to do everything they can to achieve "success" in aging at the risk of being blamed or held responsible for "failure." This can lead investigators to overlook the considerable social and biological constraints on individual aging. The grip of optimism in aging research—exemplified in successful and positive aging—threatens to obscure from our scientific lenses the difficult sides of aging and old age that must also be acknowledged or our science will yield inadequate knowledge and ineffective interventions.

■ THEORIZING LONGEVITY, HEALTH, AND WELL-BEING IN AGING

Health (or at least the absence of disease) has probably become the core metric of aging, and the varied and complex patterns of disease, disability, and mortality with age have become the central problem of researchers (O'Rand, Chapter 19). It is clear, however, that much of the research in this field, especially in epidemiology and public health, has built up descriptive accounts of incidence and prevalence of illnesses and disabilities, sorted by various subpopulation characteristics. Such reports document that one group is sicker or healthier than another but leave unexamined questions about why this may be, and thus have largely been atheoretical.

Similarly, dramatic advances in the biology of aging have led to new theories about the events that drive aging and possible interventional strategies to extend human *health span* not just longevity (i.e., added years are also functional and disease free; see Chapters 7 through 10, as well as Kennedy et al., 2014), and to minimize the period of "terminal decline" of function (Hülür, Ram, and Gerstorf, Chapter 15). These important theories, however, are largely devoid of attention to psychological and social aspects of health.

In consequence, we see research on psychological and social aspects of health as central to nurturing future theory development: first, to explain inequalities (or "disparities") in health outcomes; and second, to broaden the focus on illness and disability by emphasizing health and broader conceptions of well-being. Both of these directions are concurrent with major shifts in the ethos of health care toward prevention and personal responsibility for health and wellness.

A robust set of research programs led by social scientists has probed social inequality and its pervasive and enduring effects on health (see Chapter 19). These include: (a) the "education-health research program," which is focused on explaining the persistent relationship between years of schooling and later health; (b) the "fundamental cause program," which argues that socioeconomic status (SES) is an underlying, pervasive phenomenon that propels the aging process via multiple mechanisms over time that cannot be captured by commonly used "surface indicators" of SES; (c) the "cumulative advantage-cumulative disadvantage theory" (CAD), which draws attention to time-related processes that generate inequality and, relatedly, (d) the "cumulative inequality program," which attempts to expand theories of CAD into a broader theory of aging inequality that incorporates health and human agency, and in which health statuses also generate, and not just reflect, inequality. Each of these offers important directions for continued theory development.

Differences in social relationships and support account for health inequalities. Jaclyn Wong and Linda Waite (Chapter 18) note that theories of social capital have been central to inquiry in this area because relationships are viewed as resources on which individuals can draw to achieve their goals. Theories that stem from "main effects" models explain how relationships may lead to better health through a variety of cognitive, emotional, behavioral, and biological pathways, whereas theories that stem from "stress-buffering" models explain how relationships provide a variety of resources that can prevent damaging responses or promote adaptation to life's stressors. These, too, offer important routes to continued theory development.

It is crucial to advance theories that explain the connection among social relationships, social support, and health. In developing these it is important to not only probe close personal relationships like those between spouses or between parents and children (Uchino, Ong, Queen, and Kent de Grey, Chapter 13; Blieszner and Voorpostel, Chapter 17), but also to probe a wider range of relationships in the extended family matrix as well as social relationships and integration into larger networks beyond the family (Wong and Waite, Chapter 18).

There is a similar need to develop theories that explain how the health and well-being of elders carries consequences *for* personal and family relationships (Blieszner and Voorpostel, Chapter 17), social support (Uchino, Ong, Queen, and Kent de Grey, Chapter 13), work and retirement institutions (Hardy and Reyes, Chapter 16), neighborhoods and communities (Wahl and Oswald, Chapter 31), and political systems and the "intergenerational contract" in societies (Hudson, Chapter 25).

Within the realm of health, we want to make special note of the surge in aging research on social genomics and epigenetics, which is certain to continue growing in the future and is in need of theories to explain the interplay between genes and environments as well as the transmission of effects across multiple generations (see also Shanahan, 2013). For example, there is a need for theories that explore how social forces affect gene expression, especially in making elders more or less prone to inflammatory diseases, which are tied directly to cardiovascular and respiratory diseases of aging (Wong and Waite, Chapter 18). Similarly, the swell of research that attempts to link childhood adversity and later life outcomes is also in need of theories that explain the processes or mechanisms that bring about these effects. Here, too, biosocial research is critical to understanding the origins and trajectories of health inequalities as individuals successively encounter unequal social risks and resources over their lives (O'Rand, Chapter 19). New possibilities of integrating genomic, physiological, and clinical data with social survey data have made this line of investigation central to aging theory.

■ THEORIZING ENVIRONMENTS AND TRANSACTIONS BETWEEN AGING INDIVIDUALS AND THEIR ENVIRONMENTS

Across the disciplines that constitute gerontology, it has become increasingly recognized that understanding the environment (or "ecology," "context," "social structure," or other similar terms), and the individual's place within it, is crucial for understanding the aging process. Here, the theoretical treatment of environments and transactions between individuals and their environments remains abstract and ill specified. Further theory development must continue to probe the interplay between specific factors that are intrinsic and extrinsic to the individual. Individuals age within multiple contexts that, while they are distinct, are yet overlapping and nested, and they mutually influence each other. To make matters more complicated, contexts change over time, as do the people in them. Finally, these forces do not just impinge on individuals, but individuals also play roles in actively shaping their environments, especially to accommodate their aging.

Understanding these complex transactions between aging individuals and their environments will continue to be an important frontier for theory development. This area has seen renewed attention to a tradition within a long history—theories of "person–environment fit" or, in short, "P-E Fit"—which was especially propelled forward by the work of Powell Lawton in the 1970s. Hans-Werner Wahl and Frank Oswald (Chapter 31) provide a comprehensive explication of the varied uses of the term "environment" in gerontology, along with illustrations and common principles. They attempt to integrate both the objective and subjective environments, producing a framework that highlights the interplay between P–E "belonging" and P–E "agency" and links these processes to developmental outcomes such as identity, autonomy, and well-being.

Future theory development continues to hinge on clarifying *why* and *how* the characteristics of, and processes in, a variety of key environments shape aging experiences and outcomes. Besides traditional environments (e.g., family, residence, neighborhood and community, and work environments), new types of environments (e.g., digital media) must also be examined, as well as large-scale processes (e.g., urbanization, globalization, or upheavals in worldwide economies). There are also new frontiers to be explored in crossing aspects of the environment with human brain development, which neuroscience has long posited, but which has heretofore been explored primarily in animal models.

The social ecological model, which has a long tradition stemming especially from Urie Bronfenbrenner's (1974) classic work, *The Ecology of Human Development: Experiments by Nature and Design*, is mentioned frequently in the policy and practice literature. For example, the social ecological model is the foundation for Andersen's popular Behavioral Model of Health Services (see Montgomery, Kwak, and Kosloski, Chapter 23). Yet Nancy Morrow-Howell, in her introduction to Part V, notes how infrequently this model, with its multiple layers of factors affecting an individual situation, is fully considered in research or practice. Testing a full range of hypotheses derived from such a multilevel framework seems undoable, given the limited nature of data and the available analytic techniques. This model is fine as a heuristic, but it is so broad and lacking in the specificity required of good theory—much like life-course and life-span perspectives, which are discussed in the following section, which help to orient the development of theory but are not themselves theories.

Contemporary theories so often focus on the individual aspects of aging—what Gunhild Hagestad and Dale Dannefer (2001) once called the "microfication" of gerontology—that we lose sight of social structure. However, future theory development must keep social environments front and center in inquiry. This means more often adopting what Dannefer and Richard Settersten (2010) call the "institutional" paradigm of life-course research. The institutional paradigm emphasizes the role of more distal social forces, especially beyond immediate interpersonal relationships, that shape and even the life course. That is, understanding the life course is not just about understanding individual development over time. The life course is also a social and political construct, consisting of more or less explicitly defined age-graded stages that are created by or reified in institutions and social policies, and which reinforce cultural values and priorities (see also Settersten and Godlewski, Chapter 2).

■ THEORIZING THE LIFE COURSE AND ITS EFFECTS ON AGING

Recent years have brought a significant increase in analyses of aging as a lifelong process, fueled by the availability of longitudinal or retrospective life history data to explore these connections. The notion that aging is a lifelong process appears to now be a unifying theme across all disciplines and, indeed, it was the theme of the 2015 annual meeting of the Gerontological Society of America.

This means that, to explain aging, one must explain the influence of earlier processes and outcomes on later ones—what Dannefer and Settersten (2010) call the "personological" paradigm of life-course research (in contrast to the "institutional" paradigm, described earlier). This paradigm attempts to use key features of early life experience to predict and account for outcomes later in life, whether for individuals or for populations. This paradigm, which largely embodies a commitment to understanding time-related dynamics, is shared with life-span psychology and other longitudinal inquiry that extends across multiple life periods. The passing of time is related to aging phenomena, but many theories in this regard stop at the description stage—describing how phenomena change over time, or describing a set of earlier variables that predict later ones, but in neither case explaining why (see Chapter 2).

As researchers explore these kinds of temporal connections, more well-developed theories are needed to explain the connection between early life events and outcomes. For example, there is a great deal of interest today in connecting childhood health and SES with aging outcomes. If we attempt to link experiences that occur across seven or eight decades, there is a seemingly endless chain of possible variables to array and mechanisms to consider, but little theory to guide choices or to explain any patterns. To connect earlier and later experiences, a life-course perspective might point to critical or sensitive period models, accumulation models, or pathway models as places to start for developing substantive theories (Spini, Jopp, Pin, and Stringhini, Chapter 33).

Often, theories related to psychosocial resources and processes are aimed at understanding how these things modify associations between early-life socioeconomic factors and later-life health outcomes. With aging, the integrity and efficacy of psychological resources and processes are maintained in some domains of functioning but diminish in others. Recent theoretical work in psychology has been characterized by innovative efforts to delineate and understand mechanisms underlying different trajectories of change both within and across functional domains. For example, emotion and cognition are processes that are integrated in the brain, and they interact to produce behaviors; age-related changes in emotional processes are linked to age-related changes in cognition, and vice versa. Numerous theories are used to explain these linkages, but they focus on different underlying factors (for illustrations, see Ngo, Sands, and Isaacowitz, Chapter 12).

Examining aging as a lifelong process in conjunction with the influence of social environments has given rise to another theoretically rich theme: cumulative advantage and disadvantage (CAD) over the life course, which is again an important aspect of aging at both individual and population levels. Some of the variability among older people is due not just to individual differences that grow with age and time, but is also socially structured and due to social processes that perpetuate *inequalities* among people. The notion that benefits or liabilities cumulate with the passage of time—and therefore aging—is common to many theories.

Theories are like lenses, as we suggested in Chapter 1, and using different lenses allows researchers to see different things about the processes and experiences of aging. Most of the examples provided so far have been from researchers studying aging "objectively" from the outside, arraying variables over time, demonstrating effects, and suggesting mechanisms that link them. In contrast are theoretical advances from those adopting an "interpretive" perspective (Marshall, Martin-Matthews, & McMullin, Chapter 20). That is, aging and life-course dynamics must also be understood "phenomenologically" from the inside, probing the motivations and actions people take, and the "subjective" meanings they make from and explanations they attribute to their experiences. For example, subjective perceptions of one's social connectedness carry an independent and sizable effect on health and well-being in old age alongside the objective aspects of social relationships and networks (Wong and Waite, Chapter 18). Individuals' subjective ratings of health are relatively stable and do not necessarily represent objective health conditions; and yet, subjective health is a much better predictor of mortality in old age than objective health (Spini et al., Chapter 33). Similarly, how veterans recall (or reconstruct) their military experiences may be more important than their actual experiences in predicting the effects of their service on health and well-being in later life (Settersten, Day, Elder, & Waldinger, 2012).

References to "life course" in the research literature have grown exponentially in the last decade, with this phrase being attached to almost every topic one can conceive related to aging. Unfortunately, the term often serves as a superficial signal that a phenomenon is being examined across at least two time points. Better theorizing is needed about explanations—causal mechanisms between events and trajectories. The life-course perspective has offered valuable insights and transformed scholarship in our field, and we expect that this will only continue in the years ahead. There is a natural synergy between aging and the life course. However, it is our hope that attention to the life course will not compromise the scope and clarity of *aging*. There are questions about aging that do not entail the life course, and many more questions about the life course that do not entail aging. In theorizing connections between aging and the life course, our field becomes (potentially too) big and broad to manage. Is gerontology a field of every possible age, and every possible transition, in every possible domain of life?

Like the social ecological model described earlier, the life-course perspective in sociology (e.g., Dannefer & Settersten, 2010; Elder, Shanahan, & Jennings, 2015; Mayer, 2004) and the life-span perspective in developmental psychology (e.g., Baltes, Lindenberger, & Staudinger, 1998) are just that—orienting perspectives. They contain important concepts and propositions that can be infused into particular topic areas to advance theories. However, they are not themselves theories. Their breadth and generality mean they cannot explain with the specificity of a theory, which leads us to the need to theorize variations in trajectories of aging.

■ THEORIZING VARIATIONS IN TRAJECTORIES OF AGING

There is widespread interest in attempting to explain variability in aging—differences within and between individuals, populations, societies, and even species—rather than attempting to identify common, or universal, predictors, which was a primary focus just a few decades ago.

In the next decade, a more rigorous and nuanced explanation of variability will be central to theory development. Theories generally do not take into account the fact that individuals at all ages can show different trajectories of change (Spini et al., Chapter 33) and instead propose curves that represent an average trajectory of development (linear, curvilinear curves by age). The more we acknowledge the reality of difference and diversity, the harder it is to theorize in broad ways. Fortunately, the development of longitudinal studies and statistical methods for examining trajectories mean that aging theories can increasingly take multidirectionality and heterogeneity into account as they are formulated.

Some variability reflects intra-individual (within person) change over time at the level of the molecule, cell, system, or organism. For example, health and cognitive capacity have often been viewed in these terms, as has emotion regulation, reactivity to stimuli, self-esteem, and even personality. Even when losses in cognitive function or health can be observed for *most* individuals, there is often substantial inter-individual (between-person) differences, differences that can also grow with time—such as cumulative processes that leave individuals more unique from one another in their constellations of history and experience as they age, or like CAD processes noted earlier, in which time reinforces or amplifies earlier social and economic advantages or disadvantages, increasing inequalities among individuals or groups in later life. Research on intra- and inter-individual variability can naturally produce different results, and the resolution or integration of these differences is key to theory development.

Questions of when, in what domains of functioning, and for whom changes related to age occur are of utmost importance to theory building. There is a great need to continue developing theories that are sensitive to social diversity. Early contributions toward this goal were in the area of cohort and generation, which emphasized the effects of history and place. Feminist theorists prodded researchers to take seriously not only gender differences but also gender relations, which over time expanded to include intersections with race and ethnicity and social class.

From our perspective, a search for a single theory of aging and gender, of race or ethnicity, of social class, or of culture, is not likely to be fruitful. Instead, attention to these social dimensions of diversity must be infused into all theorizing—to build theories on particular topics that are sensitive to diversity and to the fact that it is associated with different aging processes and outcomes. Individuals have differential access to various opportunities and constraints based on various characteristics, which translate into structural inequalities that are generally outside of an individual's control. For example, in the area of health, theories must explain *why* and *how* exposure to stress is more often carried by women, members of racial/ethnic minorities, unmarried persons, and working class and poor individuals. Social capital and other coping resources are disproportionately low among these groups, which only accentuates the disadvantages they already face. Theory-based social interventions and policy initiatives are crucial in attempting to prevent or compensate for these inequalities.

■ CONCLUSION

It is clear from the evolving contents of the editions of this handbook that theory, in all disciplines, has risen in its importance and prominence in gerontology since 1988. Longstanding theoretical traditions have deepened. Important new theories have emerged in areas that reflect our dramatically changing world as well as the possibilities embodied in revolutionary leaps in technology and research methods and in investments in data. Transdisciplinary theory and research are also growing in ways that leave us excited about the table of contents of the next edition. These advances are essential to the maturation and sophistication of gerontology *as a science* because they yield stronger explanatory analyses and therefore deeper understanding and more effective interventions.

There will, however, be ongoing pressures in the academic establishment that will work against theory development as a priority in research on aging. Increased specialization and medicalization may result in theory that is so narrow in scope that it will be of little use to the field. The ready availability of Big Data may reinforce the need and temptation to publish more papers of narrow scope, and to do so quickly. Investments in Big Data may also continue to generate more descriptive studies based on correlative age comparisons without sufficient interpretation or explanation. Research funding may place such a premium on public health relevance, and on narrow health-related processes and outcomes, that knowledge accumulation and integration, and broader topics of relevance to aging, will be compromised. Theory often seems too remote or too abstract to be of relevance, too costly relative to the rewards, or beyond the scope of our manuscripts, our skills, or our time.

Advances in methods and the availability of data can risk theory development if they merely add to the heap of facts and findings. But they can also be important routes toward explanation and the development of compelling theories and ideas. As O'Rand (Chapter 19) notes, theories develop as they are applied to data and the methods used to collect and analyze data. Methods develop as well, both in response to theoretical demands and in their own right, and thereby serve to further develop theory. Theory development in the field of aging has been characterized by this pattern for more than half a century.

As Jacqui Smith notes in her introduction to Part III, the rapid expansion of publicly available data from large representative surveys—surveys that include psychological, physical, cellular, and genetic data—provides a rich platform for researchers to engage in theory-guided research and contribute new insights. Increasingly, these studies are also being linked to geographical and administrative data. The retrospective collection of life histories from participants in ongoing studies of aging will further extend current possibilities to trace antecedents to change during midlife and old age. Investments in longitudinal data are especially important in deriving knowledge of aging that reflects the dynamic, multifaceted, and interactive process it is. Smaller experimental studies are critical complements to Big Data, especially in deriving and testing theories about specific mechanisms.

We are concerned about how to counter the desire to produce different or counter intuitive findings rather than be committed to incremental and replicable research and to building on existing theories (see also Duncan, 2015; Freund, 2015), which are devalued in science. Researchers should pay more attention to previous theorizing lest they repeat the mistakes of the past or attempt to reinvent the wheel. Scientists are trained to be highly critical, but we would benefit from not rejecting out of hand insights from earlier theoretical approaches, as often seems fashionable to do. Talent and energy would better be spent refining and redeveloping, rather than ignoring or rejecting, theoretical perspectives that can help us understand contemporary experiences of aging. Theory construction is a gradual enterprise. Research provides new findings that may gradually shift theoretical perspectives within a discipline and, in the most extreme scenario, overturn existing scientific dogma. But that rests on a long process of knowledge accumulation and synthesis.

The rigor and maturity of a field are not only reflected in the ability of its theories to shape and reflect evidence-based understanding, but also to shape and reflect application (see also Hendricks, Applebaum, & Kunkel, 2010). Theories should guide interventions to improve human conditions. Theory is valuable when we attempt to apply and advance existing knowledge in order to solve problems or alleviate undesirable human conditions.

In the field of gerontology, there is a need for rigorous applied research to inform the development of many kinds of interventions, services, and policies, which is dependent on strong theory. This is a major frontier for advancing future theories of aging. The demand for quick action, coupled with limited resources, has too often meant that theory-based development, implementation, and evaluation are bypassed. The emerging science of "dissemination and intervention" (D&I) brings some hope for improvement, as it is aimed at both strengthening and shortening the "translation research gap" (Morrow-Howell, introduction to Part V). Programs and services are effective only to the extent that they are used by and improve the conditions of older adults and their families. Better theories can lead to improved outreach, targeting, enrollment, and sustained use of services in the aging network.

For the long-term intellectual vitality of our field, we hope its leaders and teachers will preach the value of theory in strong and compelling ways to ensure that publications, grants, and future generations continue nurturing the development of theory. As the scope and possibilities of our science become ever more complicated, the premium on theory will only grow.

REFERENCES

Baltes, P. B., Lindenberger, U., & Staudinger, U. M. (1998). Life-span theory in developmental psychology. In W. Damon & R. M. Lerner (Eds.), *Handbook of child psychology* (5th ed., Vol. 1: Theoretical models of human development, pp. 1027–1143). New York, NY: Wiley.

Bengtson, V. L., Silverstein, M. S., Putney, N., & Harris, S. C. (2015). Does religiosity increase with age? Age changes and age differences over 35 years. *Journal of the Scientific Study of Religion, 54*, 363–379.

Birren, J. E. (1963). Methods and models in the study of aging. In R. H. Davis & M. Neiswender (Eds.), *Aging: Prospects and issues* (pp. 1–17). Los Angeles, CA: Andrus Gerontology Center, University of Southern California.

Birren, J. E., & Bengtson, V. L. (Eds.). (1988). *Emergent theories of aging.* New York, NY: Springer Publishing Company.

Bronfenbrenner, U. (1974). *The ecology of human development: Experiments by nature and design.* Cambridge, MA: Harvard University Press.

Butler, R. N. (1974). Succesful aging and the role of the life review. *Journal of the American Geriatrics Society, 22*(12), 529–535.

Dannefer, W. D., & Settersten, R. A., Jr. (2010). The study of the life course: Implications for social gerontology. In W. D. Dannefer & C. Phillipson (Eds.), *International handbook of social gerontology* (pp. 3–19). London, UK: Sage.

Duncan, G. (2015). Toward an empirical robust science of human development. *Research in Human Development, 12*, 255–260.

Elder, G. H., Jr., Shanahan, M. J., & Jennings, J. A. (2015). Human development in time and place. In T. Leventhal & M. Bornstein (Eds.), *Handbook of child psychology and developmental science: Ecological settings and processes in developmental systems* (7th ed., Vol. 4, pp. 6–54). Hoboken, NJ: Wiley.

Flatt, M. A., Settersten, R. A., Ponsaran, R., & Fishman, J. R. (2013). Are "anti-aging medicine" and "successful aging" two sides of the same coin? Views of anti-aging practitioners. *The Journals of Gerontology, Series B, 68*(6), 944–955.

Freund, A. M. (2015). Getting at developmental processes through experiments. *Research in Human Development, 12*, 261–267.

Hagestad, G. O., & Dannefer, D. (2001). Concepts and theories of aging: Beyond microfication in social science approaches. In R. H. Binstock & L. K. George (Eds.), *Handbook of aging and social sciences* (5th ed., pp. 3–21). San Diego, CA: Academic Press.

Havighurst, R. G. (1961). Successful aging. *The Gerontologist, 1,* 8–13.

Hendricks, J., Applebaum, R., & Kunkel, S. (2010). A world apart? Bridging the gap between theory and applied social gerontology. *The Gerontologist, 50*(3), 284–293.

Kennedy, B. K., Berger, S. L., Brunet, A., Campisi, J., Cuervo, A. M., Epel, E. S., … Sierra, F. (2014). Geroscience: Linking aging to chronic disease. *Cell, 159*(4), 709–713.

Maddox, G. L. (1994). Lives through the years revisited. *The Gerontologist, 34*(6), 764–767.

Mayer, K. U. (2004). Whose lives? How history, societies, and institutions define and shape life courses. *Research in Human Development, 1,* 161–187.

Moody, H. R. (2005). From successful aging to conscious aging. In M. Wykle, P. Whitehouse, & D. Morris (Eds.), *Successful aging through the life span: Intergenerational issues in health* (pp. 55–68). New York, NY: Springer Publishing Company.

Pifer, A., & Bronte, L. (1986). *Our aging society: Paradox and promise.* New York, NY: W. W. Norton.

Rowe, J. W., & Kahn, R. L. (1987). Human aging: Usual and successful. *Science, 237*(4811), 143–149.

Rowe, J. W., & Kahn, R. L. (1997). Successful aging. *The Gerontologist, 37*(4), 433–440.

Rowe, J. W., & Kahn, R. L. (1998). *Successful aging.* New York, NY: Pantheon Books.

Settersten, R. A., Day, J., Elder, G. H., & Waldinger, R. J. (2012). Men's appraisals of their military experiences in World War II: A 40-year perspective. *Research in Human Development, 9*(3), 248–271.

Shanahan, M. J. (2013). Social genomics and the life course: Opportunities and challenges for multilevel research. In L. Waite (Ed.), *Perspectives on the future of the sociology of aging* (pp. 255–276). Washington, DC: National Academies Press.

Index